Conditioning for Strength and Human Performance

Conditioning for Strength and Human Performance

T. JEFF CHANDLER, EdD, CSCS*D, NSCA-CPT, FNSCA, FACSM
Editor in Chief, Strength and Conditioning Journal
Professor and Department Head, HPER
Jacksonville State University
Jacksonville, AL

LEE E. BROWN, EdD, CSCS*D, FNSCA, FACSM
NSCA President 2006–2009
Associate Professor
California State University, Fullerton
Department of Kinesiology
Fullerton, CA

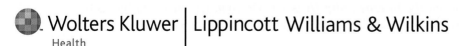
. Wolters Kluwer | Lippincott Williams & Wilkins
Health
Philadelphia • Baltimore • New York • London
Buenos Aires • Hong Kong • Sydney • Tokyo

Acquisitions Editor: Emily Lupash
Development Editors: Robyn J. Alvarez and Elizabeth Connolly
Marketing Manager: Christen Murphy
Production Editor: Eve Malakoff-Klein
Designer: Theresa Mallon
Artist: Jonathan Dimes
Compositor: Circle Graphics, Inc.
Printer: R. R. Donnelley

351 West Camden Street
Baltimore, MD 21201

530 Walnut Street
Philadelphia, PA 19106

Printed in China

Library of Congress Cataloging-in-Publication Data

Chandler, T. Jeff.
 Conditioning for strength and human performance / T. Jeff Chandler, Lee E. Brown.
   p. cm.
 Includes bibliographical references and index.
 ISBN-13: 978-0-7817-4594-9
 ISBN-10: 0-7817-4594-2
 1. Physical fitness—Health aspects. 2. Exercise—Physiological aspects. 3. Physical education and training. I. Brown, Lee E. II. Title.
 RA781.C43 2008
 613.7'1—dc22

                    2006034174

To purchase additional copies of this book, call our customer service department at **(800) 638-3030** or fax orders to **(301) 824-7390**. International customers should call **(301) 714-2324**.

Visit Lippincott Williams & Wilkins on the Internet: http://www.LWW.com. Lippincott Williams & Wilkins customer service representatives are available from 8:30 am to 6:00 pm, EST.

08 09 10

2 3 4 5 6 7 8 9 10

To my wife, Pam, for her continued love, dedication, and support.

I love you. —Jeff

For Theresa, for saving my life . . . twice. I love you. —Lee

Foreword

The ultimate goal of strength and conditioning coaches and personal trainers is to enhance human performance, both in athletes and in fitness enthusiasts. *Conditioning for Strength and Human Performance* provides the necessary knowledge base these professionals require. This text is appropriate for strength and conditioning professionals working with the general population where a major goal of a conditioning program is to enhance general health and physical fitness, as well as for professionals working in high school and collegiate athletic settings where the major goal of a conditioning program is to enhance physical performance in athletic events.

Some texts for the strength and conditioning profession claim to be based in research and science. Hearsay and popular ideas, however, often make up a significant portion of the topics covered. The contributors to *Conditioning for Strength and Human Performance* have all based the material covered in their respective chapters in research and science, which is an important aspect of the development not only of strength and conditioning professionals, but also of the profession itself.

Included in the first part of the text is information related to physiology, anatomy, and biomechanics, all presented in a clear, understandable manner. This information is necessary for the sound development of strength and conditioning programs. The remainder of the text presents chapters addressing virtually all aspects of administration of strength and conditioning programs, chapters on the various types of strength and conditioning (weight training, aerobic training), and chapters dedicated to unique aspects of strength and conditioning programs. These special topics give the reader of *Conditioning for Strength and Human Performance* sound information related to unique aspects of developing strength and conditioning programs. For example, readers will find chapters concerning spotting of resistance training exercises, plyometrics, speed and agility, the role of strength and conditioning in injury prevention and rehabilitation, ergogenic aids, and the use of implements other than traditional machines, barbells and dumbbells in strength and conditioning programs. These unique chapters are written by individuals well-known for their knowledge in these specialized areas of the strength and conditioning field.

It is important to note that the authors of the chapters in this text are a mix of sport scientists, strength and conditioning coaches, and practitioners, giving the work a balance between sound sport science information and its application in the development of strength and conditioning programs. I recommend this text to all individuals working in the strength and conditioning profession.

Steven J. Fleck, Ph.D.

Preface

Foreword

PURPOSE AND AUDIENCE

Conditioning for Strength and Human Performance is an entry-level textbook for courses covering strength training, conditioning, and personal training. This course is usually offered in the junior or senior year and has several recommended prerequisites, including anatomy and physiology, exercise physiology, and biomechanics. The textbook begins with a review of the basic science applied to training and conditioning and then moves to practical application of these basic science principles. An important option for the course instructor is a laboratory component with many activities that can be taught in the "lab" (weight room/exercise facility). The primary audience for this book consists of students in kinesiology, exercise science, athletic training programs, and preprofessional tracks such as premedicine, prephysical therapy, and prephysician assistant. Exercise science and related majors often include areas of study related to careers as a personal trainer and strength and conditioning coach.

The body of knowledge in the field of strength training and conditioning is growing rapidly. One reason we decided to produce this text was to provide students in the field with up-to-date information from this growing body of research. The field of strength training is dynamic and will continue to grow and change. Previously held beliefs will be challenged; some will stand and some will fall.

Another reason we prepared this text was to disseminate knowledge, perhaps in a somewhat different way than has been done previously. Learners have different learning styles, and we hope that we have provided learning opportunities for all types of learners.

The knowledge we have gained as professionals should not be proprietary. We do not "own" the information that we have learned, and we should freely share it with others. In fact, if the discipline of strength training and conditioning is to grow and flourish as it should, we must all take responsibility for passing on the most current body of knowledge in our field.

CHAPTER FEATURES

The pedagogical elements of the text were designed to present the basic material in a clear and concise manner as well as to challenge students to go beyond the textbook and seek information to answer more complex questions. Some students will learn best from reading and studying the figures and key terms. Some students will learn best by listening to instructors' lectures, and some will learn best from the application questions and activities recommended in the text. We encourage all students to participate in all of the activities provided, realizing that each student will learn best when information is presented in a style that suits him or her best. Since there is no universal best learning style, instructors are encouraged to use a variety of activities to disseminate the information in this text.

The text includes several pedagogical features to aid in the comprehension and retention of material. They provide numerous opportunities for students to apply the material in the context of their careers.

Key Points

Key points are succinct one- to three-sentence minisummaries. They briefly summarize the main concepts of the preceding section. Each key point is set apart as a separate paragraph in the body of the text, following the text containing the information it summarizes.

Real-World Application

These boxes contain analogies or metaphors that link theoretical concepts to practical application, or practical tips. They relate the chapter content to the real world.

Q&A from the Field

This is a simulated "ask-the-expert" column. The questions come from the point of view of a professional in a field appropriate to each chapter.

Maxing Out

These questions or activities designed to stimulate critical thinking appear at the ends of the chapters. They are based on real-life scenarios and may contain challenging content that students may not be able to answer based on the preceding chapter. They will take students above and beyond what they have just read.

Case Example

Case examples walk students through the design and implementation of a program. They are based on the following template:

1. Background
2. Recommendations/Consideration
3. Implementation
4. Results

LEARNING RESOURCES

The book comes with a CD-ROM that provides numerous opportunities for students to reinforce their learning. A set of nearly 200 quiz questions will help them to test their retention of the material. A practical exam uses video clips to demonstrate various exercises, and multiple-choice questions allow students to practice identifying exercises and ensuring proper form. Students can further apply their knowledge of the text through additional case examples and lab assignments, which put the book's content into context and provide a link to their future careers.

Instructors' resources are available on CD-ROM or via the website (http://thepoint.lww.com/Chandler). Included in the instructors' resources are the following valuable assets:

■ PowerPoint presentations by chapter
■ Test generator
■ Image bank
■ Answers to "Maxing Out" activities from the chapters

As with any first edition of a textbook, we look forward to making many improvements in future editions of *Conditioning for Strength and Human Performance*. The editors therefore encourage you, both instructors and students, to send us feedback on the usefulness of each component of the text. Together, we can continue to make a significant contribution to the field of strength training and conditioning.

Jeff Chandler and Lee Brown

Acknowledgments

In an extensive work such as this book, many individuals play critical roles. We would like to thank Robyn Alvarez, Developmental Editor, and the entire editorial staff at LWW for their dedication and hard work on this project.

Lee Brown would like to acknowledge the support of his graduate students and the faculty in the Department of Kinesiology at California State University, Fullerton. Jeff Chandler would like to acknowledge his former faculty members and students in the Division of Exercise Science, Sport, and Recreation at Marshall University, Hunting-ton, WV, and his current students and faculty in the Department of Health, Physical Education, and Recreation at Jacksonville State University, Jacksonville, AL.

We would like to acknowledge the efforts of Britt Chandler for his work in developing the ancillaries for this text.

We are fortunate to be involved with an outstanding group of colleagues in the field of strength training and conditioning. We acknowledge your contributions to the field and your continued hard work to move our discipline forward.

x

Contributors

CLINT ALLEY, MS, CSCS
Strength and Conditioning Coach
University of Charleston, Charleston, WV

JOSÉ ANTONIO, PHD, CSCS, FACSM
Chief Executive Officer
International Society of Sports Nutrition
Deerfield Beach, FL

C. ERIC ARNOLD, MS
Assistant Professor
Exercise Science Director, Exercise Physiology
  Laboratory
Marshall University
Huntington, WV

TRAVIS BECK, MPE
Graduate Assistant
University of Nebraska-Lincoln
Lincoln, NE

JOHN BERARDI, PHD, CSCS
Adjunct Assistant Professor
University of Texas at Austin
Austin, TX

JAKE BLEACHER, MS, PT, OCS, CSCS
Clinic Director
Gilbert Physiotherapy Associates
Gilbert, AZ

BRITT CHANDLER, MS, CSCS, NSCA-CPT
Sports Performance Specialist
Lexington Tennis Club/Fitness Wellness Services
Lexington, KY

JOHN M. CISSIK, MS, CSCS*D, NSCA-CPT*D
Director of Fitness and Recreation
Texas Woman's University
Denton, TX

JARED W. COBURN, PHD, CSCS*D
Associate Professor
Dept. of Kinesiology
California State University, Fullerton
Fullerton, CA

HERBERT A. DEVRIES, PHD
Emeritus Professor of Kinesiology
University of Southern California
Los Angeles, CA

TODD S. ELLENBECKER, MS, DPT, SCS,
OCS, CSCS
Clinic Director, Physiotherapy Associates Scottsdale
  Sports Clinic
National Director of Clinical Research
Scottsdale, AZ

ANDREW C. FRY, PHD, CSCS
Director, Exercise Biochemistry Laboratory
Department of Health and Sport Sciences
The University of Memphis
Memphis, TN

JOHN F. GRAHAM, MS, CSCS*D
Vice President, Performance & Preventative
  Health Services
Orthopaedic Associates of Allentown
Allentown, PA

PATRICK HAGERMAN, EDD, CSCS, NSCA-CPT
Assistant Professor of Exercise and
  Sports Science
The University of Tulsa
Tulsa, OK

ALLEN HEDRICK, MA, CSCS*D
Head Strength and Conditioning Coach
United States Air Force Academy
Colorado Springs, CO

JAY R. HOFFMAN, PHD, FACSM, CSCS*D
Professor, Chair
Department of Health and Exercise Science
The College of New Jersey
Ewing, NJ

TERRY J. HOUSH, PHD
Professor
Department of Nutrition and Health Sciences
University of Nebraska–Lincoln
Lincoln, NE

DUANE KNUDSON, PHD, FACSM
Associate Dean, College of Communication
    and Education
Professor, Department of Kinesiology
California State University, Chico
Chico, CA

WILLIAM J. KRAEMER, PHD, FACSM, CSCS
Professor
Human Performance Laboratory
Department of Kinesiology
University of Connecticut
Storrs, CT

MOH H. MALEK, MS, CSCS*D, NSCA-CPT*D
Doctoral Student/Graduate Assistant
Human Performance Laboratory
University of Nebraska-Lincoln
Department of Nutrition and Health Sciences
Lincoln, NE

RON MENDEL, PHD
President
Ohio Research Group
Wadsworth Medical Center
Wadsworth, OH

CHRISTOPHER R. MOHR, MS, RD
Owner, Mohr Results, Inc.
Louisville, KY

DANIEL P. MURRAY, MS, PT, CSCS
Adjunct Faculty
Physical Therapy Department
Bouve College of Health Sciences
Northeastern University
Boston, MA

ROBERT U. NEWTON, PHD, CSCS
Foundation Professor of Exercise and Sport Science
Associate Dean for Research and Higher Degrees

Edith Cowan University
Perth, Western Australia, Australia

STEVEN PLISK, MS, CSCS*D
Sports Performance Director
Velocity Sports Performance
Trumbull, CT

BARRY A. SPIERING, MS, CSCS
Doctoral Fellow
Human Performance Laboratory
University of Connecticut
Storrs, CT

MEG STONE, MS
Assistant Track and Field Coach
Director of the Sports Performance Enhancement
    Consortium
East Tennessee State University
Johnson City, TN

MICHAEL H. STONE, PHD, UKSCA
Laboratory Director
Kinesiology, Leisure and Sports Sciences
East Tennessee State University
Johnson City, TN

ANNA THATCHER, PT, OCS, ATC, CSCS
Physical Therapist
Achieve Orthopaedic and Sports Therapy, PC
Phoenix, AZ

JASON D. VESCOVI, PHD, CSCS
Postdoctoral Fellow
Women's Exercise and Bone Health Laboratory
University of Toronto
Toronto, Ontario, Canada

JOSEPH P. WEIR, PHD FACSM
Professor
Physical Therapy Program
Des Moines University, Osteopathic Medical Center
Des Moines, IA

ANN M. YORK, PT, PHD
Assistant Professor
Postprofessional DPT Program
Des Moines University
Des Moines, IA

TIM N. ZIEGENFUSS, PHD, CSCS, FISSN
Chief Executive Officer, Ohio Research Group
Wadsworth Medical Center
Wadsworth, OH

Reviewers

The publisher and author gratefully acknowledge the many professionals who shared their expertise and assisted in developing this textbook, helping us to refine our plan, target our marketing efforts appropriately, and set the stage for subsequent editions. We are grateful to the following reviewers:

GAIL PARR, PHD
Assistant Professor of Kinesiology
Towson University
Towson, MD

DIXIE STANFORTH
Lecturer, Department of Kinesiology
University of Texas at Austin
Austin, TX

NICHOLAS J. DICICCO, EDD
Director of Health and Exercise Science
Nova Southeastern University
Blackwood, NJ

DAVID SANDLER, PHD
Assistant Professor
Florida International University
Miami, FL

TIMOTHY HOWELL, EDD
Program Director, Athletic Training
Alfred University
Alfred, NY

User's Guide

This User's Guide introduces you to the many features of *Conditioning for Strength and Human Performance.* Taking full advantage of these features, you not only read about strength and conditioning, you become involved in activities that help you learn and put your knowledge into practice.

Each chapter is loaded with features that help you focus on the key points, deepen your knowledge, and apply your new skills.

Introductions beginning each chapter explain why the material is important to you and give you a preview of what you'll find in the chapter.

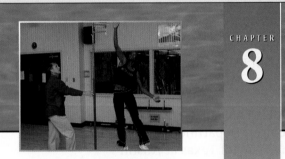

CHAPTER

8

Test Administration and Interpretation

LEE E. BROWN
DANIEL MURRAY
PATRICK HAGERMAN

Introduction

Testing and measurement are at the heart of any resistance-training program. This is where initial decisions are made regarding the exercise prescription and such issues as frequency, intensity, and volume. Testing, however, is not a one-time task but rather an ongoing method of evaluation throughout the prescribed program. In this sense, it is the beginning, middle, and end of a truly individual periodized regime. The results can be used to evaluate performance and make decisions regarding the future of a program or individual. They may also be used to predict future performance in much the same way that college entrance exam scores are used to predict an individual's probability of graduating. Last, test scores may be used in a research environment as part of an in-depth analysis of an important question. Ultimately, the outcome of this entire process is the individualized exercise prescription that will best serve each athlete or client.

Physical testing is an ongoing task to assess the status of both the athlete and the program.

147

---

150   PART 2 ■ Organization and Administration

The five major types of validity are:

1. **Face** validity states that the test is logical on the surface, as when having a person lift a weight to measure strength.
2. **Content** validity states that the test includes material that has been taught or covered; for instance, testing speed after training for speed.
3. **Predictive** validity states that test scores can accurately predict future performance. An example would be the National Football League measuring college football players prior to the draft to determine their potential.
4. **Concurrent** validity states that the test is a measure of the individual's current performance level. This happens when the test occurs shortly after training is completed.
5. **Construct** validity states that the test measures some part of the whole skill, such as measuring bench-press strength for football linemen.

Reliability

Reliability is loosely defined as repeatability. That is, the ability of a test to arrive at or near the same score upon repeated measurements in the absence of any intervention strategy. A reliable test should result in consistent scores. To accomplish this (using the new device scenario stated previously), the procedure would be to measure individuals using the new device, then allow a time delay of approximately 48 to 72 hours so no significant training effects could interfere with the results, and then measure each person a second time using the identical procedures as the first measurement. If reliability is high, then people scoring well on the first test should also score well on subsequent tests (4,5).

The rank order of participants should remain relatively constant, as in back-to-back days of hand-grip strength testing. A perfect rank order between tests would mean that each person kept his or her spot in the ordinal sequence relative to all others.

REAL-WORLD APPLICATION
Reproducing Physical Test Results in Training and Conditioning

Reproducing the results of physical tests is important to maintain the test's validity and reliability. Testing athletes in the weight room or on the field presents special challenges in terms of reproducing test data.

Why is reproducibility important in training and conditioning? It is important for a number of reasons, even though the data may not be used for research purposes.

You will make a decision about the type of program you use based on the results you obtain. If your results are not accurate, then you may be making the wrong decision and choosing a program that is not producing the results you seek. Pre- and posttesting must use reproducible procedures so that you can accurately make your decision.

Conditioning programs should focus on specific areas of weakness in a particular athlete. Those areas must be monitored on a regular basis using reproducible tests. If the tests used are not reproducible, then, once again, an incorrect decision will be made.

Inconsistent test results may not motivate the athlete to improve. We know that hard work pays off with improved scores; but if the scoring is inconsistent, we are providing bad information.

Documenting improvement in the athletes you train is an indication that you, as a conditioning coach, are doing your job. Providing your administrators with accurate testing records obtained by using reproducible tests is an important step in justifying your position.

Are there steps that the conditioning professional can take to improve the reproducibility of the test results? Of course!

- Standardize the testing procedures for every test. Have the procedures in writing and provide a copy to each data collector.
- Train the data collectors to collect the test results accurately and consistently.
- Use the same data collectors as much as possible.
- Allow the same number of trials for each test.
- Test in the same environmental conditions as much as possible. Environmental conditions are best controlled indoors, so test indoors as much as possible and practical.
- Standardize the amount and type of external motivation provided to the athlete, and keep it consistent from one testing session to the next.
- Test at the same time of day if possible.
- Always test after a day of rest if possible. Strenuous training of specific muscle groups may decrease performance on some tests.
- Maintain the same order of testing.

Control diet as much as possible. You may not be able to control diet to a great extent, but remember that it can have an effect on performance, both positive and negative.

Key Points summarize and reinforce key concepts that you need to know at the end of a section.

Real-World Application Boxes demonstrate how to apply what you learn to real-world training situations.

Figures and Charts are a fast and easy way to get a quick overview of key relationships and key information.

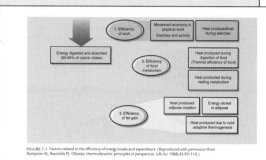

FIGURE 7.1 Factors related to the efficiency of energy intake and expenditure. (Reproduced with permission from Rampone AJ, Reynolds PJ. Obesity: thermodynamic principles in perspective. Life Sci 1988;43:93–110.)

Full Color Photographs help you learn exactly how you should perform specific training techniques.

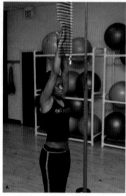
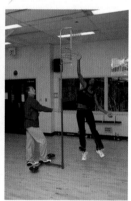

FIGURE 8.5 Countermovement vertical jump. **A.** First, determine the athlete's reach while standing on the floor. **B.** Then, have the athlete jump to determine maximum height.

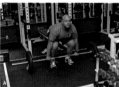
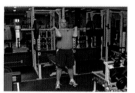

FIGURE 8.6 Power clean. **A.** Starting position. **B.** Catch.

Sequence Boxes present step-by-step instruction and illustration of exercises and movements you will use with the athletes you train.

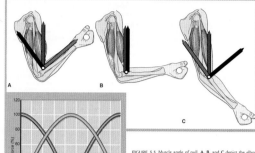

FIGURE 5.5 Muscle angle of pull. **A, B,** and **C** depict the elbow flexors at three different joint angles. The red arrow represents muscle force, the yellow arrow is the component of this force producing rotation about the joint, and the blue arrow indicates the stabilizing force (if directed toward the joint) or dislocating force (if directed away from the joint). **A.** The angle of pull is less than 90 degrees and dislocating force is evident. **B.** The angle of pull is 90 degrees and 100% of muscle force is contributing to joint rotation with no dislocating or stabilizing force. **C.** The angle of pull is greater than 90 degrees and a stabilizing force is evident. **D.** Muscle angle of pull determines percentage of muscle force contributing to joint rotation (orange line) or to dislocating and stabilizing forces (purple line).

effectiveness of the developed muscle tension. For example, when the angle of pull is 30 degrees to the long axis of the bony lever, the contractile force is only 50% efficient in terms of transfer into torque about the joint.

Strength Curve

Combination of the length-tension effect and angle of pull results in the strength curve for the particular movement. It is important to note that the **strength curve** is the net combination of all the muscles, bones, and joints involved in the movement. So for a single joint movement, like elbow extension, only the triceps brachii length and angle of pull combine to produce the strength curve. For a more complex, multijoint movement, such as bench press, all the muscles involved in shoulder horizontal adduction and elbow extension

combine to produce the strength curve for this movement. The result is a range of different-shaped strength curves for each movement. The most common is **ascending,** which describes movements such as squat and bench press. In both cases, from the bottom to the top of the lift the force-generating capacity of the musculoskeletal system increases.

Line and Magnitude of Resistance

The direction of the force that must be overcome during resistance training is termed the **line of resistance.** In training with free weights, this is always vertically down, because the resistance is the gravitational weight force acting on the barbell or dumbbell (Fig. 5.6). Using combinations of levers and pulleys, the line of resistance for a

---

least one spotter should be used to guide the exerciser in removing the resistance from its starting position and then returning it at the completion of the set to ensure that the barbell is safely removed and returned. For the safety of the exerciser and others in the immediate area as well as for equipment maintenance, exercise should be initiated with the resistance being lifted from its resting position and returned to its starting position slowly.

Resistance-Training Exercises

Power Exercises
Power Clean
Power Snatch
Power Jerk

Hip/Thigh Exercises
Back Squat
Front Squat

Dead Lift
Barbell Lunge
Stiff-Leg Dead Lift
Leg Press
Leg Extension
Leg Curl
Standing Heel Raise

Chest Exercises
Bench Press, Dumbbell
Bench Press, Barbell
Incline Press, Dumbbell
Incline Press, Barbell
Dumbbell Fly

Upper Back Exercises
Dumbbell One-Arm
   Row
Lat Pull-Down
Seated Cable Row

Shoulder Exercises
Dumbbell Seated
   Shoulder Press
Machine Shoulder Press
Barbell Upright Row
Dumbbell Prone
   Posterior Raise

Triceps Exercises
Supine Triceps
   Extension
Triceps Pushdown

Biceps Exercises
Barbell Bicep Curl
Dumbbell Seated
   Alternate-Arm
   Bicep Curl

Forearm Exercises
Wrist Curl
Reverse Wrist Curl

**Abdominal and
Lower Back Exercises**
Abdominal Crunch
Back Extension

POWER EXERCISES

Power Clean

Type of Exercise
Total body/power (explosive) exercise

Muscles Used
Gluteus maximus, hamstrings (semimembranosus, semitendinosus, biceps femoris), quadriceps (vastus lateralis, vastus intermedius, vastus medialis, rectus femoris), soleus, gastrocnemius, trapezius, and deltoids (anterior, medial, and posterior)

Starting Position
Use a standard barbell. The lifting position is identical to that for the power snatch except for the hand position. The feet are between hip- and shoulder-width apart and pointing forward or just slightly outward. Squat and grasp the barbell with a shoulder-width or slightly wider pronated hand position using a closed or hook grip. Arms are outside the knees, elbows extended and pointing outward. Stand so that the barbell is over the balls of the feet and close to the shins. Back is rigid and flat or slightly arched. Head is up or slightly hyperextended.

Chest is held up and out. Shoulder blades should be squeezed together. Trapezius and upper back should be relaxed and in a slight state of stretch. With the heels always remaining in contact with the floor, the body weight should be balanced between the balls and middles of the feet. Shoulders are slightly in front of or over the barbell (Fig. 10.1A,B).

Upward Motion: First Pull
Initiate the power clean by taking in a deep breath and holding it. Lift the barbell off the floor through forceful hip and knee extension. Maintain a constant position of the torso in relation to the floor throughout the first pull. In other words, make sure that the hips do not rise faster or before the shoulders and keep the back flat or slightly arched. The head should remain in a neutral position in relation to the spine. The shoulders should remain slightly in front of or over the barbell. The elbows should still be fully extended. During the first pull, keep the barbell as close to the shins as possible. Continue to hold your breath (Fig. 10.1C,D).

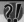

158   PART 2 ■ Organization and Administration

Q & A from the Field

The head strength and conditioning coach for the football team at our university only uses four tests for the players: the 40-yard dash, vertical jump, 1-RM squat, and 1-RM bench press. We had such a great season last year, when we won our conference championship, that the tests seem adequate, but should we be doing more?
—*graduate student intern*

Certainly we must take many things into consideration in designing a testing program. A mature, well-trained group of players might be able to continue to perform well with minimal testing. To determine the appropriate tests, we must review the basic rationale for testing athletes. Remember the primary reasons for testing:

1. To determine the fitness base of the athlete
2. To determine the performance characteristics of the better players in the sport
3. To motivate the athletes to continue to train hard

There are other possible reasons for testing. One reason might be that the S&C coach is in the process of justifying his position on the coaching staff. Good, solid data demonstrating improvement in a number of performance characteristics in the teams he trains would provide solid evidence that he is performing an important service for those athletes.

To get a total picture of the athlete's fitness base, you will probably need tests in a number of areas of performance. These areas might include the following:

1. upper-body strength
2. lower-body strength
3. upper-body endurance
4. lower-body endurance
5. upper-body power
6. lower-body power
7. aerobic capacity
8. speed
9. speed endurance
10. maximal anaerobic capacity

You may choose some tests that overlap two of these characteristics, or you may determine that a test is not appropriate for a particular sport. Maximal anaerobic capacity tests that cause a dramatic rise in lactic acid production might not be appropriate for a golfer, for example. Do recall, however, that aerobic capacity is used in recovery,

even in anaerobic sports. Remember also that we base our decisions about the type of training program needed on the testing results. In a mature, highly performing group of athletes, it is possible that the training protocols are well established and the testing data will not greatly affect the program. Thus, a minimal testing program might work in some specific situations. Spending less time testing allows more time for conditioning or practice of the sport, which might be an advantage in some situations.

In summary, there are several reasons to consider adding tests to the testing program described above. It is also possible to spend too much time and energy on testing, taking away from training time and practice time. The correct answer to your question depends on the goals of your particular testing program. Do the athletes need more motivation to train hard? Additional tests may provide the additional motivation. Is it important for the S&C coach to provide data to justify his value to the team? Additional tests may prove his importance. Do the chosen tests adequately represent the physical requirements of the sport? If not, additional tests may provide the missing data. Are the tests position-specific? In football, the physical demands of different positions can vary. A 40-yard dash may be appropriate for backs, while a 10- or 20-yard dash may be more appropriate for linemen. Matching testing to position-specific physical requirements will provide useful information. The training program should provide position-specific benefits to the individual athlete.

Every group of athletes will differ to some extent, and the philosophy of conditioning programs will vary from school to school as well. An S&C coach is constantly thinking about what he can do to keep motivation high, athletes working hard, and maintain a positive attitude toward the training. The testing program should evaluate improvement in performance that is specific to the sport of football as well as to the athlete's position. A properly designed testing program can be a key component in achieving these goals!

lete's strengths and weaknesses. It should not be used as a direct predictor of how he or she will perform on the field.

STANDING LO[...]
The standing lo[...] that measures[...]

Although the vertical jump is used to measure vertical power, the long jump is used to measure horizontal power. As another test of lower-body power, it too is a good choice for athletes requiring

Q&A from the Field is a simulated ask-the-expert column that offers you fresh insight and perspective by answering questions posed by students and professionals.

CHAPTER 17 ■ Principles of Injury Prevention and Rehabilitation   401

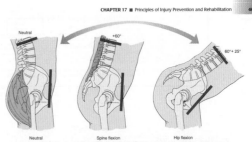

FIGURE 17.12 Muscle activity in forward bending. Bending forward is a two-part movement involving both the spine and the pelvis. Part one involves the first 60 degrees of movement, and part two involves an additional 25 degrees of forward trunk flexion.

SUMMARY

Injury prevention and rehabilitation involve a coordinated effort from various health care professionals. Strength and conditioning professionals must be aware of the stress placed on body tissues during strengthening exercises to minimize injury risk. When pain or injury does occur, activity needs to be modified and referral to an appropriate health care professional should be made as needed. Communication between sports medicine professionals is vital in transitioning an athlete from a supervised rehabilitation program to a return to sport interval program, and ultimately an independent conditioning program. Conduct-

ing preparticipation physicals, identifying muscular strength and endurance deficits, awareness of joint and body mechanics during strengthening exercises, and appropriate activity progression after injury are all ways to minimize injury risk and maximize sport performance.

MAXING OUT

1. A basketball player at a rural high school sustains an ankle sprain. There is no health care professional present at the time of the injury. What actions should be taken?
2. What muscles should be addressed by exercises in a core stabilization program?

CASE EXAMPLE
Upper Extremity

BACKGROUND

A 45-year-old recreational athlete has a goa[l of] returning to a weightlifting program for g[en]eral fitness. He states that 5 years ago he [had] shoulder surgery, due to a long history of sh[oul]

der tendonitis that began when he was in college playing baseball. He has no idea what type of lifting he should do for his upper body but feels very weak and wants to increase his strength and general fitness levels.

(continued)

Summaries at the end of each chapter highlight the most important concepts discussed in the chapter.

---

286   PART 3 ■ Exercise Prescription

MAXING OUT

1. Before you design a resistance exercise program, you must first perform a needs analysis. Perform a needs analysis for a basketball team using the questions in the "Needs Analysis" section on page 274 as a guide.
2. You are a strength and conditioning coach for a high school football team. During the season, the head football coach instructs you to design an in-season workout that lasts no longer than 45 min-

utes. You can choose resistance-training exercises. List the exercises you would choose and give a brief reason for your choices.

3. You are a strength and conditioning coach in a high school. The school is building a new weight room, and the athletic director wants to equip the weight room with various pieces of machine resistance equipment. You have a meeting with the athletic director to discuss your preference of free weights. Outline the major points you will make to the athletic director at this meeting.

CASE EXAMPLE
Designing a Resistance-Training Program for a College Football Player

BACKGROUND

You are a strength and conditioning professional at a college and have been asked to design a resistance-training program for a football player. The player is a running back entering his junior season and has 5 years of resistance-training experience including multiple-joint and Olympic-style lifts. Perform a needs analysis and design an individualized resistance-training program.

CONSIDERATIONS

Football is a high-intensity sport with short periods of play (approximately 5 seconds) interspersed with brief rest periods (approximately 30 seconds). Running backs require speed, strength, and power to be successful. This specific athlete already possesses adequate muscle mass and minimal body fat; therefore hypertrophy and/or changes in body mass are not desired. The athlete is beginning his summer break and is in a "preseason" training phase. The athlete has no injuries or health concerns.

IMPLEMENTATION

Exercise selection. Multiple-joint, large-muscle-mass exercises including power exercises should be emphasized.
Exercise order. (1) Power exercises; (2) multiple-joint large-muscle-mass exercises; (3) single-joint small-muscle-mass exercises
Loading. Power exercises: 30% to 50% of 1 RM
Strength exercises: >80% of 1 RM
Volume. Multiple sets, one to six repetitions per set
Rest intervals. Fundamental exercises: 2 to 3 minutes
Assistance exercises: 1 to 2 minutes
Frequency. Four sessions per week
Workout structure. Split routine
Muscle actions. Concentric and eccentric
Repetition velocity. Power exercises—the repetitions are to be performed as quickly as possible
Strength exercises: Volitional speed

RESULTS

Example of a week of training

MONDAY	TUESDAY	WEDNESDAY	THURSDAY	FRIDAY
Bench throws:	Hang pulls:	OFF	Incline press:	Squat jump:
4 sets	3 sets		3 sets	4 sets
3 reps	3 reps		6 reps	3 reps
30% of 1 RM (use medicine ball)	30% of 1 RM		6 RM	30% of 1 RM

Maxing Out Boxes help you use your new skills and knowledge to solve problems based on real-life scenarios.

Case Examples set forth a range of scenarios and then guide you step-by-step through the design and implementation of a training program.

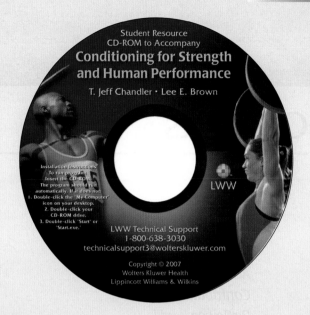

STUDENT RESOURCES

Your Student CD-ROM gives you even more opportunity to test and strengthen your understanding and practice your skills. All the features of the CD-ROM are also available on **thePoint**, http://thepoint.lww.go/chandler.

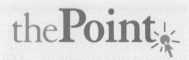

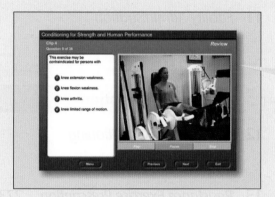

Practical Exam video clips demonstrate exercises and are followed by multiple choice questions to identify exercises and proper form.

Chandler & Brown
Conditioning for Strength and Human Performance
Chapter 9: Warm-up and Flexibility
Lab Assignment

Lab Assignment: Measuring Flexibility

Note: All flexibility testing should be done with slow, controlled movements to prevent injury and ensure accurate scoring. Circle the highest score from each test.

Sit & Reach → *Remove shoes and place feet flat against board with knees extended. Exhale as you bend forward at the waist, pushing with both middle fingers.*

    Trial 1 = _____ cm   Trial 2 = _____ cm   Trial 3 = _____ cm

Back

Extension → *Lie on your stomach with your hands to your sides and a partner holding your feet. Raise your chest up, looking directly in front of you. A third partner measures the vertical displacement of your chin.*

    Trial 1 = _____ cm   Trial 2 = _____ cm   Trial 3 = _____ cm

Back Scratch → *With one shoulder internally rotated (elbow pointed down) and one shoulder externally rotated (elbow pointed up) attempt to grasp your hands behind your back. A partner with a ruler can measure the amount of space between (-) or overlap (+) of the middle fingers.*

Lab Assignments offer suggestions for lab activities for you to practice and further develop their skills.

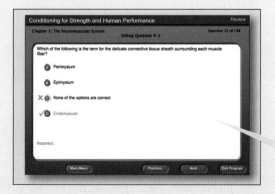

Quizzes let you evaluate your grasp of the material.

Contents

Expanded Contents

CHAPTER 7 Nutrition 123
José Antonio, John Berardi, and Christopher R. Mohr

PART 2 Organization and Administration

CHAPTER 8 Test Administration and
Interpretation 147
Lee E. Brown, Daniel Murray, and Patrick Hagerman

CHAPTER 9 Warm-up and Flexibility 166
Duane V. Knudson

CHAPTER 10 Resistance Exercise Techniques
and Spotting 182
John F. Graham

CHAPTER 11 Facility Administration
and Design 237
Steven Plisk

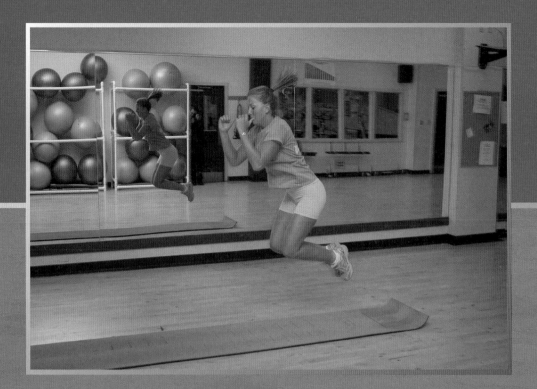

PART

1

Basic Science

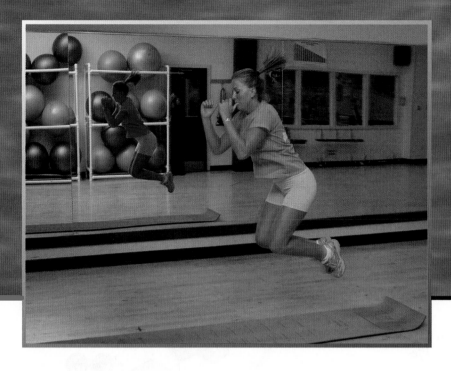

Bioenergetics

T. JEFF CHANDLER
C. ERIC ARNOLD

Introduction

Human movement requires energy, and energy is vital for athletic performance. Bioenergetics is the flow of energy in biological systems and is a key consideration during exercise. For any physical activity, energy must be generated and used by the body to accomplish the task. The source of energy influences the ability of the sprinter to complete the 100-m dash or the marathoner to complete a run. An understanding of metabolism, specifically the energy systems used during various types of exercise, is vital in developing effective activity-specific conditioning programs. With a basic knowledge of bioenergetics, the student can understand why specific chemical reactions taking place in skeletal muscles are turned on and how energy from these reactions fuels muscles during exercise.

Bioenergetics is the study of sources of energy in living organisms and how that energy is ultimately utilized.

The food we eat contains chemical energy. We store this chemical energy in our body in the forms of glycogen, fat, and protein. Ultimately, this stored chemical energy can be released to provide the energy needed to produce adenosine triphosphate (ATP). ATP is the most important source of energy supporting muscle contraction during exercise.

ATP's structure is composed of an adenine group, a ribose group, and three phosphate groups joined together (Fig. 1.1). The formation of ATP occurs by combining adenosine diphosphate (ADP) and inorganic phosphate (Pi). This process requires a substantial amount of energy that must be captured from the food we eat.

> *ATP is the high-energy molecule responsible for muscular contraction and other life-sustaining metabolic reactions in the human body.*

ATP is a high-energy molecule that stores energy in the form of chemical bonds. Energy is released when the chemical bonds that join ADP and Pi together to form ATP are broken (Fig. 1.2). The chemical energy derived from the breaking of the chemical bonds provides energy for the performance of various types of exercise.

Metabolism is the sum total of **anabolic** and **catabolic** processes. A catabolic process breaks larger compounds into smaller compounds. In metabolism, this involves the breakdown of substances such as carbohydrate for the purpose of providing fuel for the muscles during exercise. An anabolic reaction builds larger substances from smaller substances.

> *METABOLISM = CATABOLISM + ANABOLISM.*

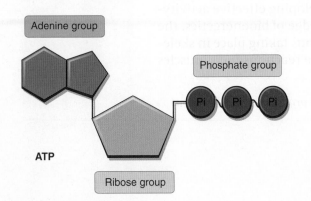

FIGURE 1.1 The basic structure of ATP. Energy is stored in the three phosphate bonds.

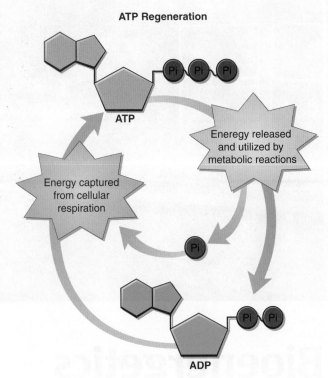

FIGURE 1.2 Regeneration of ATP. Energy is released when ATP is broken down into ADP and Pi. ATP is regenerated from ADP and energy captured from food.

ENZYMES

Enzymes are protein-structured molecules that speed or facilitate certain chemical reactions by lowering the energy of activation of a chemical reaction (7). The energy of activation is considered an energy barrier that must be overcome for a chemical reaction to occur (Fig. 1.3). Enzymes lower the **energy of activation**, or the amount of energy needed to cause a specific chemical reaction to occur. In this way, enzymes facilitate metabolic chemical reactions. The enzyme does not become a part of the product but remains intact as an enzyme.

A chemical reaction is classified as either an exergonic or an endergonic reaction. An **exergonic** reaction gives up energy and an **endergonic** reaction absorbs energy from its surroundings. During a 100-m sprint, ATP is broken down in the muscles and energy is released (exergonic reaction) and utilized by the muscles (endergonic reaction) that are actively recruited during the activity. An exergonic reaction is illustrated in Figure 1.4, where A → B is a spontaneous downhill reaction. In this example, the reactant's (A) (ATP) energy level is greater than the product (s) (ADP + Pi) (7).

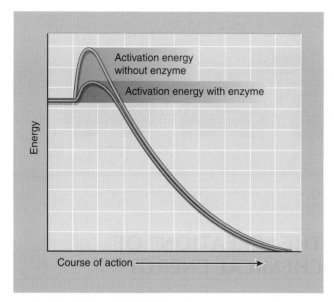

FIGURE 1.3 Energy of activation. An enzyme lowers the amount of energy that must be overcome for a chemical reaction to occur.

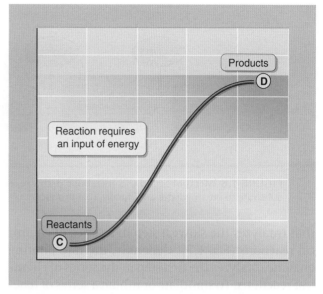

FIGURE 1.5 Endergonic chemical reaction. In an endergonic reaction, the energy level of the product(s) is greater than that of the reactant(s).

An endergonic reaction is illustrated in Figure 1.5, where C → D is a nonspontaneous uphill reaction (7). In this example, the energy level of the product(s) is greater than that of the reactant(s) (7). The C → D transition will not occur unless an enzyme is present to lower the energy of activation (7). Thus the energy of activation serves as an energy barrier to the chemical reaction (7). Box 1.1 compares a mousetrap to exergonic and endergonic reactions.

Metabolism is a series of enzyme-controlled chemical reactions for the purpose of storing or using energy. Metabolism (Fig. 1.6) begins with a substrate, which is the beginning material in the reaction. In each step, the substrate undergoes a chemical change catalyzed by enzymes and is modified; these modified compounds are referred to as intermediates. In the final step, the resulting compound is referred to as the product.

In a series of metabolic reactions, one enzyme is generally referred to as the rate-limiting enzyme. A **rate-limiting enzyme** is defined as an enzyme

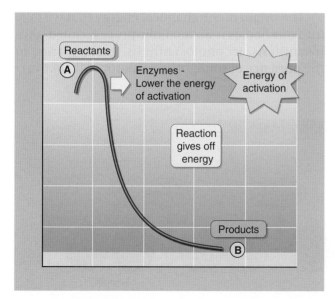

FIGURE 1.4 Exergonic chemical reaction. In such a reaction, the energy level of the reactant(s) is greater than that of the product(s).

1.1 MOUSETRAP ANALOGY

The following biochemical reaction is instrumental in muscular contraction: ATP → ADP + PI + energy (ATPase is the enzyme that catalyzes this reaction).

During muscular contraction, the bonds that link the phosphate groups in the ATP molecule are broken and liberate energy. The liberation of energy by the phosphate bonds is termed exergonic. The breaking of the bonds liberates this energy (exergonic) and fuels muscular contraction (endergonic). The mousetrap is utilized to illustrate both exergonic and endergonic biochemical reactions. Pulling the mousetrap spring back creates stored energy in the spring; when the spring is released, an exergonic reaction occurs. The endergonic reaction is illustrated by the snapping of the mousetrap (trap consuming the energy).

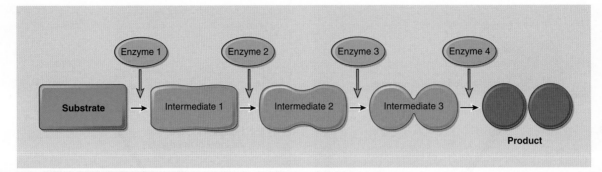

FIGURE 1.6 Metabolism. In this metabolic pathway, enzymes facilitate chemical reactions that change a substrate to intermediates and, finally, to a product.

that catalyzes the slowest step in a series of chemical reactions (Fig. 1.7). Generally, the rate-limiting enzyme catalyzes the first step in the series of chemical reactions. To stimulate or inhibit a series of reactions, a substance must affect the rate-limiting step. This is referred to as a negative feedback system, because the change that occurs is in the opposite direction from what was happening before the feedback.

Enzymes are influenced by changes in both pH and temperature. Changes in pH can influence key enzymes that control metabolic pathways. During high-intensity exercise, pH decreases within muscle, which may affect enzyme function and can slow down glycolysis, thus reducing the amount of ATP available for muscle contraction.

Temperature can have an important effect on enzymatic reactions. This effect is studied by changing the temperature in multiples of 10°C and is referred to as the **Q10 effect**. Increasing the temperature by 10°C doubles the speed of the enzymatic reaction. From a practical perspective, warming up the muscles prior to engaging in physical activity allows the athlete to take advantage of the Q10 effect.

THE "CREATION" OF CHEMICAL ENERGY

Where does energy come from? Energy is neither created nor destroyed but can be changed from one form to another. This concept reinforces the first law of thermodynamics, the physical science dealing with energy exchange, where energy is "changed" from one form to another. The first law of thermodynamics, also known as the law of the conservation of energy, can be applied to muscle contraction. It states that the increase in the internal energy of a system is equal to the amount of energy added to the system by heating plus the amount added in the form of work done on the system. During exercise, chemical energy in the form of ATP is transformed into mechanical energy in the form of muscle contraction. Without chemical energy from the breakdown of ATP, mechanical energy in the form of muscle contraction could not occur.

The origin of the chemical energy that we take into our bodies is an anabolic process called photosynthesis. In photosynthesis, green plants, in the presence of sunlight and chlorophyll, take car-

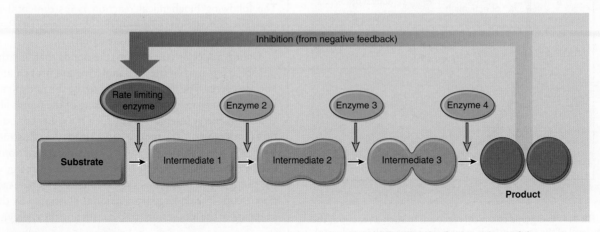

FIGURE 1.7 Inhibition of a chemical reaction. A rate-limiting enzyme is inhibited by the final product of the reaction through the negative feedback mechanism.

bon dioxide and water and change it into carbohydrate (a carbon/hydrogen/oxygen compound), with oxygen given off into the atmosphere. It is this reaction that converts the sun's energy to the chemical energy that we need to live and also replenishes the oxygen supply in our atmosphere. This carbohydrate compound formed in green plants is the basic form of energy needed by humans. Its carbon structure can be modified through anabolic reactions to form fats, which also contain carbon, hydrogen, and oxygen, and proteins, the last of which contain carbon, hydrogen, oxygen, and nitrogen.

ENERGY SYSTEMS

Three distinct yet closely integrated energy systems operate together in a coordinated fashion to provide energy for muscle contraction: the phosphocreatine system, the anaerobic glycolytic system, and the oxidative system. The phosphocreatine and anaerobic glycolytic systems provide ATP at a high rate to support muscle contraction during short bursts of high-intensity exercise such as a 200-m sprint. The amount of ATP supplied by the phosphocreatine and anaerobic glycolytic energy systems, however, is limited.

Three energy systems provide ATP for muscular work: the phosphocreatine system, the anaerobic glycolytic system, and the oxidative system.

The oxidative system predominates during low to moderate exercise intensity when oxygen is available to the muscle. At lower exercise intensities, as during walking, ATP demand is low and energy can be supplied at a high enough rate through the oxidative energy systems (19). At higher exercise intensities, ATP demand is high, and energy cannot be supplied solely by oxidative metabolism (19). Therefore, the anaerobic glycolytic system must fill this gap between the phosphocreatine system and the oxidative system. During high-intensity exercise, the supply of ATP must be derived from the phosphocreatine and anaerobic glycolytic energy systems.

It is important to note that all three energy systems are active at a given point in time but one system will predominate based on the conditions at that time (Table 1.1). Each energy system operates like a dimmer switch in that it is not completely turned off but transitioned from one system to the next based on the energy requirements of the muscle during exercise. Figure 1.8 provides a graphic representation of the overlap and timing of the major energy systems. Box 1.2 provides a summary of the transition of energy systems from one to the next.

Exercise intensity is the most important variable related to which energy system is activated to produce ATP for muscular work.

Exercise intensity, duration, and the mode of exercise play an instrumental role in determining which energy system will predominate during exercise, although exercise intensity plays the most important role in dictating which energy system is activated.

Exercise intensity is prescribed using a percentage of maximal oxygen consumption (percent $\dot{V}O_{2max}$). Maximal oxygen consumption is defined as the greatest amount of oxygen utilization that occurs during dynamic exercise and is measured in either mL/kg/min or L/min. For example, an individual may be prescribed exercise that requires 70% of his or her $\dot{V}O_{2max}$.

TABLE 1.1	THE ENERGY SYSTEMS AND THEIR APPROXIMATE CONTRIBUTIONS TO VARIOUS DURATIONS OF EXERCISE *AT MAXIMAL INTENSITY (1)*
ENERGY SYSTEM	**DURATION**
Phosphocreatine system	0–10 seconds
Phosphocreatine system and glycolytic system (slow)	10–30 seconds
Glycolytic system (fast)	30 seconds–2 minutes
Glycolytic system (fast) and oxidative system	2–3 minutes
Oxidative system	< 3 minutes and rest

Note: At submaximal intensity, each system can supply ATP for a longer time. Recovery from all types of energy expenditure is aerobic.
Source: Adapted with permission from Bassett DR Jr, Howley ET. Limiting factors for maximum oxygen uptake and determinants of endurance performance. Med Sci Sports Exerc 2000;32(1):70–84.

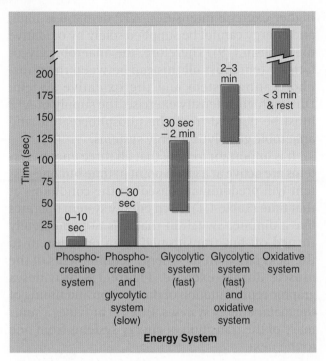

FIGURE 1.8 The energy systems and their approximate contributions to various durations of exercise at maximal intensity. Note the overlapping and timing of the various energy systems.

Understanding when a specific energy system is turned on during various activities and/or sporting events can help the strength coach to develop programs that are metabolically specific.

The Phosphocreatine System

ATP is broken down to release energy (a catabolic process) and can be regenerated from its compo-

nent parts, an adenosine group and three **phosphate groups**. Conversely, energy is required to add a phosphate group to an adenosine group, which is an anabolic process. Box 1.3 lists the characteristics of the phosphocreatine system.

When muscular energy is needed for a short time, the phosphocreatine system is capable of supplying most of the needed ATP. The phosphocreatine system will also supply energy in the beginning stages of all types of exercise. ATP is produced in the phosphocreatine system anaerobically (without oxygen present). Three basic reactions occur in the phosphocreatine system (Fig. 1.9). When physical activity is initiated, ATP stored in the muscles is utilized. All activities are initiated anaerobically, as it takes time to begin to produce ATP aerobically. The phosphocreatine system can regenerate ATP anaerobically, allowing anaerobic activity to proceed at a maximal or near maximal level, but only for a short time.

MYOSIN ATPase REACTION

The first step in the phosphocreatine system is the breakdown of ATP to ADP + Pi in the presence of the enzyme myosin ATPase. This reaction produces energy for muscle contraction anaerobically. Some ATP is stored in the muscles to perform this task. As mentioned, the initiation of all activity depends on this stored ATP. Following the initial breakdown of ATP, there are two reactions that regenerate ATP anaerobically. These reactions are often named by the enzymes that catalyze the reactions; the creatine kinase reaction and the myokinase reaction.

1.2 ENERGY SYSTEM TRANSITION

The recruitment and/or activation of energy systems during exercise are analogous to a dimmer switch that controls the level of lighting in a room. The phosphocreatine energy system is the first energy system recruited, followed by anaerobic glycolysis and oxidative phosphorylation (e.g., aerobic metabolism). The dimmer switch provides more light as you turn it up and less light as you turn it down. This relationship applies to all energy systems—the phosphocreatine, anaerobic glycolysis, and oxidative systems. As exercise progresses, the energy systems transition from one energy system to the next to provide the ATP needed to provide the energy that the muscles need to perform. As one system fades, the next system begins to take over the demand for the production of energy.

1.3 CHARACTERISTICS OF THE PHOSPHOCREATINE SYSTEM

1. It involves only one chemical step.
2. It is catalyzed by the enzyme creatine kinase (CK).
3. Its chemical reaction is very fast.
4. One ATP is generated per phosphocreatine molecule.
5. The reaction lasts for 5 to 10 seconds at maximal intensity.
6. It is anaerobic.
7. Fatigue is associated with the depletion of phosphocreatine.
8. It is the dominant energy system in speed and explosive power events.

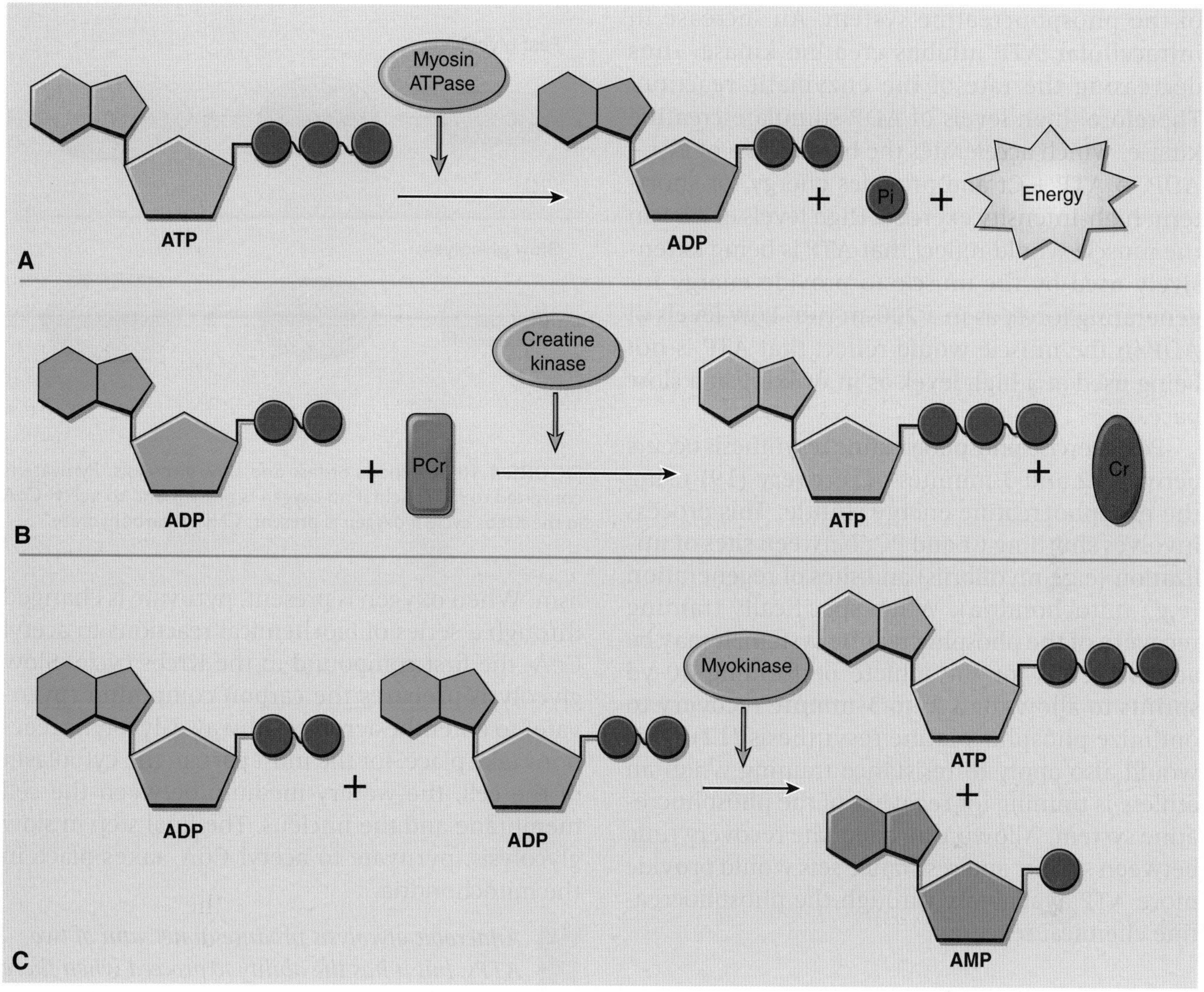

FIGURE 1.9 Reactions of the phosphagen system. **A.** Myosin ATPase reaction, **B.** creatine kinase reaction, and **C.** myokinase reaction.

CREATINE KINASE REACTION

In the creatine kinase reaction, phosphocreatine is combined with ADP in the presence of the enzyme creatine kinase to form new ATP.

MYOKINASE REACTION

A second reaction that can regenerate ATP anaerobically over the short term is the myokinase reaction, which regenerates ATP from two ADPs. This reaction results in the production of one ATP molecule and one adenosine monophosphate (AMP) molecule. The production of AMP is important to the control of metabolism, as AMP is a potent stimulator of glycolysis.

In summary, the ATP used in the phosphocreatine system starts with energy from carbohydrates (or fats or proteins), with the energy from the food stored in the chemical bonds between adenosine and phosphate (see Fig. 1.2). ATP is broken down to provide energy and can also be "recharged" anaerobically. When ATP is regenerated, energy is stored. When ATP is used for energy, energy is released. ATP is the ultimate source of energy for muscular contraction.

Regulation of Energy Production

The **energy charge of the cell (ATP/ADP ratio)** plays an integral role in regulating the phosphocreatine system. The energy charge of the muscle cell provides information on how much energy (ATP) is available in the muscle to support the activity. Increased ADP concentration in the cell stimulates creatine kinase, the key regulatory control enzyme of the phosphocreatine system. An increase in intracellular ATP inhibits creatine kinase, thus decreasing the rate of the enzymatic reaction. Therefore, high levels of ADP stimulate creatine kinase, which accelerates the breakdown of PCr + ADP → ATP + Cr and provides energy for short-term high-intensity exercise. High levels of ADP in the muscle would reflect that ATP is being extensively used by the muscle to provide energy for generating force, as in a 200-m run. Low levels of ADP in the muscle would reflect that ATP is not being used at a high level, as in walking at a slow pace.

Postexercise phosphocreatine resynthesis occurs between 2 and 3 minutes of recovery (19) using the phosphocreatine energy shuttle. This process involves shuttling Cr and PCr between sites of utilization (e.g., myofibrils) and sites of regeneration (e.g., mitochondria). When specifically training recovery of the phosphocreatine system, it may be advantageous for the athlete performing 40-yd sprints to allow for a 2- to 3-minute recovery to optimize phosphocreatine resynthesis (12). This would also apply to resistance training when an athlete is training for recovery of the phosphocreatine system. Allowing an adequate recovery time between sprints and resistance sets would provide more ATP availability through the phosphocreatine chemical reaction.

The Glycolytic System

The glycolytic system, or anaerobic glycolysis, involves the breakdown of carbohydrate anaerobically to produce energy. Fats and proteins cannot be metabolized in the glycolytic system. The carbohydrate (the substrate) comes from either blood glucose or glycogen stored in the liver or muscles. The two types of glycolysis are fast glycolysis and slow glycolysis (Fig. 1.10). Slow glycolysis is sometimes referred to as "aerobic glycolysis" (7) because pyruvate is converted to acetyl-CoA if oxygen is present and to lactic acid if no oxygen is present. Box 1.4 provides an analogy for the ATP investment and generation phases in glycolysis.

Fast glycolysis breaks down glucose (CHO) to pyruvate and eventually to lactic acid anaerobically with the net production of two ATPs. If glycogen is the substrate, one ATP is saved and there is a net production of three ATPs.

Slow glycolysis is the path the pyruvate takes if sufficient oxygen is present for aerobic metabolism. When oxygen is present, pyruvate is changed through a series of biochemical reactions to acetyl CoA, the first compound in the Krebs cycle. Slow glycolysis prepares the carbon compound (pyruvate) to enter the aerobic pathway. Glycolytic reactions take place, for the most part, in the cytoplasm of the cell, the watery medium between the cell membrane and the nucleus. The final step in slow glycolysis, pyruvate to acetyl CoA, takes place in the mitochondria.

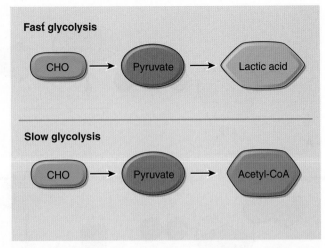

FIGURE 1.10 Reactions of fast and slow glycolysis. Pyruvate is converted to lactic acid if no oxygen is present and to acetyl-CoA in the Krebs cycle if oxygen is present. CHO = carbohydrate.

> *Anaerobic glycolysis produces a net gain of two ATPs, but it has the ability to proceed when there is no O_2 present.*

The control enzyme of the glycolytic system is phosphofructokinase (PFK). PFK is the rate-limiting enzyme that controls the rate of glycolysis. PFK

1.4 ATP INVESTMENT AND GENERATION PHASES IN GLYCOLYSIS

In the initial phases of anaerobic glycolysis, two ATPs must be invested into the system, and 4 ATPs are eventually produced, for a net gain of 2 ATPs. This investment of ATPs is like an investment in a particular stock (e.g., IBM stock), and ATP generation is like a profit gained from that particular stock (e.g., IBM stock). So a net total of 2 ATPs are generated from the metabolism of 1 glucose molecule in glycolysis. Glycolysis is similar to investing in a stock where you invest $200 and get back $400 dollars at the end of the quarter. Therefore, you have a net gain of $200, or double what you had when you initially invested in the stock.

is inhibited by high levels of ATP, phosphocreatine, citrate, free fatty acids, and a markedly decreased pH. PFK is stimulated by high concentrations of inorganic phosphate (Pi), ADP, phosphate, and ammonia and is strongly stimulated by AMP. Box 1.5 summarizes the basic characteristics of the glycolytic system.

The Oxidative System

The oxidative system aerobically oxidizes or "burns" carbohydrates (or other carbon-containing structures obtained from fat or protein). The preferred fuels for aerobic metabolism are carbohydrates and fats, but protein can be **deaminated** by removing the amino group, the nitrogenous component of the carbon/hydrogen/oxygen/nitrogen compound, and oxidizing the remaining carbon/hydrogen/oxygen compound aerobically. The oxidative system is a complex process that involves two parts: the Krebs cycle (citric acid cycle) (Fig. 1.11) and the electron transport system (ETS) (Fig. 1.12).

The Krebs cycle is a complex series of enzyme-controlled metabolic reactions. It is located in the mitochondria, the site of aerobic ATP production. The Krebs cycle plays an integral role in oxidizing carbohydrates, fats, and proteins. The electron transport chain is located in the inner membrane of the mitochondria and responsible for the aerobic production of ATP. The Krebs cycle generates elec-trons in the form of hydrogen ions shuttled through the ETS by electron carriers (FAD^+ or NAD^+). It is in the ETS that many ATP molecules are generated. Aerobic metabolic reactions take place in the mitochondria, organelles inside the cell membrane in the cytoplasm. One molecule of glucose oxidized aerobically produces 36-38 ATPs (7).

> *The aerobic system can produce many more ATPs per molecule than the anaerobic system, but it cannot produce ATP rapidly; the intensity must remain at or below steady state.*

Fats can also be oxidized aerobically to form ATP. First, fats are broken down into glycerol and free fatty acids. The free fatty acids enter the mitochondria and, through a process called beta oxidation, are degraded to acetyl CoA and hydrogen atoms. The acetyl CoA enters the Krebs cycle directly as an intermediate compound.

Although it is not a preferred source of energy, protein can be broken down and oxidized aerobically. First, proteins are catabolized into their smaller components, amino acids. Amino acids can then be deaminated. The carbon/hydrogen/oxygen portion of the compound can be converted to glucose through gluconeogenesis, pyruvate, and other Krebs cycle intermediates. The contribution of amino acids to energy production is minimal for anaerobic activities but may contribute up to 18% of the energy requirements for aerobic exercise (3). Branched-chain amino acids are the major amino acids used by skeletal muscle for energy production. The nitrogenous waste, the amino portion of the amino acid, is eliminated from the body as urea or ammonia. Ammonia is potentially a contributor to fatigue (18).

Control of the oxidative system is related to several factors. First, adequate amounts of FAD^+ and NAD^+ must be present to shuttle hydrogen ions into the ETS. A reduction in FAD^+ and NAD^+ leads to a decrease in the rate of oxidative metabolism. The ETS is inhibited by high concentrations of ATP and stimulated by high concentrations of ADP (7). Box 1.6 summarizes the characteristics of the oxidative system.

LACTATE

The lactic acid formed as a result of fast glycolysis is immediately buffered and changed into a salt called lactate. Although lactic acid is certainly associated

1.5 CHARACTERISTICS OF THE GLYCOLYTIC SYSTEM

1. Of its 18 chemical reactions, 6 are repeated.
2. It comprises 12 chemical compounds and 11 enzymes.
3. Phosphofructokinase (PFK) is the rate-limiting enzyme.
4. It is fast, but not as fast as the creatine phosphate system.
5. It uses 2 ATPs if glucose is the substrate and 3 ATPs if glycogen is the substrate.
6. It is anaerobic.
7. It functions for 1 to 2 minutes at high (not maximal) intensity.
8. Fatigue associated with decreased pH reflects an increase in hydrogen ions.
9. It is the predominant energy system in high-intensity nonmaximal exercise (e.g., an 800-meter run).

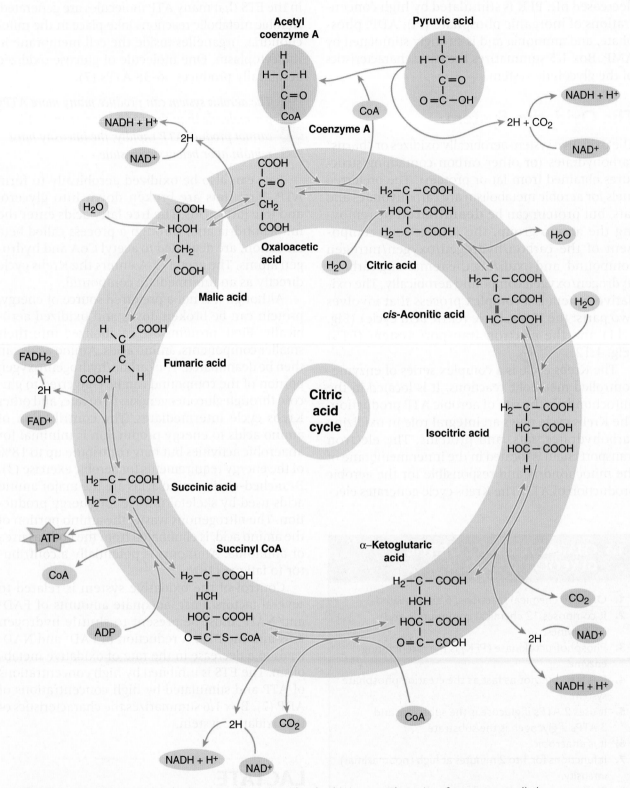

FIGURE 1.11 The Krebs cycle. Also known as the citric acid cycle, this is a complex series of enzyme-controlled metabolic reactions.

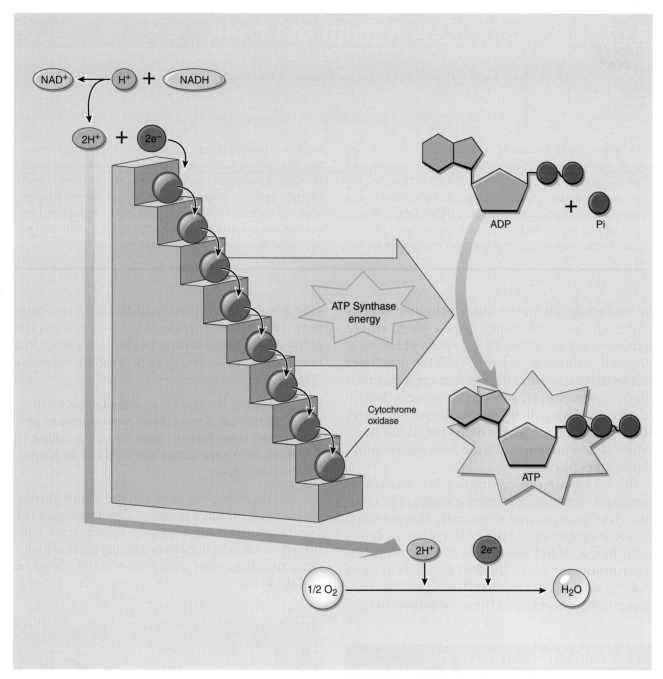

FIGURE 1.12 The electron transport system (ETS), which is responsible for the aerobic production of ATP.

with fatigue, lactate becomes a substrate that can be converted back into pyruvate and used in the Krebs cycle, particularly in the heart and in slow-twitch muscle fibers (3,8).

The lactic acid produced during heavy exercise is rapidly converted to lactate. Lactate is a useful metabolic compound that can be transported to the liver and changed to glucose in a process called "gluconeogenesis" in the liver. It can then be used by the body as fuel during recovery from exercise.

Lactate was once perceived as a metabolic waste product; however, it is now considered an important fuel source. The lactate shuttle hypothesis explained that lactate played a key role in the distribution of carbohydrate energy among various tissues and cellular compartments (6). The original lactate shuttle hypothesis was later renamed the cell-cell lactate shuttle (4), which involves the transportation of lactate produced by fast-twitch muscle fibers (type IIx) during exercise to slow-twitch muscle fibers (type 1). The lactate produced

Q & A from the Field

I have always heard that lactic acid makes you fatigued. Is that true?

Lactic acid is a by-product of anaerobic metabolism. Anaerobic exercise is by definition of high intensity, and the end product will be lactic acid. Also by definition, high intensity anaerobic exercise will lead to fatigue rather rapidly. In one sense, the production of lactic acid parallels fatigue. It may also be that molecules of lactic acid interfere with efficient muscle contraction. Lactic acid is also responsible for the immediate burning in muscle that is exercising at a high intensity. This burning is not to be confused with the delayed onset of muscle soreness that occurs over the next 24 to 48 hours, which is not due to lactic acid. The lactic acid that is produced is quickly buffered to lactate. Lactate can be transported to the liver and converted to glucose. Lactate is a useful energy source for recovery from intense anaerobic exercise.

by the fast-twitch muscle fibers is shuttled directly to the adjacent slow-twitch muscle fibers, where oxidation occurs. Some 75% to 80% of lactate is disposed of through oxidation, with the remainder converted to glucose or glycogen in a process called gluconeogenesis (5). During this process, lactate leaves the fast-twitch muscle fibers, circulates through the blood, and is delivered to the liver, where the formation of glucose from noncarbohydrates takes place.

Blood lactate can be utilized as a laboratory test to predict endurance performance. The common test incorporated to estimate this maximal steady-state speed is the lactate threshold. To determine this, a subject will run on a treadmill at various running speeds at different stages until he or she can no longer continue. During each stage, a blood sample is obtained from the subject to provide a measure of the blood lactate concentration. The lactate threshold (LT) represents the point where blood lactate begins to increase in a nonlinear fashion at a specific exercise intensity (Fig. 1.13).

> *The lactate threshold is an important factor in performance. If two athletes participating in an aerobic event have the same $\dot{V}_{O_2max}$, the athlete with the highest lactate threshold will be likely to win the race.*

The running speed at which the lactate threshold occurs is used as a predictor of performance (1). The measure of the maximal steady-state running speed is beneficial in predicting success in distance running events from 2 miles to the marathon (8–10,14–16).

1.6 CHARACTERISTICS OF THE OXIDATIVE SYSTEM

1. It comprises 124 chemical reactions.
2. It contains 30 compounds and 27 enzymes.
3. The rate-limiting enzymes are PFK, ID, and CO.
4. It functions slowly.
5. One less ATP is produced if glucose is the substrate compared to glycogen as the substrate.
6. It has a potentially limitless duration at lower intensity.
7. Fatigue of this system is associated with the depletion of fuel (muscle glycogen).
8. It is the predominant energy system in endurance events, such as marathons.

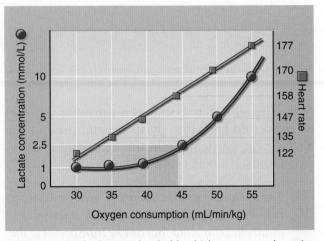

FIGURE 1.13 The lactate threshold, which represents the point where blood lactate begins to increase in a nonlinear fashion at a specific exercise intensity (18). As exercise intensity increases, blood levels of lactic acid begin to accumulate in an exponential fashion.

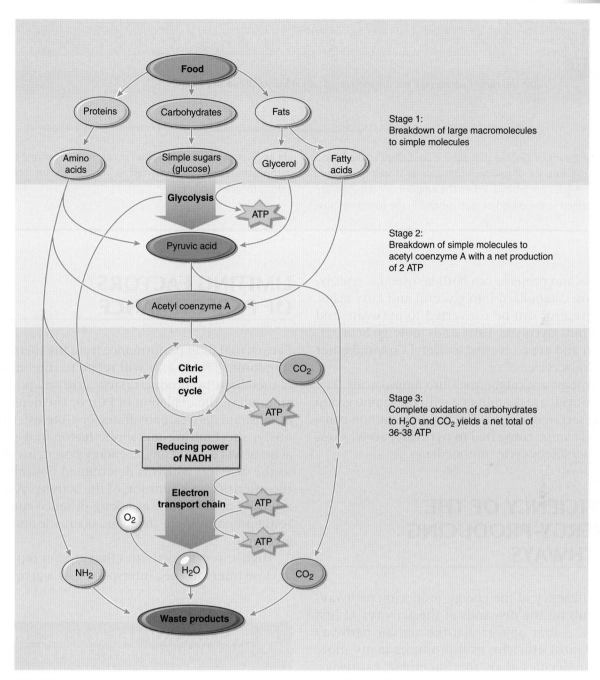

FIGURE 1.14 Summary of catabolic processes involved in the breakdown of food to energy.

SUMMARY OF CATABOLIC PROCESSES IN THE PRODUCTION OF CELLULAR ENERGY

Figure 1.14 summarizes the breakdown of food (catabolic process) for the production of energy. The food we eat is composed of fats, carbohydrates, and proteins. Carbohydrates are broken down into blood glucose, which can either be used for energy or stored as glycogen. When glycogen stores in the liver and muscles are full, the glucose is stored as fat. The glucose, through glycolysis, is converted to pyruvic acid and then into either lactic acid if no oxygen is present (fast glycolysis) or acetyl CoA if oxygen is present in the cell. The acetyl CoA then goes into the Krebs cycle and the electron transport system to produce ATP, with the eventual end products of CO_2 and H_2O.

Q & A from the Field

Are the carbohydrates we eat always stored as carbohydrate in the body?

The amount of glucose that can be contained in the blood and the amount of glycogen that can be stored in the liver and muscles are limited. When the amount of carbohydrate contained in the blood as glucose and in the liver and mus-

cle as glycogen is maximal, excess calories consumed from carbohydrates can be converted to fat. You do not have to eat fat to store body fat.

Fats and proteins can both be used for energy. Fats are catabolized into glycerol and fatty acids. The glycerol can be converted to pyruvate and enter into glycolysis. Fatty acids undergo beta oxidation and are converted to acetyl CoA and enter the Krebs cycle.

Proteins are catabolized into amino acids. The amino acids are deaminated with the amino group being secreted as urea. The resulting carbon compound can be converted to pyruvate, acetyl CoA, or other Krebs cycle intermediates.

EFFICIENCY OF THE ENERGY-PRODUCING PATHWAYS

The efficiency of the energy-producing pathways depends on the demands of the activity. At first glance, it may appear that the aerobic pathway is the most efficient, as it produces many more ATP molecules than the anaerobic pathways. Efficiency, however, can be calculated in different ways. The simplest method of looking at the efficiency of each metabolic system is relative to the task at hand. If the task is a 100-m sprint, the oxidative system is very inefficient, as it does not have the time required to produce ATP. Likewise, if the task is a marathon, the anaerobic pathways will be much less efficient, as they lack the capacity to produce ATP over a long time. Using this logic, the anaerobic energy systems are the most efficient at producing ATP immediately and the aerobic energy system is the most efficient for producing ATP over a continuous time. Box 1.7 provides an analogy to further explain the efficiency of these systems.

LIMITING FACTORS OF PERFORMANCE

Factors that limit performance from the metabolic standpoint (Table 1.2) will relate to the buildup of metabolic by-products (lactic acid and possibly ammonia), the depletion of PCr, or the depletion of substrate (fats, carbohydrates, or proteins). Obviously, the limiting metabolic factor in a given activity will depend on the energy system involved in the activity, which is determined basically by the intensity and duration of the activity. A low-intensity activity such as a long-distance run will result primarily in the depletion of muscle and liver glycogen.

High-intensity activities that are not repeated at close intervals (i.e., interspersed by a great deal

---

1.7 EFFICIENCY OF THE AEROBIC AND ANAEROBIC ENERGY SYSTEMS

Efficiency must be related to a specific task. For example, a gas-electric hybrid is more economical or efficient in terms of miles per gallon than a 4 × 4 "monster truck" for cross-country travel, but the truck is more efficient at carrying or pulling a heavy load or climbing a steep hill. Efficiency must be viewed as task-specific. The anaerobic energy systems are most efficient at producing ATP rapidly. The aerobic system is very inefficient at producing ATP if the demand is immediate. The aerobic energy system is more efficient at producing ATP over a longer duration and with a lower workload. The anaerobic system, like the truck, is inefficient at performing low-intensity work for a long time. The aerobic system, like the hybrid, is inefficient at performing at high intensity, as in pulling heavy loads or climbing a steep hill.

TABLE 1.2	METABOLIC FACTORS THAT LIMIT PERFORMANCE
ACTIVITY	**PRIMARY LIMITING FACTORS**
Marathon	Muscle glycogen, liver glycogen
High-intensity repeated (10 × 40 yd)	ATP, muscle glycogen, decreased pH
High-intensity (400 m)	Decreased pH

of rest) have essentially no metabolic limiting factors. In repeated high-intensity activities, muscle glycogen, ATP/PCr, and a decrease in pH are all possible limiting factors. The hydrogen ions given off from the buildup of lactic acid have been shown to decrease force production in skeletal muscle (13), possibly by competing with the binding sites on troponin.

OXYGEN CONSUMPTION

Oxygen consumption is the ability of the body to take in and use oxygen to produce energy. It can be estimated by using a "metabolic cart," which can measure the oxygen content of the inspired and expired air. Maximal oxygen consumption is considered a measure of **cardiorespiratory endurance**. Maximal oxygen consumption is also called $\dot{V}O_{2max}$, which can be measured in milliliters/kilogram/body weight (mL/kg/bw) or in liters/minute (L/min). $\dot{V}O_{2max}$ is measured in mL/kg/min when two individuals are being compared, because body weight influences maximal oxygen consumption. Liters per minute is used when an individual's data are just being compared from one test to another. From a practical perspective, a coach develops a training program for his or her cross-country athletes and wants to gauge its impact on their $\dot{V}O_{2max}$. Prior to starting the training program, the coach obtains a baseline measure of $\dot{V}O_{2max}$ and then the training program begins. Therefore, the coach would have his or her athletes perform a second $\dot{V}O_{2max}$ test to determine whether there had been any significant changes in their respective values.

An important addition to the $\dot{V}O_{2max}$ test would be the ability to obtain blood lactate levels during the test. The coach would have his or her athletes

run on a treadmill at various speeds and a blood lactate sample would be obtained at each stage of the protocol. Information obtained from the $\dot{V}O_{2max}$ would include:

1. At what $\dot{V}O_2$ did the lactate threshold occur?
2. At what percentage of the $\dot{V}O_{2max}$ did the lactate threshold occur?
3. At what running speed did the lactate threshold occur?
4. What heart rate (subjects would need a heart rate monitor) was achieved at the lactate threshold?

The information provided can help both the coach and the athletes to tailor a specific program based on their $\dot{V}O_{2max}$, indicating at what point and or percentage of the $\dot{V}O_2$ the LT occurred and what heart rates were achieved at the LT.

In the recovery from anaerobic work, energy (ATP) is supplied aerobically. Since it takes time for the oxidative system to begin to produce enough ATP to support an aerobic activity, all exercise is supported initially by anaerobic metabolism. The initial portion of energy supplied anaerobically is termed the oxygen deficit. After exercise, this "shortfall" must be replenished aerobically. This replenishment of the anaerobic system is termed the oxygen debt, or excess postexercise oxygen consumption (EPOC). The term *EPOC* is more accurate than *oxygen debt*. The term *debt* implies a direct replacement of the deficit or initial shortfall. EPOC supports a number of metabolic processes that are in effect postexercise. EPOC must support the following:

1. Elevated HR during recovery
2. Elevated respiration rate during recovery
3. Elevated metabolism for heat dissipation
4. Elevated metabolism for the breakdown of hormones released during exercise
5. Resynthesis of ATP and CP stores
6. Resynthesis of glycogen from lactate
7. Resaturation of body tissues (blood and muscle tissue) with oxygen (2,11,17)

Oxygen consumption, oxygen deficit, and EPOC are depicted for aerobic work in Figure 1.15A and anaerobic work in Figure 1.15B. Exercise where the oxygen supply is equal to the oxygen demand is termed steady-state exercise. In aerobic exercise, anaerobic metabolism supplies energy for the first few minutes, creating an oxygen deficit. Although part of this deficit can be paid back during the activity, the deficit must be repaid postexercise.

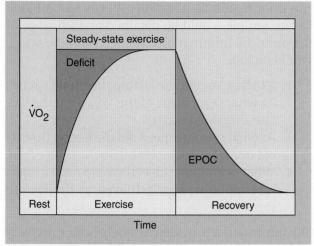

A

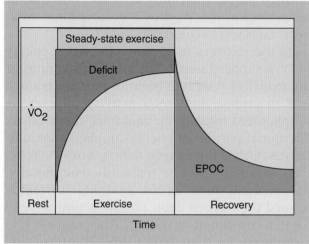

B

FIGURE 1.15 Oxygen deficit and EPOC (excess postexercise oxygen consumption). **A.** For aerobic exercise and **B.** for anaerobic exercise.

Again, the energy for this postexercise metabolic activity comes from aerobic sources. With anaerobic activity, note that the oxygen deficit is much larger because the demand for energy is greater than in the initial stage of aerobic activity.

METABOLIC SPECIFICITY

Specificity of training is a key concept in the field of training and conditioning. If training is to be specific to an actual sport or activity, then the training must focus on the same metabolic energy pathways used in the sport or activity. It is important to note that all energy systems are active to some degree all the time. And the intensity of the

activity is also a key determining factor in the energy system utilized.

The training of energy systems involves manipulating both the intensity and the duration of the activity. Metabolic specificity does not mean that *all* training is of exactly the same intensity and duration as the activity. Most activities are difficult to classify exactly in terms of intensity and duration. Box 1.8 provides examples of specificity of training.

SUMMARY

The concepts of bioenergetics are keys to understanding human performance as well as the exercise prescriptions that will enhance it. The source of energy for a specific sport or activity depends on the intensity and duration of the activity. The breakdown of food and changing it to the energy we need to move and live is a complex process. Since human adaptation to training is specific to the type of training, we must learn to train athletes in such a way that the appropriate energy system is stressed at the appropriate time and peaks at the appropriate time.

1.8 EXAMPLES OF SPECIFICITY OF TRAINING

1. If the average tennis point is 6 seconds and the average intensity is 60% of maximum, it does not mean that all training should be done for 6 seconds at 60% of maximum intensity. Some points are shorter and some are longer. Some points are more intense and some less intense. Duration and intensity, then, should be used to determine a reasonable range within which a majority of the training should fall. Progression, from general training to metabolically specific training, is also a factor.

2. Football players predominately perform short bursts of high intensity. The short burst of activity requires the phosphocreatine and anaerobic glycolytic energy systems. Devising a conditioning program that includes sprint/agility activities at 5 to 10 seconds of sustained high-intensity exercise would activate the phosphocreatine system. The anaerobic glycolytic energy system would be activated during the longer sprints (30 seconds to 2 minutes).

MAXING OUT

1. Energy system training is sport-specific and may be specific to positions within a sport. Consider a soccer player. What are some things you need to consider when planning a metabolically specific training program for a soccer player?

2. What happens to the excess carbohydrate we consume in our diet when muscle glycogen stores are full?

3. What is the fate of lactic acid produced during exercise?

REFERENCES

1. Bassett DR Jr, Howley ET. Limiting factors for maximum oxygen uptake and determinants of endurance performance. Med Sci Sports Exerc 2000;32(1):70–84.

2. Borsheim E, Bahr R. The effect of exercise intensity, duration, and mode on excess post oxygen consumption. Sports Med 2003;33(14):1037–1060.

3. Brooks GA. Amino acid and protein metabolism during exercise and recovery. Med Sci Sports Exerc 1987(5 Suppl);19:S150–S156.

4. Brooks GA. Intra- and extracellular lactate shuttles. Med Sci Sports Exerc 2000;32(4):790–799.

5. Brooks GA. Lactate shuttles in nature. Biochem Soc Trans 2002;30(2):258–264.

6. Brooks GA. The lactate shuttle during exercise and recovery. Med Sci Sports Exerc 1986;18(3):360–368.

7. Brooks GA, Fahey TD, Baldwin K. Exercise Physiology: Human Bioenergetics and Its Applications. New York: McGraw-Hill, 2005.

8. Costill D, Thompson H, Roberts E. Fractional utilization of the aerobic capacity during distance running. Med Sci Sports 1973;5(4):248–252.

9. Farrell P, Wilmore J, Coyle EF, et al. Plasma lactate accumulation and distance running performance. Med Sci Sports 1979;11(4):338–344.

10. Foster C. Blood lactate and respiratory measurement of the capacity for sustained exercise. In: Maud P, Foster D, eds. Physiological Assessment of Human Fitness. Champaign, IL: Human Kinetics, 1995.

11. Gaesser GA, Brooks GA. Metabolic bases of excess post oxygen consumption. Med Sci Sports Exerc 1984;10(1):29–43.

12. Harris RC, Edwards RHT, Hultman E, et al. The time course of phosphocreatine resynthesis during recovery of the quadriceps muscle in man. Pfluegers Arch 1976;97:392–397.

13. Hermansen L. Effect of metabolic changes on force generation in skeletal muscle during maximal exercise. In: Porter R, Whelan J, eds. Human Muscle Fatigue. London: Pitman Medical, 1981.

14. Lafontaine T, Londeree B, Spath W. The maximal steady state versus selected running events. Med Sci Sports Exerc 1981;13:190–192.

15. Lawler J, Powers S, Dodd S. A time saving incremental cycle ergometer protocol to determine peak oxygen consumption. Br J Sports Med 1987;21(4):171–173.

16. Lehmann M, Burg A, Kapp R, et al. Correlations between laboratory testing and distance running performance in marathoners of similar ability. Int J Sports Med 1983;4(4):226–230.

17. Mole P. Exercise metabolism. In: Exercise Medicine: Physiological Principles and Clinical Application. New York: Academic Press, 1983.

18. Smith SA, Montain SJ, Matott RP, et al. Creatine supplementation and age influence muscle metabolism during exercise. J Appl Physiol 1998;85(4):1349–1356.

19. Spriet LL, Howlett RA, Heigenhauser GJF. An enzymatic approach to lactate production in human skeletal muscle during exercise. Med Sci Sports Exerc 2000;32(4):756–763.

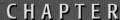

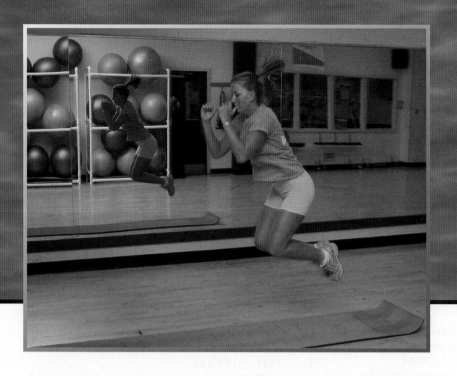

The Cardiorespiratory System

JAY R. HOFFMAN

Introduction

The primary role of the cardiorespiratory system is to meet the energy demands of the body. As energy demands increase, as might be expected during exercise, the cardiorespiratory system can compensate by increasing the amount of oxygen consumed and the volume of blood pumped into the circulation. During prolonged exercise training, physiological systems are able to adapt to increased demands. These adaptations are specific to the type of exercise stimulus presented. This chapter reviews the cardiovascular and respiratory system as well as the changes seen during acute exercise and adaptations occurring during prolonged training. Environmental factors affecting cardiorespiratory function are also discussed.

CARDIOVASCULAR SYSTEM

The cardiovascular system consists of an elaborate network of vessels comprising the circulatory system and a powerful pump (the heart) responsible for delivering oxygen and nutrients to active organs and muscles as well as removing the waste products of metabolism. The heart is a four-chambered muscular organ located in the center of the chest cavity. Its anterior border is the sternum, and it borders the vertebral column posteriorly. The lungs are situated on the heart's lateral borders. Inferior to the heart is the diaphragm.

Morphology of the Heart

The heart muscle, referred to as the **myocardium**, is similar in appearance to striated skeletal muscle. The fibers of the myocardium, however, are multinucleated and interconnected end to end by **intercalated disks**. These disks contain desmosomes, which maintain the integrity of the cardiac fibers during contraction, and gap junctions, which allow for the rapid transmission of the electrical impulse signaling for contraction. The structure of the myocardium can be thought of in terms of three separate areas: atrial, ventricular, and conductive. The atrial and ventricular areas of the myocardium function similarly to skeletal muscle in that they contract in response to electrical stimuli. In contrast to the function of skeletal muscle fibers, however, an electrical stimulus to only a single cell of either chamber will initiate an action potential that spreads rapidly to the other cells of the atrial and ventricular myocardium, resulting in a coordinated contractile mechanism. In addition, the cardiac fibers in each of these areas can function separately. The conductive tissue found between these chambers provides a network for the rapid transmission of conductive impulses, allowing for coordinated action of both the atrial and ventricular chambers.

The structural details of the heart can be seen in Figure 2.1. There is a striking difference in the anatomy and physiology of the right and left sides of the heart, which is related to their specific functions. The right side of the heart receives blood from all parts of the body (right atrium), while the right ventricle pumps deoxygenated blood to the lungs through the pulmonary circulation. The left side of the heart receives oxygenated blood from the lungs (left atrium) and pumps this blood from the left ventricle into the aorta and through the entire systemic circulation. The left ventricle is an ellipsoidal chamber surrounded by thick musculature that provides the power to eject the blood through the entire body. The right ventricle is crescent-shaped, with a thin musculature reflecting the reduced ejection pressures required of this ventricle, 25 mm Hg, compared to approximately 125 mm Hg in the left ventricle at rest. A thick solid muscular wall or **interventricular septum** separates the left and right ventricles.

Blood flow from the right atrium to the right ventricle passes through the tricuspid valve (consisting of three cusps, or leaflets, that allow only a one-directional flow of blood). The bicuspid, or mitral, valve allows blood flow between the left atrium and left ventricle. The semilunar valves, located on the arterial walls on the outside of the ventricles, prevent blood from flowing back into the heart between contractions. During systole, the cusps lie against their arterial wall attachments; during diastole, or retrograde flow, however, the cusps fall passively inward, sealing the lumen.

Cardiac Cycle

The contractile phase, in which the atria or ventricles expel the blood in their chambers, is called **systole**. The relaxation phase, in which these chambers refill with blood, is referred to as **diastole**. One complete revolution of systole and diastole is referred to as a cardiac cycle. At rest, the heart spends most of its time (approximately 60%) filling with blood (diastole) and less time (approximately 40%) expelling the blood (systole). During exercise, however, this situation is reversed, with most of the cardiac cycle spent in systole. During systole, the tricuspid and mitral valves are closed. Blood flow from pulmonic and systemic circulation, however, continues into the atria. As systole ends, the atrioventricular valves rapidly open and the blood that has accumulated in the atria flows quickly into the ventricles, accounting for 70% to 80% of ventricular filling. Three specific periods occur in diastole: during the initial third, there is rapid filling; during the middle third, referred to as diastasis, very little blood flows into the ventricle; and during the final third, ventricular filling is completed, with an additional 20% to 30% of blood pumped into the ventricle as the result of atrial systole.

The volume of blood in the ventricle at the end of diastole is called the **end-diastolic volume**

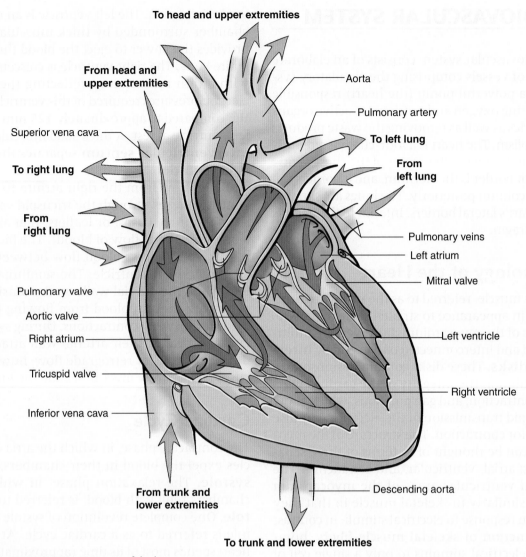

To head and upper extremities

From head and upper extremities

Aorta

Pulmonary artery

To left lung

From left lung

Superior vena cava

To right lung

From right lung

Pulmonary veins

Left atrium

Mitral valve

Pulmonary valve

Aortic valve

Right atrium

Left ventricle

Tricuspid valve

Right ventricle

Inferior vena cava

Descending aorta

From trunk and lower extremities

To trunk and lower extremities

FIGURE 2.1 Anatomy of the heart.

(EDV). During systole, two main phases occur: preejection and ejection. The preejection phase includes an electromechanical lag, which is the time delay between the beginning of ventricular excitation (depolarization) and the onset of ventricular and isovolumic contraction. The latter is the phase in which intraventricular pressure is raised prior to the onset of ejection. This part of the preejection phase occurs between the closure of the mitral valve and the opening of the semilunar valve (opening of the aortic valve). During the **ejection phase**, the blood in the ventricle is pumped into the systemic circulation through the open semilunar valve. This phase ends with the closing of the semilunar valve. The blood remaining in the ventricle at the end of ejection is referred to as the **end-systolic volume (ESV)**. The difference between EDV and ESV is called the **stroke volume**. The proportion

of blood pumped out of the left ventricle with each beat is called the **ejection fraction (EF)** and is determined by SV/EDV. The ejection fraction averages about 60% at rest. This simply means that 60% of the blood in the left ventricle at the end of diastole will be ejected with the next contraction.

> *The time spent in systole or diastole depends on whether the individual is at rest or exercising.*

Heart Rate and Conduction

A unique feature of the heart is its ability to contract rhythmically without either neural or hormonal stimulation. This autorhythmicity is due to a specialized intrinsic conduction system that consists of the sinoatrial node (SA node), internodal pathways, the atrioventricular node (AV node), and Purkinje fibers. The intrinsic conduction system of the heart can be seen in Figure 2.2.

The SA node—a collection of specialized cells capable of generating an electrical impulse—is located in the right atrium. Due to its distinctive ability, the SA node is appropriately nicknamed the pacemaker of the heart. Once an impulse leaves the SA node, it propagates leftward and downward, spreading through the atrial syncytium of first the right and then left atrium through internodal pathways merging on the AV node, which is located toward the center of the heart on the lower right atrial wall.

The AV node, or AV junction (comprising the AV node and the bundle of His), delays transmission of the impulse for a tenth of a second. This slight delay of ventricular excitation and contraction allows the atria to contract and also limits the number of signals transmitted by the AV node. This mechanism appears to protect the ventricles from atrial tachyarrhythmias. The bundle of His is found distally in the AV junction and divides into right and left segments (bundle branches), which trans-

mit the electrical impulses to the right and left ventricles, respectively. The Purkinje fibers are found on the distal tips of the right and left bundle branches and extend their fibers into the walls of the ventricles, accelerating the conduction velocity of the impulse to the rest of the ventricle. The conduction velocity of the Purkinje fibers may be fourfold faster than that at the bundle of His.

As mentioned earlier, the SA node, AV node, and Purkinje fibers are able to initiate electrical impulses spontaneously. The autonomic nervous system, however, can also influence the rate of impulse formation (referred to as **chronotropy**), the contractile state of the myocardium (**inotropy**), and the rate of spread of the excitation impulse. The sympathetic and parasympathetic nervous systems as well as certain hormones can influence cardiac contractility. The atria are well supplied with both sympathetic and parasympathetic neurons, while the ventricles are primarily innervated by sympathetic neurons. Sympathetic stimulation releases the catecholamines epinephrine and norepinephrine from sympathetic neural fibers. These

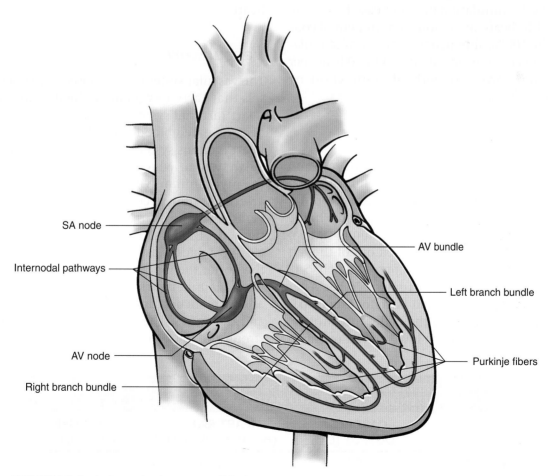

FIGURE 2.2 Intrinsic conduction system of the heart.

neural hormones accelerate heart rate by increasing the activity of the SA and increase both atrial and ventricular contractile force. An increased heart rate is termed **tachycardia**.

Parasympathetic stimulation through the vagus nerves releases the neurohormone acetylcholine, which has a depressant effect on SA node activity and decreases atrial contractile force. A decreased heart rate is termed **bradycardia**. Sympathetic stimulation may increase heart rate by over 120 beats per minute and strength of contraction by 100%, although maximal vagal stimulation may decrease heart rate by 20 to 30 beats per minute and lower strength of contraction by approximately 30% (1).

Cardiac Output

Cardiac output is the product of heart rate and stroke volume. It refers to the amount of blood pumped by the heart in 1 minute. Cardiac output responds to the energy demands of the body. In the average adult male (regardless of training status), the total volume of blood pumped out of the left ventricle per minute at rest is approximately 5 L. If an individual's resting heart rate is 70 beats per minute, stroke volume would have to be approximately 71 mL per beat. In the endurance athlete, heart rate is generally much lower at rest owing to a greater vagal tone and reduced sympathetic drive. If the heart rate of this athlete were 50 beats per minute, stroke volume would be 100 mL per beat. A comparison of the cardiac output in trained and sedentary males can be seen in Table 2.1. The mechanism that drives this particular adaptation is not entirely clear but is likely related to the increased vagal tone seen consequent to endurance training and to morphological adaptations of the heart.

Vasculature

The vascular system is composed of a series of vessels that carry oxygenated blood away from the heart (arterial system) to the tissues and return deoxygenated blood from the tissues back to the heart (venous system). The heart has its own vascular system, which is responsible for supplying the myocardium with oxygen and nutrients. The arterial system receives the blood from the left ventricle of the heart and distributes it throughout the body. Blood is first ejected from the left ventricle into a thick, elastic vessel called the aorta. From the aorta, the blood is circulated throughout the body via a network of arteries, arterioles (small arterial branches), metarterioles (smaller branches), and capillaries. The walls of the arteries are both strong and thick so as to withstand the rapid trans-

TABLE 2.1	CARDIAC OUTPUT AT REST IN SEDENTARY AND ENDURANCE-TRAINED MALES		
	CARDIAC OUTPUT (L)	HEART RATE (BEATS·MINUTE⁻¹)	STROKE VOLUME (mL)
SEDENTARY	5	70	71
TRAINED	5	50	100

port of blood under high pressure to the tissues. The thickness of these vessels prevents any gaseous exchange between them and the surrounding tissues. In addition, the arterial vascular system is innervated by the sympathetic nervous system, allowing it to be effectively stimulated to regulate blood flow. As blood reaches the tissues, it is diverted to smaller branches of the arterial system. At the end of the metarterioles (the smallest arterial vessel) are the microscopic capillaries. The capillaries are approximately 0.01 mm in diameter and their walls consist of a single layer of endothelial cells. As a result of this small diameter, the rate of blood flow decreases as the blood circulates toward and into the capillaries. In addition, there is an extensive branching of the capillary microcirculation, creating a large surface area between the capillary vasculature and surrounding tissues. The combination of a large surface area, slow rate of blood flow, and a thin layer of endothelial cells makes the capillaries an ideal place for gas exchange between the blood and the tissues.

As the blood leaves the capillaries, it enters the venous circulation. Like the arterial system, the venous system is composed of vessels of various sizes that become larger as they get closer to the heart. Deoxygenated blood leaving the capillaries enters venules (small veins), which increase the rate of blood flow (due to the smaller cross-sectional area of the venous system in comparison to the capillary system). The blood is transported back to the heart via the superior vena cava (venous blood returning from areas above the heart) and the inferior vena cava (venous blood returning from areas below the heart). The deoxygenated blood then enters the right atrium, passes through to the right ventricle, and is pumped to the lung to be reoxygenated and subsequently transported back into the left side of the heart, to be circulated through the arterial circulation.

During rest, blood flow is controlled by the autonomic nervous system and is primarily distributed to the liver, kidneys, and brain. During exercise, however, blood flow is redistributed to the exercising muscles, which may receive 75% or more of the available blood at the expense of the other organs. In combination with a greater cardiac output, the exercising muscles may receive up to a 25-fold increase in blood flow. The flow of blood to the muscles and organs at rest and during exercise is shown in Figure 2.3.

During exercise, blood flow is diverted from other organs to exercising muscles.

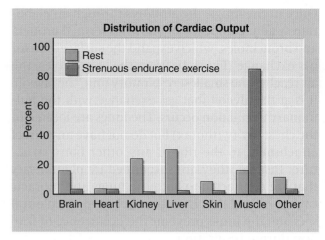

FIGURE 2.3 Distribution of cardiac output.

Blood Pressure

During each contraction, blood is pumped into the aorta from the left ventricle (systole). The pressure within the aorta under normal resting conditions reaches approximately 120 mm Hg. This measurement is referred to as the systolic blood pressure and represents the strain against the arterial walls during ventricular contraction. Since the pumping action or contraction of the left ventricle of the heart is pulsatile in nature, the arterial pressure fluctuates from an elevated level during systole to a lower level during the heart's relaxation phase, known as diastole. Diastolic blood pressure is approximately 80 mm Hg at rest and provides an indication of peripheral resistance, or the ease with which blood flows into the capillaries. As blood flows through the systemic circulation, pressure continues to fall and reaches approximately 0 mm Hg as the blood reaches the right atrium. The decrease in arterial pressure in each successive segment of the systemic circulation is directly proportional to the vascular resistance in that segment. Changes in the resistance of the systemic circulation are quite important in the regulation of blood flow.

RESPIRATORY SYSTEM

The coordination between the cardiovascular and respiratory systems provides the body with an efficient means to transport oxygen to the tissues and remove carbon dioxide. During respiration, air is breathed in (**inspiration**) through the nasal cavity or mouth. The air then travels through the pharynx, larynx, and trachea and finally into the lungs.

Once in the lungs, the air flows through an elaborate system composed of branches termed bronchi and bronchioles, which expand the surface area for gas exchange (Fig. 2.4). From the bronchioles, the air reaches the smallest respiratory unit, the alveoli. It is at the alveoli that gas exchange with the pulmonary circulation occurs. The lungs are located in the chest cavity (thorax) but do not have any direct attachment to the ribs or any other bony structure. Instead, they are suspended by pleural sacs that are connected to both the lungs and thoracic cavity. A fluid that is present between the pleural sacs and the lungs prevents the occurrence of friction during respiration.

During inspiration, the muscles of the thoracic cavity (diaphragm and external intercostal muscles) contract, causing the thorax to expand. As a result, the lungs stretch, initiating a reduction in air pressure within them. As pressure within lungs is reduced to levels below that on the outside, the pressure gradient causes air to rush into the lungs. During exercise, additional muscles (i.e., the pectoralis and sternocleidomastoid) can be recruited, causing a greater movement of the thorax and creating an even larger lung expansion.

When air is breathed out (**expiration**), the inspiratory muscles relax; during forced expiration, however, contraction of the internal intercostal and abdominal muscles causes the thorax to return to its normal position. As a result, the pressure within the lungs expands to levels above that on the outside, causing expiration to occur.

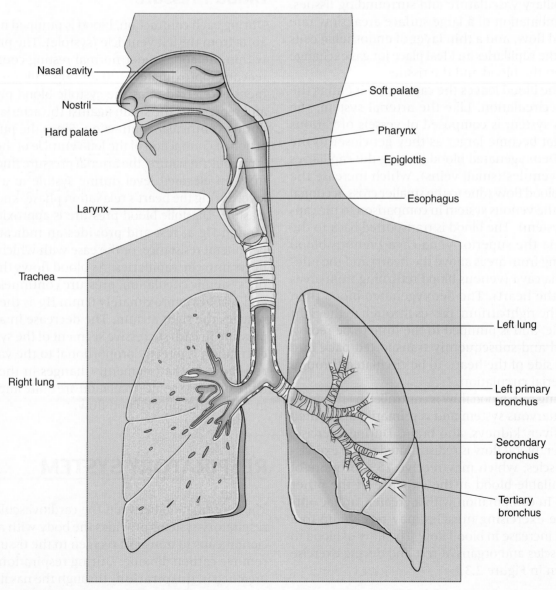

FIGURE 2.4 Anatomy of the respiratory system.

Change in pressure is the primary mechanism whereby air and gases flow into and out of the lungs and through the entire respiratory and circulatory systems. For ventilation to occur (process of inspiration and expiration), only slight changes in pressure between the lungs and the outside environment need to occur. For instance, standard atmospheric pressure is 760 mm Hg, and only slight changes in intrapulmonary pressure (pressure within the lungs) are needed to cause air to be inhaled. During ascent to altitude, this process is not as simple; it is explained in much greater detail further on.

Pressure Differentials in Gases

In addition to changes in pressure that cause inspiration and expiration, pressure differentials in the gases of the air we breathe are the primary impetus causing oxygen and carbon dioxide exchange. The air we breathe comprises a mixture of gases, each of which exerts a pressure proportional to its concentration in the mixture, known as its **partial pressure**. The air we breathe consists of 79.04% nitrogen, 20.93% oxygen, and 0.03% carbon dioxide. At sea level, where atmospheric pressure is 760 mm Hg, the partial pressure of oxygen is 159.1 mm Hg (20.93% of 760 mm Hg) and that of carbon dioxide, 0.2 mm Hg (0.03% of 760 mm Hg).

As the air reaches the alveoli, the partial pressures of the gases in the alveoli and those of the gases in the blood create a pressure gradient (Fig. 2.5). This is the basis of gas exchange. If the partial pressures of the gases on either side of the membrane were equal, no gas exchange would occur. The greater the pressure gradient, the more quickly the gases diffuse across the membrane. As inspired air moves into the alveoli, the partial pressure of oxygen (P_{O_2}) is between 100 and 105 mm Hg (this is due to the mixing of air within the alveoli). At the pulmonary capillary level, blood has been stripped of most of its oxygen by the tissues. Typically, the P_{O_2} at the pulmonary capillary level is between 40 and 45 mm Hg. As a result, the pressure gradient favors oxygen going from the alveoli to the capillary. In addition, the pressure gradient of carbon dioxide favors exchange from the capillaries to the alveoli, where it is exhaled from the body during expiration. The pressure gradient for carbon dioxide at the capillary–alveolar membrane is not as great as it is for oxygen. Nevertheless, carbon dioxide diffuses

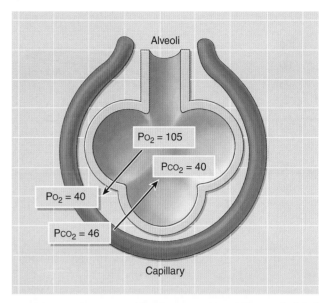

FIGURE 2.5 Pressure gradient between the capillary and alveoli within the lungs.

quite easily across the membrane, despite the low pressure gradient, owing to its greater membrane solubility as compared with that of oxygen.

> *Gas exchange occurring at the level of the capillaries and alveoli and between the capillaries and tissues results from pressure differentials that cause oxygen or carbon dioxide to diffuse from an area of high concentration to one of low concentration.*

Oxygen and Carbon Dioxide Transport

Oxygen is transported in the blood either combined with hemoglobin (98%) or dissolved in the blood plasma (2%). Each molecule of hemoglobin can carry four molecules of oxygen. The binding of oxygen to hemoglobin also depends on the P_{O_2} in the blood and the affinity between oxygen and hemoglobin. The greater the P_{O_2}, the more saturated the hemoglobin molecules are with oxygen. In addition, the temperature and pH of the blood also affect the affinity between oxygen and hemoglobin. As the pH of the blood decreases, the affinity of hemoglobin to oxygen also decreases and oxygen is released. The rightward shift of this curve is known as the **Bohr effect** (Fig. 2.6) and is important during exercise, when a greater amount of oxygen is needed in the active musculature. On the other hand, when the pH is high, as it would be in the lungs, a greater affinity exists between oxygen

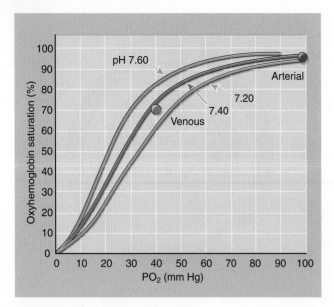

FIGURE 2.6 Bohr effect.

and hemoglobin; this helps saturate the hemoglobin molecules with oxygen.

Carbon dioxide transport in the blood occurs primarily in the form of bicarbonate ion (approximately 60% to 70%). Carbon dioxide is also transported dissolved in the plasma (7% to 10%) or bound to hemoglobin. It does not compete with oxygen, however, since it has its own binding site on the globin molecule. In contrast, oxygen's binding site is on the heme molecule. As carbon dioxide diffuses from the muscle to the blood, it combines with water to form carbonic acid. This is a very unstable acid that quickly dissociates, releasing a hydrogen ion (H^+) and forming a bicarbonate ion (HCO_3^-). The result is an increase in acidity, which in turn causes hemoglobin to lose its affinity for oxygen and increases oxygen's rate of diffusion into the tissues.

 Gas exchange is affected by changes in pH and temperature.

BLOOD

Blood is a viscous fluid made up of cells and plasma. More than 99% of the cells in the blood are red blood cells, the remainder being white blood cells. Plasma is part of the body's extracellular fluid. It is quite similar in composition to the interstitial fluid found between tissue cells, the primary difference being the amount of protein the two fluids contain (plasma contains approximately 7% pro-

tein; interstitial fluid contains about 2%). The percent of the blood that is cells is called the hematocrit. The hematocrit for the average male is approximately 42, and that for the average female approximately 38. In other words, 42% of the blood in males, as compared with 38% in females, is made up of cells. The remaining component is plasma.

CARDIOVASCULAR RESPONSE TO ACUTE EXERCISE

Oxygen consumption ($\dot{V}O_2$) is elevated during acute exercise to meet the higher energy needs of the exercising muscle. As exercise intensity increases, a greater demand for energy is met by an increase in the cardiac output and/or by a greater oxygen extraction from the vasculature (a greater a–$\bar{V}O_2$ difference). During the early stages of exercise, increases in both heart rate and stroke volume occur quite rapidly, bringing about elevations in cardiac output. Figure 2.7 demonstrates the effects varying intensities of exercise on heart rate, stroke volume, and cardiac output.

Cardiac Output

Cardiac output at rest is approximately 5 L. During maximal endurance exercise, however, cardiac output may increase up to 20 L in young, sedentary males; in young, endurance-trained male athletes, cardiac output may reach 40 L. In

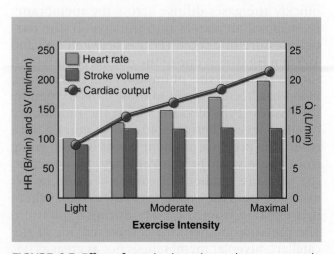

FIGURE 2.7 Effect of exercise intensity on heart rate, stroke volume, and cardiac output. HR = heart rate; SV = stroke volume; $\dot{Q}$ = cardiac output.

examining this considerable difference, we can see that the maximal heart rate for both of these individuals (assuming that both are 20 years old) will be approximately 200 beats per minute (maximal heart rate = 220 – age). Thus, a difference in stroke volume must account for the large differences in cardiac output. In our example, the stroke volume of the sedentary male would be approximately 100 mL per beat, while the stroke volume in the endurance-trained athlete may reach 200 mL per beat.

The importance of a large cardiac output for the endurance athlete is reflected by the linear relationship between cardiac output and oxygen consumption (22). This relationship is seen not only in adults but also in children and adolescents (9) and between trained and untrained individuals (43).

 Increases in cardiac output during exercise result from changes in stroke volume and heart rate.

Heart Rate

Heart rate elevation during exercise is primarily controlled by sympathetic stimulation from the brain's higher somatomotor centers. The heart rate response is directly proportional and linear to the intensity of exercise. As intensity of exercise increases, heart rate continues to increase until it reaches a plateau. It is at this point that the individual has apparently reached his or her maximal level.

Initial increases in heart rate are also related to a withdrawal of parasympathetic input. This occurs during low-intensity exercise. As exercise continues in duration or increases in intensity, greater sympathetic stimulation is seen, and this becomes the driving force in elevating heart rate. Sympathetic activation occurs from feedback mechanisms in peripheral mechanical and chemical receptors that monitor changes in pH, hypoxia, temperature, and other metabolic variables that can alter sympathetic drive.

As heart rate increases, the volume of blood pumped into the circulation also increases. This effect is limited, however: as heart rate rises above a certain level, the strength of each contraction may decrease owing to a metabolic overload. More importantly, the greater rate of contraction results in less time spent in diastole. The time between contractions becomes so reduced that there is not a sufficient time for the blood to flow from the atria to the ventricles. Thus, the total volume of blood made available to the circulation is reduced. This

is why, during artificial electrical stimulation, the heart rate is elevated only to between 100 and 150 beats per minute. Elevations in heart rate from sympathetic stimulation, however, result in a heart rate between 170 and 250 beats per minute, the difference being that sympathetic stimulation also results in a stronger systolic contraction, decreases the time during systole, and thus allows more time for filling during diastole.

 Decreases in resting heart rate probably reflect changes in sympathetic and parasympathetic stimulation.

Stroke Volume

Increases in stroke volume are accomplished early during exercise primarily through an increase in left ventricular end-diastolic volume (EDV). This rapid augmentation of stroke volume is due to the **Frank-Starling mechanism**, which is related to the increased volume of blood that returns to the heart during exercise. With a greater volume of blood returning to the heart, the ventricles become stretched to a greater extent than normal and respond with a more forceful contraction. This stronger contraction results in a greater volume of blood entering the systemic circulation with each heartbeat. This mechanism appears to occur early during exercise and at a relatively low level of exercise intensity. The Frank-Starling mechanism may cause an approximate 30% to 50% increase in stroke volume (4). As exercise continues, increases in EDV reach a plateau although exercise intensity is still at a submaximal intensity. Further increases in stroke volume are attributed to the enhanced left ventricular contractile function (controlled by enhanced sympathetic stimulation), resulting in a greater decrease in end-systolic ventricular volume.

Two mechanisms appear to be responsible for the increase in EDV during exercise. The initial mechanism involves the use of the exercising muscles as a pump to increase the rate of return of the blood to the heart. Interestingly, this would be expected to increase the pressures within the ventricular cavity during filling, thereby raising diastolic pressure. This does not occur in the healthy heart, however. In contrast, the relaxation seen in the left ventricle reduces ventricular pressure below that of the left atrium. This causes the mitral valve to open and ventricular filling to begin. As mentioned earlier, the enhanced sympathetic response during exercise increases relaxation time during diastole. During this time, the increase in size of the left ventricle causes a further reduction in pressure, creating a suctioning effect and drawing additional blood into the chamber. This facilitation of the suctioning mechanism by sympathetic drive is the secondary mechanism that contributes to the increased stroke volume; it is crucial in the recruitment of Frank-Starling mechanisms (4).

Cardiac Drift

As exercise is prolonged or when exercise is performed in a hot environment, a gradual increase in heart rate and a decrease in stroke volume may occur even when exercise intensity is maintained. This is referred to as **cardiovascular drift** and is thought to occur when, due to increased core temperature, a greater percentage of circulating blood is diverted to the skin to dissipate body heat. The greater concentration of blood at the periphery and a loss of some plasma volume to sweat results in the reduction of blood return to the heart. This decrease in EDV results in reduced stroke volume. Heart rate is then elevated to compensate for the change in stroke volume and to maintain cardiac output.

a–$\bar{V}o_2$ Difference

During rest in an individual with a normal hemoglobin concentration, each liter of blood contains approximately 200 mL of oxygen. Considering that a normal cardiac output is 5 L per minute at rest, approximately 1 L of oxygen is available to the body. Only 250 mL, or 25% of the available oxygen, however, is actually extracted from arterial blood (a–$\bar{V}o_2$ difference) during rest, leaving the remaining 750 mL of oxygen available as a reserve.

As might be expected, oxygen extraction from the arterial blood during exercise is increased. Up to 75% of the available oxygen may be used by the exercising muscles. This increase in oxygen extraction appears to be related to the intensity of exercise and may be further enhanced following endurance training programs. The body's ability to extract oxygen from the blood and the total blood volume available to the muscles is critical in determining an individual's aerobic capacity. This is reflected by the **Fick equation**:

$$\dot{V}o_{2max} = \text{maximal cardiac output} \\ \times \text{maximal a}-\bar{V}o_2 \text{ difference}$$

Interestingly, there may be very little difference between moderately trained individuals and endurance athletes in the ability to extract oxygen despite large differences in $\dot{V}o_{2max}$. Therefore, the primary factor determining aerobic capacity is probably cardiac output.

Distribution of Cardiac Output

During exercise, most of the circulating blood is diverted to the active muscles (see Fig. 2.3). The extent of this shunting depends on environmental conditions and possibly other factors, including type of exercise and fatigue. The shunting of blood is generally accomplished by diverting blood flow from organs or areas of the body that can tolerate a reduction in blood flow to the exercising muscles. Certain organs, however, such as the heart, cannot function without a normal blood flow and will not compromise their blood supply during exercise.

Blood Pressure

Blood pressure typically increases linearly during dynamic exercise, such as walking, jogging, or running. In the healthy individual, this increase is seen only in the systolic response. This response appears to be buffered to a large extent by the decrease in peripheral resistance caused by vasodilation in the vasculature of the exercising muscles (23). The decrease seen in peripheral resistance also appears to account for the minimal to no change observed in diastolic pressure. Diastolic pressure may also decrease during higher-intensity bouts of exercise.

During exercise involving the upper body only, both systolic and diastolic blood pressures are higher than when exercise is performed with only the legs (53). This is thought to occur because of the relatively smaller muscle mass and vasculature of the arms. Even when these vessels are maximally dilated, the same effect on peripheral resistance as with lower-body exercise does not appear to occur. The higher pressor response seen with upper-body exercise has important implications in determining the exercise prescription for individuals with coronary heart disease.

During resistance exercise, large increases in both systolic and diastolic blood pressures can be seen (24,25,41). During maximal efforts that involve a large muscle mass, intra-arterial blood pressures exceeding 350/250 mm Hg in healthy young men have been reported (25). The large pressor response seen during resistance training is a combination of vascular compression within contracting muscles and a Valsalva maneuver (which is performed by trying to expire air through a closed glottis). The magnitude of the pressor response is also related to the relative size of the muscle mass involved and the intensity of the effort. Blood pressure increases with each repetition in a set to failure and then drops rapidly to below resting levels after the last repetition (25,41). This is a transient decrease and is probably related to the large vasodilation of the vasculature that was occluded during muscle contraction; it may contribute to the dizziness sometimes experienced after an intense exercise session.

A major portion of the large pressor response seen during resistance training is attributed to a **Valsalva maneuver** (23). The rapid increase in intrathoracic pressure during a Valsalva maneuver results in an increase in both systolic and diastolic blood pressures (24). If the Valsalva maneuver is maintained, however, the systolic and diastolic pressures begin to drop within several seconds because diastolic filling is reduced by impaired venous return. Although often contraindicated during resistance exercise, the Valsalva maneuver may in fact be beneficial and have a protective effect in healthy resistance-trained individuals (23,32). The increase in intrathoracic pressure seen during the Valsalva maneuver provides stabilization to the spinal column and reduces left ventricular transmural pressure (afterload) (21). This contrasts with the high afterload normally expected when systolic pressure is elevated. In addition, the increase in intrathoracic pressure is also transmitted to the cerebrospinal fluid, thus reducing the transmural pressures of the cerebral vessels and preventing vascular damage at the time of peak peripheral resistance (30).

> *During exercise, systolic blood pressure increases relative to changes in exercise intensity; diastolic blood pressure, however, remains the same or decreases slightly.*

PULMONARY VENTILATION DURING EXERCISE

During submaximal exercise, ventilation increases linearly with oxygen uptake. The increase in oxygen consumption is primarily the result of an increase in tidal volume (amount of air inspired or expired during a normal breathing cycle). As the intensity of exercise increases, the increase in oxygen consumption may rely more on increasing the rate of breathing. During steady-state exercise, minute ventilation (liters of air breathed per minute) plateaus when the demand for oxygen is met by supply. The ratio of minute ventilation to oxygen consumption is termed the ventilatory equivalent and is symbolized by $\dot{V}E/\dot{V}O_2$. During submaximal exercise, the ventilatory equivalent in healthy individuals is approximately 25:1 (56); that is, 25 L of air is breathed in for every liter of oxygen. This ratio may be slightly higher in children (40) and may also be affected by the mode of exercise (swimming versus running) (29). During maximal exercise, however, minute ventilation increases disproportionately in relation to oxygen uptake, and the ventilatory equivalent may reach as high as 35 to 40 L of air per liter of oxygen consumed in the healthy adult.

CARDIOVASCULAR ADAPTATIONS TO TRAINING

Prolonged participation in exercise programs results in a number of cardiovascular adaptations specific to the type of exercise program used. Endurance training and resistance training are modes that represent two distinctly different physiological demands on the cardiovascular system. Although many of the cardiovascular adaptations observed in these training programs are similar, others are quite different. A summary of these adaptations, discussed below, is presented in Table 2.2.

Cardiac Output and Stroke Volume

Increases in $\dot{V}O_{2max}$ are characteristic of endurance training programs. These increases are generally accompanied by increases in cardiac output and improved extraction capability within skeletal muscle (increase in a–$\overline{V}O_2$ difference). Improvement in oxygen extraction is related to the greater perfusion ability of exercising muscle. Since maximal heart rates are unaffected by training and will not differ between elite endurance athletes and age-matched sedentary individuals, increases in cardiac output are primarily the result of improved stroke volume.

TABLE 2.2	CARDIOVASCULAR ADAPTATIONS TO PROLONGED ENDURANCE AND RESISTANCE TRAINING			
	ENDURANCE TRAINING		**RESISTANCE TRAINING**	
	Rest	*Exercise*	*Rest*	*Exercise*
Heart rate	D	NC	D or NC	NC
Stroke volume	I	I	I or NC	I or NC
Cardiac output	NC	I	NC	I or NC
Blood pressure				
Systolic	D or NC	D or NC	D or NC	D or NC
Diastolic	D or NC	D or NC	NC	D or NC
MORPHOLOGICAL ADAPTATIONS				
Left ventricular mass		I		I
Left ventricular diameter		I		I or NC
Wall thickness				
Left ventricle		I		I
Septum		I		I

I = increase; D = decrease; NC = no change.

Endurance training is a potent stimulus for increasing stroke volume both at rest and during maximal exercise. Increases in stroke volume are related to an enlarged ventricular chamber (referred to as **eccentric hypertrophy**) caused by a chronic increased ventricular filling, as seen during endurance exercise. This increased preload is thought to relate to the expanded plasma volume associated with such training (5,8).

Resistance training results in little to no change in cardiac output. Although significantly greater stroke volumes have been reported in elite level weightlifters compared to recreational lifters (36), the increase in stroke volume seen in these athletes appeared to be more a factor of a larger body size than training adaptation (13).

 Increases in cardiac output following prolonged endurance training result from increased stroke volume.

Heart Rate

A decrease in resting heart rate and a relative decrease in heart rate at any given submaximal $\dot{V}O_2$ is a commonly found adaptation in athletes undergoing endurance training (3,6). The decrease in heart rate during submaximal exercise is probably due to improved stroke volume and also reflective of an improved exercise economy. The mechanism regulating training-induced bradycardia is not thoroughly understood but may be related to a change in the balance between sympathetic and parasympathetic activity. In addition, a decrease in the intrinsic rate of firing of the SA-node following long-term training may also be a factor in the bradycardic response to long-term training (47).

Blood Pressure

In normotensive individuals, resting systolic or diastolic pressure is generally unresponsive to endurance training programs, although based on a number of epidemiological studies and other investigations examining exercise and hypertension, it appears that exercise is a potential stimulus for reducing both systolic and diastolic blood pressure in hypertensive individuals (48). The reduction in resting blood pressure appears to occur during endurance exercise sessions that occur between three and five times per week, are at least 30 minutes in duration, and mobilize between 50% and 70% of $\dot{V}O_{2max}$ (12,48).

During endurance exercise, the blood pressure response has been shown to decrease for a given

Q & A from the Field

Can resistance training be harmful to the heart? I heard it can cause an enlarged heart.

The heart is a muscle, and exercise, including resistance training, increases the workload on the heart. The heart can hypertrophy just like any other muscle. Body builders and weightlifters can get an enlarged heart, which by itself does not cause any heart problems. Resistance training will cause your heart muscle to thicken without enlargement of its cavity. This enables the heart to work better under the increased intrathoracic pressure that occurs with anaerobic exercise. Other causes of an enlarged heart (certain diseases) are associated with specific heart problems. Endurance exercise may decrease the size of an "enlarged heart" and has other benefits as well.

level of exercise intensity (23). This is probably related to the individual's initial level of conditioning, and well-conditioned endurance athletes must probably train at a high intensity of exercise for a long duration to see such adaptations.

Resistance training appears to result in no change or a slight decrease in resting blood pressure (18) but a significant decrease in the blood pressure response during resistance exercise at the same absolute load (31, 42). Any decrease in resting blood pressure subsequent to resistance training is probably the result of a decrease in body fat and a possible reduction in the sympathetic drive to the heart (similar to what may drive the reduction in blood pressure during endurance exercise) (15).

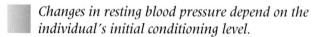

Changes in resting blood pressure depend on the individual's initial conditioning level.

Cardiac Morphology

An athlete's heart is quite large in comparison to that of a recreationally trained or sedentary individual. For many years, a debate raged as to whether this was a consequence of pathological disease or physiological adaptation. Technological advances over the past 30 years, however, have allowed for a much closer examination of the physiological adaptations of the heart in conjunction with prolonged training.

During prolonged training, the heart adapts to match the workload placed on the left ventricle to maintain a constant relationship between systolic cavity pressure and the ratio of wall thickness to ventricular radius (49). Adaptations to the morphology of the heart are governed by the law of Laplace, which states that wall tension is proportional to pressure and the radius of curvature (16). During a pressure overload, common to resistance-exercise programs, the septum and posterior wall of the left ventricle increase in size so as to normalize myocardial wall stress. During a volume overload, common to endurance-training programs, the increase is predominantly in the internal diameter of the left ventricle (increasing the size of the cavity), with a proportional increase in both the septum and posterior wall of the ventricle. Both endurance training and resistance training are at either ends of the spectrum with regard to the volume and pressure stresses placed on the heart. Most sports, however, have a parallel impact on both cavity dimension and wall thickness (51). In these sports, athletes are performing a combination of aerobic and anaerobic training, resulting in cardiovascular adaptations associated with both an enlarged diastolic cavity and increased wall thickness. In the sports that primarily emphasize a single form of training, the morphological changes in the heart may be more extreme.

Endurance-trained athletes have been shown to have a greater than normal left ventricular internal diameter, with normal to slightly thicker walls (26,34,37,51). This type of left ventricular hypertrophy is termed eccentric hypertrophy and is considered a normal physiological response to a volume overload (greater end-diastolic volumes) consistent with prolonged endurance training.

Resistance-trained athletes, on the other hand, have normal internal diameters but significantly thicker ventricular walls (14,32,34,36). This type of hypertrophy is referred to as **concentric hypertrophy** and at times may approach the levels seen in **hypertrophic cardiomyopathy**, a disease of the myocardium associated with substantial thickening of the septum and posterior wall at the expense of cavity size, thus greatly impairing left ventricular function. Importantly, the concentric hypertrophy seen in the resistance-trained athlete does not affect the internal diameter of the ventricle. In addition, the type of hypertrophy seen in cardiomyopathy is usually asymmetrical, whereas in resistance-trained or power athletes the change in wall size is generally symmetrical. Figure 2.8 compares morphological changes in the left ventricle between endurance- and resistance-trained individuals.

Left ventricular mass in highly trained athletes is on an average 45% greater than in age-matched control subjects (26). This increase in mass is related to the increases in the internal diameter of the left ventricle and the thickness of the ventricular wall. When examined relative to changes in body mass

or body surface area, the significantly greater ventricular mass is still present. Some studies have suggested that such differences are more prevalent in elite athletes than in athletes of lesser caliber (13).

 Morphological changes of the heart depend on the type of training program performed.

RESPIRATORY ADAPTATIONS TO TRAINING

For the most part, the respiratory system is not a limiting factor in providing enough oxygen to the exercising muscles. Like most other physiological systems, the respiratory system can also adapt to physical exercise to maximize its efficiency. In general, lung volume and capacity change very little

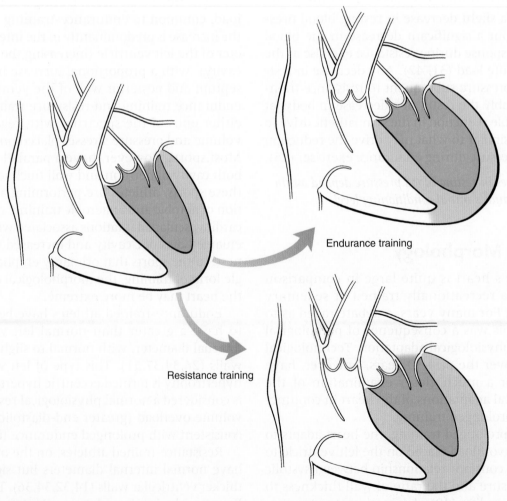

Endurance training

Resistance training

FIGURE 2.8 Caricature of morphological adaptations of the left ventricle subsequent to endurance and resistance training.

as the result of physical exercise. It does appear that during maximal exercise, vital capacity may increase slightly, but this is probably related to the slight decrease in residual volume (the amount of air remaining in the lungs following a maximal expiration) (58).

> *Respiratory capacity does not appear to be significantly affected by physical exercise.*

Ventilatory Equivalent and Minute Ventilation

Endurance training appears to reduce the **ventilatory equivalent** (i.e., the amount of air inspired at a particular rate of oxygen consumption) during submaximal exercise (17,61). As a result, the oxygen cost of exercise attributable to ventilation is reduced. This benefit may be realized by a reduction in fatigue of the ventilatory musculature and greater oxygen availability to the exercising muscles (27).

Minute ventilation also appears to decrease during submaximal exercise following prolonged endurance training, reflecting the improved exercise efficiency resulting from such training. During maximal exercise, however, endurance training appears to cause minute ventilation to increase, an effect thought to be related to increases in $\dot{V}O_{2max}$ (28). In untrained subjects, minute ventilation can increase from 120 L·min^{-1} to about 150 L·min^{-1} following training (58). In addition, minute ventilation may increase to 180 L·min^{-1} in highly trained endurance athletes and has been reported to be as high as 240 L·min^{-1} in elite rowers (58).

BLOOD VOLUME ADAPTATIONS TO TRAINING

Endurance training appears to be a potent stimulus for causing **hypervolemia** (increases in blood volume). This adaptation seems to occur within the initial 2 to 4 weeks of training and is thought to be the result of plasma volume expansion (7). As training progresses, further increases in blood volume probably result from both continued plasma volume expansion and an increase in the number of red blood cells.

The increase in plasma volume is believed to be due to increases in the fluid regulatory hormones,

antidiuretic hormone and aldosterone, that bring about an increase in fluid retention by the kidneys. In addition, exercise causes an increase in plasma proteins, primarily albumin (60). This causes a greater osmotic pull, so that more fluid is retained in the blood.

Increases in blood volume are apparently due to both plasma volume expansion and an increase in the number of red blood cells, although the expansion in plasma volume appears to be a greater contributor to this hypervolemia (19). Figure 2.9 shows the effect of prolonged endurance training on blood volume expansion and the contributions of both plasma volume expansion and increases in the number of red blood cells. Although both plasma volume and red blood cell volume increase, they do not increase proportionally. Thus, hematocrit will decrease. A reduced hematocrit will lower the viscosity of the blood and facilitate blood flow through the circulation. Reductions in hematocrit do not seem to cause a concern for low hemoglobin concentrations. In fact, hemoglobin concentrations in endurance-trained athletes are typically above normal and provide an ample supply of oxygen to meet the body's needs during exercise.

> *Increases in the number of red blood cells and plasma volume as a result of endurance training cause a reduction in hematocrit.*

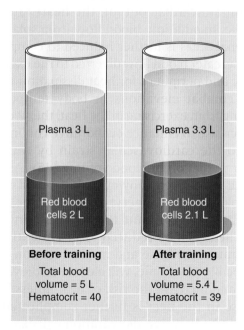

FIGURE 2.9 Effect of endurance training on blood volume, plasma volume, and hematocrit. Modified with permission from Hoffman JR. Physiological Aspects of Sport Training and Performance. Champaign, IL: Human Kinetics, 2002.

ENVIRONMENTAL FACTORS AFFECTING CARDIORESPIRATORY FUNCTION

Exercise performed under severe environmental conditions can greatly strain the cardiorespiratory system's ability to meet the body's need for oxygen. In addition to potential performance limitations, exercise under such conditions poses significant risks to the health and well-being of the individual. The discussion below focuses on the effects of exercise in the heat and at altitude on cardiorespiratory function.

Cardiorespiratory Response to Exercise in the Heat

During exercise in the heat, a large volume of circulating blood (up to 7 L/min) is diverted to the skin to help dissipate the increase in body heat (39). As blood flow to the skin increases, the peripheral vasculature becomes compliant and engorged with blood, creating blood pools (46). Blood pooling in the periphery causes a reduction in venous return and subsequently a decrease in cardiac filling. The resulting cardiovascular strain is reflected in a decrease in stroke volume. To compensate and to maintain cardiac output, the heart rate must increase. In addition, blood flow from splanchnic and renal areas is further reduced to compensate for the greater blood flow diverted to the exercising muscle and periphery for heat dissipation (39).

To combat elevations in body temperature resulting from exercising in the heat, the sweat rate will increase to enhance evaporative cooling. This adds to the cardiovascular strain by causing a greater reduction in blood volume (45). As blood volume is reduced, however, less blood will be available to the periphery; as a result, the output of sweat will decline and the body's ability to dissipate heat will be reduced. Consequently, core temperature will rise and in combination with a reduced blood volume, will elevate cardiovascular strain and increase the risk of heat illness. When exercise in the heat is further complicated by a deficit in body water, dehydration will exacerbate the physiological strain.

A body water deficit has significant implications for cardiovascular function. **Hypohydration** (an existing body water deficit) results in a reduction in plasma volume. As a consequence, less blood is available to both exercising muscle and the skin. In addition, decreases in plasma volume are associated with a reduction in stroke volume (35). To compensate and to maintain normal blood flow, the heart rate will increase. Depending on the magnitude of the body water deficit, however, the increase in heart rate may be insufficient to fully compensate for the lower stroke volume. As a result, cardiac output will also be reduced (35,44), although it does appear that cardiac output can be maintained at higher degrees of hypohydration if it occurs in the absence of a thermal strain (52).

Cardiovascular function can be compromised during exercise in the heat by the reduction in stroke volume.

Effect of Altitude on the Cardiorespiratory Response

As one ascends above sea level, the partial pressure of oxygen (Po_2) is reduced. Remember that the pressure gradient between arterial and tissue Po_2 is approximately 64 mm Hg at sea level (the difference between an arterial Po_2 of 104 mm Hg and a tissue Po_2 of 40 mm Hg). This creates a pressure gradient, causing oxygen to diffuse easily into the tissues. At altitude, however, a reduction in arterial Po_2 causes a decrease in the pressure gradient, reducing the diffusion capacity of oxygen from the vasculature into the tissue. For instance, at an elevation of 2,500 m, the arterial Po_2 drops to about 60 mm Hg while the tissue Po_2 remains at 40 mmHg, creating a pressure gradient of only 20 mm Hg. This 70% reduction in the pressure gradient causes a significant reduction in the speed at which oxygen moves between the capillaries and tissues. The reduction in the pressure gradient between the vasculature and the tissues has important implications in maintaining exercise performance during exercise at altitude. To compensate for the reduced Po_2 at altitude, breathing rate is increased. As breathing rate increases (**hyperventilation**), the partial pressure of carbon dioxide (Pco_2) in the alveoli is also reduced. As a result, the stimulus to maintain a high rate of ventilation may be removed, since Pco_2 is an integral part of the driving force behind hyperventilation.

To compensate for the reduced oxygen availability at altitude, elevations in cardiac output occur at rest and during exercise. The primary mechanism resulting in the increased cardiac output appears to be an increase in the heart rate, which has been shown to rise between 40% and 50% at rest without any change in stroke volume (54). Even during exercise, the increase in cardiac output appears to be primarily the result of an increase in heart rate. In contrast to what is normally seen during exercise at sea level, during exercise at altitude, stroke volume decreases (20). This decrease is apparently due to the reduction in plasma volume observed within a short time after arrival at altitude (50,59).

During initial exposure at altitude (observed at elevations above 3,000 m) decreases in plasma volume appear to result from both a diuresis and natriuresis (increased sodium excretion) (20). The diuresis may be explained by the large evaporative heat loss caused by ventilation of dry inspired air at altitude. The natriuresis appears to be the result of neural stimulation of the kidney to decrease the reabsorption of sodium due to the **hypoxic** (low oxygen) stimulus (20). Even during prolonged exposure to altitude, plasma volume will still remain below normal levels, and studies examining individuals residing at altitude have reported lower plasma volumes in comparison to residents of sea-level communities (57). Thus, acclimatization does not appear to have any significant effect on a return of blood volume to preexposure levels.

Changes in the partial pressure of oxygen as the result of ascending to altitude will impair gas exchange in the lungs and tissues.

CARDIORESPIRATORY CHANGES DUE TO PROLONGED EXPOSURE AT ALTITUDE

During the first few days at altitude, changes in the respiratory response are seen. Initially, the breathing rate increases, while arterial P_{O_2} decreases. After a few days at altitude, arterial P_{O_2} begins to rise as P_{CO_2} values fall, although the ventilatory rate will continue to rise as a result of changes in the ventilatory response to CO_2 levels and in the sensitivity of the carotid body. The carotid body is situated above the bifurcation of the carotid artery. It serves as a sensor of oxygen saturation in the blood, and its location is ideal for this role, since it receives a large blood supply, allowing it to respond to oxygen saturation and not to oxygen content (55). The increased sensitivity of the carotid body appears to lead to a biphasic response. The initial response may be a decrease in the hypoxic ventilatory response

during the first 3 to 5 days of altitude exposure; however, following these initial days of exposure, an increase in the ventilatory response is seen (55).

In addition to changes in the ventilatory response, another component of respiratory adaptation to altitude may be in the diffusion capacity of oxygen. Following 7 to 10 weeks of altitude exposure, diffusion capacities are reported to increase between 15% and 20% (57). Although much of this improved diffusion capacity may be accounted for by increases in hemoglobin concentrations, other studies comparing individuals permanently residing at altitude to those residing at sea level have also reported significant differences in oxygen diffusion capacity between these population groups (10). These differences may be related to the larger lung volumes developed through exposure to chronic hypoxia and the subsequent development of a greater surface area for oxygen diffusion (2).

After several weeks of altitude exposure, cardiac output remains similar to those values observed at sea level. Similar to what occurs during an acute exposure to altitude, increases in cardiac output following extended stays at elevation also appear to be primarily attributable to increases in heart rate. Stroke volume, however, continues to remain reduced (38). One of the best-known adaptations to prolonged exposure to altitude is the increase in the number of red blood cells per unit volume of blood. Exposure to hypoxic conditions results in the release of the hormone erythropoietin. **Erythropoietin** is responsible for stimulating the production of red blood cells (erythrocytes) and increases within 2 hours of exposure to altitude; it reaches a maximum rate of increase at about 24 to 48 hours (11). After 3 weeks of exposure to altitude, erythropoietin concentrations appear to return to baseline levels, but not until they have contributed to an approximately 20% to 25% increase in packed red cell volume (33). Red cell mass continues to increase even after erythropoietin returns to normal levels (33), although the mechanism that underlies this continued increase is not known. This physiological adaptation to altitude is one of the reasons why many endurance athletes live at altitude and train at sea level.

As red cell volume increases, so does the blood's hemoglobin concentration. This increase allows for a greater amount of oxygen to be carried per unit volume of blood. As red cell volume and hemoglobin concentration increase, however, the viscosity of the blood will also increase, presenting an inherent danger associated with the physiological adaptations to altitude.

SUMMARY

In this chapter we saw the effect of acute exercise on cardiac function and how the heart will compensate for the increased energy demands of exercising muscles. This compensation is manifest by changes in cardiac output, regulated in part by enhanced sympathetic drive and increased venous return. In addition, blood flow is diverted from nonexercising muscles and nonessential organs to exercising muscles, providing for the delivery of more oxygen. Differences in the acute cardiac response between endurance and resistance training programs were also discussed. Discussion also focused on the coordinated relationship between the cardiovascular and respiratory systems and the effect that both acute and prolonged training have on their function. In addition, the effects of prolonged training on both cardiovascular and respiratory adaptations were discussed, and focus was directed on how these adaptations depend on the type of training program employed. Finally, the effects of environmental stresses were reviewed. Specific discussion was directed at acute exercise in heat and at altitude. Adaptation to prolonged exposure to altitude was also briefly reviewed.

MAXING OUT

1. Using this chapter and other resources, discuss the physiological changes that occur in the athlete's body related to training at altitude.
2. You are working with an elite athlete who asks you about taking the hormone erythropoietin. She has heard that it will improve her endurance in athletic performance. Using information provided in this chapter as well as other sources, how would you describe the effects of erythropoietin on performance?
3. Using Tables 2.1 and 2.2 and other sources, compare the effects of aerobic training and resistance training on the cardiorespiratory system.

REFERENCES

1. Adamovich DR. The Heart: Fundamentals of Electrocardiography, Exercise Physiology and Exercise Stress Testing. Freeport NY: Sports Medicine Books, 1984.
2. Bartlett D, Remmers JE. Effects of high altitude exposure on the lungs of young rats. Respir Physiol 1971;13:116–125.
3. Blomqvist CG, Saltin B. Cardiovascular adaptations to physical training. Annu Rev Physiol 1983;45:169–189.
4. Bonow RO. Left ventricular response to exercise. In Fletcher GF, ed. Cardiovascular Response to Exercise. Mount Kisco, NY: Futura, 1994:31–48.
5. Carroll JF, Convertino VA, Wood CE, et al. Effect of training on blood volume and plasma hormone concentrations in the elderly. Med Sci Sports Exerc 1995; 27:79–84.
6. Charlton GA, Crawford MH. Physiological consequences of training. Cardiol Clin 1997;15:345–254.
7. Convertino VA, Keil LC, Bernauer EM, et al. Plasma volume, osmolality, vasopressin, and renin activity during graded exercise in man. J Appl Physiol: Respir Environ Exerc Physiol 1981;50:123–128.
8. Convertino VA. Blood volume: its adaptation to endurance training. Med Sci Sports Exerc 1991;23:1338–1348.
9. Cunningham DA, Paterson DH, Blimkie CJ, et al. Development of cardiorespiratory function in circumpubertal boys: a longitudinal study. J Appl Physiol 1984;56;302–307.
10. Dempsey JA, Reddan WG, Birnbaum ML, et al. Effects of acute through life-long hypoxic exposure on exercise pulmonary gas exchange. Respir Physiol 1971;13:62–89.
11. Eckardt K, Boutellier U, Kurtz A, et al. Rate of erythropoietin formation in humans in response to acute hypobaric hypoxia. J Appl Physiol 1989;66:1785–1788.
12. Fagard RH. Exercise characteristics and the blood pressure response to dynamic physical training. Med Sci Sports Exerc 2001;33:S484–S492.
13. Fleck SJ. Cardiovascular adaptations to resistance training. Med Sci Sports Exerc 1988;20:S146–S151.
14. Fleck SJ, Henke C, Wilson W. Cardiac MRI of elite junior Olympic weight lifters. Int J Sports Med 1989;10:329–333.
15. Fleck SJ, Kraemer WJ. Designing Resistance Training Programs. Champaign, IL: Human Kinetics, 1997.
16. Ford LE. Heart size. Circ Res 1976;39:299–303.
17. Girandola RN, Katch FL. Effects of physical training on ventilatory equivalent and respiratory exchange ratio during weight supported, steady-state exercise. Eur J Appl Physiol Occup Physiol 1976;21:119–125.
18. Goldberg L, Elliot DL, Kuehl KS. A comparison of the cardiovascular effects of running and weight training. J Strength Condition Res 1994;8:219–224.
19. Green HJ, Sutton J, Coates G, et al. Response of red cells and plasma volume to prolonged training in humans. J Appl Physiol 1991;70:1810–1815.
20. Honig A. Role of arterial chemoreceptors in the reflex control of renal function and body fluid volumes in acute arterial hypoxia. In: Acher H, O'Regan RG, eds. Physiology of the Peripheral Arterial Chemoreceptors. New York: Elsevier, 1983:395–429.
21. Lentini AC, McKelvie RS, McCartney N, et al. Assessment of left ventricular response of strength trained athletes during weightlifting exercise. J Appl Physiol 1993;75:2703–2710.
22. Lewis SF, Taylor WF, Graham RM, et al. Cardiovascular responses to exercise as functions of absolute and relative work load. J Appl Physiol 1983;54;1314–1323.
23. MacDougall JD. Blood pressure responses to resistive, static, and dynamic exercise. In: Fletcher GF, ed. Cardio-

vascular Response to Exercise. Mount Kisco, NY: Futura, 1994:155–174.

24. MacDougall JD, McKelvie RS, Moroz DE, et al. Factors affecting blood pressure response during heavy weight-lifting and static contractions. J Appl Physiol 1992;73;1590–1597.

25. MacDougall JD, Tuxen D, Sale DG, et al. Arterial blood pressure response to heavy resistance exercise. J Appl Physiol 1985;58:785–790.

26. Maron BJ. Structural features of the athletic heart as defined by echocardiography. J Am Coll Cardiol 1986;7:190–203.

27. Martin B, Heintzelman M, Chen HI. Exercise performance after ventilatory work. J Appl Physiol 1982;52:1581–1585.

28. McArdle WD, Glaser RM, Magel JR. Metabolic and cardiorespiratory response during free swimming and treadmill walking. J Appl Physiol 1971;30:733–738.

29. McArdle WD, Katch FI, Katch VL. Exercise Physiology. Energy, Nutrition, and Human Performance. 4th ed. Baltimore, MD: Williams & Wilkins. 1996:417–456.

30. McCartney N. Acute responses to resistance training and safety. Med Sci Sports Exerc 1999;31:31–37.

31. McCartney N, McKelvie RS, Martin J, et al. Weight-training-induced attenuation of the circulatory response of older males to weight lifting. J Appl Physiol 1993;74:1056–1060.

32. Menapace FJ, Hammer, WJ, Ritzer TF, et al. Left ventricular size in competitive weight lifters: an echocardiographic study. Med Sci Sports Exerc 1982;14:72–75.

33. Milledge JS, Coates PM. Serum erythropoietin in humans at high altitude and its relation to plasma renin. J Appl Physiol 1985;59:360–364.

34. Morganroth J, Maron BJ, Henry WL, et al. Comparative left ventricular dimensions in trained athletes. Ann Intern Med 1975;82:521–524.

35. Nadel ER, Fortney SM, Wenger CB. Effect of hydration on circulatory and thermal regulation. J Appl Physiol 1980;49:715–721.

36. Pearson AC, Schiff M, Mrosek D, et al. Left ventricular diastolic function in weight lifters. Am J Cardiol 1986;58:1254–1259.

37. Pelliccia A, Maron BJ, Spataro A, et al. The upper limit of physiologic cardiac hypertrophy in highly trained elite athletes. N Engl J Med 1991;324:295–301.

38. Reeves JT, Groves BM, Sutton JR, et al. Operation Everest II: preservation of cardiac function at extreme altitude. J Appl Physiol 1987;63:31–539.

39. Rowell LB. Human Circulation Regulation during Physical Stress. New York: Oxford University Press, 1986.

40. Rowland TW, Green GM. Physiological responses to treadmill exercise in females: adult-child differences. Med Sci Sports Exerc 1988;20:474–478.

41. Sale DG, Moroz DE, McKelvie RS, et al. Comparison of blood pressure response to isokinetic and weight-lifting exercise. Eur J Appl Physiol 1993;67:115–120.

42. Sale DG, Moroz DE, McKelvie RS, et al. Effect of training on the blood pressure response to weight lifting. Can J Appl Physiol 1994;19:60–74.

43. Saltin B, Astrand PO. Maximal oxygen uptake in athletes. J Appl Physiol 1967;23:353–358.

44. Sawka MN, Pandolf KB. Effects of body water loss on physiological function and exercise performance. In: Gisolfi CV, Lamb DR, eds. Fluid Homeostasis during Exercise: Perspectives in Exercise Science and Sports Medicine, vol 3. Indianapolis, IN: Benchmark Press, 1990:1–38.

45. Sawka MN, Knowlton RG, Critz JB. Thermal and circulatory responses to repeated bouts of prolonged running. Med Sci Sports Exerc 1979;11:177–180.

46. Sawka MN, Wenger CB, Young AJ, et al. Physiological responses to exercise in the heat. In: Marriott BM, ed. Nutritional Needs in Hot Environments. Washington, DC: National Academy Press 1993:55–74.

47. Schaefer ME, Allert JA, Adams HR, et al. Adrenergic responsiveness and intrinsic sinoatrial automaticity of exercise-trained rats. Med Sci Sports Exerc 1992;24:887–894.

48. Seals DR, Hagberg JM. The effect of exercise training on human hypertension: a review. Med Sci Sports Exerc 1984;16:207–215.

49. Shapiro L. The morphological consequences of systemic training. Cardiol Clin 1997;15:373–379.

50. Singh MV, Rawal SB, Tyagi AK. Body fluid status on induction, reinduction and prolonged stay at high altitude on human volunteers. Int J Biometeorol 1990;34:93–97.

51. Spirito P, Pelliccia A, Proschan M, et al. Morphology of the "athlete's heart" assessed by echocardiography in 947 elite athletes representing 27 sports. Am J Cardiol 1994;74:802–806.

52. Sproles CB, Smith DP, Byrd RJ, et al. Circulatory responses to submaximal exercise after dehydration and rehydration. J Sports Med Phys Fit 1976;16:98–105.

53. Toner MM, Glickman EL, McArdle WD. Cardiovascular adjustments to exercise distributed between the upper and lower body. Med Sci Sports Exerc 1990;22:773–778.

54. Vogel JA, Harris CW. Cardiopulmonary responses of resting man during early exposure to high altitude. J Appl Physiol 1967;22:1124–1128.

55. Ward MP, Milledge JS, West JB. High Altitude Medicine and Physiology. London: Chapman & Hall Medical, 1995.

56. Wasserman K, Whipp BJ, Davis JA. Respiratory physiology of exercise: Metabolism, gas exchange, and ventilatory control. Int Rev Physiol 1981;23:149–211.

57. West JB. Diffusing capacity of the lung for carbon monoxide at high altitude. J Appl Physiol 1962;17:421–426.

58. Wilmore JH, Costill DL. Physiology of Sport and Exercise. Champaign, IL: Human Kinetics, 1999.

59. Wolfel EE, Groves BM, Brooks GA, et al. Oxygen transport during steady-state submaximal exercise in chronic hypoxia. J Appl Physiol 1991;70:1129–1136.

60. Yang RC, Mack GW, Wolfe RR, et al. Albumin synthesis after intense intermittent exercise in human subjects. J Appl Physiol 1998;84:584–592.

61. Yerg II, JE, Seals DR, Hagberg JM, et al. Effect of endurance exercise training on ventilatory function in older individuals. J Appl Physiol 1985;58:791–794.

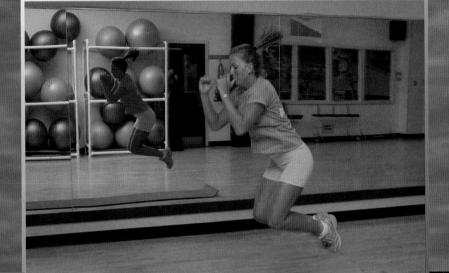

The Neuromuscular System: Anatomical and Physiological Bases and Adaptations to Training

JARED W. COBURN
TRAVIS W. BECK
HERBERT A. DEVRIES
TERRY J. HOUSH

Introduction

The nervous system can be divided anatomically into the central (brain and spinal cord) and peripheral (outside of the spinal cord) systems or functionally into the somatic (voluntary) and autonomic (involuntary) systems. The autonomic nervous system is composed of the sympathetic and parasympathetic systems, which control the involuntary functioning of various internal organs, the circulatory system (including vasoconstriction and vasodilation), and the endocrine glands. Voluntary human movement, however, is controlled by the somatic nervous system. When we decide to perform a muscle action, the electrical activity that eventually leads to muscle contraction originates in the motor cortex of the brain and travels through the central and peripheral systems to the muscle.

The nervous system controls both voluntary and involuntary functions. Voluntary human movement is controlled by the somatic nervous system, while the involuntary functioning of internal organs, circulatory system, and endocrine glands is controlled by the autonomic nervous system.

THE NEURON

A nerve cell, or **neuron**, is the basic structural unit of the nervous system. Billions of neurons are in the nervous system; usually, several neurons are interconnected by **synapses** (junctions between neurons) to form pathways for conducting nervous impulses. The neurons that conduct sensory impulses from the periphery to the central nervous system are called **sensory**, or **afferent**, neurons. The neurons that conduct impulses from the central nervous system to the muscles are called **motor**, or **efferent**, neurons. Although neurons are microscopic in diameter, one cell can be up to approximately 3 feet in length, such as a neuron that extends from the spinal cord to a muscle of the foot.

The typical motor neuron (Fig. 3.1) includes a cell body, **dendrites** (which receive impulses and conduct them to the cell body), and an **axon** (which conducts the impulses away from the cell). The cell body of the motor neuron, which innervates skeletal muscle, lies in the gray matter in the ventral horn of the spinal cord; its axon joins many axons from other motor neurons (and many sensory axons) to form a spinal nerve. Such a nerve is thick enough to be seen in gross dissection. The motor neuron branches and rebranches into many twigs, each of which innervates one muscle fiber.

One characteristic of many neurons is the presence of **myelin**, which surrounds the axon as a sheath. It is a fatty white substance produced by **Schwann cells** in the peripheral nervous system. The myelin sheath is laid down in segments along the length of the axon, resulting in gaps called **nodes of Ranvier**. In myelinated axons, the velocity whereby the action potential is conducted is increased because it jumps from one node of Ran-

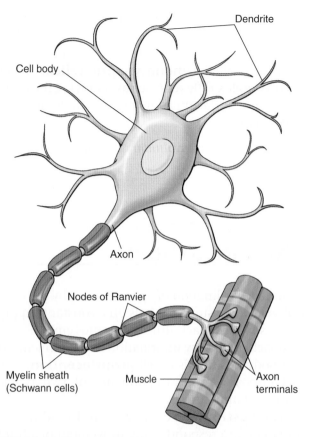

FIGURE 3.1 The neuron and its components. Each neuron consists of dendrites, a cell body, and an axon.

vier to the next. This is called **saltatory conduction**. Generally speaking, the thicker the myelin sheath around an axon, the greater the conduction velocity of an action potential.

Neurons conduct electrical impulses to and from the central nervous system.

REFLEXES AND INVOLUNTARY MOVEMENTS

A **reflex** is most simply defined as an involuntary motor response to a given stimulus. An illustration is the automatic, unthinking leg extension response when a physician taps the patellar tendon with a rubber mallet. In this simplest form, a reflex consists of a discharge from a sensory (afferent) nerve ending, with the impulses traveling over the sensory nerve fiber to a synapse in the spinal cord with a motor (efferent) neuron. When the motor neuron is stimulated to discharge, impulses travel over its axon to the muscle, causing it to move. This simple reflex arc is called the **myotatic**, or stretch reflex; because it involves only one synapse in the spinal cord, it is called a **monosynaptic reflex**. Other more complex reflexes (such as removing the hand from a hot surface) can involve multiple neurons and synapses.

> *A reflex is an involuntary response to a given stimulus.*

PROPRIOCEPTION AND KINESTHESIS

Optimal coordination of motor activity by the central nervous system depends on a constant supply of sensory feedback during the movement. This feedback of sensory information about movement and body position is called **proprioception**. The receptors for proprioception are of two types: vestibular and kinesthetic.

The **vestibular receptors** are found in the inner ear and respond to the movement of a fluid called **endolymph**. Indirectly, the inertia of the endolymph provides data to the brain regarding rotational acceleration or deceleration of movement, as in twisting or tumbling. Movement itself, however, is not recognized. For example, moving at almost the speed of sound in an airliner produces no sensation unless a change of direction or velocity occurs.

The vestibular system also includes an inner ear structure called the **utricle**, which provides data regarding positional sense. Specialized structures in the utricle respond to linear acceleration and tilting and thus are the source of data that inform us of our posture and orientation in space. For example, sensory information from the utricle is responsible for our ability to tell whether we are standing up or lying down, even with our eyes closed.

The kinesthetic or muscle sense is crucial to our ability to properly execute movement; it provides information about what our limbs or body segments are doing without our having to look. For example, most individuals have no difficulty touching their noses with their index fingers, even when blindfolded. Furthermore, one can usually make reasonably accurate guesses about the weight of an object by lifting it.

The two primary receptor structures that serve **kinesthesis** (sense of movement and body part location in space) are muscle spindles and Golgi tendon organs. Muscle spindles are large enough to be visible to the naked eye and are widely distributed throughout muscle tissue. Their distribution, however, varies from muscle to muscle. In general, muscles used for intricate movements (such as finger muscles) have many muscle spindles, while muscles involved primarily in gross movements have few.

In humans, each spindle includes from five to nine **intrafusal (IF) muscle fibers**. These IF fibers should not be confused with skeletal (extrafusal or EF) muscle fibers, which cause muscle contraction. The IF fibers of the muscle spindles are innervated by gamma motor neurons, while EF (skeletal) fibers are innervated by alpha motor neurons. Alpha motor neurons make up about 70% of the total efferent fibers; gamma motor neurons make up the remaining 30%. The structure of a muscle spindle is shown in Figure 3.2. It is important to

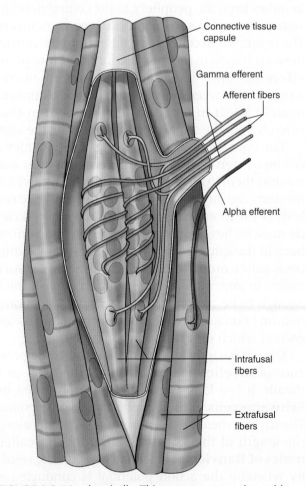

FIGURE 3.2 Muscle spindle. This sensory receptor is sensitive to stretch and helps to monitor muscle length.

note that the muscle spindles are oriented parallel to the EF fibers.

Because IF fibers lie lengthwise, parallel with the skeletal (EF) fibers, an externally applied stretch results in stretching the IF as well as the EF fibers. Thus, stretching results in a sensory afferent discharge from the muscle spindles, which leads to contraction of the muscle that was stretched. This response underlies the stretch or myotatic reflex when a physician strikes the patellar tendon.

The Golgi tendon organ (Fig. 3.3) is found in the musculotendinous junction and lies in series with the EF (skeletal) muscle fibers. Therefore, active shortening of the muscle (contraction) causes the Golgi tendon organ to discharge, while the muscle spindle discharges only when the muscle is stretched. The muscle spindle ceases to fire when contraction begins because it is in parallel with the EF muscle fibers and is thus unloaded as soon as the EF fibers shorten in contraction.

The primary functional difference between the muscle spindle and the Golgi tendon organ is that the muscle spindle facilitates contraction, whereas the Golgi tendon organ inhibits contraction, not only in the muscle of origin but also in the entire functional muscle group. Thus, the Golgi tendon

organ may provide a protective mechanism that prevents damage to muscle tissue or a joint during extreme contractions. The activity of the Golgi tendon organ that prevents overstressing the tissues is called the **inverse myotatic reflex**.

> *Proprioception involves sensory feedback about movement and body position. Kinesthesis is sometimes called muscle sense and involves the functions of muscle spindles and Golgi tendon organ.*

HIGHER NERVE CENTERS AND VOLUNTARY MUSCULAR CONTROL

Voluntary muscular activity is controlled by three primary systems: the pyramidal system, the extrapyramidal system, and the proprioceptive-cerebellar system.

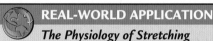

REAL-WORLD APPLICATION
The Physiology of Stretching

It has been theorized that stretching can improve performance and prevent injury. It is also important, however, to consider how to stretch. Specifically, we must consider the effect of the muscle spindle on flexibility and stretching.

A muscle that is stretched rapidly with a jerky motion will respond by contracting. The magnitude and rate of this contraction vary directly with the magnitude and rate of the movement that causes the rapid stretch. This contraction is a result of the myotatic or stretch reflex. The rapidly applied stretch causes activation of the muscle spindles located between the skeletal (extrafusal) muscle fibers. This rapid stretch causes an afferent impulse to be carried by a sensory neuron to the spinal cord, where the neuron synapses with a motor neuron. The motor neuron then carries an impulse back to the skeletal muscle, causing it to contract. The important point is that if, in an attempt to stretch the muscle, the stretch is applied with a bouncing, jerky motion, the result is activation of the myotatic reflex and a contraction of the very muscle that is the object of the attempted stretch. This can lead to less than optimal stretching at best and injury at worst.

Static stretching, on the other hand, in which the stretch is applied slowly, does not invoke the myotatic reflex. By moving slowly into the stretched position, activation of the muscle spindles is avoided. This allows the muscle to relax while being elongated, leading to a more effective stretch.

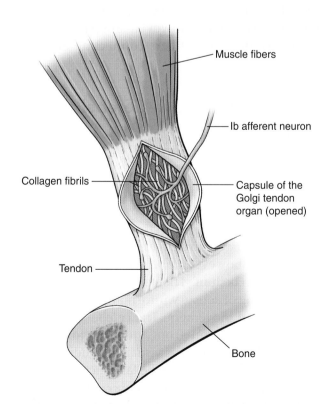

FIGURE 3.3 Golgi tendon organ. Located at the musculotendinous junction, this sensory receptor monitors tension.

The Pyramidal System

Electrical stimulation and clinical observations have been used to identify the functions of the various parts of the cerebral cortex. The most commonly used architectural map of the human cortex that relates location to function is that of Brodmann (Fig. 3.4).

The **pyramidal system** originates in large pyramid-shaped neurons found mainly in area 4, often called the motor cortex, of the Brodmann map. The axons of the motor neurons with cell bodies in area 4 form large descending motor pathways, called **pyramidal tracts**, that go directly (in most cases) to synapses with the motor neurons in the ventral horn of the spinal cord. The neurons with cell bodies in the brain are called **upper motor neurons**, while those in the spinal cord are called **lower motor neurons**. About 85% or more of the neurons of the pyramidal tract cross from one side to the other (decussate), some at the level of the medulla, others at the level of the lower motor neuron. The motor cortex is oriented by movement, not by muscle. That is, stimulation of the motor cortex results not in a twitch of one muscle but in a smooth synergistic movement of a group of muscles.

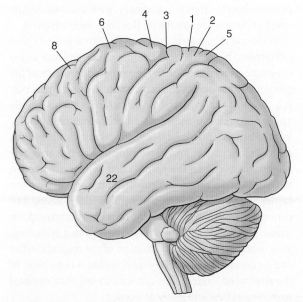

FIGURE 3.4 The areas of the human cerebral cortex involved in the pyramidal and extrapyramidal systems. The pyramidal system originates mainly in area 4 (motor cortex) of the brain and controls specific, voluntary movements. The extrapyramidal system (mainly area 6, but also areas 1 to 3, 5, 8, and 22) is concerned with large, general movement patterns and posture control.

The Extrapyramidal System

The **extrapyramidal system**, or the premotor cortex, originates primarily in area 6 of Brodmann's area. Some of the fibers descending in the extrapyramidal tracts, however, originate in other areas of the cortex, such as areas 1, 2, 3, 5, and 8.

The descending tracts from the premotor cortex are more complex than those from the motor cortex. These neurons do not synapse directly with the lower motor neurons but travel through relay stations called **motor nuclei**. The most important motor nuclei are the **corpus striatum**, **substantia nigra**, and **red nucleus**. Some neurons, however, also go by way of the pons to the cerebellum.

Important functional differences exist between the pyramidal and extrapyramidal systems. For example, electrical stimulation of area 4 produces specific movements, while stimulation of area 6 produces only gross movement patterns. Thus, it is likely that learning a new skill in which conscious attention must be devoted to the movements (as in learning a new gymnastic move, where every aspect of the movement is contemplated) involves area 4. As an individual becomes more skilled, the origin of the movement is thought to shift to area 6 (often, gymnasts do not have to concentrate on their feet but rather on very general patterns of movement). Area 4, however, still participates as a relay station, with fibers connecting area 6 to area 4.

The Proprioceptive-Cerebellar System

Kinesthesis and the vestibular system involve the sensory functions of the **proprioceptive-cerebellar system**. Typically, the pathway associated with vestibular proprioception leads directly or indirectly (via the medulla) to the cerebellum. Conscious sensory knowledge of movement from kinesthesis, however, travels via the thalamus, cortex, and cerebellum. The cerebellum is central to the gathering of sensory information on position, balance, and movement. The cerebellum receives sensory information from muscles, joints, tendons, and skin as well as visual and auditory feedback. Thus, the loss of cerebellar function can lead to the impairment of volitional movements, disturbances of posture, and impaired balance control.

Three primary systems control voluntary human movement: the pyramidal system, the extra-pyramidal system, and the proprioceptive-cerebellar system.

GROSS STRUCTURE OF SKELETAL MUSCLE

A skeletal muscle is covered by a connective tissue sheath called the **epimysium**, which lies beneath the skin, subcutaneous adipose tissue, and superficial fascia. The epimysium merges with the connective tissue of the tendon, which allows the force produced by muscular contraction to be transmitted through the connective tissues to the tendon and bone, resulting in movement.

Skeletal muscle cells or muscle fibers are oriented in bundles called fasciculi. Each fasciculus, which contains from a few muscle fibers to several hundred, is surrounded by a connective tissue sheath called the perimysium. Figure 3.5 illustrates these and other gross and microscopic structures of skeletal muscle.

The gross structures of skeletal muscle are important for transducing the force of muscular contraction to the tendon and bone, resulting in movement.

MICROSCOPIC STRUCTURE OF SKELETAL MUSCLE

Surrounding each muscle fiber is a delicate connective tissue sheath known as the **endomysium**. Thus, the endomysium surrounds a single fiber, the perimysium surrounds a fasciculus, and the epimysium surrounds the whole muscle. The force produced within a muscle fiber is transferred in series to the endomysium, perimysium, epimysium, tendon, and then bone.

The diameter of individual muscle fibers may vary from approximately 10 to 100 μm (1,000 μm = 1 mm), while the length may range from 1 mm to the length of the whole muscle. The thickness of the fiber is related to the amount of force that the fiber can produce, and each muscle has fibers of characteristic size. For example, the eye muscles

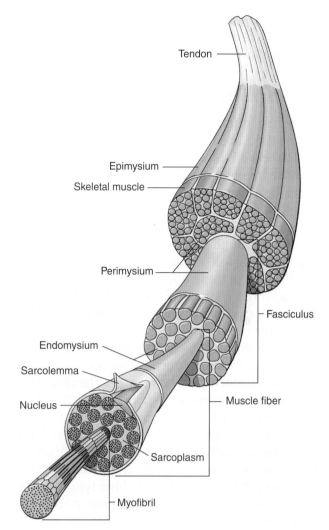

FIGURE 3.5 Muscle fibers and connective tissue sheaths. Each fiber, fasciculus, and whole muscle is surrounded by connective tissues called endomysium, perimysium, and epimysium, respectively.

have fibers with a small diameter, while the fibers of the quadriceps femoris muscles are large.

Structure of the Muscle Fiber

Each skeletal muscle fiber is surrounded by a cell membrane known as the **sarcolemma**. Situated just inside the sarcolemma are many nuclei, which direct protein synthesis within the cell. The fluid part, or cytoplasm, of the muscle cell is known as the **sarcoplasm**. Much of the sarcoplasm is occupied by column-like structures known as myofibrils. Alternating light and dark bands run the length of the myofibrils. The strict alignment of these bands from one myofibril to another is what gives the muscle fiber its characteristic striated appearance under the light microscope.

Muscle fibers may vary greatly in size and length yet have the same structures (i.e., cell membrane, cytoplasm) as other cells in the body.

Muscle Fiber Types

In the past, muscle fibers were classified based simply on their appearance. Red fibers were considered to be well suited for endurance activities, such as those involving long-term contractions. White fibers, however, were considered to be specialized for speed of contraction yet susceptible to fatigue. Recently, the identification of types of skeletal muscle fiber through the use of histochemical techniques has made it possible to examine the chemical constituents of these fibers, thereby providing the means for correlating their structure and function.

Two to as many as eight different muscle fiber types have been identified. The nomenclature for describing the various fiber types has been based on their appearance, function, biochemical properties, and histochemical properties. The older fast-twitch (white) versus slow-twitch (red) fiber-type classification system has become inadequate, since there are two subtypes of fast-twitch fibers that are physiologically and histochemically different. Thus, the new nomenclature (proposed by Peter et al.) for three different muscle fiber types is based on the function and biochemical properties of the fiber (70).

The three primary fiber types in human skeletal muscle are slow-twitch oxidative (SO), fast-twitch oxidative glycolytic (FOG), and fast-twitch glycolytic (FG) (70). These fiber types are also identified as type I, type IIA, and type IIB, respectively, by Dubowitz and Brooke (15). The former nomenclature, however, is more descriptive, since it provides information about the characteristics and functioning of the various fiber types. For example, SO fibers have a slow twitch speed and favor oxidative (aerobic) energy production, while FG fibers have a fast twitch speed and favor glycolytic (anaerobic) energy production. Table 3.1 compares the naming systems and lists the characteristics of muscle fiber types.

The basic functional unit of the neuromuscular system is the **motor unit**, which consists of a motor neuron (nerve) and all the muscle fibers that it innervates. All of the fibers within a particular motor unit are of the same type, although the fibers from different motor units are intermingled. In small muscles, a single motor unit may consist of only a few fibers; in large muscles, each motor unit may comprise several hundred fibers.

The patterns of fiber type distribution in the various muscles are related to the function(s) of the muscle. For example, postural muscles must be fatigue-resistant and therefore are usually composed mainly of SO fibers. The ocular muscles, however, do not contract for extended periods and

TABLE 3.1	CHARACTERISTICS OF MUSCLE FIBER TYPES		
NOMENCLATURE			
Older systems	Red slow-twitch (ST)	White fast-twitch (FT)	
Dubowitz and Brooke (15)	Type I	Type IIA	Type IIB
Peter et al. (70)	Slow, oxidative (SO)	Fast, oxidative glycolytic (FOG)	Fast, glycolytic (FG)
CHARACTERISTICS			
Speed of contraction	Slow	Fast	Fast
Strength of contraction	Low	High	High
Fatigability	Fatigue resistant	Fatigable	Most fatigable
Aerobic capacity	High	Medium	Low
Anaerobic capacity	Low	Medium	High
Size	Small	Large	Large
Capillary density	High	High	Low

therefore consist primarily of fast-twitch fibers. Each individual's fiber-type pattern is genetically determined, established prior to adulthood, and probably unchanging thereafter. Although training may result in significant improvements in the performance capabilities of all three fiber types, the relative proportions of slow- and fast-twitch fibers within a muscle are not altered.

Different athletic activities place different demands on skeletal muscles. Elite competitors in either endurance or sprint/power activities have extreme patterns of fiber-type distribution (i.e., mostly of the slow- or fast-twitch type). Non-athletes, however, usually have a fairly even pattern of fiber-type distribution.

Structure of the Myofibril and the Contractile Mechanism

The **sarcomere** is the functional unit of the myofibril (Fig. 3.6). It extends from one **Z line** to an adjacent Z line. The sarcomere comprises two **myofilaments** (contractile proteins), **myosin**, and **actin**, which lie parallel to one another. The myosin filament is approximately twice as thick as the actin filament and defines the length of the **A band**. It is the A band that forms the dark part of the striation effect. The actin filaments are longer than the myosin filaments and extend inward from the Z lines toward the center of the sarcomere. Within the A band is a lighter region known as the **H zone**, the area of the A band that does not contain actin filaments. The **I band** is the area between the ends

of the myosin filaments. Because it is less dense than the A band, the I band is also lighter in color. These alternating areas of greater and lesser optical density are what give skeletal muscle its characteristic "striped" or "striated" appearance.

THE SLIDING-FILAMENT THEORY OF MUSCLE CONTRACTION

The **sliding-filament theory** has been used to describe the mechanics of muscle contraction. It states the following:

1. Voluntary muscle contraction is initiated in the cortex of the brain.
2. Typically, the electrical current, or **action potential**, travels via an upper **motor neuron** and synapses with a lower motor neuron in the ventral horn of the spinal cord.
3. The action potential passes along to the end of a lower motor neuron (**end bulb**) and causes the release of the stimulatory neurotransmitter **acetylcholine (ACh)**. The intersection between a lower motor neuron and a muscle fiber is called the **myoneural junction**, or **neuromuscular junction**.
4. The ACh is released into a small gap between the motor neuron and the muscle fiber called the **synapse**. The ACh then binds to receptor sites on the muscle fiber

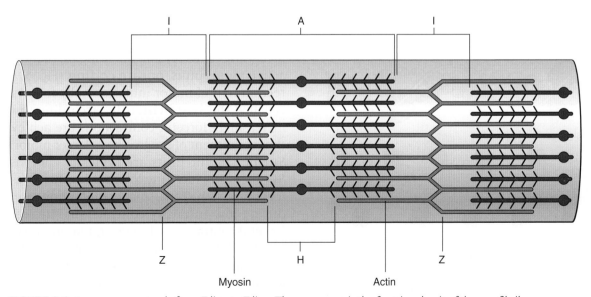

FIGURE 3.6 A sarcomere extends from Z line to Z line. The sarcomere is the functional unit of the myofibril.

membrane at a location called the **motor endplate**.

5. The binding of ACh with the receptors at the motor endplate causes an action potential to spread along the muscle fiber's sarcolemma.

6. The action potential travels along the sarcolemma and down channels that lead into the muscle fiber, called **transverse tubules**, or **t tubules**.

7. The action potential travels down the t tubules and intersects an intracellular structure called the **sarcoplasmic reticulum (SR)**. One function of the SR is to store calcium. When stimulated by the action potential, the SR releases calcium into the fiber's sarcoplasm.

8. The calcium binds to a protein called **troponin**, which is bound to another protein called **tropomyosin**. Under resting conditions, the contractile proteins actin and myosin are separated by the presence of tropomyosin. The binding of calcium to troponin changes the shape of the tropomyosin molecule and uncovers the binding sites on the actin molecule. Figure 3.7 illustrates these contractile proteins.

9. The **myosin crossbridge**, or myosin head, then binds with the binding site on the actin molecule.

10. The breakdown of **adenosine triphosphate (ATP)** to **adenosine diphosphate (ADP)** is required for muscular contraction. Multiple theories have been put forward regarding the way in which the energy lib-

erated from the breakdown of ATP contributes to muscular contraction (71). The traditional sliding-filament theory indicates that the binding of the actin and myosin filaments activates an enzyme called **myosin ATPase**, which breaks down an ATP molecule bound to the myosin crossbridge. The breakdown of ATP liberates energy that causes the myosin crossbridge to swivel toward the center of the sarcomere. As the myosin molecule swivels, it pulls the actin molecules and Z lines of the sarcomere together. This causes a shortening of the sarcomere, or muscular contraction.

11. Once the myosin crossbridge has swiveled, a fresh ATP molecule binds to it and causes the actin/myosin bond to be broken. This allows the myosin crossbridge to return to the upright position, bind to another actin binding site, and begin the contraction process again. This repeating process is called **crossbridge recycling** or **crossbridge recharging**. Figure 3.8 summarizes the sliding-filament theory of muscle contraction.

Muscle contraction is initiated by the central nervous system and generated at the molecular level through interaction of the contractile proteins actin and myosin.

GRADATION OF FORCE

The central nervous system controls the gradation of muscular force by varying the number of motor units activated, or motor unit **recruitment**, and by increasing or decreasing the firing frequency of the active motor units, or **rate coding** (Fig. 3.9). The recruitment of motor units generally follows what is called the **size principle**, according to which increasingly forceful contractions are achieved by the recruitment of progressively larger motor units. Smaller motor units are typically composed of SO fibers and have the lowest stimulus thresholds for contraction. Thus, smaller motor units are active during low-intensity contractions. Increasingly forceful contractions, however, require the recruitment of larger motor units containing fast-twitch fibers. In addition, active motor units can produce greater force by firing at higher frequencies (rate coding). The relative contributions of recruitment

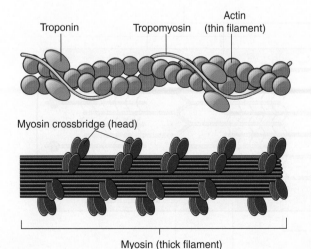

FIGURE 3.7 Contractile proteins actin, myosin, troponin, and tropomyosin. The interaction of myosin (thick filament) and actin (thin filament) allows muscle contraction to take place.

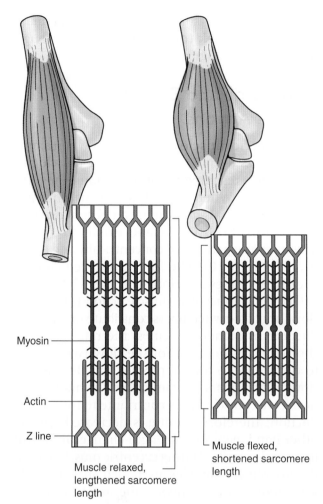

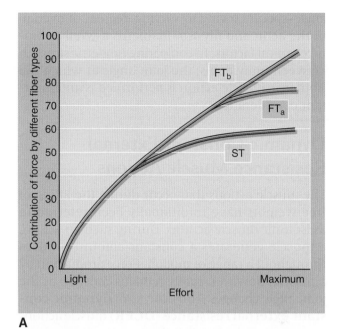

A

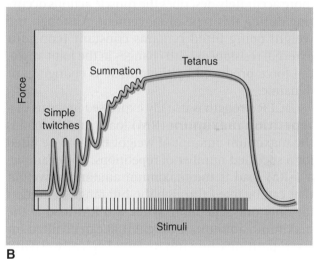

B

FIGURE 3.8 The sliding-filament theory of muscle contraction. This theory proposes that the filaments slide past each other during muscle contraction without themselves changing in length.

Myosin

Actin

Z line

Muscle relaxed, lengthened sarcomere length

Muscle flexed, shortened sarcomere length

FIGURE 3.9 Contributions of **A.** motor unit recruitment and **B.** firing rate to force production. The nervous system uses these two methods to vary the force production of whole muscles.

or rate coding to increasing force production vary from muscle to muscle. In general, large muscles with mixed fiber types, such as the quadriceps, tend to rely on recruitment to a greater degree than do small muscles, such as those in the finger, which rely more on rate coding.

> *Muscle force is modulated through two mechanisms: motor unit recruitment and rate coding. The relative contributions of these two mechanisms to force production vary in different muscles.*

TYPES OF MUSCLE ACTIONS

The term *muscle contraction* implies muscle shortening. Muscles, however, can produce force while shortening, lengthening, or maintaining a given length. The term *muscle action* is therefore more accurate and descriptive. Muscle action types include isometric, dynamic constant external resistance (DCER), isokinetic, concentric, and eccentric muscle actions.

Isometric Muscle Actions

Isometric muscle actions involve production of force without movement at the joint or shortening of the muscle fibers. Very few athletic activities involve isometric muscle actions; thus isometric strength does not predict success in sporting activities very well. Isometric strength is also joint angle–specific owing to varying degrees of overlap of the actin and myosin filaments as well as biomechanical factors. In comparing isometric strength between individuals, the joint angle at which the isometric muscle action is performed is an important consideration.

Dynamic Constant External Resistance Muscle Actions

The muscle actions that occur during the lifting of free weights have traditionally been referred to as isotonic muscle actions. During such an action, a muscle generates a constant amount of force throughout a range of motion. Force production by a muscle, however, rarely remains constant as the joint angle changes. Thus, the term **dynamic constant external resistance (DCER)** muscle actions more accurately describes the muscle actions occurring during this type of movement. Although the weight being lifted remains constant (constant external resistance) with changes in the joint angle, the force produced by the muscle is changing, or dynamic.

DCER strength is usually expressed in terms of a **repetition maximum (RM)** load. An RM load is the maximum amount of weight that can be lifted for a specified number of repetitions. For example, a 1-RM load is the maximum amount of weight that can be lifted through the full range of motion for only one repetition, while a 6-RM load is the maximum amount of weight that can be lifted for six repetitions but not seven. Typically, DCER strength testing involves a trial-and-error procedure where progressively heavier weights are attempted until the 1 RM is determined. Because strength is joint angle–specific, DCER strength is limited by the weakest point in the range of motion; therefore, the 1-RM load is the maximum weight that can be lifted at the weakest point in the range of motion.

Isokinetic Muscle Actions

An **isokinetic muscle action** is a dynamic movement that occurs at a constant velocity. Typically, isokinetic muscle actions are performed on a dynamometer, a device that accommodates the counterresistance based on the amount of torque being produced. This allows movement to occur at a constant velocity regardless of torque production. Isokinetic strength testing has advantages over both isometric and DCER testing because,

during a maximal isokinetic muscle action, maximum torque (**peak torque**) is produced throughout the entire range of motion.

Concentric and Eccentric Muscle Actions

A **concentric muscle action** occurs when a muscle produces torque (technically, the muscle produces force, resulting in torque around the joint) and shortens. When a muscle lengthens while producing torque, it is performing an **eccentric muscle action**. Both DCER and isokinetic muscle actions can be performed concentrically and eccentrically (Fig. 3.10). The force produced concentrically decreases as velocity increases. When the velocity of a concentric muscle action is low, both slow- and fast-twitch fibers contribute to force production; at higher velocities, the rate of muscle shortening is too great for the slow-twitch fibers to contribute to torque production. Because the slow-twitch fibers are "unloaded" at high velocities, fewer muscle fibers contribute to torque production; therefore, torque is decreased. On the other hand, eccentric strength changes little with increased velocity. During eccentric muscle actions, the myosin crossbridges are pulled apart from the actin molecules. In theory, the amount of force necessary to pull the myosin heads from the actin molecules is independent of the velocity.

> *The three types of muscle action are isometric, dynamic constant external resistance (DCER), and isokinetic. Isokinetic and DCER muscle actions may be performed either concentrically or eccentrically.*

NEUROMUSCULAR ADAPTATIONS TO RESISTANCE TRAINING

The following discussion focuses on neuromuscular changes resulting from prolonged resistance training.

Muscular Strength Adaptations

Training can lead to strength gains, regardless of the mode of resistance (25). Isometric, isokinetic, variable resistance, and DCER programs are all

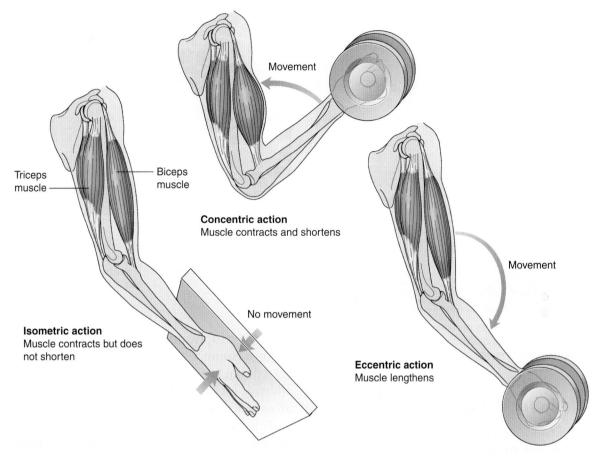

FIGURE 3.10 Types of muscle actions. Muscle may produce force while shortening, lengthening, or maintaining a constant length.

effective at eliciting strength gains assuming that scientific principles of program design are applied. Strength gains, however, tend to be sensitive to the mode of training. For example, isometric training leads to greater gains in isometric strength than isokinetic strength (25). Even within a specific mode of training, there can be specificity. For example, in training with isokinetic muscle actions, greater gains in muscular strength tend to occur at velocities closest to the training velocity (12). Thus, specificity of training must be considered if the goal of a resistance training program is to transfer the newly developed strength to other activities, such as sport, recreational, or occupational pursuits.

Strength gains resulting from resistance training tend to be specific to the type of training performed.

In terms of the absolute weight lifted, males tend to be stronger than females. This is because males are usually bigger and have more muscle mass. Females tend to be about 40% to 50% as strong as males in upper body movements and 50% to 80% as strong in lower body movements (25).

When strength is expressed relative to muscle cross-sectional area, however, there are no gender differences in muscular strength (45) (Fig. 3.11). Thus, for a given amount of muscle, males and females produce the same amount of force.

The quality of muscle is the same for men and women. In addition, men and women respond to resistance training in a similar manner.

For many athletes, the ability to develop force rapidly is as important, if not more so, as developing maximal force. It usually takes in excess of 0.3 to 0.4 seconds to generate maximal force (89). Because time is limited during many sport activities (i.e., 0.22 to 0.27 seconds during shot putting and 0.101 to 0.108 seconds during sprinting) (55,62), however, the activated muscles must exert as much force as possible in a short time. This capability can be measured by determining the **rate of force development (RFD)**. Performing "power" or "explosive" training exercises (plyometrics, cleans, pulls, weighted jumps, etc.) can increase the RFD (31).

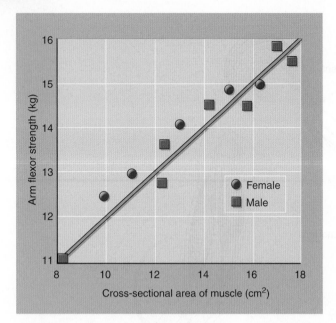

FIGURE 3.11 Muscle strength per unit of cross-sectional area of human muscle. There is no qualitative difference in strength per unit of muscle size between the genders.

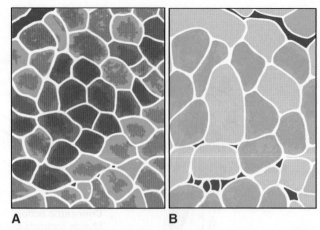

A   **B**

FIGURE 3.12 Muscle hypertrophy following resistance training. **A.** Pretraining. **B.** Posttraining. Hypertrophy results from an increased content of contractile protein (actin and myosin) in muscle.

Muscle Fiber Adaptations

Resistance training typically results in increases in muscle size and strength. These adaptations may be partially explained by muscle fiber adaptations.

HYPERTROPHY AND HYPERPLASIA

Perhaps the most obvious adaptation to resistance training is enlargement of the trained muscles. Growth in muscle size can result from an increase in the size of existing muscle fiber (**hypertrophy**) or an increase in the number of muscle fibers (**hyperplasia**).

Substantial evidence supports muscle fiber hypertrophy as the primary mechanism of increasing muscle size (4,5,16,28,35,40,78) (Fig. 3.12). This increase is primarily due to an increase in the number and size of actin and myosin filaments (26). The actin and myosin filaments are added to the periphery of the myofibrils, resulting in enlargement of existing myofibrils. Once the myofibril reaches a critical size, it splits, yielding two or more daughter myofibrils (26). Although both slow- and fast-twitch fibers increase in size, the fast-twitch fibers appear to be more responsive to resistance training (26,53).

It has been suggested that eccentric muscle actions are necessary to induce muscle hypertrophy (11). Hypertrophy, however, can occur following concentric-only training (41,65), suggesting that hypertrophy does not require eccentric muscle actions. Nonetheless, numerous studies have suggested that eccentric muscle actions may be more effective for inducing hypertrophy than concentric muscle actions (9,23,37,40,68,76).

Females respond to resistance training much like men (38). Although the absolute gains in muscle size are greater in men, the percentage increases are similar for the two genders (7,14).

Evidence from studies of laboratory animals suggests that hyperplasia may contribute to resistance training–induced increases in muscle size (6,27). Although there is some conflicting information (57,57,82), the general consensus in humans is that hypertrophy accounts for the training-induced increase in muscle size and that hyperplasia is probably of little or no significance (25).

 Hypertrophy is the primary mechanism by which muscles increase in size.

MUSCLE FIBER TRANSFORMATION

The possibility that training can alter muscle fiber types has intrigued exercise scientists and resistance training practitioners for years. The transformation of a type I (SO) fiber to a type II (FOG or FG) fiber, or vice versa, has obvious implications for strength and power performance. To date, the evidence suggests that heavy resistance training can transform only muscle fibers within a given muscle fiber type, i.e., from type IIB to IIA (53,79). Transformation of type IIB to type IIA fibers occurs rapidly with heavy resistance training (2,35,48,80).

Q & A from the Field

The head coach of our women's volleyball team is hesitant to implement a resistance training program for our team. He doesn't believe that female athletes can gain strength and muscle size, like male athletes can. My previous experience is with conditioning males athletes. Is it true that females are less trainable than males when it comes to resistance training?

—undergraduate student intern

There is every reason to believe that female athletes will adapt to resistance training in a manner similar to male athletes. The typical female athlete will be smaller, weaker, and have less muscle mass than her male counterpart. Her gains in size and strength will also be less than those of the male if expressed on an absolute basis, i.e., weight lifted in pounds. When size and strength gains are expressed as a percentage increase relative to initial values, however, the female will experience gains that are comparable to those of her male counterpart. Female muscle is of the same quality as male muscle, and is just as trainable.

The functional implication of this transformation, however, is unclear.

Nervous System Adaptations

Although muscles produce force, it is the nervous system that provides for the activation of muscle tissue. It is not surprising, therefore, that resistance training programs lead to adaptations in both the nervous and muscular systems.

EVIDENCE OF NEURAL ADAPTATIONS

Several pieces of evidence point to the role of **neural adaptations** in resistance training. For example, increases in muscular strength may occur without accompanying increases in muscular size (33,64). If there is no increase in the size of the muscle fibers producing force, the logical conclusion is that adaptations within the nervous system are responsible for the observed strength gains.

It has been shown that the early gains in strength following initiation of a resistance training program often occur in the absence of muscle hypertrophy (46,64). Previously untrained subjects may have difficulty in fully activating their motor units, and strength gains resulting from the first several weeks of resistance training have been attributed to learning to recruit those units (64). Although neural adaptations are often associated with the early phase of resistance training (46,64), one study found that 2 years of training led to significant increases in strength and power despite minimal changes in muscle fiber size in competi-tive Olympic weightlifters (33). Weightlifters compete within body-weight categories and often want to develop increased strength without changes in muscle mass that might lead to changes in body weight (25). Thus, neural adaptations are an essential mechanism of strength increase among these athletes.

Early gains in strength are due to neural factors, while long-term gains in strength are primarily due to hypertrophy.

Performing resistance training with one limb can lead to strength increases in the untrained limb on the opposite (contralateral) side of the body (22,36,42,43,65,86–88,90). This phenomenon is known as the **cross-education** or **cross-training** effect. The strength gain in the untrained limb is typically equal to or less than 60% of that in the trained limb (90). The cross-education effect demonstrates specificity of training. For example, unilateral resistance training for one leg will increase the strength of the contralateral leg but not the contralateral arm. There is also specificity with regard to muscle action type. Training with concentric muscle actions leads to greater gains in the untrained limb when tested concentrically than eccentrically (90). Theories to explain this cross-education effect include (1) neural activation of the corresponding muscles on both sides of the body, (2) activation of muscle of the contralateral limb to maintain stability during unilateral muscle actions, or (3) some unidentified spinal mechanism (36,90).

Force measured with both limbs concurrently (bilaterally) is typically less than the sum of the force developed by each limb independently (unilaterally) (13,67,86,87) (Fig. 3.13). This **bilateral deficit** may be the result of less activation to each muscle group during bilateral activation than to either muscle group activated maximally alone (44). This suggests that there is an inhibitory mechanism that limits maximal activation during bilateral muscle actions. Training with bilateral muscle actions reduces the bilateral deficit, bringing bilateral force production close to the sum of unilateral force production (19).

> *Cross education and the reduction of the bilateral deficit provide evidence of neural adaptations to resistance training.*

ELECTROMYOGRAPHIC EVIDENCE OF NEURAL ADAPTATIONS

Electromyography (EMG) records and quantifies the electrical activity in the muscle fibers of activated motor units (75) (Fig. 3.14). It reflects the number of motor units activated and their firing rates (75). Typically, isometric muscle actions are characterized by linear or curvilinear increases in EMG amplitude with torque (or force) (3,17,18, 30,60,66,77). Therefore, an increase in maximal EMG activity would reflect an increase in motor unit activation (a neural adaptation). The increase in EMG activity may result from increased numbers of active motor units (i.e., high-threshold motor units), increased motor unit firing rates, or motor unit synchronization.

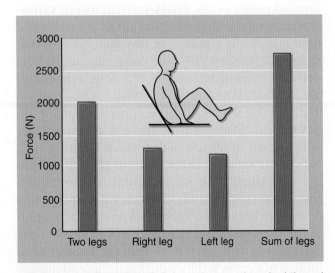

FIGURE 3.13 The bilateral deficit, showing that the bilateral force (two legs) is less than the sum of the left and right legs acting separately (sum of legs).

Numerous investigations have shown increases in EMG activity as a result of resistance training (1,37,65). Untrained individuals (those unfamiliar with a resistance training exercise) may not be able to recruit the highest-threshold motor units (types IIA and IIB) (1,37,39,40,65,74). This is indicative of an inability to fully activate the agonist muscle(s). An increase in the ability to recruit these high-threshold motor units can increase the expression of muscular strength. For example, type IIB motor units make up only about 5% of the total number of motor units of the triceps brachii, but these units contain approximately 20% of the total number of muscle fibers (21,75).

Increasing the firing rate of motor units can also affect the force produced by activated motor units. Motor units can increase their force 10-fold by altering their firing rates (73). Not surprisingly then, resistance training has been shown to increase motor unit firing rates after training (49,69,85).

Increased synchronization of motor units has been observed after strength training (24,63). The more synchronous the firing of motor units, the more motor units will be firing at any given time. Theoretically, this might lead to an increase in maximal force production, although some evidence suggests that asynchronous firing of motor units may be more effective than synchronous firing in producing force during submaximal muscle actions (56,72). Thus, the role of synchronization of motor unit firing in force production remains unclear (25,75).

> *Increased neural drive results from increased motor unit recruitment, increased motor unit firing rate, or synchronization of motor unit firing.*

A maximal muscle action of an agonist muscle or muscle group is typically accompanied by simultaneous activation of the antagonist muscle or muscle group (75). This is known as **antagonist coactivation** (or cocontraction). For example, a maximal voluntary contraction of the elbow flexors (agonists) may also involve activation of the elbow extensors (antagonists). This coactivation reduces the net torque in the intended direction, reducing performance on the strength test. Coactivation may be a strategy used to help stabilize a joint, particularly if the individual is inexperienced or uncertain about lifting a load (20). Strength training reduces coactivation of antagonist muscle groups, leading to an increase in the expression of muscular strength (8,29).

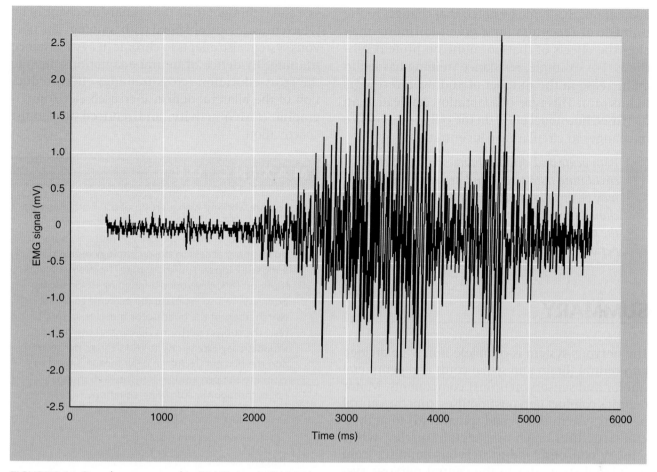

FIGURE 3.14 Raw electromyographic (EMG) signal. EMG is the recording of muscle action potentials.

Metabolic Adaptations

Some evidence points to increased fuel availability following resistance training. One study showed increases in ATP (18%), PC (25%), and glycogen (66%) levels following 5 months of heavy resistance training (59). Another study showed increased activity levels of several key enzymes involved in anaerobic energy metabolism (creatine kinase, myokinase, and phosphofructokinase) (10). Others, however, concluded that strength training does not increase ATP or PC levels (83) or lead to increased activities of enzymes associated with the phosphagen, glycolytic, or oxidative energy systems (81). Differences between studies may be due to the pretraining status of subjects, muscles examined, and variations in the design of the training programs (25).

Endocrine Adaptations

The two hormones most important for resistance training adaptations are **testosterone** and **growth hormone**. It has been shown that an acute bout of resistance exercise can increase circulating levels of these anabolic hormones (50–52), which are sensitive to program design variables such as load and rest period. Testosterone, for example, was elevated following the use of both 5-RM loads with 3-minute rest periods and 10-RM loads with 1-minute rest periods. Growth hormone, however, was highest following a 10-RM load with 1-minute rest periods between multiple sets.

Reports conflict regarding chronic changes in circulating levels of testosterone following resistance training. Some studies have reported increased resting levels of testosterone (33,80), while others have not (32,34). Discrepancies may be attributed to differences in the volume and intensity of the training programs employed (32). Circulating levels of growth hormone do not appear to change with resistance training (54,61). The cumulative effect of acute increases in growth hormone following resistance training sessions may be the most important mechanism leading to adaptations. It should be noted that changes in the number of receptors for a given hormone may alter the effects of that hormone on protein synthesis. For example, resistance training has led to an increase in the number of androgen receptors in rats (47). This type of adaptation can lead to an increased hormonal effect on the cell in the absence of changes in circulating concentrations.

> *Both acute and chronic changes in the levels of circulating testosterone and growth hormone may occur following resistance training. These changes appear to be sensitive to the design of the training program, such as load and rest period between sets.*

SUMMARY

The nervous system is complex; it may be divided into central (brain and spinal cord) and peripheral (motor and sensory neurons) components. Motor neurons conduct nervous impulses from the central nervous system (brain and spinal cord) to peripheral structures, such as skeletal muscles, while sensory neurons conduct nervous impulses from peripheral structures to the central nervous system. A reflex is an involuntary motor response to a given stimulus. Of the many types of reflexes, the myotatic (stretch) and inverse myotatic reflexes are especially important for those cultivating strength and conditioning.

The individual fibers comprising skeletal muscle are arranged into bundles called fasciculi. Each fiber, fasciculus, and whole muscle is surrounded by connective tissues called endomysium, perimysium, and epimysium, respectively. These connective tissues transmit the force of muscle contraction to the tendons, which are attached to bones and cause movement. The sliding-filament theory of muscle contraction describes how actin and myosin interact to cause contraction and thus force production.

The three muscle fiber types found in humans are slow oxidative (SO), fast oxidative glycolytic (FOG), and fast glycolytic (FG). These fiber types differ from one another based on their contractile and metabolic characteristics. The relative proportions of each fiber type differ among people, and is largely determined by genetics.

Resistance training increases muscle size and strength. *Hypertrophy* refers to an increase in cell

size and is thought to be the primary mechanism by which muscles are enlarged with training. The nervous system also adapts to chronic heavy resistance training. Evidence of neural adaptations include the cross-education (cross-training) effect, reduction of the bilateral deficit, increased electromyographic (EMG) activity, and reduced antagonist coactivation.

MAXING OUT

1. You are working with a group of track athletes who want to estimate the percentage of fast-twitch muscle fibers in their quadriceps muscles, but you do not have access to the technology required for a muscle biopsy. You know that Thorstensson and Karlsson (84) developed a fatiguing isokinetic leg-extension test to estimate the percentage of fast-twitch fibers in the quadriceps muscles. In this test, the subject performs 50 consecutive maximal isokinetic leg extensions at 180 degrees per second and the percent decline in peak torque is used to estimate the percentage of fast-twitch muscle fibers through the following equation:

   Percent fast-twitch fibers
   $$= (\text{percent decline} - 5.2)/0.9$$

   Percent decline
   $$= [(\text{initial peak torque} - \text{final peak torque})/\text{initial peak torque}] \times 100$$

   Estimate the percentage of fast-twitch muscle fibers for subjects with declines of 25, 40, 67, and 83%.

2. A previously inexperienced weight trainer has completed the first 2 weeks of a resistance training program designed to increase muscle size and strength. The athlete approaches you and expresses frustration that she does not see any sign of an increase in muscle size or fat-free body mass. Considering the time course of contributions from neural adaptations versus hypertrophy, explain to the athlete why this is normal following just 2 weeks of resistance exercise.

3. An athlete is intrigued that he is not able to exert as much force during higher- versus slower-speed concentric muscle actions despite making a maximal effort under each condition. Explain why there is a negative relationship between force and velocity for concentric muscle actions.

REFERENCES

1. Aagaard P, Simonsen EB, Andersen JL, et al. Neural inhibition during maximal eccentric and concentric quadriceps contraction: effects of resistance training. J Appl Physiol 2000;89;2249–2257.

2. Adams GR, Hather BM, Baldwin KM, Dudley GA. Skeletal muscle myosin heavy chain composition and resistance training. J Appl Physiol 1993;74:911–915.

3. Alkner BA, Tesch PA, Berg HE. Quadriceps EMG/force relationship in knee extension and leg press. Med Sci Sports Exerc 2000;32:459–463.

4. Alway SE. Characteristics of the elbow flexors in women bodybuilders using androgenic-anabolic steroids. J Strength Cond Res 1994;8:161–169.

5. Alway SE, Grumbt WH, Gonyea WJ, Stray-Gundersen J. Contrasts in muscle and myofibers of elite male and female bodybuilders. J Appl Physiol 1989;67:24–31.

6. Alway SE, Winchester PK, Davis ME, Gonyea WJ. Regionalized adaptations and muscle fiber proliferation in stretch-induced enlargement. J Appl Physiol 1989;66:771–781.

7. Brown CH, Wilmore JH. The effects of maximal resistance training on the strength and body composition of women athletes. Med Sci Sports 1974;6:174–177.

8. Carolan B, Cafarelli E. Adaptations in coactivation after isometric resistance training. J Appl Physiol 1992;73:911–917.

9. Colliander EB, Tesch PA. Effects of eccentric and concentric muscle actions in resistance training. Acta Physiol Scand 1990;140:31–39.

10. Costill DL, Coyle EF, Fink WF, et al. Adaptations in skeletal muscle following strength training. J Appl Physiol 1979;46:96–99.

11. Cote C, Simoneau JA, Lagasse P, et al. Isokinetic strength training protocols: do they induce skeletal muscle fiber hypertrophy? Arch Phys Med Rehabil 1988;69:281–285.

12. Coyle EF, Feiring DC, Rotkis TC, et al. Specificity of power improvements through slow and fast isokinetic training. J Appl Physiol 1981;51:1437–1422.

13. Cresswell AG, Ovendal AH. Muscle activation and torque development during maximal unilateral and bilateral isokinetic knee extensions. J Sports Med Phys Fit 2002;42:19–25.

14. Cureton KJ, Collins MA, Hill DW, McElhannon FM Jr. Muscle hypertrophy in men and women. Med Sci Sports Exerc 1988;20:338–344.

15. Dubowitz V, Brooke MH. Muscle Biopsy: A Modern Approach. Philadelphia: Saunders, 1973.

16. Dudley GA, Tesch PA, Miller BJ, Buchanan P. Importance of eccentric actions in performance adaptations to resistance training. Aviat Space Environ Med 1991;62:543–550.

17. Ebersole KT, Housh TJ, Johnson GO, et al. MMG and EMG responses of the superficial quadriceps femoris muscles. J Electromyogr Kinesiol 1999;9:219–227.

18. Eloranta V. Patterning of muscle activity in static knee extension. Electromyogr Clin Neurophysiol 1989;29:369–375.

19. Enoka RM. Muscle strength and its development. New perspectives. Sports Med 1988;6:146–168.

20. Enoka RM. Neuromechanics of Human Movement. 3rd ed. Champaign, IL: Human Kinetics, 2002:xix, 556.

21. Enoka RM, Fuglevand AJ. Motor unit physiology: some unresolved issues. Muscle Nerve 2001;24:4–17.

22. Farthing JP, Chilibeck PD. The effect of eccentric training at different velocities on cross-education. Eur J Appl Physiol 2003;89:570–577.

23. Farthing JP, Chilibeck PD. The effects of eccentric and concentric training at different velocities on muscle hypertrophy. Eur J Appl Physiol 2003;89:578–586.

24. Felici F, Rosponi A, Sbriccoli P, et al. Linear and non-linear analysis of surface electromyograms in weightlifters. Eur J Appl Physiol 2001;84:337–342.

25. Fleck SJ, Kraemer WJ. Designing Resistance Training Programs. 2nd ed. Champaign, IL: Human Kinetics, 1997:xi, 275.

26. Goldspink G, Harridge S. Cellular and molecular aspects of adaptation in skeletal muscle. In: Komi PV, ed. Strength and Power in Sport. Oxford, UK: Blackwell Scientific, 2003:231–251.

27. Gonyea, W. J., D. G. Sale, F. B. Gonyea, and A. Mikesky. Exercise induced increases in muscle fiber number. Eur J Appl Physiol Occup Physiol 1986;55:137–141.

28. Haggmark T, Jansson E, Svane B. Cross-sectional area of the thigh muscle in man measured by computed tomography. Scand J Clin Lab Invest 1978;38:355–360.

29. Hakkinen K, Kallinen M, Izquierdo M, et al. Changes in agonist-antagonist EMG, muscle CSA, and force during strength training in middle-aged and older people. J Appl Physiol 1998;84:1341–1349.

30. Hakkinen K, Komi PV. Electromyographic changes during strength training and detraining. Med Sci Sports Exerc 1983;15:455–460.

31. Hakkinen K, Komi PV, Alen M. Effect of explosive type strength training on isometric force- and relaxation-time, electromyographic and muscle fibre characteristics of leg extensor muscles. Acta Physiol Scand 1985;125:587–600.

32. Hakkinen K, Pakarinen A, Alen M, et al. Relationships between training volume, physical performance capacity, and serum hormone concentrations during prolonged training in elite weight lifters. Int J Sports Med 1987;8(Suppl 1):61–65.

33. Hakkinen K, Pakarinen A, Alen M, et al. Neuromuscular and hormonal adaptations in athletes to strength training in two years. J Appl Physiol 1988;65:2406–2412.

34. Hakkinen K, Pakarinen A, Alen M, Komi PV. Serum hormones during prolonged training of neuromuscular performance. Eur J Appl Physiol Occup Physiol 1985;53:287–293.

35. Hather BM, Tesch PA, Buchanan P, Dudley GA. Influence of eccentric actions on skeletal muscle adaptations to resistance training. Acta Physiol Scand 1991;143:177–185.

36. Hellebrandt FA. Cross education; ipsilateral and contralateral effects of unimanual training. J Appl Physiol 1951;4:136–144.

37. Higbie EJ, Cureton KJ, Warren GL III, Prior BM. Effects of concentric and eccentric training on muscle strength, cross-sectional area, and neural activation. J Appl Physiol 1996;81:2173–2181.

38. Holloway JB, Baechle TR. Strength training for female athletes. A review of selected aspects. Sports Med 1990;9:216–228.

39. Hortobagyi T, Devita P. Favorable neuromuscular and cardiovascular responses to 7 days of exercise with an eccentric overload in elderly women. J Gerontol A Biol Sci Med Sci 2000;55:B401–410.

40. Hortobagyi T, Hill JP, Houmard JA, et al. Adaptive responses to muscle lengthening and shortening in humans. J Appl Physiol 1996;80:765–772.

41. Housh DJ, Housh TJ, Johnson GO, Chu WK. Hypertrophic response to unilateral concentric isokinetic resistance training. J Appl Physiol 1992;73:65–70.

42. Housh, DJ, Housh TJ, Weir JP, et al. Effects of unilateral concentric-only dynamic constant external resistance training on quadriceps femoris cross-sectional area. J Strength Cond Res 1998;12:185–191.

43. Housh, DJ, Housh TJ, Weir JP, et al. Effects of unilateral eccentric-only dynamic constant external resistance training on quadriceps femoris cross-sectional area. J Strength Cond Res 1998;12:192–198.

44. Howard JD, Enoka RM. Maximum bilateral contractions are modified by neurally mediated interlimb effects. J Appl Physiol 1991;70:306–316.

45. Ikai M, Fukunaga T. Calculation of muscle strength per unit cross-sectional area of human muscle by means of ultrasonic measurement. Int Z Angew Physiol 1968;26:26–32.

46. Ikai M, Fukunaga T. A study on training effect on strength per unit cross-sectional area of muscle by means of ultrasonic measurement. Int Z Angew Physiol 1970;28:173–180.

47. Inoue K, Yamasaki S, Fushiki T, et al. Rapid increase in the number of androgen receptors following electrical stimulation of the rat muscle. Eur J Appl Physiol Occup Physiol 1993;66:134–140.

48. Kadi F, Thornell LE. Training affects myosin heavy chain phenotype in the trapezius muscle of women. Histochem Cell Biol 1999;112:73–78.

49. Kamen G. Resistance training increases vastus lateralis motor unit firing rates in young and old adults. Med Sci Sports Exerc 1998;30:S337.

50. Kraemer WJ, Fleck SJ, Dziados JE, et al. Changes in hormonal concentrations after different heavy-resistance exercise protocols in women. J Appl Physiol 1993;75:594–604.

51. Kraemer WJ, Gordon SE, Fleck SJ, et al. Endogenous anabolic hormonal and growth factor responses to heavy resistance exercise in males and females. Int J Sports Med 1991;12:228–235.

52. Kraemer WJ, Marchitelli L, Gordon SE, et al. Hormonal and growth factor responses to heavy resistance exercise protocols. J Appl Physiol 1990;69:1442–1450.

53. Kraemer WJ, Patton JF, Gordon SE, et al. Compatibility of high-intensity strength and endurance training on hormonal and skeletal muscle adaptations. J Appl Physiol 1995;78:976–989.

54. Kraemer WH, Staron RS, Hagerman FC, et al. The effects of short-term resistance training on endocrine function in men and women. Eur J Appl Physiol Occup Physiol 1998;78:69–76.

55. Lanka, J. Shot putting. In: Zatsiorsky VM, ed. Biomechanics in Sport: Performance Enhancement And Injury Prevention. Oxford, UK, and Malden, MA: Blackwell Science, 2000:435–457.

56. Lind AR, Petrofsky JS. Isometric tension from rotary stimulation of fast and slow cat muscles. Muscle Nerve 1978;1:213–218.

57. MacDougall JD, Sale DG, Alway SE, Sutton JR. Muscle fiber number in biceps brachii in bodybuilders and control subjects. J Appl Physiol 1984;57:1399–1403.

58. MacDougall JD, Sale DG, Elder GC, Sutton JR. Muscle ultrastructural characteristics of elite powerlifters and bodybuilders. Eur J Appl Physiol Occup Physiol 1982;48:117–126.

59. MacDougall JD, Ward GR, Sale DG, Sutton JR. Biochemical adaptation of human skeletal muscle to heavy resistance training and immobilization. J Appl Physiol 1997;43:700–703.

60. Matheson GO, Maffey-Ward L, Mooney M, et al. Vibromyography as a quantitative measure of muscle force production. Scand J Rehabil Med 1997;29:29–35.

61. McCall GE, Byrnes WC, Fleck SJ, et al. Acute and chronic hormonal responses to resistance training designed to promote muscle hypertrophy. Can J Appl Physiol 1999;24:96–107.

62. Mero A, Komi PV. Force-, EMG-, and elasticity-velocity relationships at submaximal, maximal and supramaximal running speeds in sprinters. Eur J Appl Physiol Occup Physiol 1986;55:553–561.

63. Milner-Brown HS, Stein RB, Lee RG. Synchronization of human motor units: possible roles of exercise and supraspinal reflexes. Electroencephalogr Clin Neurophysiol 1975;38:245–254.

64. Moritani T, Devries HA. Neural factors versus hypertrophy in the time course of muscle strength gain. Am J Phys Med 1979;58:115–130.

65. Narici MV, Roi GS, Landoni L, et al. Changes in force, cross-sectional area and neural activation during strength training and detraining of the human quadriceps. Eur J Appl Physiol Occup Physiol 1989;59:310–319.

66. Nonaka H, Mita K, Akataki K, et al. Mechanomyographic investigation of muscle contractile properties in preadolescent boys. Electromyogr Clin Neurophysiol 2000;40:287–293.

67. Oda S, Moritani T. Maximal isometric force and neural activity during bilateral and unilateral elbow flexion in humans. Eur J Appl Physiol Occup Physiol 1994;69:240–243.

68. O'Hagan FT, Sale DG, MacDougall JD, Garner SH. Comparative effectiveness of accommodating and weight resistance training modes. Med Sci Sports Exerc 1995;27:1210–1219.

69. Patten C, Kamen G, Rowland DM. Adaptations in maximal motor unit discharge rate to strength training in young and older adults. Muscle Nerve 2001;24:542–550.

70. Peter JB, Barnard RJ, Edgerton VR, et al. Metabolic profiles of three fiber types of skeletal muscle in guinea pigs and rabbits. Biochemistry 1972;11:2627–2633.

71. Pollack GH. Muscles and Molecules: Uncovering the Principles of Biological Motion. Seattle: Ebner, 1990.

72. Rack PM, Westbury DR. The effects of length and stimulus rate on tension in the isometric cat soleus muscle. J Physiol 1969;204:443–460.

73. Sale D, Quinlan J, Marsh E, et al. Influence of joint position on ankle plantarflexion in humans. J Appl Physiol 1982;52:1636–1642.

74. Sale DG. Neural adaptation to resistance training. Med Sci Sports Exerc 1988;20:S135–S145.

75. Sale DG. Neural adaptations to strength training. In: Komi PV, ed. Strength and Power in Sport. Oxford, UK: Blackwell Scientific, 2003:281–314.

76. Seger JY, Arvidsson B, Thorstensson A. Specific effects of eccentric and concentric training on muscle strength and morphology in humans. Eur J Appl Physiol Occup Physiol 1998;79:49–57.

77. Shinohara M, Kouzaki M, Yoshihisa T, Fukunaga T. Mechanomyogram from the different heads of the quadriceps muscle during incremental knee extension. Eur J Appl Physiol Occup Physiol 1998;78:289–295.

78. Shoepe TC, Stelzer JE, Garner DP, Widrick JJ. Functional adaptability of muscle fibers to long-term resistance exercise. Med Sci Sports Exerc 2004;35:944–951.

79. Staron RS, Johnson P. Myosin polymorphism and differential expression in adult human skeletal muscle. Comp Biochem Physiol B 1993;106:463–475.

80. Staron RS, Karapondo DL, Kraemer WJ, et al. Skeletal muscle adaptations during early phase of heavy-resistance training in men and women. J Appl Physiol 1994;76:1247–1255.

81. Tesch PA, Komi PV, Hakkinen K. Enzymatic adaptations consequent to long-term strength training. Int J Sports Med 1987;8(Suppl 1):66–69.

82. Tesch PA, Larsson L. Muscle hypertrophy in bodybuilders. Eur J Appl Physiol Occup Physiol 1982;49:301–306.

83. Tesch PA, Thorsson A, Colliander EB. Effects of eccentric and concentric resistance training on skeletal muscle substrates, enzyme activities and capillary supply. Acta Physiol Scand 1990;140:575–580.

84. Thorstensson A, J. Karlsson J. Fatiguability and fibre composition of human skeletal muscle. Acta Physiol Scand 1976;98:318–322.

85. Van Cutsem M, Duchateau J, Hainaut K. Changes in single motor unit behaviour contribute to the increase in contraction speed after dynamic training in humans. J Physiol 1998;513 (Pt 1):295–305.

86. Weir JP, Housh DJ, Housh TJ, Weir LL. The effect of unilateral eccentric weight training and detraining on joint angle specificity, cross-training, and the bilateral deficit. J Orthop Sports Phys Ther 1995;22:207–215.

87. Weir JP, Housh DJ, Housh TJ, Weir LL. The effect of unilateral concentric weight training and detraining on joint angle specificity, cross-training, and the bilateral deficit. J Orthop Sports Phys Ther 1997;25:264–270.

88. Weir JP, Housh TJ, Weir LL. Electromyographic evaluation of joint angle specificity and cross-training after isometric training. J Appl Physiol 1994;77:197–201.

89. Zatsiorsky, V. M. Biomechanics of strength and strength testing. In: Komi PV, ed. Strength and Power in Sport. Oxford, UK: Blackwell Scientific, 2003:439–487.

90. Zhou S. Chronic neural adaptations to unilateral exercise: mechanisms of cross education. Exerc Sport Sci Rev 2000;28:177–184.

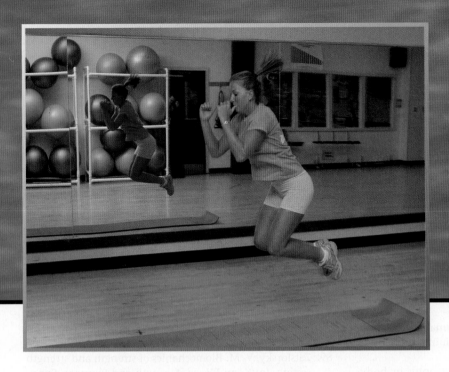

The Skeletal System

T. JEFF CHANDLER
CLINT ALLEY

Introduction

The living skeleton is much more than the calcified bones we study in anatomy. It is a dynamic system with living cells that continually remodel bone, and it responds through adaptation to the demands placed on it by training and conditioning. Specific protocols of loading and unloading bone tissues cause unique adaptations to bones, ligaments, tendons, and cartilage. **Ligaments** connect one bone to another. **Tendons** connect muscle to bone, and **cartilage** protects the ends of bones. This chapter discusses the anatomy, physiology, and response to training of the skeletal system.

The bones of the skeletal system provide the internal framework of the body; that is, they comprise the levers and articulations that enable us to move. A **lever** is a rigid bar that moves around an axis of rotation. **Articulations**, where one bone meets another bone, allow movement and serve as the axes around which movement occurs. Bones function to protect our vital organs from trauma; they also produce blood cells, including the red blood cells that transport oxygen to our tissues. In addition to all this, bones serve as depositories for the minerals we need to remain healthy.

STRUCTURE OF THE SKELETAL SYSTEM

The human skeleton is divided into two major parts, axial and appendicular (Fig. 4.1). The axial skeleton consists of the skull, vertebral column,

sacrum, coccyx, ribs, and sternum. The appendicular skeleton can be subdivided into the pectoral and the pelvic girdles. The pectoral girdle includes the clavicle and scapula. The pelvic girdle is made up of the coxal bones of the hip. The bones of the appendicular skeletal system form articulations or joints that allow movement when forces are applied by muscles.

> *The skeletal system is composed of an axial skeleton and an appendicular skeleton.*

The body's movement is general in nature (both angular and linear) and can range from locomotion and gross positioning to adept manipulations of the hands and feet.

Bone Tissue

One way to classify bones is by their appearance (Fig. 4.2). The long bones (femur, tibia, humerus, and radius) determine most of the length of the

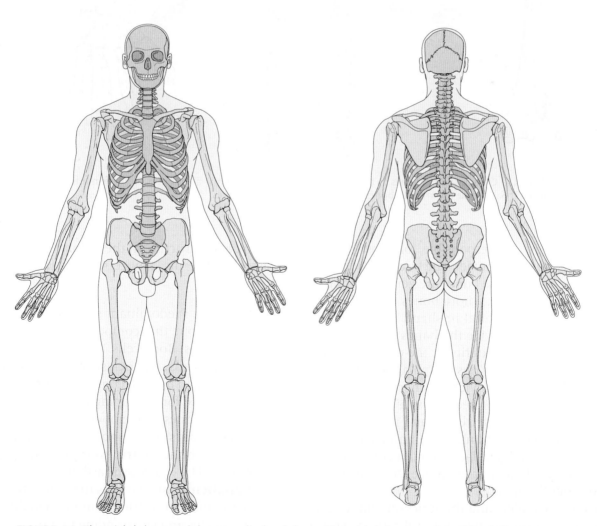

FIGURE 4.1 The axial skeleton and the appendicular skeleton. The axial skeleton consists of the skull, spine, and ribs. The appendicular skeleton consists of the appendages, shoulder girdle, and hip girdle.

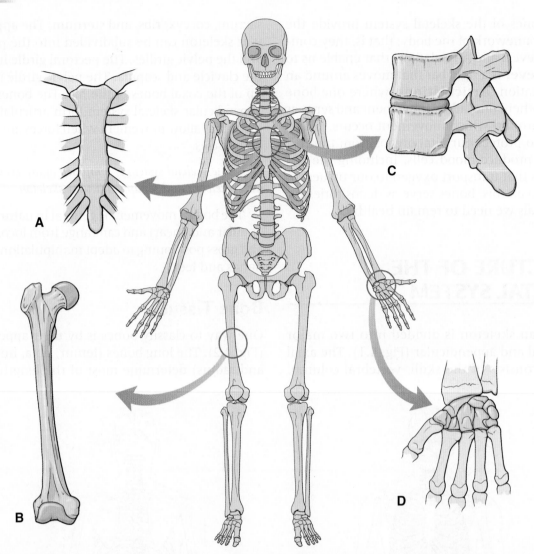

FIGURE 4.2 Classification of bones by their appearance. **A.** The sternum is a flat bone. **B.** The femur is a long bone. **C.** The vertebrae are irregular bones. **D.** The carpals are short bones.

arms and legs, are responsible for most of our mature height, and provide one location for blood cell production. These bones are generally longer than they are wide. Short bones (carpals and tarsals) are more cubical in shape. Several adjacent short bones provide the hands and feet with a flexible base for dexterity at the distal articulations. The flat bones (ribs, scapula, bones of the skull and sternum) provide another site for blood cell production and protect the vital organs. Last, irregular bones (the vertebrae and maxilla) have different shapes depending on their functions. They may provide multiple facets for articulation and muscular attachment or unique leverage, depending on their location.

To better understand the function and nature of bone and its relation to physical activity, let us first look at its structure at the cellular level and at its associated terms. Figure 4.3 illustrates these structures.

1. **Osteons**: Predominant structures found in cortical bone that compose the matrix.
2. Osteocytes: Bone cells. There are two types of bone cells, osteoclasts and osteoblasts, both located in the lacunae. **Osteoclasts** are responsible for reclaiming calcium for metabolic processes and removing damaged bone. **Osteoblasts** are responsible for depositing new bone matrix to replace the bone removed by osteoclastic activity.
3. **Canaliculi**: Small canals that allow the dissemination of nutrients and metabolites to osteocytes and surrounding tissue.

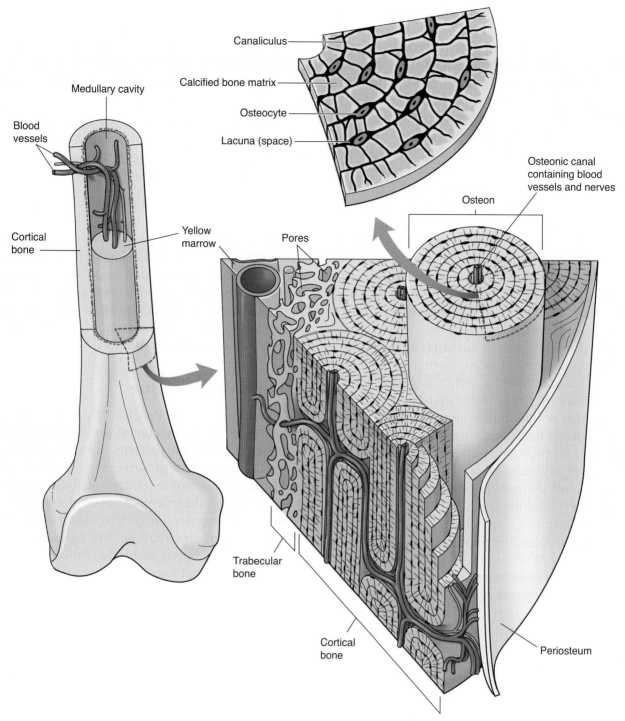

FIGURE 4.3 Longitudinal cross-section of a mature long bone. Osteonic canals run longitudinally through long bones. Osteocytes are arranged in concentric circles around the osteonic canal.

4. **Lacunae**: Small spaces at the centers of canaliculi, which house the osteocytes.
5. **Osteonic canal**: A longitudinal canal at the center of the osteon, which provides for the passage of nutrients and metabolic wastes. The osteonic canals house arterioles and venules, which carry blood and nourishment

to the bone tissue. Osteonic canals are interconnected by perforating canals running perpendicular to them.

In a magnified cross-sectional view of a mature long bone, the osteonic canals run parallel to the shaft of the long bone and are surrounded by a calcified concentric matrix that fuses them together. Much like the annular concentric rings you see in a cross-cut tree, the concentric rings travel outward from the osteonic canal. Canaliculi are strategically placed to disperse fluid to the surrounding tissue. The osteocytes residing in the lacunae are distributed throughout the concentric rings to support the metabolism of specific portions of the bone. All the concentric rings surrounding an osteonic canal form an osteon.

There are two types of bone relative to porosity. **Cortical bone** is highly mineralized and dense, having a low porosity. This type of bone is found in the shafts of long bones and most small, short, irregular bones that are regularly subjected to compressive stresses. **Trabecular** bone is less mineralized, is more porous, and is therefore less dense. It is found at the ends of long bones and is encased in cortical bone, which provides certain advantages in enabling movement. Cortical bone is denser and thus contains more minerals, which add to its weight and rigidity. Because trabecular bone is located at the ends of long bones, the weight at the end of the bone is decreased, thus reducing the force that muscles must generate to move the lever. If the entire skeleton were composed of cortical bone, movement would be impaired due to the weight of the bones.

Bone tissue is continually being reabsorbed and reformed, and exercise is a key stimulus to this process. When bone is optimally stressed, osteoblasts deposit minerals, primarily calcium phosphate, on the collagen matrix. **Collagen** is a tough flexible protein found in other connective tissue as well as bone. Particularly in preadolescents and to some extent in adolescents, bone is more flexible because less calcium phosphate has been deposited on the collagen matrix. The **periosteum** is a tough, fibrous outer covering of bone. As we age, our bones continue to grow in circumference because new bone is being developed underneath the periosteum.

Epiphyseal discs are the site at which bone increases in length. Long bones continue to grow in length up to the time of epiphyseal closure. Prior to epiphyseal closure, bone tissue in this region is more prone to injury from abnormal stresses. Injuries to the epiphysis prior to closure can cause cessation of bone growth (in length), which can lead to a limb-length discrepancy. Although resistance training is a concern in this regard, an appropriately designed resistance training program controls the stresses applied to the skeletal system more closely than does participation in many sports and activities.

Bone tissue is living tissue that is constantly being remodeled. Several factors—including hormonal status, nutritional status, and exercise—determine bone density.

Appropriately applied forces will strengthen the skeletal system. It may be that building bone density in youth will help to maintain bone density throughout life. Many of the skeletal problems associated with aging are related to decreases in bone density. Some of these problems may be related to hormonal or nutritional status. Some problems may be related to our failure to attain maximum bone density as we mature to adulthood.

Ligamentous Tissue

Ligaments are composed of tough, fibrous tissue with little elasticity. Ligaments prevent joints from moving in abnormal patterns. By their arrangement, they may allow movement in one plane only or restrict movement in an abnormal direction. In a joint that is inherently lax, as in the shoulder, numerous ligaments function to stabilize the joint in various planes of motion. The ligaments may also serve to fix a bone to another bone where little or no movement is intended, as in the acromioclavicular joint.

Cartilage

Articular cartilage (Fig. 4.4) covers the ends of long bones and reduces friction at the joint while it is moving under pressure. In basic composition, the structural components consist of a dense mesh of collagen fibrils, proteoglycan macromolecules (PGs), and water, creating a stiff gel-like substance. The tissue is semi-transparent, with four distinct layers:

1. The articular surface, which is superslick. This layer greatly reduces friction between two articulating bone surfaces.
2. The middle zone, composed of collagen fibrils and fluid-swollen proteoglycans.

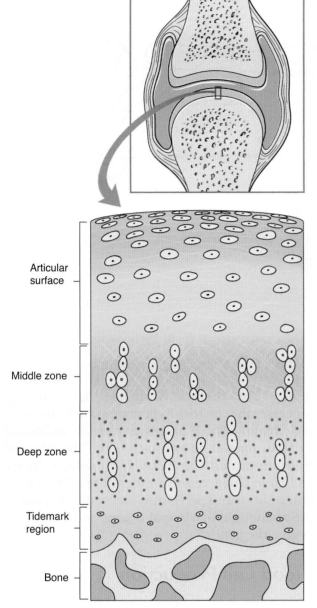

Articular surface

Middle zone

Deep zone

Tidemark region

Bone

FIGURE 4.4 Layers of articular cartilage. Articular cartilage covers the ends of long bones.

3 and 4. The deep zone and the tidemark region, where the cartilage matrix meshes with the actual bone structure.

By maintaining the fluid content in the tissue at normal levels, the protective and friction-reducing properties of cartilage are retained (22). Damage to the cartilaginous tissue results in eventual deterioration of the joint and an increased potential for injury (14).

Articulations

Articulations are where bones join together. At articulations, contact is maintained by cartilage and forces associated with movement of the joint. This arrangement allows bone growth, conversion of angular to linear motion, and dexterity at distal extremities; it also provides for fusion, support summation, and motion as dictated by the location, type, and function of the articulation.

Articulations can be classified by the type of connective tissue used to form the articulation. We have synarthrosis joints, amphiarthrosis joints, and diarthrosis joints. Each type of articulation has specific characteristics in terms of the amount of movement allowed. A description of the classifications is as follows (Fig. 4.5):

1. Synarthrosis: Immovable joints, bound tightly by fibrous tissue.
2. Amphiarthrosis: Slightly movable joints, cartilaginous.
3. Diarthrosis: Freely movable joints, synovial.

FUNCTIONS OF THE SKELETAL SYSTEM

The bones of the skeleton provide structure, allow movement, and provide protection for our organs as well as other physiological functions. Let's examine each of these functions in more detail.

Structure and Protection

Without bones, we would be incapable of standing, sitting, or moving in general. The length of our long bones determines the length of our body segments. For example, the talus, calcaneus, tibia, and femur make up the length of the leg and allow for ankle and knee flexion, extension, and gross compensation for surface irregularities so that we may stand erect. We can walk on an irregular or uneven surface because the foot can compensate for the slope with this adaptable base of support.

Movement

Bones provide both a proximal and distal insertion for muscles, allowing movement when sufficient tension is developed in the muscle that crosses a

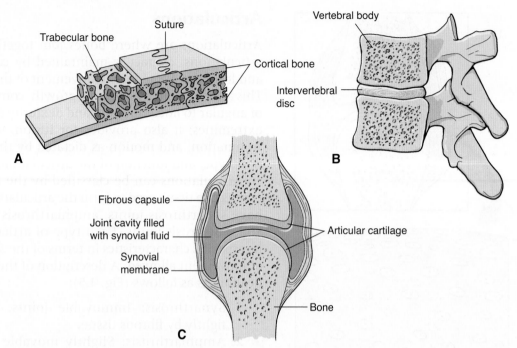

FIGURE 4.5 Types of articulations. **A.** A cranial suture is a synarthrotic joint. **B.** The shoulder is an amphiarthrotic joint. **C.** The knee is a diarthrotic joint.

joint. The **proximal insertion** is closer to the trunk, and the **distal insertion** is farther from the trunk. The bones of the appendicular skeleton and to a lesser degree the axial skeleton are arranged as sets of levers with reciprocally shaped surfaces that allow maximal contact to be maintained at the joint during movement. Joints function as axes of rotation around which torque is generated by muscle force.

> *The structure of the skeletal system allows it to perform one of its essential functions: movement.*

The bones of the skeleton act as a mechanical framework for movement and the attachment of muscles. The irregular bones of the spine (the vertebral bodies) are specifically engineered to bear the summed weight of the body superior to a specific vertebral articulation. Vertebral bodies distribute weight over a large surface area to distribute increasing pressures at each descending vertebral level. The legs, in particular the femur and tibia, are structured such that the cortical portion of the bone resists compressive forces from the weight of the entire body superior to them. The hips can experience as much as six times body weight during normal stair climbing (6). The bones support as much as five times their weight in soft tissue in the normal adult.

One function of the skull and vertebral column is to protect the brain and spinal cord from injury. The thoracic vertebrae have spinous processes that restrict hyperextension in the thoracic region. These processes provide additional surfaces for muscular attachment. The ribs and sternum protect the heart, liver, spleen, lungs, and large blood vessels in the thorax. The vertebral column and pelvis also mechanically protect the abdominal or visceral organs and to a lesser degree the genitalia.

Blood Cell Production

The spongy bone houses the red marrow, which produces the blood cells. The production of red and white blood cells is a result of differentiation of mature blood stem cells that reside primarily in the flat bones of the skull, ribs, sternum, and the ends of the long bones. As the spleen naturally destroys damaged red blood cells (RBCs), these cells must be continually replaced. Every second, the body produces over 2 million RBCs (17).

GROWTH OF THE SKELETAL SYSTEM

Bone changes in size and functional characteristics via two processes: 1) normal growth, and 2) remodeling due to applied loads. Normal growth is largely a function of migration of the epiphysis, resulting in an increase in bone length and diameter prior to skeletal maturity. Chondrocytes secrete a matrix of cartilage and minerals that then deposit themselves on the matrix, stiffening and strengthening it. This process is passive and takes time. Figure 4.6 depicts the epiphyseal region of a long bone.

The second mechanism, remodeling, is a result of the stresses and strains (or lack thereof) applied to the skeletal system through daily activity or planned exercise. In this process bone adapts to stresses due to osteoclastic and osteoblastic activity, which serves to strengthen bone to withstand the applied forces. Remodeling is more active in the maintenance of bone integrity; it increases and decreases the bone's circumference in relation to activity level. It is here that we have the greatest opportunity to generate bone adaptation to training. By loading in an exercise/training format, we can influence this adaptation and thus the strength of bone.

Primary Bone Growth in the Epiphysis

At birth, the skeletal system is composed of a cartilaginous framework that has the general form of the skeleton but is not distinguished in proportion, specific structure, or definitive landmarks. In the first stage of growth, calcification of the cartilage framework begins. Development of the periosteum is evidenced by the periosteal bone collar along the center of the shaft and the development of **articular cartilage** at the ends of the femur. The collar appears as ring of calcified bone around the shaft at approximately the midline. A short time later, the periosteal bone collar becomes the primary ossification center and epiphyseal capillaries develop in the bone's proximal and distal ends.

Soon the ossification (calcium deposition) of the **diaphysis** or shaft of the bone becomes evident at the center of the shaft, and the epiphyseal plates or growth centers are apparent at the ends of the heavily mineralized centers. As the epiphyseal discs lay down new bone, they migrate toward the distal ends. Still later, additional growth centers originate at both ends, forming the unique structural features of a long bone. The secondary ossification centers lay down spongy bone, which is covered by articular cartilage. As this growth in length is taking place, the layer on the surface just beneath the periosteum is adding to the circumference of the bone in response to the compression, shear, tension, and torsional loading imposed by movement and exercise. Long bones reach their final length in early adulthood, when the epiphyseal discs are completely closed. Figure 4.7 illustrates the transition of bone from cartilaginous to fully ossified.

Chondrocytes are active cells that specialize in the generation of the protein cartilage framework or matrix. In human growth, they synthesize and secrete matrix into the extracellular space (1). Chrondrocyte hypertrophy is an active process

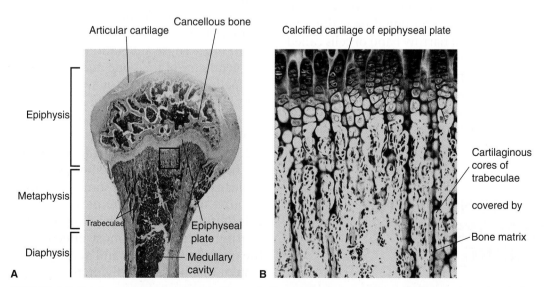

FIGURE 4.6 Epiphyseal growth region. **A.** The end of a long bone covered by cancellous bone and articular cartilage. The epiphyseal disc separates the epiphysis from the metaphysis. **B.** A magnified section of the metaphysis undergoing calcification of the cartilaginous matrix. From Cormack DH. Essential Histology. 2nd ed. Philadelphia: Lippincott Williams & Wilkins, 2001. With permission.

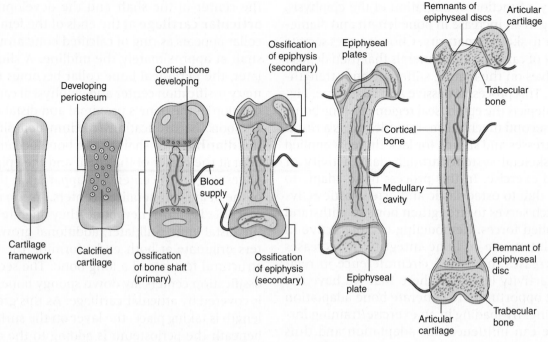

FIGURE 4.7 Prior to ossification, bone begins as a cartilaginous framework.

resulting in increased amounts of intercellular material, including mitochondria and endoplasmic reticulum. Increases in the height of the chondrocyte column height are responsible for 44% to 59% of longitudinal bone growth, the remainder being due to matrix synthesis and chondrocyte proliferation. The rate of differentiation of mesenchymal stem cells into chondrocytes is a factor that regulates the synthesis of the matrix and thus the rate of bone growth (1). In addition to the collagen matrix being laid down, osteoclasts and osteoblasts are being differentiated near the epiphysis, where there is a narrow band of cells called the "proliferating region" of the growth plate. Here, chondrocytes multiply and secrete matrix materials, causing migration of the active growth center toward the proximal and distal ends of the long bones. The matrix material is the template for ossification.

ADAPTATIONS OF THE SKELETAL SYSTEM TO LOADING

Loads applied to the skeletal system cause adaptations to occur that are specific to the type of load.

Wolff's Law

Adaptation to training can be defined according to Wolff's law, which states that "the densities, and to a lesser extent, the sizes and shapes of bones are determined by the magnitude and direction of the acting forces applied to bone."

Growth in circumference acts to distribute the compressive forces over an increased cross-sectional area and thus reduces the amount of pressure per square unit of the bone's cross-sectional surface. In animal experiments, growth in regions of higher stresses and strain has been shown to occur (16). These adaptations can actually change the geometry of the bone and thus the response to a repetitive movement or strain. Increased thickness in the direction of force application and bending serves to better accommodate repeated flexion. Bones, like muscles, adapt to progressive overload. If we increase the load, we increase flexion in the bone. Figure 4.8 demonstrates how bone under axial load "bends," stimulating the deposition of bone underneath the periosteum at the specific location where the bending occurred. Weight-bearing exercises are most effective in ensuring the overall health (size and density) of the skeletal system in a healthy individual.

The response of bone tissue to stress is specific to the type of stress applied.

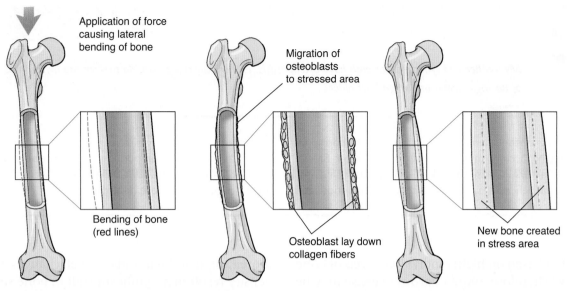

Application of force causing lateral bending of bone

Migration of osteoblasts to stressed area

Bending of bone (red lines)

Osteoblast lay down collagen fibers

New bone created in stress area

FIGURE 4.8 Wolff's law. If the load and speed of movement are high enough, bone will "bend" under an axial load. This stimulates the deposition of calcium in the specific location of the stress. Therefore, bone responds to "bending" by getting thicker in the direction of the load.

Because the diameter of the bone is enlarged through growth at the outer surface, the space in the center of the bone—required for the marrow, nerves, and blood supply—is not reduced. Since these functions are essential to healthy bone, hypertrophy on the external surfaces does not reduce the functional interior space but does allow increasing load accommodation.

Minimal Essential Strain

Minimal essential strain (MES) is the minimal volume and intensity of loading required to cause an increase in bone density. Approximately 10% of the strain required to fracture the bone is considered the threshold at which new bone formation is triggered (8). The interaction of matrix strain and fluid flow may actually be the interacting source of the remodeling signal in bone tissue (12). Whether the stress comes from exercise or the work environment, bone remodeling will occur if the stress triggers the osteoblasts to migrate to the strained region of bone. Box 4.1 provides an analogy to illustrate the concept of bone remodeling.

An exercise program that does not reach the level of minimal essential strain will be ineffective at promoting bone density.

MES varies by age and individual. An obese person will have greater loads placed on the skeletal system in normal daily activities than his or her lighter peers. The obese individual, however, will also likely be less active.

Bone density decreases with age, beginning in the third decade. The amount of strain needed to start the remodeling process may occur in the elderly with a decreased load. In a younger, more active population, the requirements of MES should

4.1 BONE REMODELING ANALOGY

Imagine the strength of an I-beam increased proportionally by increases in thickness of specific portions of the beam. The increases in thickness of the vertical portion of the beam simulate an increase in rigidity from increased bone mineral density (BMD). As you can see there is an increased difficulty of bending the I-beam on the right versus the left. If bone strength is increased due to increased BMD as a result of remodeling, then the minimal essential strain (MES) would increase as the bone got stronger.

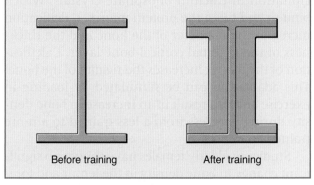

Before training   After training

Q & A from the Field

My mother and grandmother both have osteoporosis. Is there anything I can do to decrease my chances of having osteoporosis when I get older?

Heredity is certainly a risk factor. In females, the hormonal changes that accompany menopause are a risk factor. Several lifestyle factors increase the risk of osteoporosis: smoking, nutritional deficiencies, excessive alcohol consumption, and the lack of weight-bearing exercise. Everyone loses some bone density as they age. It is important to maximize bone density when you are younger with a weight-bearing exercise program designed to improve bone density.

be higher based on higher individual levels of bone density. Therefore, more rigorous exercise may be required to achieve MES in a young, active population. Although stresses applied to bone and subsequent remodeling are ongoing, bone continues to increase in diameter. The total stress required to initiate new bone growth by remodeling is increased if the bone is stronger.

Training Adaptations to the Skeletal System

The response of bone to applied forces is specific to the applied forces. Strain activation changes a small section of exterior bone from the normal state to a state of remodeling. The location of the adaptation is underneath the outer layer of the bone—in the periosteum. The activated area of bone begins resorption, or the removal of the damaged bone by osteoclasts. This will take 1 to 3 weeks. Next is a reversal from primarily osteoclastic activity to osteoblastic activity, which takes another 1 to 2 weeks. Osteoblasts start forming new bone by producing matrix in the now cleared resorption area, which takes approximately $3\frac{1}{2}$ months.

Mineralization of bone takes place by the precipitation of calcium phosphate crystals, which bind to and fill in the protein matrix. Calcification increases the diameter of the bone and the thickness of the external cortical bone layer. Calcification of the matrix increases the rigidity of the bone. This adaptation can be stimulated by loading in exercise and can result in an increase in bone density during progress from a less trained to a more trained condition.

Studies in elderly females have shown no significant change in bone density in the femur and forearm after a resistance training period of 5 months or more (20). In animal studies, small changes in bone density result in a significant shift in bone strength (16). In all cases, care should be taken in training the elderly and the untrained so as to reduce the risk of injury. In these populations, acute loading may require less resistance than that perceived to result in the damage or failure of bone.

THE SKELETAL SYSTEM AND HEALTH

Although balanced growth, proper mineralization, and good training are important indicators of good health, pathologies can occur as a result of specific disorders of or stresses on the skeletal system. This section discusses loss of bone mass, improper alignment, structural damage, and repair of bone.

Bone Density and Health

Peak bone density is an indicator of long-term skeletal health. It is generally accepted that those who achieve a higher peak bone mass are less at risk for osteoporotic fracture later in life. **Osteoporosis** is a disease characterized by a loss of bone density; it is insidious in that it presents no signs or symptoms until the fracture of a bone that has lost its mineral density occurs. Three distinct populations are at higher risk for osteoporosis: (1) postmenopausal women after about age 50, (2) both men and women after about age 70, and (3) young female athletes who also have eating disorders, in whom it is a component of the female athletic triad (discussed later in this chapter).

We know that the appropriate dose of physical activity can increase bone mineral density (BMD) throughout our lives (13). Consider the person who achieves higher peak bone density and a larger calcium depot reserve to begin with. As he or she ages, the individual with higher bone density will likely be less prone to developing osteoporosis.

If the bone mineral reserve was small to begin with, reductions in bone mineralization and decreases in strength would reach a critical state more rapidly. Reduced bone mineralization and thus the structural integrity of the bone makes the elderly more susceptible to bone breakage. A broken hip in an elderly individual can occur as a break at the neck of the femur under the normal load of locomotion, causing the person to fall. In normal locomotion, the stress on bone can be two to three times that of body weight. These breaks occur because the bone density and strength at a vital load-bearing point are diminished due to increased relative osteoclastic activity.

The higher the bone density achieved in the active years, the better the ability to maintain bone density through the aging process into the regression period. Attention given to diet and exercise in the early years may make the functional difference in the later years (19). Although new bone formation can occur at any time of life, the greatest gains are attained in the preadolescent and adolescent years. Adults who started engaging in load-bearing sports before puberty had 22% greater bone min-

eral content than did a control group. This is compared with a similar group of adults who first started participating in load-bearing activities in adulthood; although these individuals also had increased bone mineral content, it was only 8.5% greater than that in the control group (19). In the case of the female athletic triad, at the time in life when bone mineral density should be peaking, these athletes are intentionally starving their systems and thus greatly reducing their probability of good bone health in their later years.

Spinal Alignment Maladies

The spinal maladies presented below are related to an improper or exaggerated spinal curve. An exaggerated thoracic curve, the curve of the vertebrae associated with the ribs and cervical area, is called kyphosis. This malady can result in a gross "head forward" posture or "hunchback." Another spinal deformity is the curvature of the lumbar vertebrae called lordosis. Both lordosis and kyphosis occur primarily in the sagittal plane.

A lateral curvature of the spine that can be life-threatening in extreme cases is scoliosis, which can occur simultaneously in the frontal and transverse planes (3), resulting in a far more complex diagnosis (Fig. 4.9). This curve is not a mere exaggeration but rather should not exist and serves no

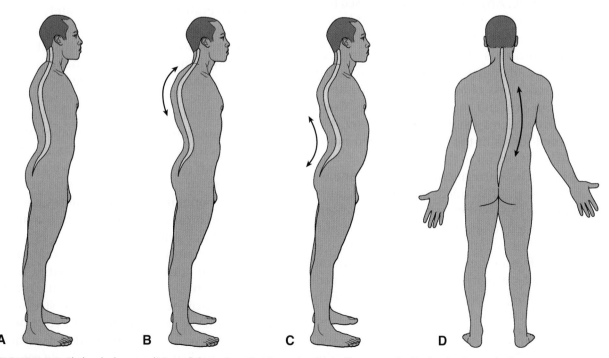

FIGURE 4.9 Skeletal abnormalities of the spine. **A.** Normal spinal alignment. **B.** Kyphosis. **C.** Lordosis. **D.** Scoliosis.

function. In an exercising population, we should be aware of these maladies and the restrictions they may impose on the individual. Exercise programs that accommodate or minimize the effects of these disorders should be considered as much as possible.

Female Athletic Triad

The female athletic triad is a disease predominantly found in females whose sport, training, or competition is enhanced by a reduced ratio of body fat to lean body mass. Its components are osteoporosis, disordered eating (usually anorexia nervosa), and amenorrhea. Long-distance runners and gymnasts seem particularly susceptible to this malady, although it is also possible that young girls choose these sports to hide their disorder. Addiction to exercise caused by endorphin addiction has been also been proposed as a cause of this behavior. Often these athletes attempt to improve their performance by reducing body fat. Reduced body fat improves performance by modifying the strength-to-weight ratio, increasing power, and reducing total workload. When this process is carried to extremes, the female athletic triad can occur.

The three factors that make up this disorder are described as follows:

1. An eating disorder (normally anorexia nervosa) generally accompanied by a distorted body image. An anorexic athlete will see herself as fat even when she has starved herself to a dangerously low level.
2. Osteoporosis is the loss of bone mineral density and destruction of associated matrix materials. Loss of bone tissue can compromise health and make bone brittle. Competitive athletes generate much greater than normal forces in the body, and their bones may not hold up to these forces.
3. Amenorrhea (irregular or complete absence of menses). The athlete reduces nutritional intake to the point where not enough essential fat is left to produce enough female hormones. Estrogen is the major hormone responsible for the balance of osteoclastic and osteoblastic activity. If the athlete cannot produce enough estrogen, osteoclastic activity rises and bone tissue is lost.

A heavy training load (frequently self-imposed) is usually a part of a competitive athlete's training program. The female athlete triad is probably an interaction of overtraining, poor diet, and lack of adequate body fat from which to produce the required hormones to generate the menstrual cycle. It may also be driven by psychological factors, including the desire to be thin (2).

Different types of female athletes were compared in and out of season, looking at factors related to the female athletic triad. Long-term exposure to decreased estrogen levels was nearly associated linearly with decreased bone mineral density. A prolonged exposure to decreased estrogen locally generates compounds that cause an environment favoring the formation of osteoclasts and inhibiting apoptosis in osteoclasts when signaled (4). A lack of tone (normal resting muscle tension) in the muscles, in spite of a high-level training state, can be a key indicator of abnormality. In essence, these athletes starve themselves yet continue to train hard in an effort to improve their performance.

EXERCISE PRESCRIPTION TO PROMOTE BONE DENSITY

Now that we understand the mechanisms of bone growth, the next step is creating training programs that will provide maximal bone growth, bone density, and overall health. To adequately test bone strength, we might remove the bone from the body and measure the forces that cause it to break. Because this is not possible, we have to depend on studies in animals and cultured bone cells to understand the characteristics and responses to stimuli exhibited in these situations. The current studies do not define the exact number of repetitions, sets, percentage of RM, speed, and frequency of loading, nor do they provide us with a "magic" combination or formula. Generally, when we examine a population of nonathletes compared with a population of athletes, we find major differences in bone mineral densities.

In racquet athletes, we find increased bone density in the dominant arm compared to nondominant arm (11). Elevated activity levels in the athlete provide musculoskeletal stresses that improve BMD over that of the less active population (13). Currently, we cannot describe the best way to accomplish the desired goal. We can, how-

Q & A from the Field

I have heard that swimming is not a good activity to promote bone density. Is this true? Why? It seems like it would be a very good activity for bone density.

Swimming, or any activity in the water, takes place in a semiweightless environment. Astronauts lose bone density through prolonged exposure to a weightless environment.

Because swimming is not a weight-bearing activity, it does not provide the minimal stimulus to bone to stimulate growth.

---

ever, provide some insight into the possible results of specific training programs and their effect on bone density.

Loading Speed

Studies have been done to determine the effect of purposely slow training on bone density. Static loading has repeatedly been shown to produce little or no significant effect on new bone growth. Dynamic loading, on the other hand, has been shown to produce significant increases in new bone formation (9).

> *Bone cells are extremely sensitive to changes in hydrostatic pressure. Training movements and loads that maximize fluctuations in hydrostatic pressure within the bone cells will stimulate bone growth.*

This occurs primarily because dynamic loading causes fluctuations in fluid pressure within the lacunar-canalicular system. Bone cells are very responsive to these fluctuations. We can presume that to stimulate new bone growth, our movements must be dynamic in nature.

Rate and Frequency of Loading

Bone responds most effectively to exercises that are dynamic and involve rapid loading (9). The frequency of an exercise also affects the rate of bone formation. A runner who runs with a stride frequency of 90 cycles per minute will form more bone in the pelvis and lower extremities than will someone who runs with a slower cadence of 60 cycles per minute.

> *Dynamic exercise at a high loading rate stimulates bone development. Deliberately slow movements probably will not promote bone adaptation to the same extent as dynamic movements.*

Direction of Loading and Response

In animal experiments using rats, a process of loading the right ulna was applied to the right side of the animal, with the left side unstressed and used as control (16). Data were gathered after a 16-week application of loading. Before and after, dual x-ray absorptiometry (DEXA) tests were conducted. A modest increase of 5.4% bone mineral density was found. After DEXA, the ulnae were removed and tested for strength in the direction of the loading protocol. It was determined that the increase in maximal amount of force that the bone could support before failing was 64%. So a relatively small increase in bone mineral density can translate into a much greater increase in strength to failure. The majority of bone growth took place consistent with the direction of loading. In keeping with Wolff's law, the stimulus of loading actually changed the geometry of the bone.

> *Training programs that utilize a variety of movement and loading patterns will probably stimulate bone development to a greater extent.*

Intensity of Exercise

Load-bearing activities that place an axial load on the skeleton will induce greater bone formation. Along these lines, exercises such as running or jumping will elicit greater bone formation than will

Q & A from the Field

What is the best activity to promote bone density throughout the entire skeletal system?

At present, it would appear that moderate- to high-intensity resistance training using a variety of exercises and movement patterns would cause maximum adaptation of the skeletal system. Exercises should load the body axially, such as the bench press for the upper body or the squat for the lower body. Other activities do not stimulate bone density in the entire skeleton. Jogging causes some increase in bone density in the hips but not in the upper body. Tennis may stimulate increases in bone density in the dominant arm but not in the nondominant arm.

walking (10). Dynamic weight-bearing exercises (such as the sport of weightlifting and the Olympic-style lifts) load more of the skeleton per repetition than do, say, arm curls. In animal experiments, the majority of new bone formation (greater than 95%) is stimulated by the first 40 repetitions of an exercise (23). Additional repetitions do not significantly increase the amount of bone that is formed.

> *Exercises that place an axial load on the skeletal system are probably superior, in terms of improving bone density, to exercises that do not place an axial load on the skeleton.*

Short bouts of exercise followed by rest are better than prolonged workouts (18). The androgen receptors in the body that stimulate new bone growth experience desensitization after a period of time. They need a recovery period before they can be stimulated again to promote bone growth.

Bone takes about 6 to 8 hours to recover its ability to stimulate new bone (18). After the androgen receptors that regulate new bone growth become saturated, they are again available after 6 to 8 hours of rest. Because more receptors are available, full stimulation from the new bout of exercise may result. If a second training session starts before this recovery period, the formation of new bone may be compromised slightly.

Frequency of Training

It appears it is better to add workouts to the training schedule rather than to extend existing workouts as long as there is enough rest between sessions. Rats that were trained to make 120 jumps five times a week experienced twice as much bone

growth in their limbs as did another group that was trained to make 300 jumps twice a week (10). The same number of jumps distributed over a greater number of workouts significantly increased the development of new bone.

Vibration

With space travel, it was learned that astronauts lost bone density while in space (21). On the long-duration flights on Mir in the 1990s, cosmonauts lost as much as 20% of their bone density. In a weightless environment, as in space, axial loading of the skeletal system due to gravity does not occur. One of the contemplated remedies for this problem is vibration. Some information suggests the use of vibration as an alternative or supplemental method of training to maximize or maintain bone density.

When we look at the sensitivity of mature osteocytes to changes in hydrostatic pressure and increased osteoblastic activity, vibration would change the direction and flow of intracellular fluid at a rapid rate. Would the rate be adequate to inspire new bone growth and if so, what rate would be optimal?

Experimentation to combat the effects of microgravity using vertical vibrational loading to promote bone strength and BMD gains is ongoing (22). Therapeutic applications of vibration to improve or maintain bone density are being investigated in rehabilitation settings (5).

One study used a vibrating platform to manipulate rats with removed ovaries. Hormonal changes after menopause are thought to be at least partly responsible for bone loss in females. Over a 12-week period, the experimenters evaluated the effect of vibration in regard to bone loss and compared the experimental condition to a control condition (7). The results showed less bone loss over a 5-week period in the vibration-trained group compared to the control group.

> *Vibration as a stimulus for bone growth may promote bone density and prevent its loss under specific conditions.*

Some important factors in vibration research include harmonic resonance dynamics, frequency modulation, consistent loading and stimulus application, and study length. Harmonic resonance occurs at certain frequencies of vibration. At some frequencies, tissue damage may occur. Frequency modulation is associated with the construction and application of sonic vibration. The mechanism of applying mechanical vibrational loading must be quantifiable and repeatable.

SUMMARY

Mechanisms within the human body cause adaptation of skeletal tissue in response to imposed stresses (15). Dynamic loading stimulates bone growth. The rate and frequency of loading in animal models has a direct effect on bone growth. Stressing the bone in multiple directions will strengthen bone specifically in that direction. Modest changes in BMD can represent large changes in bone strength. Short bouts with high-intensity loads are probably superior in promoting bone strength. Vibration will promote bone density in certain populations under specific conditions.

Frequent, short, dynamic exercises followed by 6 to 8 hours of rest appear to be optimal for the maintenance of bone health in athletes and others. The rest allows the osteoclastic activity to become more prominent than osteoblastic activity. This should be considered in planning training programs or practice sessions where multiple sessions are performed in one day.

MAXING OUT

1. A nonathletic female expresses concern to you that she may be at risk of bone density disorders as she gets older. Design a conditioning program to promote maximal bone density in this individual.

2. You believe that a female athlete on the track team is at risk for osteoporosis and that she may possibly have an eating disorder complicating the situation. What steps should you take to deal with this situation appropriately?

3. An athlete in a collision sport has a history of bone injuries, primarily stress fractures. He is accustomed to hard training and is experienced in a variety of lifting techniques. He is currently not injured. Plan a resistance training program for this athlete to promote maximal bone density.

REFERENCES

1. Ballock RT, O'Keefe RJ. Current concepts review: the biology of the growth plate. J Bone Joint Surg 2003; 85a(4):715–726,
2. Bemben DA, Torey D, Buchanan, et al. Influence of type of mechanical loading, menstrual status, and training season on bone density in young women athletes. J Strength Cond Res 2004;8(2):220–226.
3. Burwell RG. Aetiology of idiopathic scoliosis: current concepts. Pediatr Rehabil 2003;6(3–4);137–170.
4. Chan GK, Duque G. Age-related bone loss: old bone, new facts. Gerontology 2002;48:62–71.
5. Cheung JT, Zhang M, Chow DH. Biomechanical responses of the intervertebral joint to static and vibrational loading: a finite elemental study. Clin Biomech 2003;9:790–799.
6. Costigan PA, Deluzio KJ, Wyss UP. J. Gait Posture Aug 2002;16(1):31–37.
7. Flieger J, Karchaolis T., Khaldi L, et al. Mechanical stimulation in the form of vibration prevents post-menopausal bone loss in ovariectomized rats. Calcif Tissue Int 1998;63: 510–514.
8. Frost H. From Wolff's law to the Utah paradigm: insights about bone physiology and its clinical applications. Anat Rec 262;398–419.
9. Hert J, Liskova M, Landa J. Reaction of bone to mechanical stimuli. 1. Continuous and intermittent loading of the tibia in rabbits. Folia Morphol (Praha) 1971;19;290–300.
10. Hsieh YF, Turner CH. Effects of load frequency on mechanically induced bone formation. J Bone Min Res 2001;16: 918–924.
11. McClanahan BS, Harmon-Clayton K, Ward, KD, et al. Side-to-side comparisons of bone mineral density in upper and lower limbs of collegiate athletes. J Strength Cond Res 2002;16(4):586–590.
12. Nauman E, Wesley C, Chang W, et al. Microscale engineering applications in bone adaptation. Microscale Thermophys Eng 1998;2;139–172.
13. Nutter J. Physical Activity increases bone density. NSCA J 1986;8(3):67–69.
14. Olsen S, Oloyede A. A finite element analysis methodology for representing the articular cartilage structure. Comp Meth Biomech Biomed Eng 2002;5(6):377–386.
15. Platen P, Chae E, Antx R, et al. Bone mineral density in top level male athletes of different sports. Eur J Sport Sci 2001;1:5.

16. Robling AG, Hinant FM, et al. Improved bone structure and strength after long term mechanical loading is greatest is loading is separated into short bouts. J Bone Min Res 2002;17:1545–1554.
17. Rothenberg E, Lugo JP. Differentiation and cell division in the mammalian thymus. Dev Biol 1985;112:1–17.
18. Rubin C, Lanyon L. Regulation of bone formation by applied dynamic loads. J Bone Joint Surg 1985;66-A;397–402.
19. Silverwood B. Pediatr Nurs 2003;15(5):27–29.
20. Simpkin A, Ayalon J, Leichter I. Increased trabecular bone density due to bone loading exercises in postmenopausal osteoporotic women. Calcif Tissue Int 1987;40:59–63.
21. Shackelford LC, Oganov V, LeBlanc A, et al. Bone mineral loss and recovery after shuttle-Mir flights. Available at www.hq.nasa.gov/osf/station/issphase1sci.pdf. Accessed June 24, 2006.
22. Teshima R, Nawata J, et al. Effects of weight bearing on the tidemark and osteochondral junction of articular cartilage. Acta Orthop Scand 1999;70(4):381–386.
23. Torvinen S, Kannua P, Sievanen H, et al. Effect of 8-month vertical whole body vibration on bone, muscle performance, and body balance: a randomized controlled study. 2003.
24. Umemura Y, Ishiko T, Yamauchi M, et al. Five jumps per day increase bone mass and breaking force in rats. J Bone Min Res 1997;12:1480–1485.

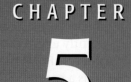

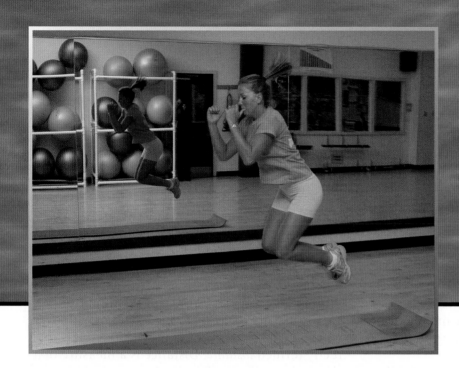

Biomechanics of Conditioning Exercises

ROBERT U. NEWTON

Introduction

Biomechanics is the science of applying mechanical principles to biological systems such as the human body. It has much to offer the field of strength and conditioning. A basic knowledge of biomechanics is essential for the specialist involved in testing and training people, because mechanical principles dictate the production of movement and the outcomes in terms of performance. As we will see, the human body is made up of a series of biological machines that allow it to produce the incredible range of movement involved in sport, training, dance, and everyday activities. For the sake of simplicity, some of the biomechanical concepts are explained with slight variations from the strict mechanical definitions. In the strength and conditioning field, it is more important to convey meaning and for the concepts to be understood than to be pedantic about the terminology.

The purpose of this chapter is to convey some key biomechanical concepts essential for understanding how we produce movement, how various exercise machines function and interact with the performer, and how tests and equipment are used to assess performance. All sporting movement results from the application of forces generated by the athlete's muscles working the bony levers and other machines of the skeletal system. Human movement is incredibly complex in all the myriad of activities in which we participate, but this is perhaps most eloquently expressed in the extraordinary exploits of athletes. For example, jumping vertically into the air is a common movement that most of us perform without thought, but the underlying mechanical phenomena that contribute to jumping are numerous and complex. The comprehension and application of biomechanics play an integral role in the work of the strength and conditioning specialist and make for more effective and safer exercise program designs. This process occurs at several levels:

■ Biomechanics knowledge increases understanding of how a particular movement is performed and the key factors that limit performance.
■ A major aspect is technique analysis, because a greater understanding of movement brings with it a better ability to identify inefficient and/or dangerous techniques.
■ The range of equipment available for strength and conditioning is considerable and expanding. Biomechanical analysis will differentiate useful and well-designed equipment from that which is potentially dangerous or undesirable. An understanding of biomechanics also permits the design of new equipment and exercises based in science.
■ From a biomechanical perspective, the athlete can be seen as a machine with neural control and feedback, mechanical actuators, biological structures with certain properties, and interaction with the environment and equipment. This brings with it an excellent understanding of the factors limiting performance and the mechanisms of injury. The result is better design of training programs.

BIOMECHANICAL CONCEPTS FOR STRENGTH AND CONDITIONING

It is important to develop a foundation understanding of some key mechanical variables and relationships so that we can explore in more detail the biomechanical concepts of strength and conditioning exercise, performance testing, and test interpretation.

> *Being able to conceptualize several key mechanical quantities will greatly enhance our understanding of strength and conditioning as a science.*

We all experience the passing of **time** in the fact that we remember what we have just experienced and know that events will occur in the future. Time is measured in various units, but principally seconds, minutes, hours, days, months, and years are used in strength and conditioning to represent different quantities of time.

The term *distance* has a slightly different meaning than *displacement,* but the two are usually used interchangeably. In strength and conditioning, we are usually referring to the length of path over which the body or an object moves, and this is correctly termed *distance.* Distance is a measure of a change in position or location in space and has two forms, linear and angular. Linear distance is usually measured in meters (m) and is the length of the path traveled. Angular distance refers to how far an object has rotated and is usually measured in degrees. You may also see angular distance measured in radians. A radian is equal to approximately 57 degrees.

Velocity (often termed *speed*) is the rate of change of distance over time. It is calculated as the distance moved divided by the time it takes to cover that distance; it is expressed in units of meters per second (m/s) (metric system) or feet per second (f/s) (imperial system). Box 5.1 shows this calculation using the example of sprint running.

Acceleration is the rate of rate of change of velocity with time. It refers not only to changes

5.1 CALCULATING AVERAGE VELOCITY DURING SPRINT RUNNING

In a running event, average velocity over the course of the race will determine the winner. The athlete who starts the fastest certainly has an advantage, but the runner with the fastest average velocity will finish first. In this example, an athlete is completing a 40-m sprint. We have electronic timing lights at 10, 20, and 30 m from the starting light gate. The average speed over the last 10 m could be used as an indication of maximum running speed. Let's assume the times and distances are as follows:

Distance	10	20	30
Time	1.741	2.890	3.995

Velocity is change in distance over change in time. Therefore, velocity = (30–20)/(3.995–2.890) = 10/1.105 = 9.05 m/s.

in how fast the movement is but also to change of direction. The change of running direction in performing a cutting maneuver requires an acceleration other than zero, even though the speed of movement might be maintained. Acceleration is calculated as the change in velocity divided by the time over which this occurred. The measurement units are usually meters per second per second (m/s/s) (metric system) or feet per second per second (f/s/s) (imperial system).

It should be noted that both *velocity* and *acceleration* refer not just to linear motion but also to angular motion or rotation.

Mass is the quantity of matter that makes up a given object. This sounds like quite an abstract concept, but fortunately it is easy to measure because we often equate mass with weight. The two concepts are not the same, however, because weight is actually the force generated by gravity (defined below) acting on the mass.

Inertia is the resistance of an object to changes in its state of motion. In other words, if the object is stationary, it will resist being moved. If it is already moving, it will resist changes in the direction or speed of movement. Inertia in linear terms is measured in kilograms and is functionally the same as mass. For example, a sprinting football player who weighs 120 kg is much harder to stop than a gymnast who weighs 50 kg.

Force can be most easily visualized as a push or pull for linear force or a twist for a rotating force (termed *torque*). Force is measured in units called newtons (N) or newton meters (N.m) in the case of torque. To produce a change in motion (acceleration), there must be application of a force or torque. The amount of change that results depends on the inertia of the object. To calculate the total force of resistance at a given time point, the following formula is used:

$$F = m(a + g)$$

where

F = force
m = mass of barbell or dumbbell
a = instantaneous acceleration
g = acceleration due to gravity (9.81 m/s/s)

Torque is calculated as the force applied multiplied by the length of the lever arm:

$$T = F \times d$$

Gravity is a specific force produced because of the enormous size of the planet Earth. The mass of Earth creates an attractive force on all objects near it; that is why, when you throw a ball into the air, it falls back to the ground. The most common form of resistance training uses this principle. Weight training is lifting and lowering objects against the force of gravity.

Momentum is the quantity of motion that an object possesses. It is calculated as the velocity multiplied by the mass. This concept has relevance to strength and conditioning from a range of aspects, including injury mechanisms and assessment of performance. For example, it is often useful to express sprinting ability not just in terms of time or velocity but also of momentum: an athlete with mass of 100 kg running at 10 m/s has considerably more momentum than an 80-kg athlete running at the same velocity. In collision sports such as rugby or football, it is momentum that usually determines the outcome.

Work is calculated as the force applied multiplied by the distance moved. It is a useful concept in strength and conditioning. For example, in coaching, the volume of a weight-training workout is most accurately calculated as the amount of work completed. Work is measured in units called joules (J).

Power is the rate of doing work and can be calculated as work divided by the time over which the work is done. Power can also be calculated as the force applied multiplied by the velocity. Power is measured in units called watts (W), although it is also frequently expressed in horsepower (hp), whereby 1 hp = 745.7 W. Box 5.2 shows the calculation of work and power using the example of weight training.

Friction is the force that resists two surfaces sliding over each other. The concept is important for strength and conditioning because we use this friction in exercise equipment (e.g., the Monarch cycle ergometer), and it is also a factor in weight training (e.g., as when chalk is applied to the hands). Friction is a force and is therefore measured in newtons; it is related to the nature of the two surfaces and the force pressing them together. It should be noted that friction is the interaction between both surfaces. For example, a smooth-soled basketball shoe has excellent grip on the polished wooden floor of the court but has little grip on a grassed soccer field. An example that illustrates how increasing the force pushing two surfaces together affects friction is provided by the Monarch cycle ergometer, which is commonly used for exercise testing and training. When you adjust the tension on the belt around the wheel, the belt is pushed

5.2 CALCULATING WORK AND POWER DURING WEIGHT TRAINING

Calculation of work and power can be very important in designing training and conditioning programs. Total work is useful in planning the overall volume and intensity of training in a periodized conditioning program. For the training program to be specific to the power output of the sport or activity, calculating power is another useful measurement. Let's use the example of a bench press to demonstrate the calculation of work and power. If the mass of the bar is 80 kg, then the gravity force that this equates to is 784 newtons (N) (80 × 9.81). During the repetition, if the lifter moves the bar through a distance of 0.70 m, the work completed is approximately 549 joules (J) (80 × 9.81 × 0.7). Now let's assume that the lift is completed in 1.5 seconds. The average power output during the lift can be calculated as work divided by time, which equals 366 watts (W) (549/1.5). A training program would likely be designed to incorporate a variety of power outputs progressing to sport-specific movement velocities as competition approaches.

harder onto the wheel rim, so that friction increases and so does the force required to push the pedals.

FORCE-VELOCITY-POWER RELATIONSHIP

Owing to the structure of muscle and how it lengthens and shortens while developing tension, the amount of force that can be produced is related to the velocity at which the muscle changes length (Fig. 5.1).

Most sports require the application of maximal power output rather than force. An understanding of the mechanical quantity of power and factors contributing to its generation is invaluable to the strength and conditioning specialist.

The following discussion assumes that the muscle is being maximally activated; several important points for strength and conditioning arise from this phenomenon:

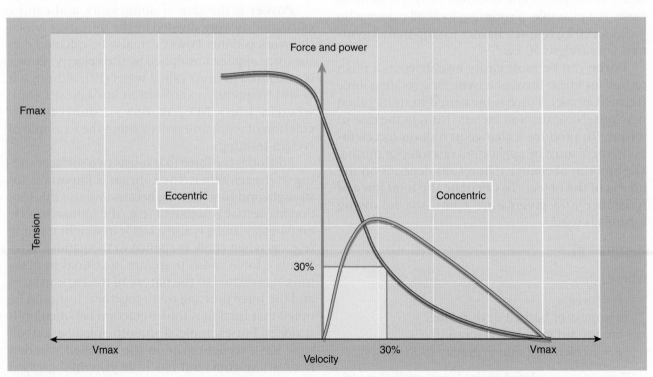

FIGURE 5.1 The force–velocity–power relationship for muscle. Force (purple line) is lowest during fast concentric muscle contraction and increases as the velocity of concentric contraction slows to zero or isometric. As the velocity becomes negative (eccentric), force continues to rise but then plateaus or may even decrease at fast eccentric contractions. The interaction of force and velocity results in a power curve (orange line) that peaks around 30% of isometric force and maximum shortening velocity. Fmax = maximum force; Vmax = maximum velocity.

1. The lowest tension can be developed during **concentric** (shortening) contractions.
2. When the velocity is zero, this is termed an *isometric contraction,* whereby the muscle is generating tension but no movement is occurring. Greater tension is developed during **isometric** contractions than during concentric contractions.
3. Negative velocities indicate that the muscle is lengthening while developing tension; this is termed **eccentric** contraction. Muscle can generate its greatest tension while it is lengthening. Note that at faster velocities of lengthening, the force no longer increases and may even decrease slightly, most likely due to reflex inhibition.
4. Positive power can be produced only during concentric contractions, and the faster the velocity of muscle shortening, the less force the muscle can develop. When the muscle is contracting against a high external load, force is high but velocity slow. If the load is light, then high contraction velocity can be achieved but force is low. Because of this interplay of force and velocity, the product of the two is maximized at a point in between. In fact, power output is greatest when the muscle is shortening at about 30% of the maximum shortening velocity. This by definition corresponds to a force of approximately 30% of that produced during an isometric contraction.

We observe this phenomenon regularly in the weight room. For example, in squatting heavier loads, the speed of movement decreases. For maximal lifts, the velocity might be very slow—in fact, approaching zero velocity in certain phases of the range of motion as the lifter tries to maximize the force applied. Also, in performing training aimed at increasing power output, lighter loads tend to be used but moved at much faster velocities—e.g., 30% to 50% of isometric maximum.

MUSCULOSKELETAL MACHINES

The muscles develop tension, and this is applied to the bones to produce or resist movement. Essentially these systems are a form of **machine**, taking the tension developed by the muscle and converting it to motion of a bone around a joint. The human body holds many examples of such machines; when these are accurately controlled by the computer that is our nervous system, the result is the bewildering array of human movements that we observe each day. In this case the musculoskeletal machines function to change high-force production and a small range of change in muscle length into low-force but fast velocity and range of motion at the other end of the bone to which the muscle attaches.

Lever Systems

The most common musculoskeletal machine in the body is the **lever system** in which a muscle pulls on a bone that may rotate about a joint. A lever is a common machine in everyday use, e.g., using a screwdriver to open a can of paint or a tire lever to dislodge a hubcap. In these examples, the length of the force arm is much greater than that of the resistance arm. Thus, pushing on the lever with, for example, 100 N, results in 1000 N applied on the paint lid to push it open. But note that the handle end of the screwdriver must move through 10 times the distance of the blade end under the lid. This trade-off of distance and force is called **mechanical advantage**. Interestingly, the musculoskeletal machines of the human usually work at a mechanical disadvantage in terms of force but at an advantage in terms of distance moved and thus potential velocity. We are designed for speed rather than high force production (Fig. 5.2).

> *The musculoskeletal system is designed for speed and range of motion rather than high force production.*

Three possible types of levers can be observed in the human body. Class of lever is based on the arrangement of the axis of rotation (A: pivot point or joint center), the resistance (R: point of application of the resistance force), and the force (F: muscle attachment and thus point of application of the muscle force). A good way to remember the three classes of lever is by the acronym ARF, because its summarizes the three possible lever arrangements or classes (Fig. 5.3). In a first-class lever, the axis of rotation (A) is in the middle. In a second-class lever, the resistance arm (R) is in the middle. In a third-class lever, the force arm (F) is in the mid-

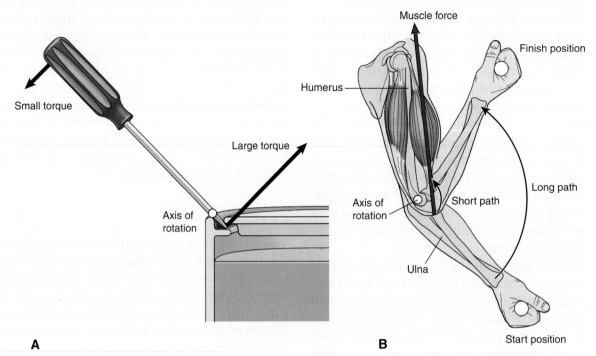

FIGURE 5.2 Examples of basic lever systems designed for high force or high range and speed of movement. **A.** A long lever (a screwdriver) is used to create torque to pry open the lid on a paint can. A large range of movement and less force at the long end results in high torque but limited range of movement applied to the object being moved. **B.** In elbow flexion, a small shortening of the muscle results in a large displacement at the hand; however, much higher force is required by the muscle to produce torque at the elbow and movement at the hand.

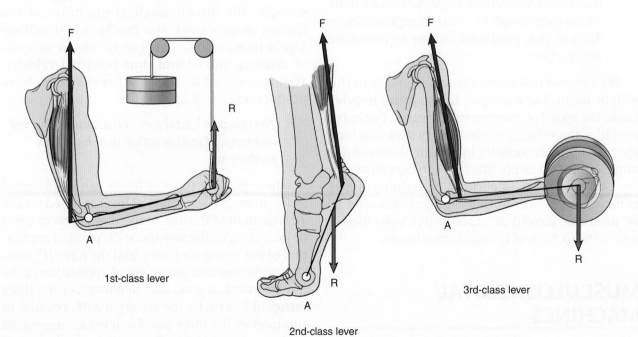

FIGURE 5.3 Arrangement of axis of rotation (A), force arm (F), and resistance arm (R) for the three different classes of lever.

dle. In the human body, the third-class lever is the most common because it is the best design for large range and speed of motion. First class is the next most common because, depending on whether the axis of rotation is closer to the force arm or the resistance arm, first-class levers can favor either force production or range of motion. Second-class levers are the least common in the human because such an arrangement always results in mechanical advantage and thus reduced speed and range of motion. Remember, we are designed for speed and range of motion, not force production.

Wheel-Axle Systems

Wheel-axle systems occur only at ball-and-socket joints, so that the hip and shoulder are particularly important examples and commonly involved in strength and conditioning. When either of these joints is moving in internal or external rotation, the muscles and bones are working as a wheel-axle system. When the tendon of the agonist muscle wraps partially around the end of the bone, muscle tension will tend to rotate the bone about its long axis, like the axle in an automobile. Let's examine the example of the shoulder joint being internally rotated. The tendon of the pectoralis major muscle inserts on the humerus, and when the shoulder is externally rotated, the tendon is partially wrapped around the bone. Muscle shortening internally rotates the humerus, forearm, and hand. If the elbow is flexed, the hand will travel through a much greater distance than the upper arm; hence the system acts as a machine trading force production at the proximal end of the humerus for greater distance and velocity of movement at the hand.

BIOMECHANICS OF MUSCLE FUNCTION

A number of key aspects of how muscle functions are important for understanding the biomechanics of strength and conditioning.

Force or power applied is determined by a complex range of neural and mechanical interactions within the muscle, between muscle and tendon, and between muscle and the machines of the skeleton.

Length-Tension Effect

Muscle generates tension by the interaction of myosin and actin filaments in a mechanism discussed in a previous chapter. This process results in the muscle being able to generate different quantities of tension at varying lengths. This is termed the **length-tension effect**, being an inverted "U" relationship such that greatest tension is produced when the muscle is at or near its resting length and substantially less contractile tension can be developed when the muscle is stretched or shortened above or below this length. The actual force output of the muscle is slightly different from this because, as the muscle stretches beyond the resting length, another force increases in contribution—the elastic recoil of the stretched muscle and tendon (Fig. 5.4).

Muscle Angle of Pull

Muscles pull on the bones to produce movement, resist movement, or maintain a certain body position. This force acting on the bony levers generates a twisting force, termed **torque**. The muscle force is most efficiently converted to torque when the angle at which the force is applied is at 90 degrees to the long axis of the bone. At angles other than perpendicular, only a portion of the muscle force is directed to producing joint rotation, with the remainder tending to either pull the joint together (**stabilizing force**) or apart (**dislocating force**) (Fig. 5.5). Muscle angle of pull has a very large impact on the

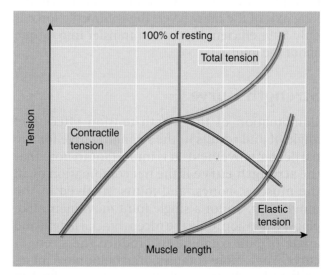

FIGURE 5.4 Length tension effect for skeletal muscle, showing both contractile tension and elastic components.

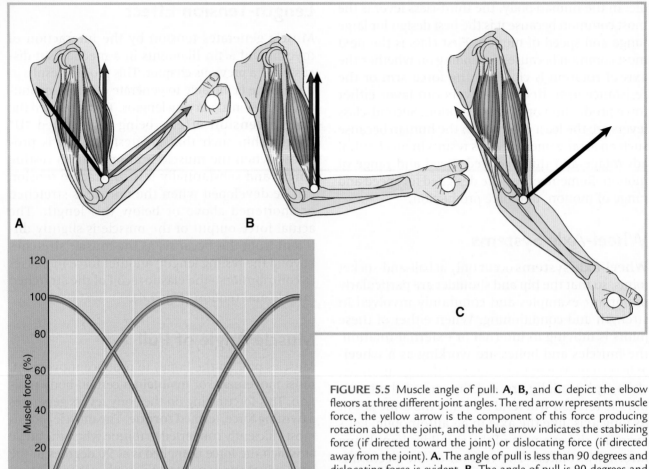

FIGURE 5.5 Muscle angle of pull. **A, B,** and **C** depict the elbow flexors at three different joint angles. The red arrow represents muscle force, the yellow arrow is the component of this force producing rotation about the joint, and the blue arrow indicates the stabilizing force (if directed toward the joint) or dislocating force (if directed away from the joint). **A.** The angle of pull is less than 90 degrees and dislocating force is evident. **B.** The angle of pull is 90 degrees and 100% of muscle force is contributing to joint rotation with no dislocating or stabilizing force. **C.** The angle of pull is greater than 90 degrees and a stabilizing force is evident. **D.** Muscle angle of pull determines percentage of muscle force contributing to joint rotation (orange line) or to dislocating and stabilizing forces (purple line).

effectiveness of the developed muscle tension. For example, when the angle of pull is 30 degrees to the long axis of the bony lever, the contractile force is only 50% efficient in terms of transfer into torque about the joint.

Strength Curve

Combination of the length-tension effect and angle of pull results in the strength curve for the particular movement. It is important to note that the **strength curve** is the net combination of all the muscles, bones, and joints involved in the movement. So for a single joint movement, like elbow extension, only the triceps brachii length and angle of pull combine to produce the strength curve. For a more complex, multijoint movement, such as bench press, all the muscles involved in shoulder horizontal adduction and elbow extension

combine to produce the strength curve for this movement. The result is a range of different-shaped strength curves for each movement. The most common is **ascending**, which describes movements such as squat and bench press. In both cases, from the bottom to the top of the lift the force-generating capacity of the musculoskeletal system increases.

Line and Magnitude of Resistance

The direction of the force that must be overcome during resistance training is termed the **line of resistance**. In training with free weights, this is always vertically down, because the resistance is the gravitational weight force acting on the barbell or dumbbell (Fig. 5.6). Using combinations of levers and pulleys, the line of resistance for a

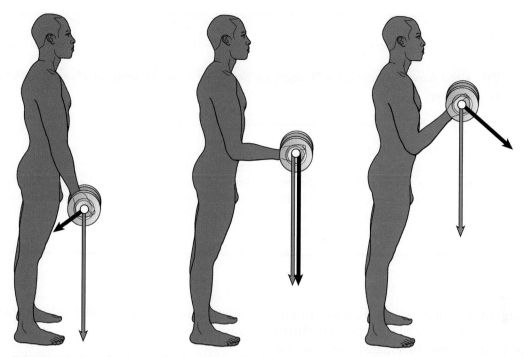

FIGURE 5.6 Line of resistance for the arm curl. The blue arrow represents the resistance vector and the yellow arrow the component producing torque about the joint. The length of the yellow arrow indicates the amount of resistance force applied. Note that the resistance torque is maximized when the forearm is horizontal and considerably less at higher or lower angles.

given exercise can be in any direction. For example, for a lat pulldown machine, a pulley is used to reverse the direction of the downward gravitational force of the weight stack to provide a vertically upward force. Similarly, pulleys are used in a seated rowing machine to direct the line of resistance horizontally.

For essentially linear movements, such as squat, shoulder, and bench press, the resistance of a free weight stays constant except for changes in velocity. As we have already seen, force is equal to mass times (a + g). The result is that when the velocity of movement is constant, acceleration is zero; so the resistance is simply the weight force of the barbell. In increasing velocity at the start of the lift (positive acceleration), however, the resistance to overcome is higher than the weight force alone. At the top of the lift, when velocity is decreasing (negative acceleration), the resistance to be overcome is actually less than the weight force of the barbell.

The changes in magnitude of resistance become even more complex for rotational movements, such as arm curls or knee extensions with free weights. The resistance torque about the joint will change in sine-wave fashion, so that it is greatest when the limb is horizontal and zero when the limb is vertical.

Sticking Region

Combining the strength curve with the line of resistance for a given movement results in varying degrees of difficulty through the range of motion. Even though the external resistance might be constant, some parts of the lift are more difficult than others. This is termed the **sticking region** and is the point in the movement where the lift is most likely to fail. For example, in a standing elbow flexion (arm curl) exercise using a dumbbell, the sticking region is at around 90 to 110 degrees of joint angle. Interestingly, this is a region of high torque capability in the strength curve, but it is also where the resistive torque generated by the dumbbell is at the peak. For the bench press, the sticking region is 5 to 10 cm off the chest. Because this is a linear lift, the line and magnitude of resistance do not change appreciably; but at this point the strength curve is at a low point because of the inefficient angle of pull for the pectoralis major.

Muscle Architecture, Strength, and Power

Muscles in the human body have a range of designs, or architectures, specific to the functional demands

Q & A from the Field

If the elbow flexors are strongest at 90 degrees of flexion, why is the "sticking point" in the midrange of the movement?

The elbow is strongest in flexion at 90 degrees because the length of the force arm (the perpendicular distance from the muscle insertion to the axis of rotation) is maximal at 90 degrees. However, the resistance arm, the perpendicular distance from the point of force application to the axis of rotation, is also greatest in the midrange of the motion for an isotonic exercise. Although the mechanical advantage of the elbow flexors is greatest at 90 degrees, the increasing length of the resistance arm in a heavy isotonic exercise overcomes this advantage. The sticking point will occur somewhere near 90 degrees of flexion.

---

required. The two main divisions are fusiform and pennate, and each has several subtypes. **Fusiform** muscles (e.g., the biceps brachialis) have muscle fibers and fascicles running in parallel to a tendon at origin and insertion. Fusiform muscles have longer fiber length and are able to generate a good range of shortening and, in particular, a higher velocity of shortening. The architecture of **pennate** muscles involves muscle fibers running obliquely into the tendon. Such a structure allows more muscle fibers to be packed into the muscle, and this favors higher force output.

The angle at which the muscle fibers are aligned relative to the tendon is termed the **pennation angle**, and this also has an impact on the relative ability of the muscle in terms of force versus power production. A higher pennation angle favors force production, although a lower angle allows the muscle to produce a greater range of motion and velocity of contraction. It is important for the strength and conditioning specialist to understand these concepts of muscle architecture and pennation angle because of their implications for function and thus performance. Of particular interest is that the pennation angle can be altered by training. For example, one study demonstrated changes in muscle pennation angle in as little as 5 weeks of resistance training (9). Heavy resistance training leads to an increase in pennation angle and thus increased strength capacity. Higher-velocity ballistic training produces adaptations of decreased pennation angle and thus increased velocity and power output. The fact that such changes occur in as little as 5 weeks of training has considerable importance for the periodization of training program design.

Multiarticulate Muscles, Active and Passive Insufficiency

Many muscles of the body are multiarticulate: they cross more than one joint and therefore can produce movement at each of the joints they cross. This arrangement has great benefits in terms of efficiency and effectiveness of muscle contraction. Two attributes, however, should be considered for strength and conditioning. A muscle can shorten by only a certain amount, typically to 50% of its resting length. The result is that if the muscle is already shortened about one joint, it cannot contract very forcefully to produce movement over the other joint that it crosses. This is termed **active insufficiency** and has significance for resistance training. In selecting certain exercises, one can change the emphasis on a given muscle group. For example, in training the calf muscles, ankle plantarflexion can be performed with the knee extended (standing calf raise) or flexed (seated calf raise) and switch the training emphasis from the gastrocnemius to the soleus. In a standing calf raise, the gastrocnemius is lengthened over the knee joint and is therefore the primary muscle producing the ankle plantarflexion. In a seated calf raise, however, the gastrocnemius is already shortened about the knee joint and cannot contribute much force about the ankle. The soleus becomes the prime mover in this case.

Similarly, a muscle can be stretched only to a certain extent. Multiarticulate muscles are lengthened over all the joints they cross. If a given muscle is already in a lengthened state to allow movement to the end of range for one joint, it may not be able to be lengthened further to permit full range of motion at the other joint it crosses. This is termed **passive insufficiency**. For an application of this principle to exercise, we will again use the gastrocnemius and soleus. To adequately stretch the muscles of the calf, one has to perform two stretches: one with the knee extended, which tends to place the gastrocnemius on stretch, and the other with the knee bent to stretch the soleus. As soon as you bend the knee, the gastrocnemius is no longer fully lengthened about the knee and so can allow more dorsiflexion of the ankle. The soleus then becomes the limiting muscle and is thus effectively stretched.

BODY SIZE AND SHAPE AND POWER-TO-WEIGHT RATIO

To understand individual differences in strength and power, it is important to understand body size and shape. For example, a long trunk and short arms and legs favor powerlifting and weightlifting performance because the shorter lever lengths permit greater force production if all else is equal. Fast speed of movement (e.g., throwing or kicking), however, is more easily achieved by an athlete who has longer relative limb lengths. In general the greater the athlete's body size and mass, the greater his or her strength capability, because absolute strength is very much dependent on total muscle mass and cross-sectional area. In many sports, relative strength and power are more important than absolute measures. These measures are strength-to-weight and power-to-weight ratio, respectively, and are simple measures to calculate. For example, relative strength for a given movement is simply the 1 RM divided by body mass. If we assume a 1-RM squat of 120 kg at a body mass of 80 kg, the relative strength for this movement is 1.5. In any sport where projection of the body is important (e.g., vertical jumping, sprinting), the athlete's power-to-weight ratio is a critical measure because it determines the amount of acceleration and thus

the peak velocities that can be achieved. For example, an athlete who produced 6,000 W in a vertical jump at a body mass of 100 kg has a power-to-weight ratio of 60 W/kg.

BALANCE AND STABILITY

It is useful to have an understanding of the biomechanics of balance and stability in analyzing strength and conditioning movements. **Balance** is the process of controlling the body position and movements in either static or dynamic equilibrium for a given purpose. **Stability** is the ease or difficulty with which this equilibrium can be disturbed. Because all exercises require balance, manipulating stability can affect the degree of difficulty and risk of injury or can be used to introduce a different training stimulus—e.g., balance training.

Being able to alter stability by modifying the exercise is useful for making the task more challenging, altering balance demands, or reducing difficulty and improving safety.

Factors Contributing to Stability

Stability is determined by:

1. **The base of support**, or the physical dimensions of the area defined by the points of support. For example, in performing the military press exercise, the base of support is the area defined by the rectangle enclosing both feet. If the feet are placed farther apart, the base of support is larger and stability is greater. If the split position is adopted, the area increases even further, particularly in the anteroposterior plane (Fig. 5.7). When the athlete is seated on a bench with his or her feet wide apart, the area and thus the stability is even greater.
2. The mass of the object or body. Heavier objects are inherently more stable because the inertia (resistance to change in state of motion) and gravitational weight force are higher. For example, the placement of weight plates on a smith machine or power rack makes the device more stable.
3. Height of the center of mass. The center of mass can be thought of as a point about

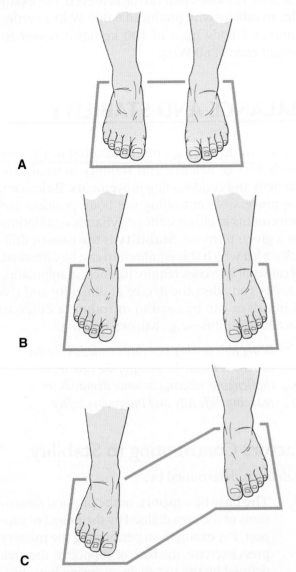

A

B

C

FIGURE 5.7 Base of support for standing feet spread (narrow and wide stance) versus split position. Shifting from **A.** narrow to **B.** wide stance greatly increases stability in the side-to-side directions. **C.** Moving to the split position increases stability in the forward and backward directions.

which the mass of the body or object is evenly distributed. For a human standing with his or her arms at the sides, it is in the center of the body roughly 5 cm below the navel. Raising the arms over head lifts the center of mass; bending at the hips and knees lowers it. The higher the center of mass, the less stable the object.

4. Location of the center of mass relative to the edges of the base of support. If a line dropped down from the center of mass is close to an edge of the base of support, the body will have low stability in that direction.

With this knowledge the strength and conditioning specialist can alter the body position and equipment used to increase or decrease stability. For example, if an older person is having difficulty maintaining balance while performing arm curls, seating him or her on a bench will make the exercise easier by increasing the base of support and lowering the center of gravity. If an athlete is unstable in performing the triceps press-down exercise, for example, spreading the feet and splitting them one forward and one back and bending slightly at the knees will provide much better stability.

In some instances, less stability is desirable to increase the balance demands of the task. This can be achieved for the dumbbell shoulder press, as one example, simply by standing on one leg.

Initiating Movement or Change of Motion

When an athlete attempts to accelerate quickly or to change direction, he will decrease his stability in the direction of movement. This means that any given force he exerts in that direction will result in rapid acceleration. For example, in starting the sprint, the athlete leans far forward over the hands so that the line of gravity falls very close to the front edge of his base of support.

STRETCH-SHORTENING CYCLE

Almost all human movement involves a preparatory or "windup" action in the opposite direction followed by the intended movement. This sequence involves a lengthening and stretching of the muscles used to produce the movement, followed by a shortening, and so has been termed the **stretch-shortening cycle (SSC)**. This is an important biomechanical phenomenon of the neuromuscular system that has importance for strength and conditioning because such an action is performed to some extent in all training exercises. In fact, some exercises, such as plyometrics, are designed specifically to develop SSC ability. The preparatory movement involves eccentric muscle contraction, and this phase potentiates the subsequent concentric movement by about 15% to 20%. That is, movements performed without prestretching produce 15% to

20% less power output than true SSC movements. Some six mechanisms are proposed to explain this phenomenon, but the predominant factor is that a higher level of force (termed *preload*) can be generated at the start of the concentric movement if pre-stretching is performed. Although the stretch reflex and storage and recovery of elastic strain energy have also been frequently touted, the role of these two mechanisms is probably less important, particularly in short-duration ballistic movements such as squat, vertical jump, and throwing.

The SSC is inherent in almost all sporting movements, and this mechanism is critical for producing high force and power.

BIOMECHANICS OF RESISTANCE MACHINES

The variety of equipment developed for strength and conditioning is quite remarkable. These devices are designed to change the direction of resistance and in some cases vary the magnitude of resistance through the range of movement. Most use the gravitational weight force, but there are also a plethora of machines that use elastic, hydraulic, and aerodynamic drag or pneumatic resistance. How these machines interact with the human body is determined by biomechanical principles. Although some have been well designed, others have not incorporated good biomechanics; the result has been poor effectiveness or even risk of injury. Following is a discussion of the predominant resistance machine designs.

Understanding the mechanics underlying a piece of resistance training or conditioning equipment will assist in initial purchase decisions as well as exercise selection.

Free Weights

Working against the inertia and gravitational weight force of a freely moving mass such as a dumbbell or barbell represents the simplest but perhaps most often used form of resistance training (Fig. 5.8). The biomechanics of such equipment are similarly straightforward, with the resistance acting vertically downward at all times. The force can be calculated as $F = mg$, where m = mass and g = acceleration due to gravity (9.81 m/s/s). When the

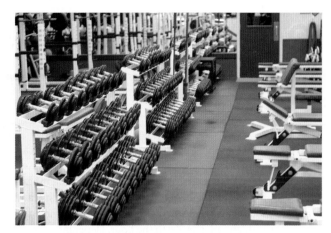

FIGURE 5.8 Free-weight equipment.

weight is also being accelerated, an additional resistance due to the inertia of the object exists; this extra force can be calculated as $F = ma$. For rapid movements, this component of the resistance to movement can become quite large—for example, in the clean and jerk or snatch. Remember that when the weight is decreasing in velocity of movement, the acceleration is negative and the resistance to overcome is actually reduced. This contributes to why the top part of a squat or bench press requires less effort than the earlier concentric phase.

Gravity-Based Machines

A disadvantage of free weights is that the line of resistance is always vertically downward. A second problem is that the resistance is constant—that is, the weight force of the dumbbell or barbell. This does not match the strength curves for various movements, and as such the amount of weight that can be lifted is limited to that which can be successfully moved through the sticking region previously discussed. For this reason several machines using various techniques have been developed, all using the gravitational weight force but modifying the resistance curve to more closely match the strength curve for the movement. Figure 5.9 shows an example of a gravity-based machine. The biomechanics of these techniques are discussed below.

PULLEYS

The most basic modification was to build machines that allowed the weight force to be redirected. Early versions used standard weight plates, but later ones incorporated cables and pulleys to provide vertically upward or horizontally directed resistance.

Q & A from the Field

Is the full squat exercise dangerous from a biomechanical perspective?

Any resistance training exercise performed improperly can cause injury. This increased risk of injury risk may be related to excessive volume, excessive resistance, poor form, inflexibility, or fatigue. With adequate strength and flexibility, any athlete should be able to squat safely to the point where the tops of the thighs are parallel to the floor. Depending on the demands of the sport, some athletes may benefit from squatting below this "parallel" position. Squats done appropriately do not affect the stability of the knee joint negatively. The squat exercise is important to both the general population and athletes because of its functionality and similarity to athletic movements and activities of daily living.

PIN-LOADED MACHINES

To overcome the problems of shifting weight plates on and off these early machines, a weight stack was incorporated with a pin used to select the resistance. This improved ease of use, helped to keep the weight room tidier, and reduced the risk of injury from lifting weight plates on and off the machines.

LEVERS AND CAMS

The next problem to overcome was the mismatch of the resistance profile to the strength curve for the movement. For example, in the bench press using free weights or in constant-resistance machines, the load lifted is limited to what can be moved through the bottom part of the range. Once the load is off the lifter's chest, the effort required decreases as the ascending strength curve exceeds the constant-resistance load by an increasing proportion. In this scenario, the neuromuscular system is not stressed as much in the upper part of the range of motion

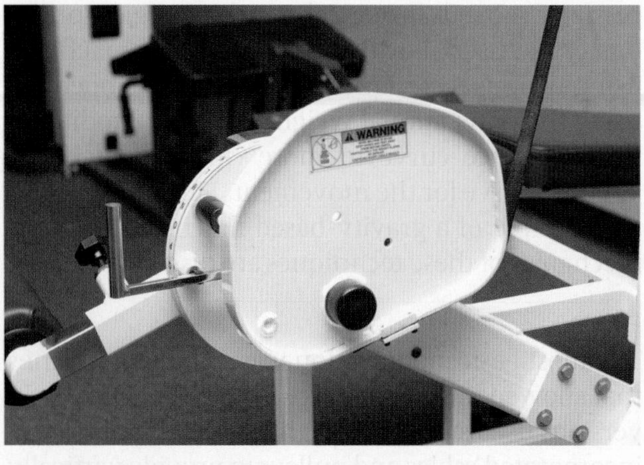

FIGURE 5.9 A cam-based resistance machine is a type of gravity-based machine.

and the intensity is limited by the sticking region. To overcome this problem, a range of **variable resistance** devices were developed. The initial designs involved sliding levers; an example would be the universal variable resistance machine. The principle was simple: as bench- or leg-press movement proceeded from the bottom to the top position, the lever arm would slide out, changing the point of application of the load on the weight stack and increasing the moment arm and thus the amount of resistance to be overcome by the lifter.

Later examples used **variable-radius cams**; for example, Nautilus, to achieve the same result. In this case a cable or chain wrapped around a cam with a changing radius alters the length of the resistance arm and thus the amount of resistance that the lifter must overcome. Using biomechanical principles, the cams could be designed to match the strength curve for various training exercises.

One of the most recent implementations of the variable-resistance concept in resistance training is the Hammerstrength range of equipment. The biomechanics of this equipment is quite simple though effective. The weight plates are placed on horns located at the end of a lever. In the bottom position, the lever is rotated out of the horizontal and, as in the case of the concepts discussed earlier regarding line of resistance, not all of the weight force of the plates is directed against the lifter. As the lift is executed, the lever arm moves toward the horizontal, so that the vertically downward weight force moves closer to 90 degrees to the lever arm and the amount of load transferred to the lifter increases, matching more closely the strength curve for the movement.

Hydraulic Resistance

Hydraulic resistance devices use a hydraulic ram and the resistance of oil (hydraulic fluid) being forced though a small aperture (Fig. 5.10). Two different technologies are used. One involves flow control, for which the size of the aperture is adjusted, thus changing the velocity at which the fluid can flow and therefore the speed of movement. As greater force is exerted against the machine, the resistance increases to match, since the fluid is incompressible and the velocity of flow is somewhat independent of the pressure. The second type uses a pressure-release-valve configuration. The valve is initially held closed by a tensioned spring, but when a force greater than the valve resistance is applied, the valve opens, allowing the fluid to flow. This technology provides a more constant resistance, similar to that of free weights, compared to the quasi-constant velocity of flow-control systems.

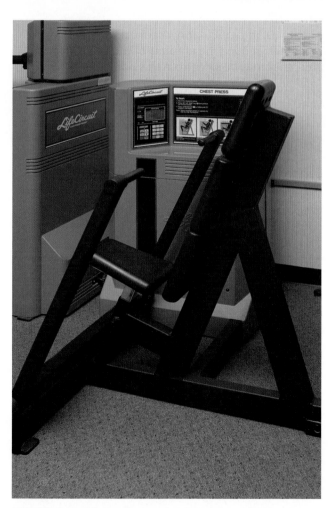

FIGURE 5.10 A hydraulic-based resistance machine.

It is important to note that both systems are passive and thus provide a purely concentric exercise mode. This equipment has found a niche in the design of circuit training programs and also for use with special populations because muscle soreness is reduced (no eccentric phase), the equipment is easy to use, and no momentum is built up, thus reducing the risk of injury.

Pneumatic Resistance

Pneumatic resistance equipment uses air pressure to provide resistance to both concentric and eccentric exercise. A pneumatic ram similar to an enormous syringe is preloaded to a certain pressure, using compressed air. The higher the pressure, the greater the resistance provided. When the movement is performed, the ram compresses the air even further, increasing pressure and thus resistance. This provides an ascending resistance curve that matches the ascending strength curve of most human movements reasonably well. On the return movement, the athlete is working to control the speed of the expanding gas, so these machines allow eccentric as well as concentric phases.

Elastic Resistance

Examples range from equipment as simple as the Theraband to devices such as the VertiMax. All use the resistance developed when an elastic material such as rubber or bungee cord is stretched. Such devices also provide an ascending resistance curve because elastic tension is greater the more the material is deformed. They also allow for eccentric exercise as the muscles act to control the speed of elastic recoil.

MACHINES VERSUS FREE WEIGHTS

It is an interesting biomechanical discussion to compare the advantages and disadvantages of machines versus free weights for resistance training. Clearly each has benefits, and it is really a matter of understanding the biomechanical principles that apply to each and then selecting the equipment and exercises appropriate to the individual. An evaluation is included in Table 5.1.

TABLE 5.1	BIOMECHANICAL COMPARISON OF MACHINE VERSUS FREE WEIGHTS
FREE WEIGHTS	**MACHINES**
Lower stability requires greater balance control; this may have added training effect.	Higher stability makes exercise easier for novices and certain populations where demands of balance control may be risky or compromise strength gains.
Line of resistance is constant and vertically downward.	Line of resistance can be altered to any plane and direction.
Resistance force is constant and proportional to the mass and does not necessarily match the strength curve for a specific movement.	Resistance force can be varied through the use of levers and cams in an attempt to match strength curve.
Resistance is more specific to the free masses that must usually be manipulated in sport performance and tasks of everyday living.	Controlling the plane of movement, varying the resistance, and changing the line of resistance reduces specificity of training.
Although not matching strength curves, the *free,* three-dimensional movement of free weights does allow for wide variation in weight, height, sex, and lever length.	Even the best application of biomechanics can only approximate the average person, and deviations in height, weight, sex, and lever length result in a considerable mismatch of machine and body mechanics.
Lifting free weights, particularly in a standing position, requires considerable activation of muscles acting as fixators and stabilizers, which increases training efficiency and strengthens muscles in these important roles.	Although less activation of muscles other than the agonists is required when using machines; this allows concentration on the agonist muscles for greater activation.
Both eccentric and concentric phases of free weight lifts can generate considerable momentum, which the lifter must control at the end of range to avoid injury.	Machines, in particular hydraulic and pneumatic machines, reduce the amount of momentum generated; that may be safer from this point of view.
Require more effort in loading the bar, lifting plates on and off, and lifting barbells and dumbbells from the rack. All requires effort and may be a source of injury if not performed with good ergonomics.	Load is easily selected and changed.
Not biomechanical but administratively, free weights require more effort to keep orderly and tidy.	Easy to keep a tidy and safe exercise environment.
If a lift cannot be completed, some exercises such as bench and squat are difficult to escape from under the bar.	Weight stack just drops back and stops if lifter cannot complete or fails the attempt.

SUMMARY

Biomechanics has considerable application in understanding many aspects of strength and conditioning. From an appreciation of the determinants of friction and how an athlete can develop force against the ground to the design principles of the wide array of resistance equipment available, biomechanics knowledge will enable the strength and conditioning professional to increase his or her effectiveness and safety.

MAXING OUT

1. You want to incorporate some Olympic lifting into the strength and conditioning program for the volleyball team. The problem is that the athletes are having real trouble learning to perform the lifts correctly. How could biomechanics be used to help you teach the athletes?
2. The football coach has told you that he wants his players completing only single-joint exercises on pin-loaded resistance machines and at slow

speed. His rationale is that he does not want the athletes injured in the weight room. From your biomechanics knowledge, you don't believe that such a program is optimal, but you have to convince the coach. Write a discussion paper outlining the basis for also using ground-supported, multijoint movements, including high-speed exercises such as jump squats and Olympic lifts.

REFERENCES

1. Baker D, Nance S. The relation between running speed and measures of strength and power in professional rugby league players. J Strength Cond Res 1999;13(3):230–235.
2. Baker D, Newton RU. Acute effect on power output of alternating an agonist and antagonist muscle exercise during complex training. J Strength Cond Res 2005;19(1):202–205.
3. Baker D, Newton RU. Methods to increase the effectiveness of maximal power training for the upper body. Strength Cond J 2005;27(6):24–32.
4. Berthoin S, Dupont G, Mary P, Gerbeaux M. Predicting sprint kinematic parameters from anaerobic field tests in physical education students. J Strength Cond Res 2001;1(1):175–180.
5. Blazevich AJ, Gill ND, Bronks R, Newton RU. Training-specific muscle architecture adaptation after 5-wk training in athletes. Med Sci Sports Exerc 2003;35(12):2013–2022.
6. Blazevich AJ, Jenkins DG. Predicting sprint running times from isokinetic and squat lift tests: a regression analysis. J Strength Cond Res 1998;12(2):101–103.
7. Brown LE, Whitehurst M. The effect of short-term isokinetic training on force and rate of velocity development. J Strength Cond Res 2003;17(1):88–94.
8. Brown LE, Whitehurst M, Findley BW, et al. Effect of repetitions and gender on acceleration range of motion during knee extension on an isokinetic device. J Strength Cond Res 1998;12(4):222–225.
9. Carlock JM, Smith SL, Hartman MJ, et al. The relationship between vertical jump power estimates and weightlifting ability: a field-test approach. J Strength Cond Res 2005;18(3):534–539.
10. Corn RJ, Knudson D. Effect of elastic-cord towing on the kinematics of the acceleration phase of sprinting. J Strength Cond Res 2003;17(1):72–75.
11. Cronin JB, Hansen KT. Strength and power predictors of sports speed. J Strength Cond Res 2005;19(2):349–357.
12. Cronin JB, McNair PJ, Marshall RN. Force-velocity analysis of strength-training techniques and load: implications for training strategy and research. J Strength Cond Res 2003;17(1):148–155.
13. Deane RS, Chow JW, Tillman MD, Fournier KA. Effects of hip flexor training on sprint, shuttle run, and vertical jump performance. J Strength Cond Res 2005;19(3):615–621.
14. Doan BK, Newton RU, Marsit JL, et al. Effects of increased eccentric loading on bench press 1 RM. J Strength Cond Res 2002;16(1):19–13.
15. Dugan EL, Doyle TLA, Humphries B, et al. Determining the optimal load for jump squats: a review of methods and calculations. J Strength Cond Res 2004;18(3):668–674.
16. Hall SJ. Basic Biomechanics. 4th ed. New York: McGraw-Hill, 2003.
17. Hori N, Newton RU, Nosaka K, McGuigan MR. Comparison of different methods of determining power output in weightlifting exercises. Strength Cond J 2006;28(2):34–40.
18. Hori N, Newton RU, Nosaka K, Stone MH. Weightlifting exercises enhance athletic performance that requires high-load speed strength. Strength Cond J 2005;27(4):450–455.
19. Jones K, Bishop P, Hunter G, Fleisig G. The effects of varying resistance-training loads on intermediate–and high–velocity-specific adaptations. J Strength Cond Res 2001;15(3):349–356.
20. Kawamori N, Newton RU. Velocity specificity of resistance training: actual movement velocity versus intention to move explosively. Strength Cond J 2006;28(2):86–91.
21. Kreighbaum E, Barthels KM. Biomechanics: A Qualitative Approach for Studying Human Movement. 4th ed. Boston: Allyn & Bacon, 1996.
22. Livingstone C, White AA, Panjabi MM. Biomechanics in the Musculoskeletal System. Philadelphia: Elsevier, 2000.
23. Lockie RG, Murphy AJ, Spinks CD. Effects of resisted sled towing on sprint kinematics in field-sport athletes. J Strength Cond Res 2003;17(4):760–767.
24. McBride JM, Triplett-McBride T, Davie A, Newton RU. A comparison of strength and power characteristics between power lifters, Olympic lifters, and sprinters. J Strength Cond Res 1999;13(1):58–66.
25. McBride JM, Triplett-McBride T, Davie A, Newton RU. The effect of heavy- vs. light-load jump squats on the development of strength, power, and speed. J Strength Cond Res 2002;16(1):75–82.
26. McGinnis PM. Biomechanics of Sport and Exercise. 2nd ed. Champaign, IL: Human Kinetics, 2004.
27. Newman MA, Tarpenning KM, Marino FE. Relationships between isokinetic knee strength, single-sprint performance, and repeated-sprint ability in football players. J Strength Cond Res 2004;18(5):867–872.
28. Newton RU, Dugan E. Application of strength diagnosis. Strength Cond J 2003;24(5):50–59.
29. Newton RU, McEvoy KI. Baseball throwing velocity: a comparison of medicine ball training and weight training. J Strength Cond Res 1994;8(3):198–203.
30. Nordin M, Frankel VH. Basic Biomechanics of the Musculoskeletal System. 3rd ed. Philadelphia: Lippincott Williams & Wilkins, 2001.
31. Robertson GE, Caldwell GE, Hamill JN, et al. Research Methods in Biomechanics. Champaign, IL: Human Kinetics, 2004.
32. Walsh M, Arampatzis A, Schade F, Brüggemann G-P. The effect of drop jump starting height and contact time on power, work performed, and moment of force. J Strength Cond Res 2004;18(3):561–566.
33. Zatsiorsky V. Kinetics of Human Motion. Champaign, IL: Human Kinetics, 2002.
34. Zatsiorsky VM. Science and Practice of Strength Training. Champaign, IL: Human Kinetics, 1995.

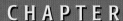

CHAPTER

6

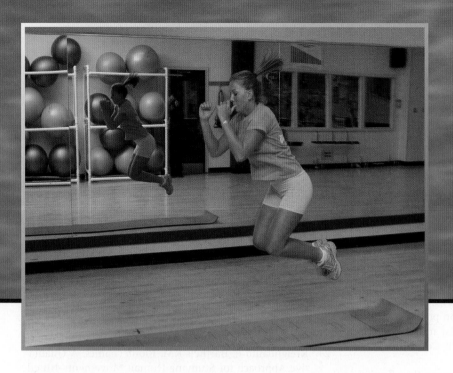

Training Responses and Adaptations of the Endocrine System

ANDREW C. FRY

JAY R. HOFFMAN

Introduction

The human body is designed to provide amazing control of its physiological systems during physical exercise and sport performance. Each of these physiological systems is closely regulated and coordinated. The optimal result is an improvement in performance. As with each of the other physiological systems, the hormonal system is closely controlled and responds to exercise and physical activity to assure optimum results. But what exactly is this hormonal, or endocrine, system? How does it work? How can it influence the other systems of the body? Perhaps of most importance to this chapter, how does the endocrine system respond to the short-term requirements of a single bout of exercise, and how does it adapt to the chronic stresses of a long-term training program?

THE ENDOCRINE SYSTEM

The endocrine system helps to maintain homeostasis in the body by regulating hormonal functions. This occurs through the communication between chemicals in the body that regulate different physiological actions. These chemicals are called messengers; they are secreted into the bloodstream and travel to their respective binding sites. Once they have arrived at the designated binding site, they promote changes in cellular functions.

What Are Hormones?

Our first challenge is to define the term *hormone*. For the purposes of this chapter, a **hormone** is a chemical compound that is secreted into the circulation to regulate a biological function at a distant site in the body. A hormone is secreted directly into the bloodstream from a tissue known as an endocrine gland. These glands contain specialized cells designed to create and release their respective hormones. A **neurohormone** is very similar except that it is released from a nerve ending into the circulation. Regardless of the source, the hormones and neurohormones travel to various parts of the body until they reach their target tissues. Once arriving, they can bind, or attach, to specialized receptors on or in the cells of the target tissues. In this manner, hormones are able to influence how the target tissues function.

> *Hormones are chemical compounds secreted by endocrine tissues and transported via the circulation.*

Endocrine Tissues

Numerous hormones and neurohormones are involved in the proper functioning of a healthy system. Hormones are chemical compounds that are produced by endocrine tissues and typically released into the circulation. Neurohormones are types of hormones that also function as neurotransmitters in the nervous system. Of particular interest for this chapter are those hormones that specifically respond to physical exercise and sport performance. Obviously, numerous endocrine tissues in the body participate in this process, whether it involves the short-term or sudden **acute** responses to a single bout of exercise or the long-term **chronic** adaptations to regular exercise and training. Figure 6.1 illustrates the endocrine glands and tissues responsible for the hormones and neurohormones discussed in this chapter. These are the tissues that produce the primary hormones examined in this chapter. In general, these tissues release their hormonal products into the circulation, whereby they are transported to their target sites throughout the body. In studying the endocrine and neuroendocrine systems, it is important to be familiar with the various endocrine tissues as well as the normal blood concentrations of the hormones, as listed in Table 6.1 (67,69).

Although those in the medical profession and the related health sciences often use conventional units of measure, scientific reporting requires the use of the measurements defined by the **Système Internationale (SI)**. The SI system is universally recognized by scientists all over the world and provides a logical and systematic method for quantification (69).

Hormonal Transportation Routes

Although most of the hormones discussed in this chapter are released into the circulation for transport to their respective targets, other methods of transport exist. Some hormones never leave their tissue; others never leave their cells. Figure 6.2 illustrates the autocrine, paracrine, endocrine, and neuroendocrine hormonal transport routes.

AUTOCRINE

When hormones or neurohormones are synthesized in their respective cells, not all are released into the circulation. Certain of these chemical compounds never leave the cell. Instead, they remain within the cell and influence the activity of the cell in some manner. These are called **autocrine** hormones (58). An example of this is insulin-like growth factor-1 (IGF-1). IGF-1 is produced in many cells of the body and is responsible for many of the actions of growth hormone. IGF-1 can be measured from the circulating blood, but some IGF-1 never leaves the cell. Although circulating amounts of this hormone are still important, they do not account for the IGF-1 that never leaves the cell and functions in an autocrine manner.

PARACRINE

Some hormones leave their endocrine cells but never enter the circulation. Instead, they travel to

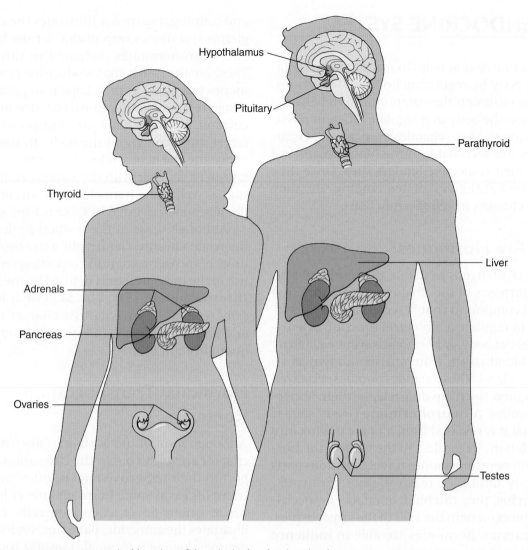

FIGURE 6.1 Anatomical location of the principal endocrine glands.

adjacent cells, where they exert their influence on cellular activity. These are called **paracrine** hormones (14). As with an autocrine system, circulating amounts of these paracrine chemical compounds may be important, but they do not account for the portion that never enters the circulation.

ENDOCRINE

This chapter is concerned primarily with endocrine and neuroendocrine mechanisms. The term **endocrine** refers to hormones that are released into the bloodstream or lymph system to control growth, metabolism, mood, and reproduction; **neuroendocrine** refers to hormones that are released into the bloodstream or lymph system following stimulation of the nervous system. Once the chemical compound is released, it travels via the circulation and eventually reaches its target tissue

or is broken down to its metabolic by-products. Although many factors influence the concentrations of these hormones in the blood, it is still essential to measure their concentrations in blood to fully understand their roles in physiological function.

Once produced, most hormones enter the circulation for transport (endocrine), some travel to adjacent cells (paracrine), and some never leave the cell (autocrine).

Types of Hormones

As might be expected, hormones come in different chemical forms (Fig. 6.3). Basically, three chemical structures account for the hormones that most interest us (55).

TABLE 6.1	TYPICAL ADULT SERUM CONCENTRATIONS IN BOTH SYSTEM INTERNATIONALE (SI) AND CONVENTIONAL UNITS (67,69)		
VARIABLE		**SI UNIT**	**CONVENTIONAL UNIT**
Testosterone (4 p.m.)	Men	10–35 nmol/L	3–10 ng/mL
	Women	<3.5 nmol/L	<.1 ng/mL
Cortisol (4 p.m.)		50–410 nmol/L	2–15 µg/dL
Growth hormone	Men	0–5 µg/L	0–5 ng/mL
	Women	0–10 µg/L	0–10 ng/mL
Insulin-like growth factor I	Men	0.45–2.2 kU/L	0.45–2.2 U/mL
	Women	0.34–1.9 kU/L	0.34–1.9 U/mL
Insulin (fasting)		35–145 pmol/L	5–20 µU/mL
Glucagon		50–100 ng/L	50–100 pg/mL
Epinephrine (resting, supine)		170–520 pmol/L	30–95 pg/mL
Norepinephrine (resting, supine)		0.3–2.8 nmol/L	15–475 pg/mL
Antidiuretic hormone		2.3–7.4 pmol/L	2.5–8.0 ng/L
Aldosterone		< 220 pmol/L	< 8 mg/dL
Thyroxine (T_4)		51–42 nmol/L	4–11 µg/dL
Triiodothyronine (T_3)		1.2–3.4 nmol/L	75–220 ng/dL
Calcitonin		< 50 ng/L	< 50 pg/mL
Parathyroid hormone		10–65 ng/L	10–65 pg/mL

STEROID HORMONES

First are the **steroid hormones**, which all share the same four-carbon-ring structure and affect growth and the development of the sex organs. All steroid hormones are made from a cholesterol molecule, which is called a **precursor molecule**. Depending on the endocrine tissue involved, the cholesterol molecule is converted by **enzymes** (proteins serving as catalysts in mediating and speeding a specific chemical reaction) into the final steroid hormone that is to be released. Different endocrine glands have different hormonal enzymes that determine which steroid hormone will be produced. Since the steroid hormones are formed from cholesterol, they are **lipophilic** ("lipid-loving"), which means that they can pass through the lipid membrane of a cell. Pharmaceutical forms of steroids, which are orally ingested or injected (and are called **exogenous** steroids—that is, coming from outside the body), are typically variations of the hormones naturally produced by the body (which are known as **endogenous** steroids). This chapter deals only with the body's own natural production of these hormones.

PEPTIDE HORMONES

A second group of hormones comprises the **peptide hormones**, which consist of chains of **amino acids**, the building blocks of protein. Small chains (of less than 20 amino acids) are simply termed *peptides;* larger chains are called *polypeptides*. These hormones can be quite long, as exemplified by growth hormone, which is 191 amino acids long. The shapes of these polypeptides are often determined by their amino acid sequences and by the existence of bonds between certain amino acids. These bonds cause the peptide to configure into the specific shape required for the hormone to function optimally. If any alteration occurs in the chain of amino acids, the hormone's function may be affected. This can occur when one or more of the amino acids in the chain are replaced with a different amino acid or if the peptide chain is cut, resulting in a smaller peptide chain. Sometimes these altered forms of the hormone still have a function, but it is often different from that of the original hormone. Peptide hormones are more prone to **degradation**, or breakdown of a complex compound into simpler compounds, in the circulation

Autocrine

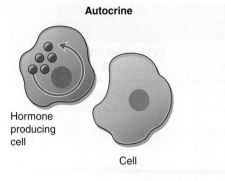

Hormone
producing
cell

Cell

Paracrine

Hormone
producing
cell

Receptor cell

Endocrine

Capillary

Hormone
producing
cell

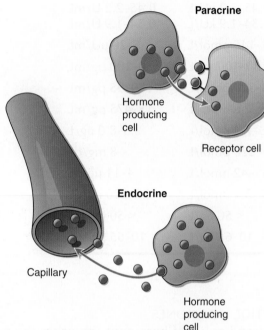

Neuroendocrine

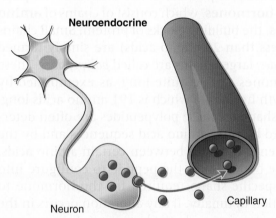

Neuron

Capillary

FIGURE 6.2 Autocrine, paracrine, endocrine, and neuroendocrine transport routes of hormones.

than steroid hormones. Additionally, peptide hormones are **lipophobic** ("lipid-hating"), meaning that they are repelled by lipids and cannot readily pass through the cell membrane. As such, they require a receptor at the membrane permitting them to act.

AMINE HORMONES

The last group of hormones are the **amine hormones**, characterized by an amine ring. Since amine hormones are derived from amino acids, they are sometimes classified as protein hormones. These hormones are found as either hormones or neurohormones and can be produced and secreted by either endocrine tissues or nerve endings. Some of these compounds also function as neurotransmitters in the nervous system. The typical precursor molecule of amine hormones is the amino acid tyrosine. In the event that tyrosine is not available in adequate quantities, phenylalanine can be converted to tyrosine and then used for the **synthesis**, or creation, of an amine hormone. Some amine hormones—such as epinephrine (also known as adrenaline) and norepinephrine (noradrenaline)—break down rapidly in the circulation. As such, they must exert their influence on target tissues rapidly. Amine hormones are lipophobic; therefore, like peptide hormones, they require a membrane receptor.

> *The three types of hormones—steroid, peptide, and amine—are each synthesized differently.*

Hormone Production

As shown in Figure 6.4, each of the three types of hormones is produced in a different manner. A cursory understanding of how one's body makes these hormones can give us a greater appreciation of the complex role they play in human performance.

PRODUCTION OF STEROID HORMONES

As mentioned earlier, the synthesis of the different types of steroid hormones is dependent on the various enzymes present in the particular endocrine gland (10,36). The first step is the conversion of cholesterol to pregnenolone in the mitochondria of the cell. This is called the **rate-limiting** step in the process, since the subsequent steps occur more readily. Once the stimulus for steroid hormone synthesis arrives at the endocrine cell, the process begins with this first step to pregnenolone. Pregnenolone is then transported to the endoplasmic reticulum, where it is converted via several enzymatic steps into the desired steroid. For some of the steroid hormones, additional processing occurs back in the mitochondria. Once the final hormone is completed, it can diffuse through the cell membrane, which consists of two lipid layers. Owing to

Type of Hormone	Examples

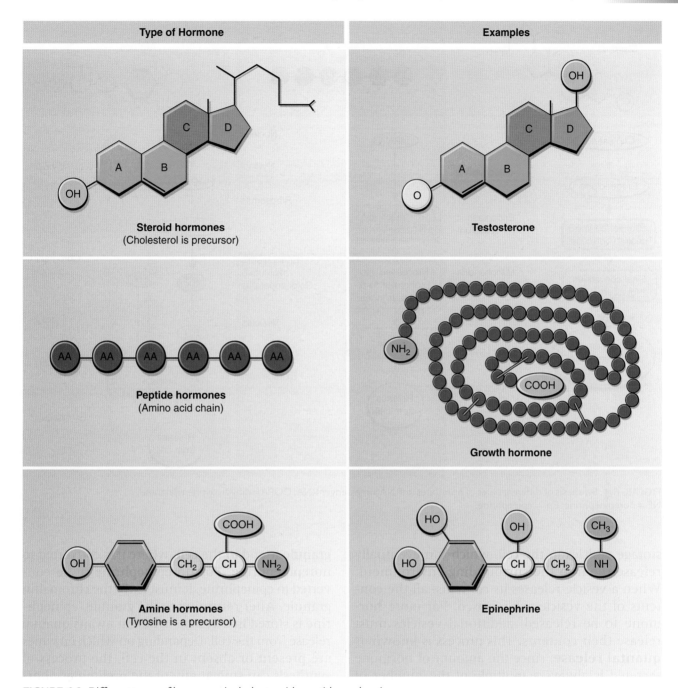

FIGURE 6.3 Different types of hormones include steroid, peptide, and amine.

the hormone's ability to exit the cell easily, these hormones are not stored but rather produced as needed.

PRODUCTION OF PEPTIDE HORMONES

Peptide hormones are synthesized when the appropriate signal for hormone production results in **messenger RNA (mRNA)** being produced in the cell nucleus (36). The mRNA serves as the code indicating which amino acids are needed and in what order. The mRNA is transported to the ribo-somes, where the appropriate amino acids are brought and assembled into a precursor molecule in a procedure called **translation**. The precursor molecules are then transported to the endoplasmic reticulum and the Golgi tendon organ for further modification; this process is termed **post-translational processing**. This often includes splicing the precursor amino acid chain into smaller molecules. Since peptide molecules are **lipopho-bic** (repelled by lipids), they cannot pass through the cell membrane. To be released, they must enter

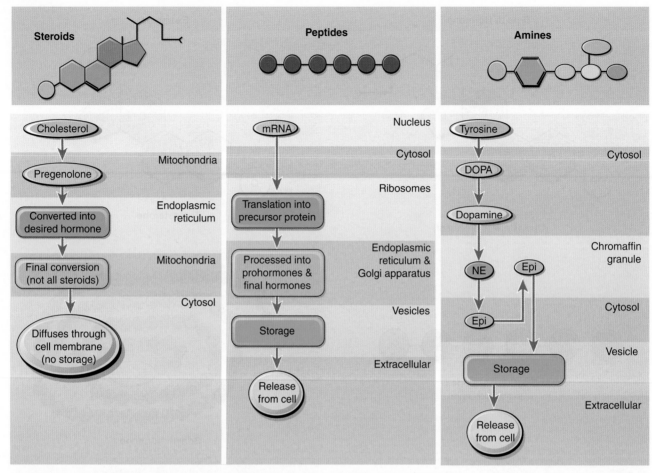

FIGURE 6.4 Synthesis of different types of hormones. mRNA = messenger RNA; DOPA = dihydroxyphenylalanine; NE = norepinephrine; Epi = epinephrine.

storage vesicles in the cell, which can eventually release them to the surrounding environment. When a vesicle releases its contents, all the contents of the vesicle are released. For more hormone to be released, additional vesicles must release their contents. This process is known as **quantal release**, since the amount of hormone secreted is always a multiple of the number of vesicles involved.

PRODUCTION OF AMINE HORMONES

Amine hormones are produced in **chromaffin cells** found in various tissues in the body (48). These cells are named based on their ability to take up chromium when stained. One family of amine hormones and neurohormones are the **catecholamines** (i.e., epinephrine, norepinephrine, dopamine, etc.). As mentioned earlier, the precursor molecule tyrosine enters the cytosol of the cell, where enzymes ultimately convert it to dopamine. Dopamine then enters the chromaffin

granule found in the cell, where it is converted to norepinephrine. For norepinephrine to be converted to epinephrine, it must leave the chromaffin granule. After returning to the granule, epinephrine is stored in a vesicle, where it awaits quantal release from the cell. Depending on which enzymes are present or absent in the cell, the process of synthesis can stop at any of the preliminary hormones. Other amine hormones, such as the thyroid hormones, are produced in the follicular cells of the thyroid gland. These hormones follow a different process for synthesis but are still characterized by amine rings.

Hormonal Transport and Binding Proteins

Once hormones are released into the circulation, they must be transported in a timely fashion to the tissues where they are to act. One problem the hormones encounter is **metabolism**, or their degradation. Numerous factors can prevent hormone molecules from ever reaching their targets because of degradation. The time it takes for a hormone to be partially metabolized in the circulation, or for half of it to be degraded, is called its **half-life ($T_{1/2}$)**. Some hormones have a half-life measured in seconds, while the half-lives of others are measured in minutes or hours. To preserve a hormone for longer periods, the hormonal molecule may be protected by becoming attached to a **binding protein**, which preserves the hormone and assists in its transport (Fig. 6.5) (54). Hormones such as steroid and thyroid hormones are bound to these **transport proteins**, while amines and protein hormones are not. **Albumin**, a binding protein made in the liver that helps to maintain blood volume in the arteries and veins, can bind numerous different hormones but does not exhibit a high **affinity** (attraction) to any of them. Regardless, the hormone-binding protein complex can move through the circulation without the hormone being degraded. The problem with this system is that the hormone is unable to bind to its target tissue until it is released from the binding protein. When this happens, the hormone is considered **biologically active**, or available for use during metabolism. The portion of the hormone not bound to a binding protein is called the percent **free hormone**, while the **total hormone concentration** includes both the free and the bound portions. Typically, when binding proteins are used, most of the circulating hormone is bound

to a transport protein. For example, only approximately 1% to 2% of the total testosterone in the circulation is free testosterone, or not bound to its binding protein.

> *Binding proteins protect the hormone (bound hormone), but the hormone is biologically active only when it dissociates from the binding protein (free hormone).*

Factors Affecting Circulating Concentrations

The concentration of hormones in the blood can be extremely variable, depending on the hormone and on a number of contributing factors (44).

HORMONE PRODUCTION AND RELEASE

At first, it would seem that the primary factor would simply be how much hormone is being produced by the endocrine gland. Although this is certainly one factor, the process is much more complicated (Table 6.2). Three sites in the body can contribute

TABLE 6.2	FACTORS AFFECTING HORMONE CONCENTRATIONS
SITE	**FACTOR**
Endocrine cell	Hormone synthesis Hormone release
Circulation	Method of transport to target tissue Binding proteins Hormonal concentration • Total • Free • Bound Fluid (plasma) shifts Venous pooling Hepatic (kidney) clearance rates Extrahepatic clearance rates Degradation of hormones
Target tissue Receptors	Binding affinity Maximal binding capacity Sensitivity
Intracellular	Second-messenger systems Nuclear receptor adaptations

Source: Reproduced with permission from Kraemer WJ. Endocrine responses and adaptations to strength training. In: Komi PV, ed. Strength and Power in Sport. Oxford, UK: Blackwell, 1992:291–304.

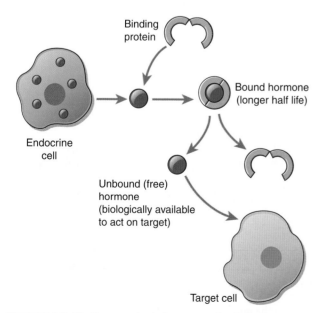

FIGURE 6.5 Binding proteins help protect circulating hormones.

to the circulating concentrations. These include the endocrine cell, the circulating blood, and the target tissue. At the endocrine cell, it is not only is the rate of hormonal synthesis that matters; additional factors are how much hormone is released and how quickly this occurs.

HORMONAL TRANSPORT IN THE CIRCULATION

In the circulation, the binding proteins can affect the availability of a hormone at its target tissue (54). Additionally, hormones are degraded in various tissues, thus affecting how much hormone arrives at the target site. Hepatic clearance is a particularly large factor in this process, but other tissues are involved as well. Concerning exercise, after a vigorous effort, blood may pool in the venous circulation, resulting in less of the hormones circulating to the target tissue. One of the largest factors during exercise is **plasma fluid shifts** (66). Plasma is the fluid portion of blood; during physical exercise, this fluid leaves the blood. This alone can result in a higher hormonal concentration. Contributing factors to this fluid shift include fluid loss via sweating, due to increased arterial pressures and postural changes. Plasma volume shifts of more than 15% have been reported for long-term aerobic exercise as well as resistance exercise. This response is augmented when the exercise occurs in a hot, humid environment.

HORMONAL ACTIVITY AT THE TARGET CELL

At the target tissue, the properties of the hormone receptors are critical factors (40). **Receptors** are the cellular structures to which the hormones bind,

resulting in the appropriate action at the cell. The number of receptors (**receptor density**) available, how readily the hormone attaches to the receptor (**affinity**), and how sensitive the receptor is to the hormone can vary. Furthermore, **postreceptor activity** can vary. This involves the role of the **signaling pathways** that tell the cell how to respond once the hormone has bound to the receptor. Some of these signals are initiated at the receptors in the cell membrane, while some are initiated in the cell nucleus, depending on the hormone.

Hormones affect their target tissues by binding to hormone-specific receptors. Binding at these receptors initiates the specific cellular responses to the hormone.

Trophic Hormones and Pulsatility

For a hormone to be secreted by its endocrine gland, the gland must receive some type of signal. The signal for many hormones is a **trophic hormone** from another endocrine gland or from the nervous system (39). When increased concentrations of a hormone are required, the body detects this need and causes the trophic hormonal signal to be increased. This signal is not based simply on the hormone's concentration. Instead, trophic hormones are released in a **pulsatile** fashion (Fig. 6.6) (63). This means that the hormone is released in periodic bursts. The trophic signal is increased either by increasing the frequency of the pulses or by increasing their magnitude or amplitude. Needless

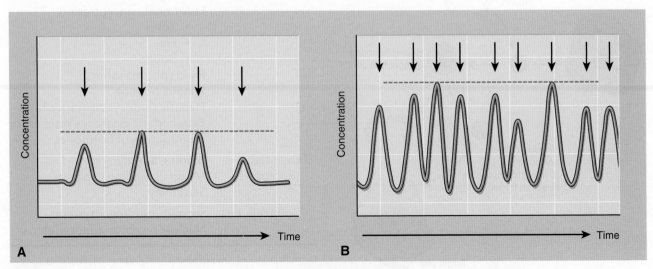

FIGURE 6.6 Pulsatility. Trophic hormones increase their signal by increasing the number and magnitude of pulses. Each arrow indicates a trophic hormone pulse. **A.** A basal trophic signal. **B.** An amplified trophic signal. Note that the signal is amplified by both increasing the frequency and the magnitude of pulses.

to say, to properly study these signals, many blood samples must be taken to measure pulse frequency and amplitude. For example, the primary trophic hormone for testosterone in males is luteinizing hormone (LH), which is released from the anterior pituitary gland. In turn, luteinizing hormone is regulated by LH-releasing hormone (LH-RH) from the hypothalamus. As such, the control of our hormones is very complex and highly dependent on the signaling pattern of the trophic hormones.

Circulating concentrations are often regulated by trophic hormones that signal the synthesis and release of the hormones. This system is synchronized by a negative-feedback system that can detect the current blood concentrations.

Hormonal Rhythms

Many hormones present different blood concentrations at different times of the day (12). In biological systems, hormonal variations occur over a number of time periods [e.g., hourly, less than every 24 hours, every 24 hours, or at different times of the year (seasonally)]. Of particular interest to this chapter are the **circadian rhythms**, or daily cycles of physiological processes, also known as the **diurnal variation**. Figure 6.7 illustrates an example of the diurnal variation for cortisol. As shown, baseline concentrations can be quite high late in the typical sleep cycle and early in the morning. Therefore, any interpretation of the hormonal responses to exercise and sport must consider

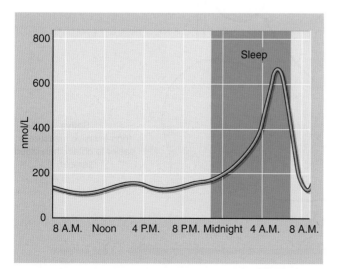

FIGURE 6.7 Examples of the variations of concentrations of cortisol during a typical day. The shaded area indicates a typical sleep cycle. (Modified with permission from Goodman HM. Basic Medical Endocrinology. New York: Raven Press, 1998:103.)

where the baseline values were prior to the physical activity (31,60). Many researchers simply avoid the times of day when hormonal concentrations are elevated (e.g., early morning for cortisol). In addition, when hormonal levels are being studied over a long time, as in a training study, the time of day the blood samples are taken must be kept constant to minimize the effect of diurnal variations.

Hormone concentrations are influenced by the time of day and by anticipation of an impending stressor, such as exercise or competition.

Anticipatory Responses

The hormonal response occurring in anticipation of impending exercise or sport is termed the **anticipatory response** (48). The body possesses a number of hormones collectively called **stress hormones**. These hormones help the body to get ready for a stressful experience, whether it involves physical activity, cognitive stress, or both. They are part of the **fight-or-flight** response (8). All biological systems have methods of responding and dealing with stressful situations, whether they involve fighting the threat or fleeing from it. Experienced athletes are very familiar with the "pre-game jitters" they encounter prior to an important competition. Similar feelings are also common in other scenarios, such as taking exams, public speaking, and musical recitals. In examining the hormonal responses to physical activity, it is important to separate the responses due to stressful anticipation from those due to the actual physical activity. The catecholamine (epinephrine) that is particularly sensitive to an anticipatory response is illustrated in Figure 6.8, although cortisol can also exhibit an anticipatory response. Blood sampling must be performed prior to the anticipatory response to determine the actual resting baseline value. It should be noted that some individuals will exhibit an anticipatory response to the actual process of taking a blood sample with a needle. In these cases, the sample must be taken when the needle has previously been inserted (i.e., via an intravenous catheter), after the individual has had time to relax and return to baseline.

Biocompartments

The typical method of measuring hormonal concentrations involves venous blood sampling. Most hormones of interest are released directly into the circulation; thus, this is often the most sensitive

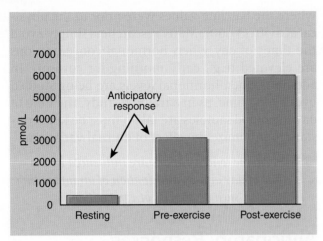

FIGURE 6.8 Example of the anticipatory response of epinephrine to a stressful lifting task. The difference between resting and pre-exercise concentrations represents the anticipatory response for the impending exercise. [Reproduced with permission from Fry AC, Kraemer WJ, van Borselen F, et al. Catecholamine responses to short-term high-intensity resistance exercise overtraining. J Appl Physiol 1994;77(2):941–946.]

way to measure the endocrine responses. Information on hormonal activity, however, can be collected from other sites, or **biocompartments**, in the body (64). Since hormones are ultimately degraded to their metabolic by-products, urine may be sampled to indirectly determine the quantity

of hormone produced over a period of time. For example, when true baseline or resting levels are of interest, **nocturnal urine measures** are analyzed for the hormonal by-products. In this manner, the total amount of hormone produced during the sleep hours (when one is most at rest) can be estimated. Another common biocompartment is saliva, which may also be analyzed to determine hormonal concentrations, since **salivary concentrations** are related to blood concentrations. A limitation with salivary samples is that this measure is less sensitive to slight fluctuations in blood concentrations, and it takes longer to respond to physical activity. On the other hand, both urine and saliva are obtained **noninvasively**, meaning that they can be obtained without breaking the skin, so they are easier to collect than samples gathered by **invasive methods**, which necessitate an incision or puncture (Figure 6.9).

Receptors and Cell Signaling

When a hormone molecule arrives at its target tissue, it interacts with the tissue by binding at a protein receptor. Receptors come in many different configurations, each hormone having a receptor specific to it. This is known as **receptor specificity**

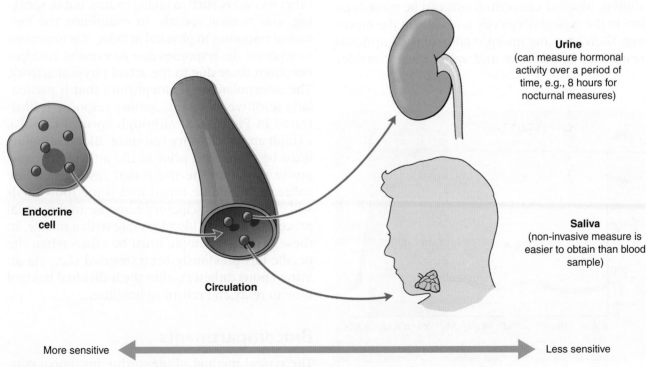

FIGURE 6.9 Hormonal levels can be determined by sampling from either blood (whole, serum, or plasma), or urinary or salivary biocompartments. Sensitivity of the sample to hormonal fluctuations decreases when not taken from the circulation.

(10,40). This specificity has been described as being analogous to a lock and key. Just as the lock can be opened with only one particular key, one hormone can bind to only one type of receptor, resulting in the optimal desired response. In some cases, however, other similar hormones can also bind to the receptor, although the results may be slightly different or smaller in magnitude. This **cross-reactivity** exists when more than one hormone can bind at a particular receptor. Cellular receptors are a favorite site of action for many of the pharmaceutical drugs in use today. These drugs act as **analogues** to the natural chemicals of the body, meaning they are similar enough that they are able to bind to their respective receptors. Since they are not identical to the body's endogenous hormones, neurohormones, and neurotransmitters, they can result in a number of unwanted side effects. Regardless, modern science has been able to constantly improve on the specificity of these drugs, resulting in their amazing effectiveness. Receptors are often located in the cell membrane,

where the circulating hormones have ready access for binding (Fig. 6.10). Steroid receptors, however, are located within the cell nucleus, since steroids can easily enter the cell due to their lipophilic nature. Regardless of the location of the receptor, as soon as a hormone binds to its receptor, the activity of the cell is modified in some manner.

SECOND-MESSENGER SYSTEMS

Figure 6.10 illustrates several of the second-messenger systems used by membrane-bound receptors. We see in this figure that several different types of hormones can interact with the **adenylate cyclase–cyclic adenosine monophosphate (cAMP) system** (24,40). When hormone A (H_a) binds to its receptor, the **stimulating G protein (G_s)** activates adenylate cyclase to produce cAMP from adenosine triphosphate (ATP). This, in turn, causes a kinase to modify an enzyme in the cell to either increase or decrease its activity. Other hormones, on the other hand, work in an opposite manner by activating an **inhibiting**

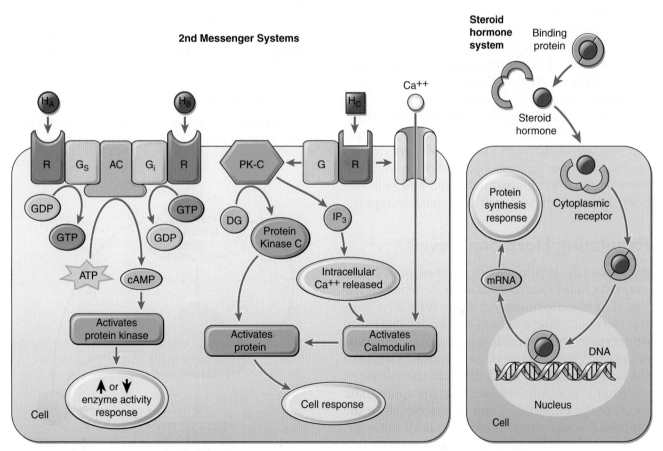

FIGURE 6.10 Hormonal intracellular signaling systems. H_{abc} = different hormones; R = receptor; G_s = stimulating G protein; G_i = inhibiting G protein; AC = adenylate cyclase; GDP = guanosine diphosphate; GTP = guanosine triphosphate; ATP = adenosine triphosphate; cAMP = cyclic adenosine monophosphate; PK-C = protein kinase C; DG = diacyl glycerol; IP_3 = inositol triphosphate.

G protein (G_i), which turns off the adenylate cyclase activity. Other hormones (H_c) bind to receptors associated with a different second-messenger system, the **diacyl glycerol (DG)-inositol triphosphate (IP_3) system** (38,40). Activation of DG results in a protein-activated cell response, while production of IP_3 releases calcium from storage sites within the cell. This calcium activates **calmodulin**, which, in turn, results in a protein-activated cell response. An alternative mechanism of action is a receptor-activated **influx** of calcium from outside the cell. As with IP_3, this activates calmodulin, which ultimately produces the desired cell response.

NUCLEAR INTERACTIONS

Steroid hormones work in a completely different manner (5,10,25). Since they can readily pass through the cell membrane, they are able to enter the **cytosol**, where they are bound to a **chaperone protein**, sometimes called a **cytoplasmic receptor**. This protein escorts the steroid to the cell nucleus, where it can bind to a site on the cell DNA. This initiates a process called **transcription**, which results in the coded signal for the production on a cellular protein. This signal leaves the nucleus in the form of **messenger ribonucleic acid (mRNA)**. At the ribosomes, the protein is assembled from the various amino acids, resulting in the desired cell response. Regardless of which system is used, each hormone binds to its target receptor, which activates a cascade of events resulting in the proper cell response. Although complex, these systems work amazingly well and help our body deal with stresses such as exercise and sport.

Regulating Hormonal Levels

As previously mentioned, the increase or decrease in production of many hormones depends on the signal of trophic hormones (39). When the central nervous system detects a need for increased or decreased hormonal levels, it signals a trophic endocrine gland to increase or decrease its signal to the target endocrine gland. The pulsatile nature of the trophic hormone release sends the appropriate signal to the endocrine gland of interest. Once the hormonal concentrations increase, both the regulating endocrine gland in the central nervous system and the trophic endocrine gland detect these increased concentrations and decrease their signals. This regulatory mechanism is called a **negative-feedback system**, which operates very much like a thermostat in a house. When the house's temperature is too high or too low, the thermostat signals the furnace to either turn on or off to maintain the desired temperature. This regulatory mechanism is also known as **cybernetic regulation** (Fig. 6.11). The previously described system for regulating testosterone in males is a good example of negative-feedback regulation. Circulating concentrations of testosterone are detected by both the hypothalamus, which produces LH-RH, and the anterior pituitary, which produces LH. This causes the signal to the testes to be altered, depending on whether more or less testosterone is needed. In this manner, the body is able to closely control the levels of hormones found in the circulating blood.

HORMONES VITAL TO EXERCISE

Although many hormones and neurohormones are responsible for the healthy functioning of the human body, the following section identifies the primary hormones of interest for this chapter.

Testosterone

Testosterone is a steroid hormone produced primarily by the **Leydig cells** in the male **testes**. Cir-

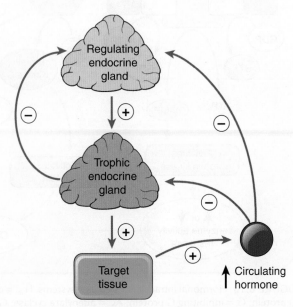

FIGURE 6.11 Example of negative feedback regulation of circulating hormones. + = upregulation; − = downregulation; ↑ = increased.

culating testosterone in females is about 10% of that in males and is derived from the **ovaries**, the female sexual glands—which produce estrogen, testosterone, and progesterone—and the adrenal cortex. During maturation, testosterone contributes to many of the male sexual characteristics associated with development. Testosterone is regulated by the **hypothalamic-pituitary axis**. In this regulatory structure, the hypothalamus detects circulating concentrations of testosterone and secretes LH-RH. This, in turn, stimulates release of LH from the anterior pituitary, which functions as the primary stimulus for the release of testosterone from the testes. This process takes up to 15 minutes to occur, so faster responses are probably due to direct innervation of the testes or to sympathetic nervous activity via circulating epinephrine or norepinephrine. Once released, testosterone is bound to **sex-hormone-binding globulin (SHBG)**, its binding protein. Perhaps the cellular effect of most interest for this chapter is the anabolic effect in skeletal muscle.

Cortisol

Cortisol is a steroid hormone secreted by the outer layer of the adrenal glands (**adrenal cortex**). It is sometimes called a **stress hormone**, since it is released when the individual experiences either physical or psychological stresses. Cortisol's principal role is to ensure the availability of energy. In this role, cortisol increases the production of glucose from either fat or protein in the liver, a process called **gluconeogenesis**, decreases glucose uptake, increases glycogen production in skeletal muscle, and causes amino acids to be mobilized from skeletal muscle. Because of this breakdown of protein into amino acids, cortisol is often termed a **catabolic hormone**. Circulating levels of cortisol are detected by the hypothalamus, which secretes **corticotropin-releasing hormone (CRH)**, a polypeptide hormone involved in the stress response. CRH then stimulates the anterior pituitary to release **adrenocorticotropic hormone (ACTH)**, which in turn signals the adrenal cortex to produce and release cortisol.

Testosterone/Cortisol Ratio

The ratio between testosterone, an **anabolic hormone** that causes the synthesis of molecules into more complex molecules, and cortisol, a catabolic hormone, has been used as a hormonal indicator of training stress (18). This can be considered for both a single aerobic training session and for a long-term training phase. With a single stressful exercise session, testosterone either increases initially or decreases. On the other hand, cortisol increases to a greater extent. The net result is that the ratio decreases. The more stressful the session, the more the ratio decreases. The ratio will also decrease over time in performing a stressful phase of training involving multiple sessions. As the individual tapers or backs off the training, the ratio returns to initial levels. As such, this ratio has been used as a marker of training stresses, and some have advocated its use to monitor recovery. Some have also advocated using the ratio between **free testosterone**, the portion of circulating testosterone not bound to SHBG, and cortisol as a more sensitive indicator. This idea is based on the fact that free testosterone is the actual hormone that is biologically available to exert its actions at the target tissue.

Growth Hormone

Growth hormone is a polypeptide hormone consisting of 191 amino acids and two disulfide bonds. It is produced and secreted from the anterior pituitary gland in a pulsatile fashion. Concentrations of growth hormone are increased by its trophic hormone, GH-RH, and decreased by **GH-inhibiting hormone (GH-IH)**, both from the hypothalamus. Many variations of growth hormone appear to exist, because various forms of the original peptide are produced. This makes growth-hormone data difficult to interpret at times. Many of the actions of growth hormone occur because of its effect on insulin-like growth factors. Although growth hormone is often most associated with its growth properties (including skeletal muscle), it also exerts tremendous influence on the metabolic system and energy availability. It increases muscle uptake of amino acids as well as the breakdown of lipids via **lipolysis**. The net result is that amino acids are preferentially used for anabolic purposes by muscle, and glycolytic energy sources are spared in favor of lipid energy sources.

Insulin and Glucagons

Insulin and glucagons are considered together, since their actions are so closely associated. Insulin is a 51-amino-acid peptide hormone produced by the **beta cells** of the **pancreas**, the organ that secrets both insulin and glucagon. Insulin consists of a 21–amino acid A-chain and a 30–amino acid B-chain connected by two disulfide bonds. Glucagon is also a polypeptide chain but is only 29 amino acids long. It is produced by the **alpha cells** of the pancreas. Insulin and glucagons are released in response to increasing or decreasing blood glucose levels, respectively. Increasing concentrations of insulin prompt circulating glucose to be taken up by the following:

1. Adipose cells for conversion to triglycerides
2. Liver cells for conversion to glycogen
3. Skeletal muscle cells for conversion to glycogen

The net result is control of rising blood glucose levels and storage of energy for future use. On the other hand, glucagon results in the exact opposite responses. Triglycerides are metabolized in adipose tissue, and amino acids and glycogen are metabolized in the liver. These collectively increase circulating glucose during times of high energy needs, such as exercise and sport. Both insulin and glucagon are also under control by epinephrine and norepinephrine from the sympathetic nervous system, causing insulin to decrease and glucagon to increase.

Epinephrine

Epinephrine, sometimes called adrenaline, is an amine neurohormone. Although it serves as a **neurotransmitter** in the central nervous system and transmits signals between the synapses of nerve cells, our interest is in its role in the circulation. Blood-borne epinephrine comes from **chromaffin cells** in the center portion (medulla) of the adrenal glands. Upon neural stimulation, the adrenal medulla dumps its contents into the renal vein, resulting in a very rapid epinephrine response. Furthermore, the adrenal medulla is completely surrounded by the adrenal cortex; thus, the medulla is constantly exposed to cortisol. This interaction with cortisol is critical for maintaining resting levels of epinephrine. When it is released into the circulation, epinephrine interacts with a variety of **alpha and beta receptors** in many different tissues of the body. Epinephrine is responsible for many of the **"fight-or-flight" responses** previously discussed. These physiological responses to stress prepare the body to either fight or flee from an impending threat and include increased arousal and cardiac output, altered blood-flow patterns, enhanced muscle contractions, and greater energy availability.

Norepinephrine

Norepinephrine, also known as noradrenaline, is also an amine neurohormone. Unlike epinephrine, which is derived primarily from the adrenal medulla, most of the circulating norepinephrine comes from **spillover** from sympathetic nervous system synapses. In this manner, norepinephrine is sometimes considered an indicator of sympathetic nervous system activity. The adrenal medulla also produces some norepinephrine, but this is usually less than 20% of the epinephrine released.

Aldosterone

Aldosterone is a steroid hormone secreted by the adrenal cortex. It is a key player in fluid regulation, responding to decreased blood pressures due to lowered blood fluid volumes. To counter this problem, aldosterone acts at the kidneys to keep sodium from being excreted. When sodium is retained, fluid is also retained, thus helping to counter the previously detected fluid loss. This response is not rapid and requires 30 minutes or more to go into effect. Small amounts of fluid loss are termed *hypohydration*, while larger losses are called *dehydration*. This can occur due to lowered fluid intakes and/or exercise in a hot environment.

Antidiuretic Hormone

Antidiuretic hormone (ADH) is a peptide hormone secreted by the posterior pituitary under hypothalamic control. Also known as arginine vasopressin, ADH responds to hydration status as does aldosterone; however, the mechanisms behind ADH are somewhat different. The concentration of proteins in the blood is known as the blood's osmolality, and this increases when fluid leaves the plasma portion of blood. This change in osmolality is readily detected in the arterial and venous circulation, resulting in a rapid ADH response. With ADH stimulation, the kidneys more readily take up fluid that would normally have been excreted. ADH is also a strong vasoconstrictor. In this manner, blood pressures are maintained even when blood fluid levels are depressed.

Thyroid Hormones

The thyroid hormones thyroxine (T_4) and tri-iodothyronine (T_3) are secreted by the thyroid gland. They are derived from tyrosine and contain either four or three iodine molecules respectively. They are regulated by thyrotropin, also known as thyroid-stimulating hormone (TSH) from the pituitary gland. T_4 is secreted in greater quantities than T_3, but much of T_4 is converted throughout the body to the more potent T_3. The thyroid hormones are basically responsible for increasing the body's metabolic rate and enhancing the action of other hormones.

Calcium-Regulating Hormones

Two hormones are essential for regulating calcium concentrations in the circulation. These are calcitonin from the thyroid gland and parathyroid hormone from the parathyroid gland. As calcium levels in the blood are detected, calcitonin is released to stop calcium from being taken from bone and to increase the excretion of calcium in the kidneys. Conversely, parathyroid hormone works in an opposite fashion. When blood calcium levels are low, release of parathyroid hormone stimulates bone to release calcium and inhibits excretion of calcium in the kidneys. Since the largest pool of calcium in the body is found in the skeletal system, it has been speculated that alterations of these hormones may be critical for the skeletal adaptations to physical exercise.

EFFECTS OF EXERCISE ON THE ENDOCRINE SYSTEM

As with any other system of the body, the endocrine system responds and adapts to the stresses placed on it. This includes sport training and other forms of exercise and physical activity. In this manner, the body adapts to the stress and ultimately produced enhanced performances or at least a tolerance for current activity levels (57). Although the hormonal response is not the only adaptation the body makes to exercise, it is certainly critical, since these hormones interact with so many other tissues and systems of the body. Our task now is to see exactly how these hormones respond and adapt and how this influences the training prescription we administer.

Acute and Chronic Training Adaptations

Regular training and physical activity result in an adaptation of the body to accommodate the stress. Hormonally, this can lead to the upregulation or downregulation of different hormones, depending on the types of physical activity and the physiological system involved. **Upregulation** refers to an increase in the number of receptors on the surface of target cells, making the cells more sensitive to a hormone or other molecule; **downregulation** is a decrease in the number of receptors on the surface of target cells, making the cells less sensitive to a hormone or other molecule. On one hand, these changes can be quite simple—they either increase or decrease the circulating concentrations found in the blood—although the changes can be more complex. Figure 6.12 illustrates an example of how some hormones can both increase and decrease in response to chronic (long-term) training (42,68). Prior to training, individuals can exercise only up to a certain work rate owing to their untrained status. As they increase their exercise intensity, the hormonal response increases accordingly. After long-term training has resulted in an increased capacity to exercise, they can exercise at a higher work rate. Now, when they exercise at the same absolute work rate as they did before training, they require less hormonal response to do the same activity. On the other hand, when they

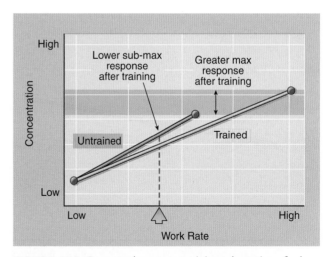

FIGURE 6.12 Common long-term training adaptations for hormonal responses to an exercise session. Note the decreased hormonal response at an absolute submaximal work rate after long-term training (indicated by the large arrow) but the increased hormonal response at maximal work rates. The trained individual is capable of exercising at higher work rates.

exercise at their maximal capacity, they can produce a greater hormonal response, thus permitting the greater work rate. In this manner, one becomes more efficient during submaximal exercise while at the same time being capable of functioning at much higher intensities. In general, acute responses to exercise are determined immediately or shortly after completing the exercise bout. These values represent the hormonal response to a single exercise session. On the other hand, chronic hormonal responses are often determined from changes in resting hormonal concentrations. These values represent the long-term concentrations that are continuously exposed to the target tissue. Of course, as shown in Figure 6.12, chronic adaptations can sometimes also alter the acute response to exercise.

Responses and Adaptations of Hormones to Endurance Exercise

The following section addresses the primary hormones of interest for this chapter and how they acutely respond to different intensities and durations of aerobic exercise. Where available, the chronic responses to long-term training are also included. Please note that the figures for each hormone indicate representative values and responses, which may vary between individuals and with different testing conditions.

> *During aerobic activities, most hormones increase as intensity and duration increase. Some important exceptions, however, should be noted.*

TESTOSTERONE AND ENDURANCE EXERCISE

During aerobic exercise, testosterone increases in an intensity-dependent manner. Low intensities of exercise elicit little or no response and maximum or near-maximum intensities result in a significant elevation (Fig. 6.13). During prolonged aerobic exercise, testosterone exhibits a biphasic response (11). Provided that the intensity is great enough, testosterone concentrations increase initially. If the duration of the exercise is long enough, concentrations decrease. Examples of this are the depressed testosterone levels reported after events such as a marathon. Because the amounts of testosterone in females are small, little or no response is observed (3). Sometimes long-term endurance training has been associated with lower concentrations of testosterone, but this may be simply due to the effects of the huge volumes of training reported for these individuals. Testosterone is inversely related to training stress; as training stress increases, testosterone levels are lowered.

In females, instead of testosterone, the primary sex-related hormones of interest are progesterone and the estrogens (estradiol, estrone, and estriol). As with testosterone, these hormones increase somewhat in an intensity-dependent manner (4).

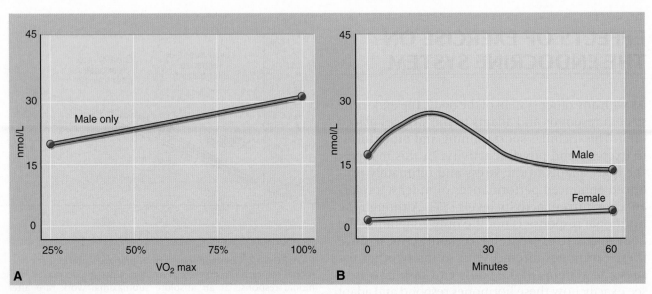

FIGURE 6.13 Responses of circulating concentrations of total testosterone to aerobic activities (3,11). **A.** Typical responses for men at different aerobic intensities (% $\dot{V}O_{2max}$). **B.** Testosterone concentrations during 60 minutes of high-intensity endurance exercise for both men and women.

The phase of the menstrual cycle, however, can influence the responses. Likewise, the use of hormonally based oral contraceptives can alter these responses.

CORTISOL AND ENDURANCE EXERCISE

During aerobic exercise, cortisol increases, for the most part, in an intensity-dependent manner (23,59). At very low intensities, cortisol is not increased and may actually decrease slightly due to the very low stress on the metabolic systems at these intensities. Intensities greater than 50% of $\dot{V}O_2$max result in elevations of cortisol due to the energy requirements needed to perform at these levels (Fig. 6.14). A similar response is observed for prolonged aerobic exercise, with cortisol levels increasing with the duration of exercise (7). The long-term training response includes lower cortisol concentrations (68), reflecting the body's ability to more effectively utilize the energy substrate available.

TESTOSTERONE/CORTISOL RATIO AND ENDURANCE EXERCISE

Because of the extremely high volumes of training that endurance athletes often perform, this hormonal ratio is often depressed among endurance athletes (50–52). This does not have to be the case, however, since this ratio can rebound when training volume decreases.

GROWTH HORMONE AND ENDURANCE EXERCISE

Since growth hormone is closely tied to energy availability, circulating concentrations are positively related to exercise intensity (23,59). Very large increases in growth hormone levels are observed at maximal intensities of aerobic exercise. In a similar manner, the levels of growth hormone increase with increasing durations of aerobic exercise (49). Long-term training results in a more efficient metabolic system; thus lower concentrations of growth hormone are produced when exercise is performed at the same absolute intensity. On the other hand, maximal efforts result in a greater growth hormone response in trained individuals (23) (Fig. 6.15).

INSULIN, GLUCAGON, AND ENDURANCE EXERCISE

During aerobic exercise, insulin decreases, thus minimizing the uptake of blood glucose when it is needed for energy. Glucagon increases, however, thus permitting glucose to become available for energy. In this manner, these two hormones work in concert to properly regulate glucose availability during physical activity (23,59). After long-term training, the decrease in insulin is less pronounced, most likely due to the almost nonexistent change in glucagon. Glucose uptake becomes less dependent on insulin, since chronic training results in increased activation of membrane glucose transport proteins, which regulate the transport of glucose

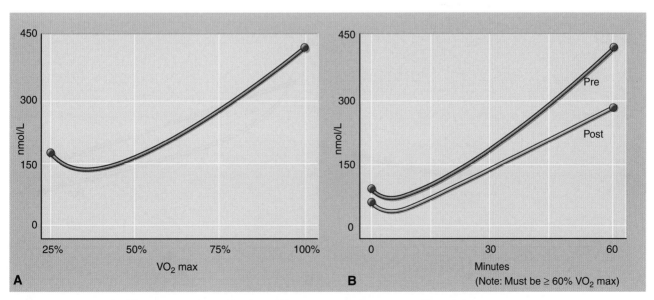

FIGURE 6.14 Responses of circulating concentrations of cortisol to aerobic activities (7,23,57,66). **A.** Typical responses at different aerobic intensities (% $\dot{V}O_{2max}$). **B.** Cortisol concentrations during 60 minutes of endurance exercise at ≥ 60% $\dot{V}O_{2max}$. *Pre* and *post* refer to before and after long-term training.

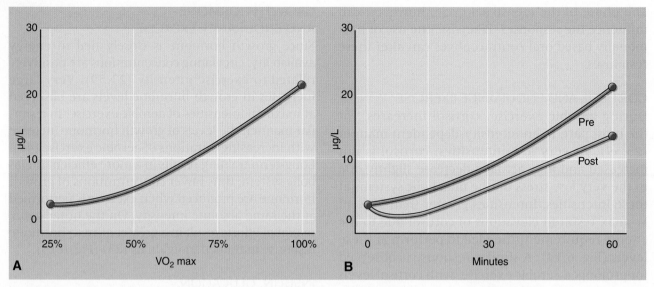

FIGURE 6.15 Responses of circulating concentrations of growth hormone to aerobic activities (23,47,57). **A.** Typical responses at different aerobic intensities (% $\dot{V}O_{2max}$). **B.** Growth hormone concentrations during 60 minutes of high-intensity endurance exercise. *Pre* and *post* refer to before and after long-term training.

across the plasma cellular membrane. In addition, chronic training results in a decreased response of the sympathetic nervous system; thus, levels of insulin are decreased and glucagon increases to a lesser extent. Figure 6.16 shows the responses of insulin to aerobic activities; Figure 6.17 shows the responses of glucagon to aerobic activities.

EPINEPHRINE AND ENDURANCE EXERCISE
Compared to other hormones, the catecholamines exhibit extremely large responses to physical exer-

cise. Epinephrine is particularly susceptible to an anticipatory response (20,22). In response to aerobic exercise, concentrations of epinephrine increase in an intensity-dependent manner (9,43) (Fig. 6.18), although the responses at low intensities are sometimes minimal. Furthermore, concentrations increase with increasing duration of aerobic exercise (23,41). Long-term aerobic training results in an increased ability to secrete epinephrine at maximal intensities. On the other hand, absolute submaximal intensities result in lower

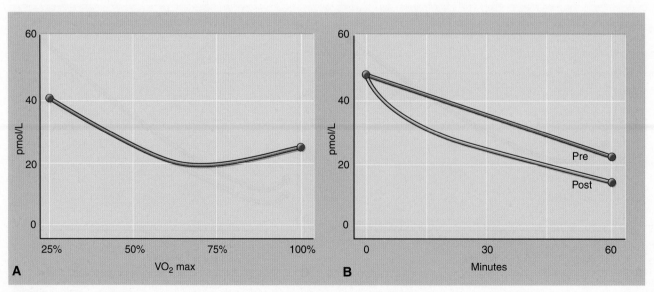

FIGURE 6.16 Responses of circulating concentrations of insulin to aerobic activities (23,57). **A.** Typical responses at different aerobic intensities (% $\dot{V}O_{2max}$). **B.** Insulin concentrations during 60 minutes of high-intensity endurance exercise. *Pre* and *post* refer to before and after long-term training.

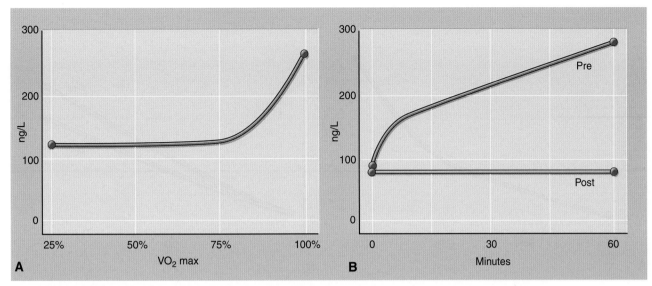

FIGURE 6.17 Responses of circulating concentrations of glucagon to aerobic activities (23,57). **A.** Typical responses at different aerobic intensities (% $\dot{V}O_{2max}$). **B.** Glucagon concentrations during 60 minutes of high-intensity endurance exercise. *Pre* and *post* refer to before and after long-term training.

concentrations after training, indicative of a more efficient system (see Fig. 6.12). The receptors for epinephrine are very sensitive to circulating concentrations and will readily decrease in number or responsiveness if epinephrine levels remain elevated for too long a time (2).

NOREPINEPHRINE AND ENDURANCE EXERCISE
Although epinephrine and norepinephrine appear to respond similarly, they are primarily derived from different sources and their responses to exercise are not absolutely identical. As such, they represent different physiological phenomena. Norepinephrine increases in an aerobic intensity-dependent manner, with greater intensities eliciting larger responses (9,43). Also like epinephrine, norepinephrine increases with longer duration aerobic exercise (23,41) (Fig. 6.19). Long-term training will result in greater norepinephrine concentrations with maximal exercise; absolute submaximal exercise will produce smaller concentrations, again indicative of a more efficient system (see Fig. 6.12).

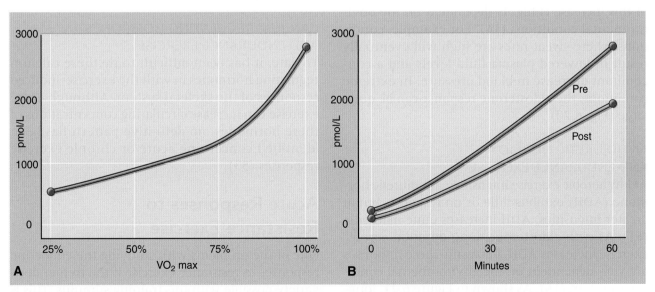

FIGURE 6.18 Responses of circulating concentrations of epinephrine to aerobic activities (9,23,40,42). **A.** Typical responses at different aerobic intensities (% $\dot{V}O_{2max}$). **B.** Epinephrine concentrations during 60 minutes of high-intensity endurance exercise. *Pre* and *post* refer to before and after long-term training.

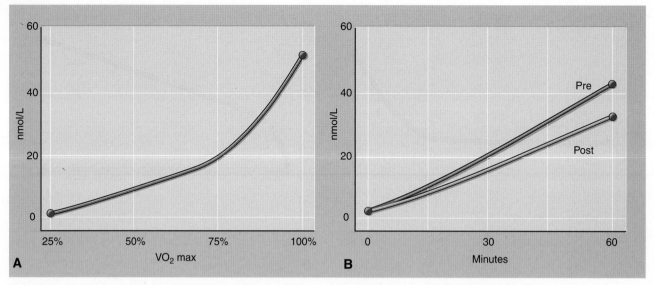

FIGURE 6.19 Responses of circulating concentrations of norepinephrine to aerobic activities (9,23,40,42). **A.** Typical responses at different aerobic intensities (% $\dot{V}O_{2max}$). **B.** Norepinephrine concentrations during 60 minutes of high-intensity endurance exercise. *Pre* and *post* refer to before and after long-term training.

If exercise results in excessive elevation of the catecholamines for extended periods of time, the physiological system responsible (sympathetic nervous system) can become exhausted, resulting in impaired performances (18). This has implications for overtraining, discussed further on.

ALDOSTERONE AND ENDURANCE EXERCISE

As with many hormones, aldosterone increases during aerobic exercise in an intensity-dependent manner (61). Although aldosterone will increase during long-duration aerobic exercise, the extent of this increase is highly dependent on the environmental conditions (16). For example, conditions where sweat rates are high will eventually result in lowered plasma fluid levels and a concomitant decrease in blood pressure. In extreme conditions, the aldosterone response can be quite large (Fig. 6.20).

ANTIDIURETIC HORMONE AND ENDURANCE EXERCISE

At low aerobic exercise intensities, antidiuretic hormone (ADH) exhibits little or no response, but at greater intensities, ADH increases quite markedly (61). As with aldosterone, long-duration aerobic exercise increases ADH, but again, these responses are very dependent on the environmental conditions present (16). As shown in Figure 6.21, long-term aerobic training results in lowered ADH responses at the same absolute exercise intensity, while the response increases at the same relative intensity.

THYROID HORMONES AND ENDURANCE EXERCISE

Although the thyroid hormones are undoubtedly critical for health, their responses to exercise are reportedly quite variable (53), and little is known concerning their responses and adaptations to acute and chronic exercise. Some evidence exists that the thyroid hormones decrease during stressful phases of training, but these data are not definitive.

CALCIUM-REGULATING HORMONES AND ENDURANCE EXERCISE

To date, it has been difficult to tie these calcium regulating hormones in with the exercise-induced responses of the skeletal system. Although acute exercise can increase circulating concentrations of these hormones, no definitive pattern has been identified concerning acute or chronic exercise responses (53).

Acute Responses to Resistance Exercise

One of the problems with studying the endocrine responses to resistance exercise is the tremendous variety possible with this training stimulus. This is best illustrated by the five acute training variables for resistance exercise (15,17). They are as follows:

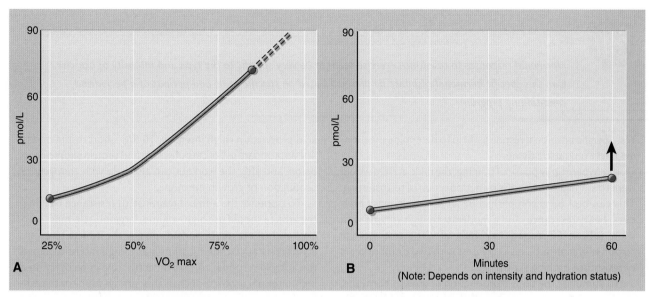

FIGURE 6.20 Responses of circulating concentrations of aldosterone to aerobic activities (16,59). **A.** Typical responses at different aerobic intensities up to 80% V̇O₂max. The dotted line indicates expected values for greater intensities. **B.** Aldosterone concentrations during 60 minutes of high-intensity endurance exercise. Note that the aldosterone response is highly dependent on the exercise intensity and the existing hydration status of the individual.

1. Choice of exercise
2. Order of exercise
3. Volume of exercise
4. Intensity (or load) of exercise
5. Interset rest intervals

These five variables represent all of the possible variables for a single weight-training session. Needless to say, each of the variables includes many options. When all five variables are considered, the number of possible combinations becomes

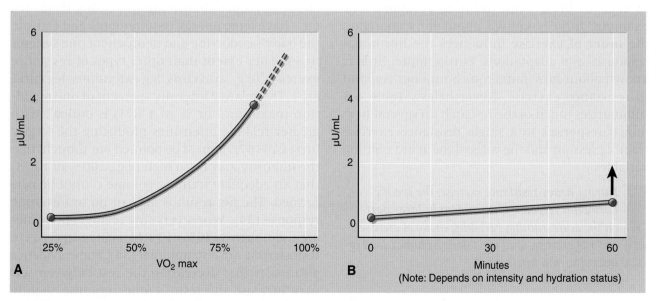

FIGURE 6.21 Responses of circulating concentrations of anti-diuretic hormone to aerobic activities (16,59). **A.** Typical responses at different aerobic intensities up to 80% V̇O₂max. The dotted line indicates expected values for greater intensities. **B.** Antidiuretic hormone concentrations during 60 minutes of high-intensity endurance exercise. Note that the aldosterone response is highly dependent on the exercise intensity and the existing hydration status of the individual.

Q & A from the Field

Hormonal responses to resistance exercise seem to be very specific to the type and intensity of exercise. Can this specific hormonal response be planned based on specific goals and periods of a periodized conditioning program?

_____

Yes. Specific hormonal responses help to determine the training effect on muscle tissue.

In a hypertrophy phase of training, the male athlete would want to stimulate the body's own production of testosterone. This can best be accomplished by large muscle-mass exercises, heavy resistance, and a moderate to high volume with short (about 60-second) rest intervals. The testosterone response in male athletes is greatest with two or more years of resistance training experience.

To stimulate the body's production of growth hormone, use resistance-training protocols that stimulate high lactic

acid production (high intensity, 10 RM, short rest periods). The appropriate use of carbohydrate and protein supplements before and after the workout can also help with endogenous production of growth hormone.

To optimize the adrenal response to resistance training, the athlete should use high-volume, large-muscle-mass exercises with short rest periods. Exposing the athlete to a variety of resistance-training stimuli at a high intensity allows the adrenal response to take an active role in recovery. In a high-intensity protocol such as this, always monitor the athlete for signs of overtraining.

---

extremely large, thus representing the huge number of stimuli resistance exercise can present. When the long-term program is added to this, the characteristics of the training program can almost be overwhelming. Regardless, much progress has been made concerning the effect of the acute training variables on the subsequent hormonal responses. Unfortunately, many questions remain unanswered concerning the hormonal responses to each of these acute training variables. For example, little is known about how changing the order of exercise influences the hormonal responses and adaptations. Furthermore, little is known about how numerous hormones respond to resistance exercise. Nevertheless, Table 6.3 summarizes much of the research on several hormonal responses to a single resistance exercise training session and the roles of the acute training variables.

> *During heavy resistance exercise, the specific hormonal response is dependent in large part on the acute training variables; choice of exercise, order of exercise, total repetitions (volume), load or intensity, and interset rest.*

TESTOSTERONE: ACUTE RESPONSE TO RESISTANCE EXERCISE

Testosterone readily increases during a weight-training session but requires at least a moderate

training volume as measured in total repetitions (13,27,47,65). Sessions that utilize large-muscle-mass multijoint exercises appear to elicit larger responses that those using just small-muscle-mass exercises (35,45). Additionally, exercise sessions that incorporate high-power exercises such as the Olympic weightlifting movements (snatch, and clean and jerk) can also produce considerable increases in testosterone (45). These types of exercises (e.g., squats, bench presses, cleans, dead lifts, etc.) have large energy requirements and activate the body's endocrine and neuroendocrine systems to a greater extent than other types of resistance exercises (e.g., arm curls, leg extensions, leg curls, etc.). The relative intensity (percent of one repetition maximum, or % of 1 RM) is critical, with greater relative intensities producing the largest increases (47). It must be pointed out though, that the intensity may be so high (e.g., 100% of 1 RM) that an adequate training volume cannot be performed. The net result is little or no testosterone response (34). When very low relative intensities are used, such as 40% of 1 RM, acute responses of testosterone are also minimal (35). Some evidence also exists that decreasing the rest between sets may increase the testosterone response slightly (47). Again, it should be pointed out that too short a rest interval may mean that the loads have to be decreased below the critical level for a significant testosterone response.

TABLE 6.3	KNOWN EFFECTS OF THE ACUTE WEIGHT TRAINING VARIABLES ON SEVERAL HORMONAL RESPONSES TO A SINGLE EXERCISE SESSION (13,1,27,28,34,35,44,45,47,56,62,65)			
ACUTE TRAINING VARIABLE	TESTOSTERONE	CORTISOL	GROWTH HORMONE	LACTATE
Choice of Exercise	↑ With large muscle mass exercises and high power exercises, moderately high volumes necessary	↑ With large muscle mass exercises and high power exercises, ↑ usually with full body training session	↑ With large muscle mass exercises and high power exercises, ↑ with free weights > ↑ with machines	↑ With large muscle mass exercises and high power exercises
Volume of exercises	Variable responses, depends on other factors	↑ With increasing volume. Note: Volume can be low if intensity is high enough	↑ With increasing volume. Note: GH response related to total work	↑ With increasing volume
Intensity of exercise	↑ With increasing relative intensity (% of 1 RM)	↑ With increasing relative intensity (% of 1 RM). Note: Cortisol ↑ > testosterone ↑	↑ With increasing relative intensity (% of 1 RM). Note: Volume must be high enough	Too high an intensity → smaller HLa response
Interset rest intervals	↓ Rest may ↑ testosterone (responses are variable)	↑ With decreasing rest intervals	↑ With decreasing rest intervals	↑ With decreasing rest intervals

↑ = increases; ↓ = decreases; RM = repetition maximum, > = greater than.

CORTISOL: ACUTE RESPONSE TO RESISTANCE EXERCISE

Compared to testosterone, cortisol tends to exhibit a larger acute response to resistance exercise (47). As with testosterone, cortisol responds most when large-muscle-mass, multi-joint exercises are performed and when high-power exercises are used (45). Owing to the metabolic requirements, cortisol levels will increase when total-body training sessions are performed. Cortisol responds in a relative intensity- and volume-dependent manner (47). When interset rest intervals are decreased, cortisol responses are also increased, again most likely due to the metabolic requirements of the session (47). It should be noted that some dietary supplements have been promoted with claims that they decrease the cortisol response to exercise. Although cortisol is a catabolic hormone, it also serves an important role in the remodeling of muscle tissue. As such, decreasing or eliminating the cortisol response may not be desirable.

GROWTH HORMONE: ACUTE RESPONSE TO RESISTANCE EXERCISE

The use of large-muscle-mass, multijoint exercises as well as high-power exercises is again critical for a large growth hormone response (45,47). Some evidence exists that free weights may produce a larger response than machine exercises, but this may simply be related to the muscle mass involvement (56). The relative intensity and the volume of exercise are positively related to the growth hormone response as well (47,62). The interset rest interval is extremely important, with very short rest intervals eliciting extremely large acute growth hormone responses (47).

LACTATE: ACUTE RESPONSE TO RESISTANCE EXERCISE

Although not a hormone, lactate provides insight on the metabolic characteristics of different weight-training sessions. In general, protocols that use large muscle mass, multijoint, and high-power exercises, with large training volumes and short interset rest intervals produce the largest lactate responses (28,45,47). If the relative intensity is too great, however, the volume that can be performed becomes too low, thus compromising the lactate response.

Long-Term Adaptations to Resistance Exercise

Table 6.4 lists the long-term (chronic) responses to heavy resistance exercise (29–32). In general,

TABLE 6.4	HORMONAL EFFECTS OF LONG-TERM NORMAL RESISTANCE EXERCISE TRAINING (5,29–32,37,46,53)
HORMONE	**EFFECTS**
Testosterone	Slight increase
Cortisol	Slight decrease
Growth hormone	Slight decrease
Insulin	Increase
Glucagon	Decrease
Epinephrine	Max intensity: increase Submax intensity: decrease
Norepinephrine	Max intensity: increase Submax intensity: decrease
Antidiuretic hormone	Slight decrease (depends on the environmental conditions)
Aldosterone	Slight decrease (depends on the environmental conditions)
Thyroxine	No known change
Triiodothyronine	No known change
Calcitonin	No known change
Parathyroid hormone	No known change

resting concentrations of these hormones are not always altered, but differences in the acute responses to a resistance-training session can occur. In some cases the response increases, indicating an enhanced capacity of the involved endocrine glands. In other cases, the response decreases, indicating greater efficiency of those hormones. At present, the responses of a number of hormones are not known.

Long-term hormonal adaptations to training are more subtle than the acute response to a single session, but they can provide an important training adaptation.

Overtraining and the Endocrine System

Although a properly designed training program is desirable for optimal results, sometimes the exercise program is improperly prescribed, resulting in maladaptations or overtraining. Overtraining occurs when training volume and/or intensity is excessive and results in prolonged decreases in performance (17,18). Short-term performance decrements are sometimes referred to as overreaching and are often part of a planned training program

(e.g., two-a-day training sessions for many sports). As might be expected, the endocrine system has been implicated in the maladaptations occurring during overtraining. It has been suggested that monitoring certain hormones may permit monitoring of the training stresses, thus avoiding the onset of an overtrained state (1). What is not often appreciated is that different types of overtraining appear to elicit different hormonal responses (18).

Overtraining occurring from activities that emphasize aerobic endurance is often characterized by very high training volumes (50–52). Table 6.5 indicates that, except for the stress hormone cortisol, most hormonal responses eventually decrease. The decrease in catecholamines appears to be reflective of exhaustion of the sympathetic nervous system. High volumes of resistance exercise exhibit many of the same endocrine characteristics (17,18,21). Perhaps the most commonly cited variable for monitoring overtraining is the testosterone/cortisol ratio (1). In general, this appears to be indicative of the collective training stresses, although changes in this ratio can often occur when overtraining is not present. Therefore, one cannot diagnose overtraining using this variable alone. It appears that subsequent exposures to high volume resistance-exercise overtraining may per-

TABLE 6.5	ENDOCRINE RESPONSES TO OVERTRAINING (1,17,18,50–52)		
HORMONE	**AEROBIC OVERTRAINING**	**HIGH-VOLUME RE OVERTRAINING**	**HIGH-INTENSITY RE OVERTRAINING**
Testosterone	Decrease	Decrease	NC or slight increase
Cortisol	Increase	Increase	NC
Tes/Cort	Decrease	Decrease	NC
Growth hormone	Increase → decrease	NC	NC
Epinephrine	Decrease	Decrease?	Increase
Norepinephrine	Decrease	Decrease?	Increase

RE = resistance exercise.

mit the body to adapt to the stress, resulting in avoidance of overtraining (21,22).

Contrary to many of the common characteristics of aerobic overtraining or high-volume resistance exercise, high-intensity resistance-exercise overtraining exhibits a much different endocrine profile. In general the steroid hormones and growth hormone are often unaffected. In fact, some studies have shown an increase in testosterone, the exact opposite of other types of overtraining (19). The catecholamines actually exhibit increased responses to exercise (20,22). It is believed that the sympathetic nervous system is still attempting to preserve performance and has not yet reached a state of exhaustion as previously described for other types of overtraining.

Using the Endocrine System to Monitor Training

A critical issue for many coaches and athletes is monitoring the physiological effects of the training program. This can be relevant for either the individual training session or for the longer-term effects of a phase of the training cycle. Obviously, obtaining blood samples from an athlete is often easier said than done, and having the blood analyzed may be even more difficult. An alternative might be to collect salivary or urine samples, but the analyses are still time-consuming and expensive. Regardless, much valuable information may be attainable if this information is accessed.

It has been proposed that levels of fatigue, recovery, and overtraining may sometimes be monitored by tracking hormonal responses and adaptations to training.

TRAINING EFFECT OF A SINGLE SESSION

The hormonal response to a single training session can help the coach determine whether the desired training stimulus is being applied (64). The responses of testosterone, cortisol, and growth hormone can help determine the anabolic characteristics of the training stimulus. It has even been suggested that the thyroid hormones and insulin be also monitored for this reason, since they have also been associated with anabolic responses of muscle.

TRAINING INTENSITY OF A SINGLE SESSION

It has been suggested that supporting information on whether proper training intensities have been applied can be deduced from the acute hormonal profiles. If hormonal responses are typically monitored, then it may be possible to evaluate whether the prescribed intensity is appropriate based on the responses of intensity-dependent hormones (64).

A training session may be designed that optimizes or minimizes the anabolic hormonal responses.

DIAGNOSING FATIGUE

All coaches and athletes would like to know how well the training program is being tolerated (17,18,64). When the training becomes excessive, it is critical to detect this problem before it turns into a long-term overtraining syndrome. To properly do this, hormonal variables must be measured on a regular basis to determine normal values for each individual. Possible variables to monitor include testosterone, cortisol, the testosterone/cortisol ratio, and the catecholamines. It is important to remember that just because some of the endocrine variables change, this does not mean that overtraining has occurred or that excessive fatigue exists. It may, however, serve as a warning of impending problems.

MONITORING RECOVERY

Once normal hormonal levels have been determined for an individual, it is possible to find out when a fatigued individual returns to prefatigue states (64). Any hormone or neurohormone that responds to training stress may have to return to normal levels for that individual before physiological recovery is considered complete. This may be a critical step in assessing whether a periodized training program has been designed to adequately permit recovery during certain phases of the training.

OPTIMIZING THE TRAINING PROGRAM

The ultimate challenge for the reader of this chapter is to utilize the information provided in designing a strength and conditioning program. Such a program will, of course, depend on the desired goals determined for the specific purpose of the training. Although numerous physiological systems of the body must be considered, insight on the development of training programs can be deduced from the endocrine data available.

Goal: Muscle Hypertrophy

In designing a program where muscle hypertrophy is a primary objective, it will be important to design the training stimulus to optimize the anabolic hormone response. For example, growth-hormone responses are optimized when large-muscle-mass exercises are used with approximately 10-RM loads, while rest intervals are kept fairly short (1 minute or less). Additionally, some work with relatively heavy loads is necessary to optimize the acute testosterone response.

Goal: No Muscle Hypertrophy

Some sports may require an individual to maintain a certain body weight (e.g., weight-class sports, activities where a large body mass is not desired). In designing a program for such individuals, it may be wise to minimize the anabolic hormone

response. For example, avoiding large-muscle-mass exercises may minimize some of the growth-hormone response to a training session. Of course, this is also dependent on the intensities and rest intervals prescribed. In some cases, large-muscle-mass, multijoint exercises are necessary for the purposes of the training. In such instances, allowing longer rest intervals will definitely minimize the growth-hormone response.

Goal: High-Power Performance

It has been suggested that optimal power performances occur when resting testosterone concentrations are relatively high (6). If this is the case, the training program must permit a long-term elevation in resting testosterone levels. One method of doing this is by decreasing the training stresses (i.e., decreasing volume and/or intensity) during the taper phase (33). Additionally, chronic utilization of high relative intensities using high-power, large-muscle-mass exercises may contribute to slight elevations of long-term resting levels of testosterone (32).

Goal: Peak Performance

If a performance peak is desired, the preceding training taper must permit the resting concentrations of certain hormones to be adequately recovered. In this case, decreasing the volume-load (reps times weight) can result in elevations of resting testosterone and increases in the testosterone/cortisol ratio (33).

Goal: Avoiding Overtraining

Although many factors can contribute to overtraining and the accompanying decreases in performance, several easily administered training variables can help (17). When training volumes and volume loads have been high, small but critical decreases in either volume or relative intensity can result in the avoidance of overtraining. Although not always the case, high volumes of resistance exercise typically depress resting testosterone and the testosterone/cortisol ratio. Simply providing a day of recovery each week, or at least a sharp decrease in volume (and usually intensity), may avoid such a problem. Such an alteration in training volume is easy to administer but often ignored.

SUMMARY

The endocrine system comprises complex interactions of hormones and neurohormones with each other and other physiological systems. Proper responses of the endocrine system are essential for optimal adaptations to a training program. Although you may not have the ability to measure and analyze these variables, a thorough understanding of how the body responds and adapts to the stresses applied is imperative for developing truly effective programs and understanding why they are effective. Last, understanding how the endocrine system responds to the various acute training variables makes it possible to design a training prescription that provides an optimal hormonal environment for the desired results.

MAXING OUT

1. Using this text and other resources, review the hormonal response to resistance training in both men and women and explain how they differ.
2. Using this text and other resources, explain the hormonal response to prolonged endurance exercise.
3. Use this text and other resources to discuss overtraining relative to hormone levels in the body. Can monitoring of hormonal levels be used to predict overtraining?

REFERENCES

1. Adlercreutz H, Harkonen M, Kuoppasalmi K, et al. Effect of training on plasma anabolic and catabolic steroid hormones and their response during physical exercise. Int J Sports Med 1986;7;S27–S28.
2. Atgie C, D'Allaire F, Bukowiecki LJ. Role of beta1 and beta3 adrenoceptors in the regulation of lipolysis and thermogenesis in rat brown adipocytes. Am J Physiol 1997;273:C1136–C1142.
3. Baker ER, Mathur RS, Kirk RF, et al. Plasma gonadotropins, prolactin, and steroid hormone concentrations in female runners immediately after a long-distance run. Fertil Steril 1984;38:38–41.
4. Bonen A, Ling WYU, MacIntyre KP, et al. Effects of exercise on the serum concentrations of FSH, LH, progesterone, and estradiol. Eur J Appl Physiol 1979;42:15–23.
5. Borer K. Exercise Endocrinology. Champaign, IL: Human Kinetics, 2003:45.
6. Bosco C, Tihanyi J, Viru A. Relationship between field fitness test and basal serum testosterone and cortisol levels in soccer players. Clin Physiol 1996;16:317–322.
7. Brandenberger G, Follenius M. Influence of timing and intensity of muscle exercise on temporal patterns of plasma cortisol levels. J Clin Endocrinol Metab 1975;40: 845–849.
8. Cannon WB. Bodily changes in pain, hunger, fear, and rage. New York: Appleton, 1922.
9. Christensen NJ, Galbo H, Hansen JF, et al. Catecholamines and exercise. Diabetes 1979;28:58–62.
10. Clark JH, Schrader WT, O'Malley BW. Mechanisms of action of steroid hormones. In: Wilson JD, Foster DW, eds. Williams Textbook of Endocrinology. 8th ed. Philadelphia: Saunders, 1992:35–90.
11. Cumming DC, L. A. Brunsting LA III, Strich G, et al. Reproductive hormone increases in response to acute exercise in men. Med Sci Sports Exerc 1986;18:369–373.
12. Czeisler CA, Klerman EB. Circadian and sleep-dependent regulation of hormone release in humans. Rec Progr Horm Res 1999;54:97–130.
13. Fahey TD, Rolph R, Moungmee P, et al. Serum testosterone, body composition, and strength of young adults. Med Sci Sports 1976;8:31–34.
14. Feyrter F. Ueber die These von den peripheren endokrinen Druesen. Wien Zeitschr Inn Med 1946;27:9–38.
15. Fleck SJ, Kraemer WJ. Designing Resistance Exercise Programs. 2nd ed. Champaign, IL: Human Kinetics, 1997.
16. Francesconi RP, Sawka MN, Pandolf KB, et al. Plasma hormonal responses at graded hypohydration levels during exercise-heat stress. J Appl Physiol 1985;59:1855–1860.
17. Fry AC. Overload and regeneration during resistance exercise. In: Lehmann M, Foster C, Gastmann U, et al, eds. Overload, Performance Incompetence, and Regeneration in Sport. New York: Kluwer Academic/Plenum, 1999.
18. Fry AC, Kraemer WJ. Resistance exercise overtraining and overreaching: neuroendocrine responses. Sports Med 1997;23(2):106–129.
19. Fry AC, Kraemer WJ, Ramsey LT. Pituitary-adrenal-gonadal responses to high-intensity resistance exercise overtraining. J Appl Physiol 1998;85(6):2352–2359.
20. Fry AC, Kraemer WJ, van Borselen F, et al. Catecholamine responses to short-term high-intensity resistance exercise overtraining. J Appl Physiol 1994;77(2):941–946.
21. Fry AC, Kraemer WJ, Stone MH, et al. Endocrine and performance responses to high volume training and amino acid supplementation in elite junior weightlifters. Int J Sport Nutr 1993;3(3):306–322.
22. Fry AC, Kraemer WJ, Stone MH, et al. Endocrine responses to over-reaching before and after 1 year of weightlifting training. Can J Appl Physiol 1994;19(4): 400–410.
23. Galbo H. Hormonal and Metabolic Adaptation to Exercise. New York: Thieme-Stratton, 1983.
24. Gilman AG. G-proteins and regulation of adenyl cyclase. JAMA 1989;262:1819–1825.
25. Glass CK. Differential recognition of target genes by nuclear receptor monomers, dimers, and heterodimers. Endocrinol Rev 1994;15:391–407.
26. Goodman HM. Basic Medical Endocrinology. New York: Raven Press, 1988:103.
27. Gotschalk LA, Loetbel DD, Nindl BC, et al. Hormonal responses of multi-set versus single-set heavy resistance exercise protocols. Can J Appl Physiol 1997;22(3): 244–255.
28. Guezennec Y, Leger L, Lhoste F, et al. Hormone and metabolite response to weight-lifting training sessions. Int J Sports Med 1986;7:100–105.
29. Hakkinen K. Neuromuscular and hormonal adaptations during strength and power training. J Sports Med Phys Fit 1989;29:9–24.

30. Hakkinen K, Pakarinen A, Alen M, Komi PV. Serum hormones during prolonged training of neuromuscular performance. Eur J Appl Physiol 1985;53:287–293.

31. Hakkinen K, Pakarinen A, Alen M, et al. Daily hormonal and neuromuscular responses to intensive strength training in 1 week. Int J Sports Med 1988;9:422–428.

32. Hakkinen K, Pakarinen A, Alen M, et al. Neuromuscular and hormonal adaptations in athletes to strength training in two years. J Appl Physiol 1988;65(6):2406–2412.

33. Hakkinen K, Pakarinen A, Alen M, et al. Relationships between training volume, physical performance capacity and serum hormone concentrations during prolonged training in elite weight lifters. Int J Sports Med 1987; 8(Suppl):61–65.

34. Hakkinen K, Pakarinen A. Acute hormonal responses to two different fatiguing heavy-resistance protocols in male athletes. J Appl Physiol 1993;74(2):882–887.

35. Harber MP, Fry AC, Rubin JC, et al. Skeletal muscle and hormonal adaptations to circuit weight training. Scand J Med Sci Sports 2004;14(3):176–185.

36. Hebener JF. Genetic control of hormone function. In: Wilson JD, Foster DW, eds. Williams Textbook of Endocrinology. 8th ed. Philadelphia: Saunders, 1992:9–34.

37. Hoffman J. Physiological Aspects of Sport Training and Performance. Champaign, IL: Human Kinetics, 2002:15–26.

38. Hokin LE. Receptors and phosphoinositide-generated second messengers. Annu Rev Biochem 1985;54:202–235.

39. Houk JC. Control strategies in physiological systems. FASEB J 1988;2:97–107.

40. Kahn CR, Smith RJ, Chin WW. Mechanism of action of hormones that act at the cell surface. In: Wilson JD, Foster DW, eds. Williams Textbook of Endocrinology. 8th ed. Philadelphia: Saunders, 1992:91–134.

41. Kinderman W, Schnabel A, Schmitt WM, et al. Catecholamines, growth hormone, cortisol, insulin, and sex hormones in anaerobic and aerobic exercise. Eur J Appl Physiol 1982;49:389–399.

42. Kjaer M, Galbo H. Effect of physical training on the capacity to secrete epinephrine. J Appl Physiol 1988;64:11–16.

43. Kotchen TA, Hartley LH, Rice TW, et al. Renin, norepinephrine, and epinephrine responses to graded exercise. J Appl Physiol 1971;31:178–184.

44. Kraemer WJ. Endocrine responses and adaptations to strength training. In: Komi PV, ed. Strength and Power in Sport. Oxford, UK: Blackwell, 1992:291–304.

45. Kraemer WJ, Fry AD, Warren BJ, et al. Acute hormonal responses in elite junior weightlifters. Int J Sports Med 1992;13(2):103–109.

46. Kraemer WJ, Koziris LP. Olympic weightlifting and power lifting. In: Lamb DR, Knuttgen HG, Murray R, eds. Physiology and Nutrition for Competitive Sport. Carmel, IN: Cooper Publishing, 1994:1–54.

47. Kraemer WJ, Marchitelli L, McCurry R, et al. Hormonal and growth factor responses to heavy resistance exercise. J Appl Physiol 1990;69(4):1442–1450.

48. Landsberg L, Young JB. Catecholamines and the adrenal medulla. In: Wilson JD, Foster DW, eds. Williams Textbook of Endocrinology. 8th ed. Philadelphia: Saunders, 1992:621–705.

49. Lassare C, Girard F, Durand J, Reynaud J. Kinetics of human growth hormone during submaximal exercise. J Appl Physiol 1974;37:826–830.

50. Lehmann M, Foster C, Netzer N, et al. Physiological responses to short- and long-term overtraining in endurance athletes. In: Kreider RB, Fry AC, O'Toole ML, eds. Overtraining in Sport. Champaign, IL: Human Kinetics, 1998: 19–46.

51. Lehmann, M, Gastmann U, Petersen KG, et al. Training-overtraining: performance, and hormone levels, after a defined increase in training volume vs training intensity in experienced middle- and long-distance runners. Br J Sports Med 1992;26:233–242.

52. Lehmann M, Gastmann U, Baur S, et al. Selected parameters and mechanisms of peripheral and central fatigue and regeneration in overtrained athletes. In: Lehmann M, Foster C, Gastmann U, et al, eds. Overload, Performance Incompetence, and Regeneration in Sport. New York: Kluwer Academic/Plenum, 1999:7–26.

53. McMurray RG, Hackney AC. Endocrine responses to exercise and training. In: Garrett WE, Kirkendall DT, eds. Exercise and Sport Science. Philadelphia: Lippincott, Williams & Wilkins, 2000:135–164.

54. Mendel CM. The free hormone hypothesis: a physiologically based mathematical model. Endocr Rev 1989;10: 232–274.

55. Ojeda SR, Griffin JE. Organization of the endocrine system. In: Ojeda SR, Griffin JE, eds. Textbook of Endocrine Physiology. New York: Oxford University Press, 1988:3–16.

56. Schilling BK, Fry AC, Ferkin MH, Leonard ST. Hormonal responses to free-weight and machine exercise [abstract]. Med Sci Sports Exerc 2001;33(5 Suppl):S270.

57. Selye H. The Stress of Life. New York: McGraw-Hill, 1956.

58. Sporn MB, Todaro GJ. Autocrine secretion and malignant transformation of cells. N Engl J Med 1980;303:878–880.

59. Sutton JR, Farrell PA, Harber VJ. Hormonal adaptations to physical activity. In: Bouchard C, Shephard RJ, Stephens T, et al, eds. Exercise, Fitness, and Health. Champaign, IL: Human Kinetics, 1990:217–257.

60. Thuma JR, Gilders R, Verdun J, Loucks A. Circadian rhythm of cortisol confounds cortisol responses to exercise: implications for future research. J Appl Physiol 1995;78(5): 1657–1664.

61. Tidgren B. Hjemdal; P. Theodorsson E, et al. Renal neurohormonal and vascular responses to dynamic exercise in humans. J Appl Physiol 1991;70:2279–2286.

62. Vanhelder WP, Radomski MW, Goode RC. Growth hormone responses during intermittent weight lifting exercise in men. Eur J Appl Physiol 1984;53(1):31–34.

63. Veldhuis JD, Johnson LM. Cluster analysis: a simple, versatile, and robust algorithm for endocrine pulse detection. Am J Physiol 1988;250:E486–E493.

64. Viru A, Viru M. Biochemical Monitoring of Sport Training. Champaign, IL: Human Kinetics, 2001:61–65.

65. Weiss LW, Cureton KJ, Thompson FN. Comparison of serum testosterone and androstenedione responses to weightlifting in men and women. Eur J Appl Physiol 1983;50(3):413–419.

66. Wilkerson JE, Gutin B, Horvath SM. Exercise-induced changes in blood, red cell, and plasma volumes in man. Med Sci Sports 1977;9:155–158.

67. Wilson JD, Foster DW, eds. Williams Textbook of Endocrinology. Philadelphia: Saunders, 1992: inside front cover.

68. Winder, WW, Hickson RC, Hagberg JM, et al. Training-induced changes in hormonal and metabolic responses to submaximal exercise. J Appl Physiol 1979;46:766–771.

69. Young DS. Implementation of SI units for clinical laboratory data. Ann Intern Med 1987;106:114–128.

Nutrition

JOSÉ ANTONIO
JOHN BERARDI
CHRISTOPHER R. MOHR

Introduction

Nutritional intake is essential to optimizing the performance adaptations initiated in the gym, on the track, or on the field. Of the modifiable factors contributing to optimal exercise performance, nutritional intake is one of the most easily utilized. Although training adaptations can take weeks to occur, several acute nutritional manipulations—such as caffeine ingestion (57), carbohydrate supplementation during endurance exercise (63,64), glucose-electrolyte beverage consumption while training in hot environments (95,139), or creatine supplementation (72,134)—have a much more rapid impact on performance. Habitually meeting macro- and micronutrient needs during periods of heavy training can improve muscle protein turnover (the breakdown of old tissue and the rebuilding of new, more functionally adapted tissue) (12–14,22, 35,102,111,129) as well as the function and recovery of the nervous system (19,42,84), immune system (17,18,92), and musculoskeletal system (62,68, 77,83,93,100,101,114). Strength and conditioning professionals must impress on their athletes the importance of understanding how to appropriately fuel the body for the demands of specific training for programs and sports. Those coaches who do not will limit their own efficacy in terms of helping their athlete to improve.

ENERGY NEEDS

Energy balance is the relationship between energy ingested and energy expended. It is an important determinant of exercise performance, body composition, training adaptation, and optimal physiological functioning in athletes (117) and in the general exercising population. Unfortunately, many people have an overly simplistic view of energy balance. It is often incorrectly assumed that total energy intake is predominantly related to weight gain or loss. For example, if an athlete wants to lose body fat or overall mass, eating less will produce a negative energy balance. Figure 7.1 lists the factors involved in both caloric intake and caloric expenditure. Our body absorbs 90% to 95% of the calories taken in, so caloric intake is not 100% efficient. Many factors relate to energy expenditure, some of which are not affected by diet and exercise.

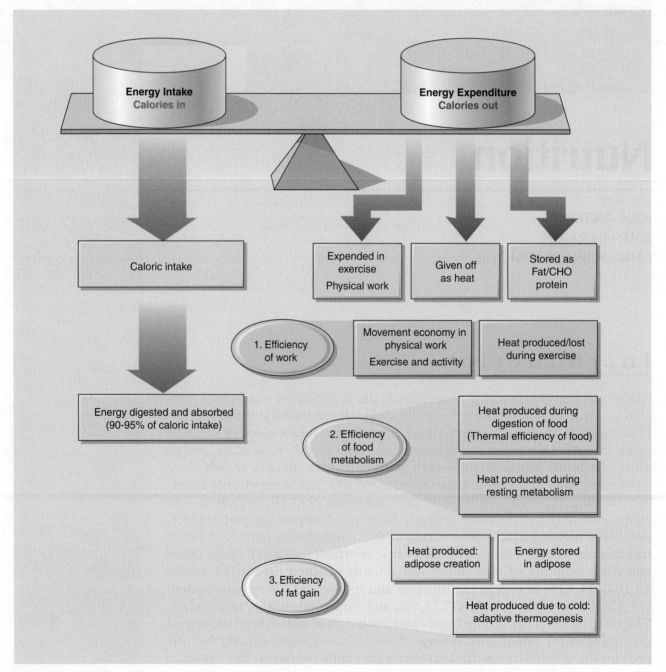

FIGURE 7.1 Factors related to the efficiency of energy intake and expenditure. (Reproduced with permission from Rampone AJ, Reynolds PJ. Obesity: thermodynamic principles in perspective. Life Sci 1988;43:93–110.)

Figure 7.2 demonstrates the relationship between energy intake and energy consumption. This relationship determines how energy intake will affect body mass and composition. Decreasing caloric intake will slow the athlete's metabolic rate and muscle mass will be compromised (10), with a negative effect on performance. Optimal performance and health are related to total energy intake, metabolic rate, tissue turnover, and muscle mass (27,117).

Since the micronutrient content of the diet is closely related to energy intake, decreases in energy consumption may lead to nutrient deficiencies. Therefore, athletes should eat nutrient-dense foods to increase the ratio of nutrients ingested to energy ingested. **Nutrient density** is the amount of nutrients (carbohydrate, protein, fat, vitamins, minerals) per unit of energy in a given food. For example, athletes who habitually eat sugary breakfast cereals in an attempt to increase carbohydrate intake would benefit from exchanging these cereals for a combination of fruits, vegetables, and a whole

grain like oatmeal. These latter foods are not only more nutrient-dense but they also have more fiber and a lower glycemic index, which means that they cause less of an increase in blood sugar than more refined carbohydrates. **Glycemic index** is a term that describes how rapidly and how long a specific carbohydrate increases blood glucose. Foods with a glycemic index greater than 100 raises blood glucose more rapidly, whereas foods with a glycemic index of less than 100 raise blood glucose more slowly. In addition, high-fiber and low-glycemic carbohydrates play a role in improving health and body composition. Table 7.1 lists the glycemic indexes of common sources of carbohydrates.

Athletes must find ways to consume more food energy while maintaining an optimal body composition and body mass for their specific activity. Although it may seem counterintuitive to suggest that an individual can lose fat mass while eating more food, taking advantage of appropriate food selection and strategic nutrient timing can accomplish both goals (11,44,45,49,54,78,83,111,116,

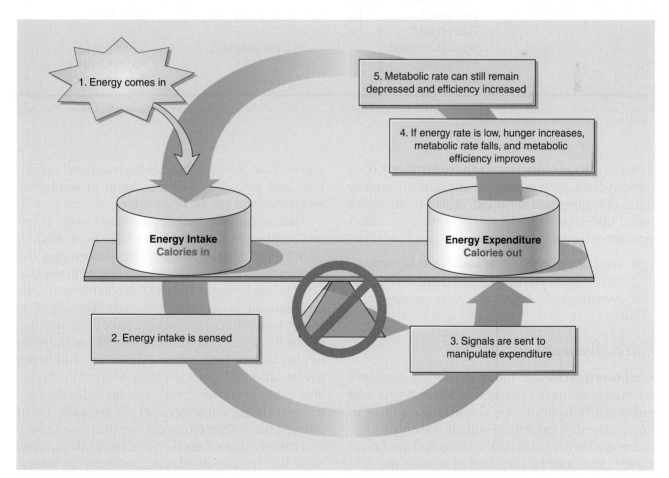

FIGURE 7.2 The relationship between energy intake and expenditure. This relationship determines how energy intake will affect body mass and composition.

TABLE 7.1	THE GLYCEMIC INDEX OF COMMON SOURCES OF CARBOHYDRATES		
GLYCEMIC INDEX	**SOURCE**	**GLYCEMIC INDEX**	**SOURCE**
Extremely high (greater than 100)	Cake, doughnut Waffles Gatorade Bagel Pretzels Corn flakes cereal Cheerios Rice Chex cereal Rice Krispies cereal Watermelon Popcorn Jellybeans	Moderately high (60–80)	Cranberry juice cocktail Tomato juice Vanilla ice cream Banana Grapes Orange Baked beans Chicken nuggets Spaghetti Chocolate milk Power bar
Glycemic standard = 100% High (80–100)	Bread, white Angel-food cake Pound cake Bran muffin Pastry Coca-Cola (250 mL) Orange juice Pineapple juice Corn chips Oat bread Pita bread Special K cereal Pineapple White rice	Moderate (40–60) Low (less than 40)	Apple Apple juice Super supreme pizza (Pizza Hut) All-bran cereal Skim milk Yogurt Peanut M&Ms Butter beans Split peas Chickpeas Kidney beans Peanuts

Source: Adapted with permission from Foster-Powell K, Holt SHA, Brand-Miller JC. International table of glycemic index and glycemic load values: 2002. Am J Clin Nutr [Special Article] 2002;76:5–56.

118,134). Examining each **macronutrient** (i.e., carbohydrate, protein, and fat) and how to optimize times of feeding will allow individuals to develop a better understanding of how these strategies affect strength athletes.

Total energy intake is the single most important dietary factor governing the adaptive response of strength-power athletes to exercise training.

Carbohydrate Intake

Carbohydrates are foods that are commonly referred to as sugars, starches, cellulose (fiber), and gums. Carbohydrates are the primary source of energy for physical activity and are the only source of energy for the brain and nervous system. Structurally, they can be classified as mono-, di-, tri-, and polysaccharides. The smallest carbohydrates are the single-unit monosaccharides, like glucose

and sucrose. Polysaccharides such as starch, cellulose, and glycogen are long chains of saccharide molecules and can be quite large.

Dietary carbohydrate intake has become a controversial topic. Carbohydrates have been demonized in the media, with some challenging the high-carbohydrate suggestions inherent in the U.S. Food Guide Pyramid and the Canadian Food Guide and instead suggesting low-carbohydrate diets (123). Some short-term studies have demonstrated that a lower carbohydrate intake leads to better overall weight loss, losses in body fat, and better preservation of muscle mass. Moreover, favorable changes in triglycerides and high-density lipoprotein (HDL) cholesterol (137) typically occur when carbohydrate intakes are decreased. Very low carbohydrate diets (i.e., ketogenic diets), however, will reduce an athlete's total energy intake, impair intense exercise performance, reduce work capacity, suppress immune function, and increase perception of effort during normal exercise tasks (59,75,76,89). These data lead to the suggestion that although athletes could potentially benefit from a slight reduction in carbohydrate intake during rest periods and training periods of low volume/intensity, it is generally not recommended that strength-power athletes restrict carbohydrate to less than 10% of total energy intake.

Although some authors recommend that as much as 70% of the diet come from carbohydrates, this amount may displace dietary protein and fat and also make fat loss more difficult, particularly if more refined carbohydrates are chosen rather than whole grains. Instead of a chronic high-carbohydrate diet, a better strategy might be to emphasize carbohydrate type (e.g., whole grain versus refined carbohydrates) and timing (before, during, and after a workout).

The data are clear that carbohydrates are important in an athletic population. Higher-carbohydrate diets can lead to increased concentrations of muscle glycogen and may therefore delay fatigue (60,106), prevent exercise-stress-induced immunosuppression (15,16,18), and—when combined with protein during the exercise and postexercise periods—stimulate an increase in muscle protein synthesis and glycogen resynthesis (62,74,91, 105,131). Athletes, however, often consume the wrong types of carbohydrates at the wrong times. Rather than simply ingesting large amounts of "empty" calories during the day, athletes should replace their high-glycemic-index, nutrient-devoid carbohydrate choices with lower-glycemic, high-fiber carbohydrate choices. The term **empty calorie** refers to a food that offers no nutritional value other than energy itself. Foods such as legumes; whole grains; minimally processed breads, pastas, and other grains; fruits; and vegetables are digested more slowly and provide more continuous energy throughout the day. By substituting better carbohydrate choices and timing carbohydrates appropriately, athletes will be better able to manage daily energy fluctuations, ingest their daily recommendation of fiber, lose fat while preserving muscle mass, and reduce the chances of developing the micronutrient deficiencies that are common in athletic populations (60). On the contrary, higher-glycemic carbohydrates can be ingested after exercise to promote recovery and glycogen storage—a source of rapid energy when it is most needed (during training and competition). This is the time when the large insulin response that accompanies

the ingestion of high-glycemic carbohydrates may lead to an improvement in muscle recovery. By following these recommendations, athletes may be better able to manage body composition while enhancing recovery.

> *Different types of carbohydrates confer different physiological responses. The majority of one's caloric intake should be derived from the consumption of unprocessed, high-fiber carbohydrates.*

Protein Intake

Protein is composed of individual amino acids, which join together to form peptide chains. Although the structure of each peptide chain is unique, the overall peptide structures collectively are known as proteins. Of the 20 amino acids, 9 are indispensable or **essential** (the term *essential* as it relates to nutrition describes nutrients that you must consume, because your body does not make them endogenously); that is, they must come from the diet. As a result of the essentiality of these amino acids, protein, unlike carbohydrate, must be present in the diet. The **RDA** (recommended dietary allowance) for dietary protein in sedentary individuals is 0.8 g of protein per kilogram of body mass. Very few athletes are at risk for a true protein deficiency, although some scientists have suggested that athletes may need more protein than their sedentary counterparts (1.5 to 2.0 g/kg body mass). Whether or not this is true and athletes actually *need* more protein (to prevent a negative nitrogen status and protein wasting) has been debated extensively and inconclusively (29,80,81,108–110). More important for sports nutrition is the question of optimization.

Many athletes may benefit from a higher dietary protein intake (23,24,26,31,34,44,77,79,81,85,115) that exceeds their calculated protein needs. Certain populations will have higher protein needs: young athletes who are still growing, athletes training for strength and muscle mass, athletes in contact sports, and women who are pregnant. At times, more than one of these situations may be present in the same athlete, thus further increasing his or her protein needs.

Athletes will often self-select a protein intake that is higher than conventionally recommended. In seeking to optimize an athlete's protein intake, a simple rule of thumb is to plan the athlete's diet from the foundation of 1g of protein per pound of body mass (2.2 g/kg body mass). This is easier for the athlete to understand and monitor and provides a small safety factor to ensure adequate protein intake. Once the protein intake is fixed, carbohydrate and fat intakes must be added to meet total daily energy needs. The best way to optimize an athlete's protein intake would be to experiment with a variety of levels of dietary protein and assess outcomes in terms of personal performance and body composition to determine which intake leads to the best response. Nutritional strategies should always be evaluated using an outcome-based approach.

In addition to experimenting with overall protein intake, it is important to make sure that a large percentage of daily protein comes from complete protein sources (proteins that contain all the essential amino acids). Even if an adequate total daily protein intake is ingested, if the protein is from an incomplete protein source (e.g., rice, grains, etc.), the athlete may experience suboptimal adaptation to training. This situation can be improved by either ensuring that most of the dietary protein is from complete protein sources (e.g., animal proteins, including eggs and dairy products) or by consuming enough total energy with sufficient amounts of incomplete proteins. Animal proteins are important not only as sources of complete protein but also because they provide a number of highly bioavailable nutrients, such as B vitamins, zinc, and iron, of which deficiency is more prevalent in an athletic population. Finally, no current evidence shows that healthy individuals would experience harm due to a higher-protein diet (25,103,121).

Strength-power athletes need more protein than the RDA. Moreover, no evidence exists that the consumption of protein at levels two to three times the RDA is harmful to otherwise healthy individuals.

Fat Intake

Despite years of antifat sentiment, especially among athletes, it has becoming clear that dietary fat is essential to the athlete's nutrition program. The three main types of dietary fatty acids are saturated fatty acids, monounsaturated fatty acids, and polyunsaturated fatty acids (omega-3 and omega-6 fats are both types of polyunsaturated fatty acids). **Fatty acids** are the main storage form of fat.

Triglycerides are formed from a glycerol skeleton with three *fatty acids* attached. Each of the three types of fats offers unique benefits. In the past, a simplistic view of fat was adopted because coaches and athletes believed that dietary fat made you fat; however, research has demonstrated this to be false (138). In fact, some fats (known as essential fatty acids) are absolutely necessary for survival. In addition, the right kinds of dietary fat can improve body composition by promoting fat loss (8,56,73,96,124). Furthermore, certain fats can improve training hormonal status (46,107), increase the body's ability to store glycogen (43), increase the body's ability to burn fat (43,56,124), and improve overall health by providing anti-inflammatory, anticarcinogenic, antioxidant, and antithrombotic effects (53,122). With this list of benefits, it should be clear that fat avoidance is both difficult and nonproductive. Although the American Dietetic Association recommends that less than 30% of the diet of a sedentary individual should come from fat, research suggests that athletes should ingest approximately 30% of the diet as fat as long as the individual proportions of fatty acids are distributed appropriately. For optimal health and performance, a balanced approach toward fat consumption is warranted; approximately 10% of dietary energy should come from saturated sources (e.g., whole-fat dairy, animal fats, etc.), approximately 10% from monounsaturated sources (many vegetable fats, especially olive oil), and approximately 10% from polyunsaturated sources (predominantly vegetable fats, especially flaxseed and fish oils). Of the polyunsaturated fats, approximately 50% should come from omega-6 fatty acids and approximately 50% from omega-3 fatty acids. It is important to realize that the distribution of fatty acids in the diet is as important as the absolute amount of fat. Therefore, athletes should pay attention to both.

A final consideration related to fat consumption is trans fat. **Trans fats** are artificial fats created when polyunsaturated vegetables oils (high in omega-6 fatty acids) are combined with hydrogen molecules to increase shelf life and stabilize the polyunsaturated oil. This process makes nonhydrogenated fat similar to saturated fat (which is naturally saturated with hydrogen), which can produce "bad" LDL cholesterol and potentially lead to heart disease. According to the *American Journal of Clinical Nutrition,* over 30,000 deaths per year are attributed to the consumption of trans fat (3,120). Consumption of trans fats leads to the inhibition of several critical enzymatic processes in the body, blood lipid abnormalities, and an increased risk of cardiovascular disease (3). Unfortunately, trans fats are found in many processed foods. Any food that lists hydrogenated or partially hydrogenated fats on the ingredient list contains trans fats.

 It is important that athletes consume predominantly unsaturated fats. Both athletes and the general population should limit (but not eliminate) saturated fats in their diets.

TRAINING NUTRITION

During and after training and competition, the energy demands of the body are high (32,115,130), fluid needs increase (36,41,69,95,139), insulin sensitivity and glucose tolerance are dramatically improved (33,55,61,97,98), and skeletal muscle is primed for anabolism as long as amino acids are provided (22,83,105,110,128,129). Nutrition during and after exercise should focus on providing carbohydrate energy, preventing dehydration, stimulating glycogen resynthesis, and stimulating increases in skeletal muscle protein synthesis. As indicated, during the workout and postworkout periods, insulin sensitivity and glucose tolerance are improved and the efficiency of glycogen storage is highest. This makes the postworkout period the best time to ingest a larger amount of carbohydrate. In addition, since a large increase in insulin can facilitate a greater glycogen resynthesis and muscle protein synthesis, higher-glycemic-index carbohydrates (i.e., sports drinks containing glucose or glucose polymers) should be ingested during these times. By providing a large amount of carbohydrate during this critical period, fewer carbohydrates can be ingested during the remainder of the day while also achieving better control of body composition and promoting maximal recovery. As a starting point, athletes could begin by ingesting liquid carbohydrate-protein supplements immediately prior to (128) or during exercise (63,95) as well as immediately after exercise (62,83,105,128,131,132) so as to promote recovery. To facilitate fluid replacement as well as rapid energy delivery, the two beverages should be diluted to 8% to 12% concentrations (80 to 120 g of substrate per 1000 mL of water) and should provide approximately 0.8 g of

carbohydrate and 0.4 g protein per kilogram of body mass. It is important to experiment with differing amounts of energy to determine the best composition for each individual athlete. Box 7.1 provides tips for achieving good nutrition.

NUTRIENT TIMING

An exciting new avenue of research is the area of **nutrient timing**, the specific time at which you consume certain nutrients to enhance the adaptive response to exercise. Certainly, we know that the composition of the food you ingest is important for promoting gains in muscle protein; however, the timing of nutrient consumption may be just as important.

> **7.1 SEVEN SIMPLE TIPS FOR ACHIEVING GOOD NUTRITION**
>
> 1. Eat about six meals each day. For instance, this would include breakfast, a midmorning meal, lunch, a midafternoon meal, a postworkout meal, dinner, and another meal before bedtime. On days you do not train, obviously skip the postworkout meal.
> 2. The bulk of your food should come from unprocessed carbohydrate foods (e.g., vegetables of all kinds, oatmeal, brown rice, yams, sweet potatoes, etc.).
> 3. Protein should be consumed; approximately 2 g of protein per kilogram of body weight; a more practical and easy-to-remember method is 1 g of protein per pound of body weight. (There is no harm in consuming this amount of protein.)
> 4. Unsaturated fats such as fish fat, fats from nuts and legumes, and olive oil are to be emphasized, but you still need to consume saturated fat (e.g., from beef, eggs, etc.) on occasion.
> 5. Always consume a postworkout carbohydrate-protein shake that consists of a high-glycemic carbohydrate and fast-absorbing protein (e.g., whey).
> 6. Limit your intake of processed carbohydrate. Simple or high-glycemic carbohydrates, however, should be consumed as part of your pre-, during-, and/or postworkout beverage.
> 7. Not including the window before, during, and after a workout, try limiting your consumption of liquid calories (e.g., soda, beer, etc.).

In a two-part study, scientists examined the effects on hormone response of a carbohydrate-only drink (1.2 g/kg per hour), and 0, 0.2, or 0.4 g/kg per hour of a protein hydrolysate and amino acid mixture(131). Eight male cyclists were tested under different dietary conditions in which they consumed these beverages every 30 minutes for 5 hours after a glycogen-depletion bike ride. They found that the beverages that contained 0.2 and 0.4 g of protein produced significantly superior insulin responses compared to the carbohydrate drink only. It is possible that the addition of protein to carbohydrates produces a superior anabolic effect through the insulin response. Additionally, the investigators took muscle biopsies from the athletes' thigh muscles to determine which beverages were best for replacing used glycogen. Again, the addition of protein to the carbohydrate beverage improved glycogen replacement.

In another study, subjects cycled intensely for 2.5 hours to fully deplete the muscle glycogen levels in their thigh muscles (62). Subjects supplemented immediately and 2 hours postexercise with the following:

- Group 1: carb-pro-fat (80 g carb, 28 g pro, 6 g fat)
- Group 2: carb-fat (108 g carb, 6 g fat)
- Group 3: carb-fat (80 g carb, 6 g fat)

Note that the beverages groups 1 and 2 consumed were isoenergetic, meaning they contained the same number of calories. After 4 hours of recovery, the investigators found that the greatest amount of muscle glycogen was replenished in group 1. Thus, the replacement of some carbohydrate with protein may expedite muscle glycogen repletion postexercise.

Other investigations have yielded similarly interesting results. Postexercise supplementation with added protein improved time to exhaustion during a test of endurance (116). Older men who consumed a protein supplement (10 g protein, 7 g carbohydrate, 3 g fat) immediately after training (12-week resistance training program, 3 days per week), had much better gains in strength, muscle fiber size, and lean body mass compared to the group who ingested the supplement 2 hours after training (49). It has been suggested that the availability of amino acids is more important than the availability of energy immediately postexercise to promote the repair and synthesis of muscle protein (82).

Other health benefits may attend ingesting protein immediately postexercise. In a study of healthy male recruits in the U.S. Marine Corps, subjects received a postexercise supplement during their 54-day basic training period, which was either a placebo (0 g carbohydrate, 0 g protein, 0 g fat), control (8, 0, 3), or protein supplement (3,8,10,50). The protein-supplemented group had an average of 33% fewer total medical visits, 28% fewer visits due to bacterial/viral infections, 37% fewer visits due to muscle/joint problems, and 83% fewer visits due to heat exhaustion compared with the placebo and control groups. Muscle soreness immediately postexercise was significantly reduced on both days 34 and 54 by protein supplementation but not by the placebo or control supplements.

Some evidence suggests that nutrient timing affects body composition (45). In one study, 17 slightly overweight men were put on a 12-week program consisting of mild caloric restriction (17% reduction) and a light resistance-exercise training program utilizing dumbbells. One group ingested a protein supplement (10 g protein, 7 g carbohydrate, 3.3 g fat, and 33% of the RDA for vitamins and minerals) immediately after exercise. The other group did not consume a supplement. Protein and energy intake were the same for both groups, and protein intake met the RDA. Both groups lost an equal amount of fat; however, the protein-supplemented group maintained fat-free mass (FFM), while the group that did not supplement lost FFM.

Although most studies have examined postworkout nutrition, some data are available that compare preworkout supplementation as well (129). Researchers compared the anabolic response of consuming a combination of an essential amino acid (6 g) plus carbohydrate (35 g sucrose) before versus after heavy resistance exercise. Phenylalanine uptake across the leg (a measure of muscle protein anabolism) over a 3-hour period was 160% greater when the amino acid/carbohydrate supplement was taken before versus after a workout. Thus, consuming the proper nutrients before exercise may possibly be more anabolic and facilitate recovery better than waiting until after exercise.

To optimize the adaptive response to exercise, all strength-power athletes should consume a carbohydrate-protein postworkout beverage. This may also be beneficial to the general exercising public to promote gains in lean muscle mass.

Carbohydrate-Protein Ratio

Controversy exists as to the correct or ideal combination of carbohydrate and protein consumed post-workout. It is difficult to make direct comparisons between investigations due to differences in subject population, treatment duration, the type of exercise performed, and nutrients ingested, etc. One can extrapolate from these studies, however, to suggest that timing may be as important (if not more so) as nutrient composition. For instance, you will find a carbohydrate-to-protein ratio of about 3:1 (approximately three times more carbohydrate than protein) and as low as 0.7:1 (30% less carbohydrate than protein) comparable for promoting recovery. Furthermore, the energy content of recovery supplements varies from 500 kcal to as little as 100 kcal. Therefore, sports nutritionists should consider each athlete individually to determine the most effective nutrient combinations for that person.

VITAMIN AND MINERAL INTAKE

Few studies have examined the micronutrient (vitamins and minerals) intakes of strength-power athletes. Clearly, however, suboptimal consumption of certain vitamins and minerals may predispose the individual to a number of diseases. For instance, according to one study,

> Suboptimal folic acid levels, along with suboptimal levels of vitamins B_6 and B_{12}, are a risk factor for cardiovascular disease, neural tube defects, and colon and breast cancer; low levels of vitamin D contribute to osteopenia and fractures; and low levels of the antioxidant vitamins (vitamins A, E, and C) may increase risk for several chronic diseases. Many people do not consume an optimal amount of all vitamins by diet alone. Subsequently, it appears prudent for all adults to take vitamin supplements, particularly with the mounting evidence of effectiveness from randomized trials (52).

At this moment it is not clear that consuming extra or supplemental vitamins can improve athletic performance. Some intriguing data on nutrient intakes in strength-power athletes, however, suggest a potential benefit of supplementing with specific micronutrients. One study compared nutrient intake data with blood lipids and anthropometric data in competitive male and female bodybuilders (6). Protein, fat, and carbohydrate intake provided 40, 12, and 48%, respectively, of total caloric intake. Vitamin C intake was less than 200 mg daily. Another study found that the average daily caloric intake (about 4,469 kcal), protein intake (about 252 g), as well as vitamin and mineral intakes of steroid-using bodybuilders greatly exceeded the U.S. RDA (70). Interestingly, however, vitamin B_6 intake in German strength and speed-power athletes was below the German RDA in more than 30% of the athletes surveyed (112).

Regardless of what the composite data may be regarding the average macro- or micronutrient intakes of athletes, one could certainly argue that these data are unimportant in counseling individual athletes. To assess whether an individual athlete is meeting his or her dietary needs, it is of no utility to draw conclusions based on the scientific literature. This is because each individual must have his or her food intake separately analyzed to determine whether alterations in a particular nutrition program may be of benefit.

> *It is impossible to determine an individual's macro- or micronutrient needs based on a composite picture derived from survey studies in the scientific literature.*

Vitamin E

Vitamin E is a fat-soluble vitamin that may have beneficial effects in athletes. For example, in one study, 12 weight-trained men were divided into two groups: one group received 1200 IU of Vitamin E once per day for 2 weeks while the control group received a cellulose-based placebo pill (90). Plasma creatine kinase (CK) levels (an indirect marker of muscle fiber injury) increased significantly in both groups after 24 and 48 hours; at 24 hours, however, the increase in CK was less in the vitamin E–supplemented group than in the placebo group. Plasma malondialdehyde (MDA), an indicator of free-radical interaction with cellular membranes, was elevated in both groups; however, MDA levels remained higher for a longer time in the placebo group. Thus, vitamin E may lessen the injury sustained by skeletal muscle fibers as a result of heavy resistance exercises; moreover, its antioxidant effects may be of potential benefit to athletes.

Other studies show a neutral effect of vitamin E supplementation. Young, healthy men performed about 240 maximal isokinetic eccentric muscle contractions (0.52 rad.s^{-1}) after supplementing with a placebo (safflower oil) or 1,200 IU of vitamin E daily for 30 days. These investigators found no differences in Z-band disruption, isometric and concentric torque, or serum CK values between the groups (7).

Furthermore, no effects of vitamin E supplementation (1200 IU for 3 weeks in non-resistance-trained men) were found on recovery responses to repeated bouts of resistance exercises. According to the investigators, "Vitamin E supplementation was not effective at attenuating putative markers of membrane damage, oxidative stress, and performance decrements after repeated bouts of whole-body concentric/eccentric resistance exercise" (4).

Vitamin C

Vitamin C is a water-soluble vitamin that is needed for collagen formation and may have beneficial effects for active individuals through its effects on cortisol and via an antioxidant effect.

Twenty-four physically active young subjects who ingested either vitamin C (400 mg), vitamin E (400 mg), or a placebo for 21 days before and 7 days after performing 60 minutes of box-stepping exercise were examined (65). The investigators tested the function of the triceps surae muscles and found that, compared to the placebo group, no significant alterations in maximal voluntary contraction (MVC) were found immediately after exercise; however, the recovery of MVC was superior in the vitamin C group during the first 24-hours after exercise. According to the study's authors, ". . . prior vitamin C supplementation may exert a protective effect against eccentric exercise-induced muscle damage." No effects were observed in the vitamin E–supplemented group.

One study had 16 male subjects randomized to a placebo or vitamin C group (125). These subjects performed a prolonged 90-minute intermittent shuttle-running test, and supplementation commenced after the cessation of exercise. That is, immediately after exercise, the subjects drank a 500-mL beverage containing 200 mg of vitamin C (or placebo) dissolved in solution. Later that same day and for the next 2 days, the subjects again consumed their treatment drinks. As a result, it was found that vitamin C supplementation had no effect on postexercise CK concentrations, muscle soreness, or muscle function of the leg extensors and flexors. Thus, in this investigation, short-term vitamin C supplementation had no effect. Other work by the same investigators found that the acute ingestion of 1 g of vitamin C 2 hours prior to exercise (90-minute intermittent shuttle running) was ineffective as an ergogenic aid (126). It should be noted that the aforementioned studies were very brief. It must be considered, then, whether they have relevance to "real-world" conditions in which athletes supplement with vitamin C (or other nutrients) for weeks, months, and perhaps years.

Certainly, longer or prolonged consumption of vitamin C must be further examined. In one study, 16 male subjects consumed either vitamin C (200 mg twice daily for 2 weeks) or placebo. Subjects performed 90 minutes of intermittent shuttle running 14 days after supplementation commenced. As a result, it was found that vitamin C did have beneficial effects on muscle soreness, muscle function, and plasma concentrations of serum malondialdehyde (127). A dose of 1,500 mg of vitamin C taken daily for 7 days before a 90-km marathon race, on race day, and for 2 days after the race has been found to attenuate increases in serum cortisol, adrenaline, and anti-inflammatory polypeptides (99). Whether this observation also applies to strength-power athletes is unclear.

Based on the very limited data on vitamins C and E, one can reasonably conclude that supplementation may have beneficial effects on a subset of individuals. There appear to be no deleterious effects on any of the parameters measured in published studies.

Minerals

Magnesium is an essential mineral that regulates neuromuscular, cardiovascular, immune, and hormonal function (20). Exercise may deplete magnesium, which—combined with inadequate intake—may impair energy metabolism. In a study investigating the effects of magnesium supplementation on strength development during a double-blind, 7-week strength training program, both groups involved gained strength; however, the magnesium-supplemented group demonstrated significantly better performance compared to the control group in absolute torque, relative torque adjusted for body weight (T/BWT), and rel-

Q & A from the Field

How does dehydration affect the strength-power athlete and what recommendations would you give to prevent the harm caused by fluid loss?

Dehydration refers to both hypohydration (being dehydrated prior to exercise) and to exercise-induced dehydration (i.e., that which develops during exercise). Inadequate fluid intake can adversely affect muscle metabolism, the regulation of body temperature, cardiovascular function (increased heart rate), and perceived exertion (more rapid development of fatigue).

Negative effects on performance have been demonstrated with modest (< 2% of body weight) dehydration. In one investigation, college wrestlers were actively dehydrated (4.9% of body weight), after which their upper body isokinetic performance was measured (136). There was a decrease in strength of 7.6% for lat pulldowns, 6.6% in chest push, and 12% in shoulder-press repetitions. In contrast, lower body musculature was not significantly affected by the 4.9% loss.

Many athletes are reluctant drinkers during exercise and do not ingest fluid at rates equal to their fluid loss. To promote proper hydration for athletes' optimal health and performance, follow these recommendations (39):

1. Athletes are advised to drink 14 to 22 oz of fluid 2 hours prior to exercise to promote adequate hydration and allow time for the excretion of excess ingested water.
2. During exercise, athletes should start drinking early into the workout and at regular intervals. If training continues for over 1 hour, a carbohydrate-containing beverage should be ingested at a rate of 30 to 60 g/hour to maintain oxidation of carbohydrates and delay fatigue.
3. Immediately after exercise; athletes should consume 16 to 24 oz of fluid for every pound of body weight lost during exercise. All athletes (strength, power, or endurance) need to maximize their fluid intake and employ behavioral strategies before, during, and after exercise to enhance their training and competitive performances. (Courtesy of Jennifer Hofheins, MS, RD, LD, of The Ohio Institute of Health & Human Performance.)

---

ative torque adjusted for lean body mass (T/LBM) when "before" values were used as the covariate.

The effects of 8 weeks of chromium supplementation in 36 weight-training men were also examined (88). Chromium supplementation increased serum chromium concentration and urinary chromium excretion. Nonetheless, there was no effect on body composition and strength. The preponderance of evidence suggests that chromium is ineffective as an ergogenic aid (30,86). It should be noted that the form of chromium(chloride versus picolinate) made no difference.

Zinc is a mineral required for the activity of more than 300 enzymes (47). Recently, it has been recognized that zinc may play an important role in thyroid hormone metabolism. The effects of zinc supplementation in athletes have been studied previously. Moreover, chronic exercise can have long-term effects on zinc metabolism (40). It has been reported that runners have lower plasma zinc levels than controls. One consequence of low serum zinc levels could be a reduction in muscle zinc concentrations, possibly resulting in a reduction in

endurance capacity. Zinc may also be acting directly at the membrane level; changes in extracellular zinc levels have been reported to influence the twitch-tension relationship in muscle. If one consumes an adequate diet rich in zinc, it is likely that zinc supplementation may be of no consequence to skeletal muscle or hormonal function. If one's diet is inadequate (e.g., vegetarians or individuals on low-energy diets), however, zinc supplementation may be considered.

Several reviews are available on mineral metabolism and exercise (38,48,86,87).

An examination of the scientific literature shows that vitamin and mineral supplementation either has a neutral or positive effect on various health and performance indexes in exercising individuals. As a strategy, it would make sense to consume a multivitamin as an "insurance policy" against poor eating habits. Eating a diet rich in unprocessed, high-fiber carbohydrates, lean meats, and other high-quality protein sources should form the basis of one's energy intake.

DIETS

Little research is available regarding dietary manipulation to improve performance relative to strength and size in comparison to improving performance in the endurance athlete (5). A number of different theories, beliefs, and recommendations from health professionals are available regarding the proper way to fuel the body for better performance. Although an infinite number of dietary prescriptions are available, essentially they fall into four overall categories: diets very high in carbohydrate and very low in fat (e.g., Pritikin and Ornish); high in carbohydrate and low in fat (e.g., the USDA MyPyramid food guide system, Fig. 7.3); very low in carbohydrate and high in protein and fat (e.g., Atkins or South Beach diets); and moderate in carbohydrate and higher in protein (e.g., Zone diet). Table 7.2 compares these approaches. Most people have their own dietary beliefs that may have worked for them or the athletes they train; significant scientific support exists, however, for each of the approaches mentioned above.

Eating disorders are a major concern with athletic and exercising populations. As exercise professionals, we must be aware of these disorders and be able to address the issue appropriately. This includes a basic understanding of the disorders and of the team approach to treatment (Box 7.2).

Very High Carbohydrate, Very Low Fat Diets

Carbohydrates are the sugars and starches and represent the primary macronutrient consumed by Americans. When we consider the dietary needs of a strength athlete, carbohydrates should be the base of a sound nutritional program. Carbohydrates provide the major source of energy for the athlete through the breakdown of glycogen (the storage form of carbohydrate) during exercise (1,9). Moreover, it is well established that an increased carbohydrate intake will delay fatigue (60,106) and can enhance postexercise protein synthesis alone (21) (though not to the same extent as amino acids) or synergistically when combined with protein during recovery (105,131). Although carbohydrates are a crucial part of a sound nutritional program for the strength athlete, they do not play the same role with the endurance athlete who uses up glycogen stores more rapidly

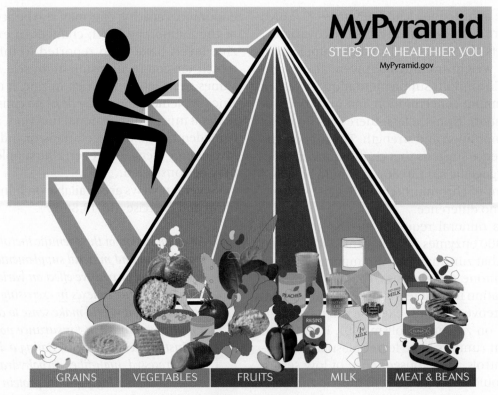

FIGURE 7.3 The USDA MyPyramid food guide system.

TABLE 7.2   COMPARISON OF POPULAR DIETS

MEAL PLAN	DIETARY RECOMMENDATIONS	COMMENTS
Ornish and Pritikin plans	≥ 80% Carbohydrate 10% Protein ≤ 10% Fat	Strength athletes do not need such a high carbohydrate intake. Fortunately there is at least a distinction made and high-quality carbohydrates are recommended with these two plans. Both the protein intake and fat intake are too low to elicit the positive benefits that these two macronutrients provide, which has been demonstrated through various research studies.
The Food Guide Pyramid (FGP)	55% to 60% Carbohydrates 12% to 15% Protein <30% Fat	Also a bit too high in carbohydrates for the strength athlete. Without the guidance of a nutrition professional, one might assume that all carbohydrates are created equal and therefore overconsume refined carbohydrates by following the FGP. The FGP also places fat in the "use sparingly" category, when we know that different types of fats are clearly linked to health benefits and positive changes for the strength athlete. Another problem with the FGP is that it does not differentiate between protein sources high in saturated fat (e.g., ground beef) versus those that are lean (e.g., whey protein powders) or contain healthy fat (e.g., salmon).
Zone diet	40% Carbohydrate 30% Protein 30% Fat	Following this diet will not provide the strength athlete with adequate energy to build lean body mass. This diet was not originally intended for strength-power athletes. However, if the energy intake is increased following a 40:30:30 plan, it should provide adequate protein, healthy carbohydrate, and unsaturated fat.
Atkins diet	Low-carbohydrate (25 to 90 g/day; the typical recommendation is 35 to 40 g) Fat and protein make up the rest of the diet. No types of fat are out of the question.	Strength athletes do not have the same macronutrient needs as endurance athletes; however, performance will be shortchanged by almost eliminating regular consumption of carbohydrates, particularly the high-fiber, low-glycemic variety. In addition, although consensus exists in much of the scientific community about strength athletes' increased protein needs above the RDA, increasing protein at the expense of unprocessed carbohydrates is not warranted. Unprocessed carbohydrates should make up the bulk of one's nutrition program.

through lower-intensity, continuous aerobic activities. Some scientific evidence suggests that carbohydrate supplementation prior to and during high-volume resistance training results in the maintenance of muscle glycogen concentration, which potentially could result in the maintenance or increase of performance during a training bout (58). Additionally, the ingestion of carbohydrates following resistance exercise may enhance muscle glycogen resynthesis, which may result in a faster time of recovery from resistance training, thus possibly allowing for a greater training volume. It is unlikely

7.2 EATING DISORDERS

Eating disorders are often related to disorders of self-image, self-concept, and self-esteem. They are not uncommon among athletic and exercising populations. Disordered eating is one component in the female athletic triad (discussed in Chapter 4). Additionally, compulsive exercise can be a component of some eating disorders.

Three eating disorders are discussed briefly below.

COMPULSIVE OVEREATING

Compulsive overeating is an "addiction" to food. Compulsive overeaters use food and eating to help with daily stresses and problem solving. Individuals who are compulsive overeaters tend to be overweight. They are aware of their inability to control their eating and may be particularly sensitive to comments about their weight or diet. Because obesity is a major health concern in today's society, we should be aware of the potential role compulsive overeating may play in this disorder.

ANOREXIA NERVOSA

The person with anorexia may perceive himself or herself as fat or may be afraid of becoming fat. This individual probably has an emotional disorder, and reacts by controlling his or her eating behaviors.

Signs of anorexia may include obsessive exercise; calorie counting or fat-gram counting; self-induced vomiting and the use of diet pills, laxatives, or diuretics; and a persistent concern with body image. Individuals with anorexia may go through periods of bulimia and their body weight is generally below average.

BULIMIA NERVOSA

The primary symptoms of bulimia are episodes of binging and purging. The individual will eat a large quantity of food in a relatively short time and then induce vomiting or take laxatives, often related to the guilt of overeating. The episodes of binging and purging may be related to feelings of anger, depression, stress, or anxiety. Individuals suffering bulimia may be aware of their eating disorder and usually enjoy discussing food and diet. They may also be overweight, or their weight may fluctuate greatly.

SUMMARY

Similarities can be found among various eating disorders, the most common being some form of emotional disorder. With anorexia and bulimia, it may seem to be nothing but an obsessive concern over body image. For many of these individuals, deeper emotional issues may need to be resolved.

Young female athletes in sports such as gymnastics are considered to be at high risk for eating disorders, specifically anorexia or bulimia. Rather than causing the disorder, it may be that some sports attract anorexic/bulimic athletes, enabling them to hide their condition. A team approach to treatment should be considered that potentially involves the coach/exercise professional, the parents, a physician, a nutritionist, a psychologist, and perhaps others. This is not a disorder the exercise professional can or should try to handle alone.

---

that resistance training depletes muscle glycogen to the same extent as endurance training.

As is seen in Table 7.2, very high carbohydrate, very low-fat diets, such as those developed by Pritikin and Ornish, recommend a macronutrient composition of approximately 80% carbohydrate and 10% protein while advocating less than 10% fat (71). Both of these approaches are supported by a number of scientific studies (2,113) in terms of positively modulating health outcomes (e.g., heart disease, lipid values, blood pressure, etc); no direct research, however, supports their applicability to strength athletes. In fact, these diets may be contraindicated if the goal is to cause hypertrophy or increase speed or another variable that an athlete participating in a high-intensity sport may desire, since these diets are low in both protein and fat. Although diets very high in carbohydrate and low in both protein and fat may suit the needs of a patient with heart disease, owing to the increased intake of fibrous carbohydrates and reduced intake of saturated fat, the limited amounts of protein and fat recommended will not benefit the strength athlete.

Macronutrient manipulation is commonly used by strength athletes to positively influence the hormonal milieu (testosterone, growth hormone, insulin, etc.), with the intention of favoring hypertrophy. As discussed earlier, dietary fat has been shown by a number of studies to correlate with serum sex hormones (46,135,107), improve body composition by promoting fat loss (8,73), improve overall health by providing anti-inflammatory effects (66,122), and even increase the body's ability to store glycogen (43). These facts, together with the known health benefits and increases in hormone concentrations from resistance training itself (94), demonstrate the importance of consuming adequate amounts of dietary fat (i.e., > 10% recommended with these plans).

Let's use the example of a 150-lb strength-trained athlete who needs 2,500 kcal/day. Using the 80%/10%/10% (carbohydrate/protein/fat, respectively) model of Ornish or Pritikin, this individual would be getting approximately 500 g of carbohydrate per day or about 7.3 g of carbohydrate per kilogram per day and about 63 g of protein and fat per day (that is, about 0.9% of protein and 0.4% of fat per kilogram per day). Obviously consuming a diet that replaces much of the dietary fat and protein with carbohydrate makes it impossible to obtain adequate levels of either fat or protein. As discussed earlier, the strength-trained athlete needs more than the RDA for protein each day [from 1.5 to 2.0 g/kg per day (14)], which is clearly much higher than the 0.9 g/kg per day the individual in our example would consume. Similarly, considering that glycogen is not depleted to the same extent in a strength athlete as it is in an endurance athlete, such a high intake of carbohydrate on a regular basis is unnecessary. Consequently, such a diet is not recommended for the otherwise healthy strength-training athlete.

High-Carbohydrate, Low-Fat Diets

Coming on the heels of the very high carbohydrate plans described above, high-carbohydrate, low-fat diets, such as that of the Food Guide Pyramid (FGP), recommend a macronutrient composition of approximately 55% to 60% carbohydrates, 12% to 15% protein, and less than 30% fat. Table 7.3 lists recommended foods that contain each macronutrient. The quantity of foods recommended from each block of the FGP is dependent on the activity level of an individual; however, again, no specific energy recommendation is provided. Using the FGP model, the same 150-lb athlete from above who needs 2,500 kcal/day would have to consume approximately 340 to 375 g of carbohydrate (~5–5.5 g CHO/kg/day), 75 to 90 g of protein (about 1.1 to 1.3 g/kg per day) and 83 g of fat (~1.2 g/kg per day).

Like the diet prescriptions described earlier, one shortcoming with the USDA FGP is that we

TABLE 7.3	RECOMMENDED SELECTIONS FOR EACH MACRONUTRIENT	
CARBOHYDRATE	**PROTEIN**	**FAT**
Oatmeal	Lean red meat	Fish oil
Oat bran	Poultry (skinless, white meat)	Olive oil
Brown rice	All seafood	Flax oil
Whole-wheat pasta	Low-fat/fat-free cottage cheese	Nuts (e.g., almonds, peanuts, etc.)
Yams/sweet potatoes	Eggs	Peanut butter
Red potatoes	Protein powders composed of whey, casein, or combinations thereof	Avocado
All vegetables		
All fruits		
Quinoa		
Legumes		
Lentils		
Whole-grain bread (e.g., pumpernickel, rye)		
Low-fat/fat-free dairy		
Buckwheat		

Note: some foods, such as legumes, lentils, dairy, and peanut butter cross over into other categories (i.e., lentils also have protein). They are placed in the category of the macronutrient that is most abundant.

have an individual in this example who would find it difficult to obtain adequate levels of protein (1.5 to 2.0 g/kg protein per day for most strength training athletes) by following the USDA's guidelines. Another limitation of the FGP is its lack of specificity when it comes to carbohydrate and fat recommendations. There is no argument that carbohydrates are used as a form of energy. In fact, they are the primary source of energy of your brain and skeletal muscles. Not all carbohydrates are alike, however. Although the FGP does emphasize a carbohydrate-based diet, it stops short of differentiating among the various types of carbohydrate. Processed carbohydrates such as white rice and pasta should be limited (not eliminated). Knowing the benefits of the other macronutrients during strength training, namely protein and fat, it would be wise to replace the refined carbohydrates in the diet with lean proteins and healthful fats. Instead, the FGP places protein near the very top, with dietary fat in the "use sparingly" category at the pinnacle of the pyramid. Separating the various types of proteins (e.g., red meat versus salmon) and fat (e.g., butter versus olive oil) is the best approach to developing a sound nutritional program for athletes.

Low-Carbohydrate, High-Protein Diets

A number of diets fall into this category. The one most commonly discussed and researched is the Zone. Barry Sears, its originator, recommends a 40/30/30 ratio (carbohydrates/protein/fat, respectively) (119), which he states will support even the most competitive athletic endeavors. The intention of this specific ratio of macronutrients is to control the body's ratio of insulin to glucagon, ultimately enhancing performance and the ability to mobilize body fat. Although no specific studies used this particular diet with strength athletes, one recent review (37) and one short-term study measured endurance performance utilizing the Zone diet (67). Both publications came to similar conclusions: athletes should not implement the Zone diet in their practices.

Energy intake is the most important component of any dietary strategy. Without adequate energy the body cannot rebuild, repair, or recuperate from training. One study demonstrated, through diet records, that at the end of the 7-week study period, subjects following the Zone diet con-

sumed 1994 ± 438 kcal/day (51). Considering that these were active male subjects with a mean age of 26 years, this energy intake is much too low to support any type of athletic endeavor. It is impossible to enhance strength and performance if the body is not being fed what it needs. Going back to our previous example of the 150-lb athlete needing 2,500 kcal/day, he would take in 250 g of carbohydrate per day (3.7 g CHO/kg/day), about 188 g of protein per day (about 2.75 g of protein per kilogram per day), and about 83 g fat (about 1.2 g of fat per kilogram per day).

One positive aspect of this plan is that it provides a bit more protein than the previously mentioned diets. With this low-energy diet, the protein is particularly important so as to prevent the loss of muscle tissue. In addition, the Zone recommends consuming most carbohydrates as whole-grain carbohydrates to reduce the insulin surge associated with refined carbohydrates. Finally, Sears also separates fats into their various components and recommends increasing the intake of more healthful fats over saturated fats. This macronutrient model is closer to what we would recommend on a daily basis for strength athletes; energy needs, however, must be met first to optimize the training adaptations of the strength-power athlete.

Low-Carbohydrate, High-Fat, High-Protein (Ketogenic) Diets

Carbohydrates were recently demonized with a resurgence of books on low-carbohydrate diets. These types of diets are essentially intended for weight loss; they are, however, increasing in popularity in athletics as well. Looking at the Atkins diet (one of the most popular low-carbohydrate plans) as a model, it recommends that one consume 25 to 90 g of carbohydrate each day, with the low end of the scale as the "induction phase" when someone first begins the program and then working up to the higher end of the scale as time progresses and the individual ultimately reaches his or her goal. With this plan, both fat and protein make up the remaining energy, meaning that intakes of both macronutrients are unlimited and rather high. Our previously mentioned 150-lb athlete who consumed 2,500 kcal/day in the induction phase would have an intake of 25 g of carbohydrate. By dividing protein and fat equally to meet the remaining energy needs in this example, we would provide 300 g of protein (about 4.5 g/kg per day) and about

133 g of fat (about 1.95 g/kg per day). This amount of protein is not only extremely high but unnecessary. The amount of fat in this diet plan is relatively high (e.g., no limit on intake), particularly since Atkins claims that saturated fats are no more hazardous to your health than unsaturated and polyunsaturated fats.

Scientists have begun to measure the effects of low-carbohydrate, high-fat diets on exercise performance (28,51,133). The assumption here is that although glycogen is the storage form of dietary carbohydrates, drastically reducing carbohydrates will cause only a transient negative effect on energy levels, since fat and protein metabolites can ultimately be used as sources of energy. All of the research in this area has been conducted on endurance athletes, because carbohydrates and glycogen are more crucial in terms of endurance performance. Eliminating or drastically reducing carbohydrates is more likely to be detrimental to endurance activity than it is to strength activities.

With strength training, the ultimate goal is typically hypertrophy, speed, and/or power. As discussed, protein is necessary for building muscle mass, and dietary fat is correlated to the production of serum sex hormones. It is obvious that the Atkins diet will provide an abundant amount of both protein and dietary fat. Unfortunately, with this diet, the purpose of high intakes of protein and fat is to displace dietary carbohydrate. Although not as important in short-duration, high-intensity activities, the drastic reduction of dietary carbohydrate and subsequently glycogen stores will hinder performance. Furthermore, the Atkins diet (and similar diets) is low in total energy. No matter what the macronutrient ratio or combination, total energy is ultimately the most important factor in an athlete's diet.

Another consideration for many strength trainers is the effect of the diet on body composition, whether with regard to esthetics and/or performance. Research has demonstrated that a diet lower in carbohydrate and higher in fat and protein may in fact have positive effects on body composition. Authors on the low-carbohydrate side of the fence suggest that this positive change (e.g., loss of body fat) is due to the lack of insulin surges caused by dietary carbohydrates. As yet, no long-term data demonstrate the superiority of one diet of this type over another, and the studies to date supporting high-fat diets were all of short duration (aside from one 12-month study, which showed no signifi-

cant changes in body weight versus the higher-carbohydrate diet at the completion of the 12 months). It should be noted that it is virtually impossible to scientifically study the effects of a diet in the long term (i.e., more than 1 year). Thus, comparisons between and among diets are relegated to short-term studies that represent small windows of time.

Another limiting factor to regularly displacing dietary carbohydrate with fat and protein is the lack of variety in the foods allowed, making a low-carbohydrate lifestyle difficult to follow for a long time. The lack of variety also limits the intake of micronutrients, phytochemicals, antioxidants, and other beneficial components of food, which are all correlated with a lower incidence of various diseases. A healthy athlete is an athlete who can continually train harder and ultimately perform better. Also consider the previously discussed studies demonstrating that carbohydrates at specific times before, during, and after workouts may enhance protein synthesis, recovery, and ultimately growth (62,49,129). Drastic reductions in carbohydrate intake will not allow athletes to take advantage of this window of opportunity, when insulin levels are high from resistance exercise and muscle cells are in need of exactly those nutrients that are shuttled in more rapidly with the ingestion of high-glycemic carbohydrates. Consequently, the suggestion that a low-carbohydrate, high-fat diet can enhance performance is unsound and not based on science.

> *It is virtually impossible to make blanket dietary recommendations for high-performance athletes without first determining their current food intake. The placement of severe restrictions on certain macronutrients, however, is probably not the best approach.*

SUMMARY

Various experts on sports nutrition may provide different answers to the same question based partly on science, anecdote, and personal experience. Blanket dietary recommendations are difficult to make because so many factors affect the optimal diet. Not only is resistance training itself important, but training history, performance goals (e.g., hypertrophy versus power versus changes in body composition), program design, individual responses to training and diet, and acute versus chronic adaptations to training will all play a role in nutritional recommendations.

A few basic nutritional principles can apply to all athletes. First, athletes must try to ingest as much energy as possible while achieving optimal body mass and composition for their respective sports. To do so, they should focus on ingesting approximately 1g of protein per pound of body weight. This recommendation simplifies the calculations necessary to determine needs, and the value can be adjusted based on established outcome measures. Dietary carbohydrate and fat energy should balance out the remainder of the diet with a higher proportion of carbohydrate than fat. The primary sources of carbohydrates should be primarily low-glycemic-index carbohydrates to provide sufficient fiber and abundant nutrients. The intake of high-glycemic-index carbohydrates should be limited to the periods before, during, and after exercise. Fat intake should be substantial (approximately 30% of total energy), with special attention to balancing saturated, monounsaturated, and polyunsaturated fats. Finally, nutrient timing through the consumption of energy (preferably in liquid form to facilitate absorption and ease of use) during and after exercise is critical to improving training response and recovery.

Dietary recommendations should be specific to the current training modality and should be regularly adjusted to meet an athlete's changing needs. Seeking the assistance of a qualified registered dietitian or sports nutritionist will allow the athlete to achieve the desired goals in a healthful but timely manner.

MAXING OUT

1. Sue, a long-distance runner who is competitive in the half-marathon to marathon (26.2-mi) distance, asks for your advice regarding her nutrition program. She currently eats five to six meals per day with an emphasis on lean proteins; healthy fats from nuts, fish, and olive oil; and unprocessed carbohydrate. At 5 ft, 5 in tall, weighing 115 lb and 25 years of age, she consumes approximately 2,300 calories per day. Her mileage ranges from 50 to 70 mi/week. She feels, however, that she is not recovering as quickly as she would like. What questions would you ask her and what nutrition advice might she need that is simple yet effective?

2. As a strength coach, you have identified a particular female athlete who seems to be exhibiting the symptoms of anorexia/bulimia. Her weight fluctuates on a weekly to monthly basis. She is cycling between periods of normal weight and periods of being underweight. Her teammates characterize her as emotional and easily upset. You have observed her eating a meal on only two occasions. Under close observation, she left for the rest room immediately after eating; therefore, you suspect induced vomiting.

3. A 16-year-old male athlete is concerned that he is not getting enough protein. He is participating in football, is training to increase muscle mass, and, because of his age, you know he is also still growing. His body weight is 100 kg. Calculate the grams of protein he should be consuming each day.

REFERENCES

1. Ahlborg B, et al. Muscle glycogen and muscle electrolytes during prolonged physical exercise. Acta Physiol Scand 1967;70:129–142.
2. Aldana SG, Greenlaw R, Thomas D, et al. The influence of an intense cardiovascular disease risk factor modification program. Prev Cardiol 2004;7(1):1;19–25.
3. Ascherio A, Willett WC. Health effects of trans fatty acids. Am J Clin Nutr 1997;66:1006S–1010S.
4. Avery NG, Kaiser JL, Sharman MJ, et al. Effects of vitamin E supplementation on recovery from repeated bouts of resistance exercise. J Strength Cond Res 2003;17(4):801–809.
5. Batheja A, Stout JR. Food: The Ultimate Drug. In: Antonio J, Stout JR, eds. Sports Supplements. Philadelphia: Lippincott Williams & Wilkins, 2001.
6. Bazzarre TL, Kleiner SM, Ainsworth BE. Vitamin C intake and lipid profiles in competitive male and female bodybuilders. Int J Sport Nutr 1992;2(3):260–271.
7. Beaton LJ, Allan DA, Tarnopolsky MA, et al. Contraction-induced muscle damage is unaffected by vitamin E supplementation. Med Sci Sports Exerc 2002;34(5):798–805.
8. Beermann C, Jelinek J, Reinecker T, et al. Short term effects of dietary medium-chain fatty acids and n-3 long-chain polyunsaturated fatty acids on the fat metabolism of healthy volunteers. Lipids Health Dis 2003;2:10.
9. Bergstrom J et al. Diet, muscle glycogen and physical performance. Acta Physiol Scand 1967;71:140–150.
10. Berthoud HR. Multiple neural systems controlling food intake and body weight. Neurosci Biobehav Rev 2002;26:393–428.
11. Bielinski R, Schutz Y, Jequier E. Energy metabolism during the postexercise recovery in man. Am J Clin Nutr 1985;42:69–82.
12. Biolo G, Declan Fleming RY, Wolfe RR. Physiologic hyperinsulinemia stimulates protein synthesis and enhances transport of selected amino acids in human skeletal muscle. J Clin Invest 1995;95:811–819.

13. Biolo G, Maggi SP, Williams BD, et al. Increased rates of muscle protein turnover and amino acid transport after resistance exercise in humans. Am J Physiol 1995;268: E514–E520.

14. Biolo G, Tipton KD, Klein S, et al. An abundant supply of amino acids enhances the metabolic effect of exercise on muscle protein. Am J Physiol 1997;273: E122–E129.

15. Bishop NC, Blannin AK, Walsh NP, et al. Nutritional aspects of immunosuppression in athletes. Sports Med 1999;28:151–176.

16. Bishop NC, Gleeson M, Nicholas CW, et al. Influence of carbohydrate supplementation on plasma cytokine and neutrophil degranulation responses to high intensity intermittent exercise. Int J Sport Nutr Exerc Metab 2002;12:145–156.

17. Bishop NC, Walsh NP, Haines DL, et al. Pre-exercise carbohydrate status and immune responses to prolonged cycling: I. Effect on neutrophil degranulation. Int J Sport Nutr Exerc Metab 2001;11:490–502.

18. Bishop NC, Walsh NP, Haines DL, et al. Pre-exercise carbohydrate status and immune responses to prolonged cycling. II: Effect on plasma cytokine concentration. Int J Sport Nutr Exerc Metab 2001;11:503–512.

19. Blomstrand E. Amino acids and central fatigue. Amino Acids 2001;20:25–34.

20. Bohl CH, Volpe SL. Magnesium and exercise. Crit Rev Food Sci Nutr 2002;42:533–563.

21. Borsheim E, Cree MG, Tipton KD, et al. Effect of carbohydrate intake on net muscle protein synthesis during recovery from resistance exercise. J Appl Physiol 2004; 96:674–678.

22. Borsheim E, Tipton KD, Wolf SE, et al. Essential amino acids and muscle protein recovery from resistance exercise. Am J Physiol Endocrinol Metab 2002;283: E648–E657.

23. Bos C, Benamouzig R, Bruhat A, et al. Short-term protein and energy supplementation activates nitrogen kinetics and accretion in poorly nourished elderly subjects. Am J Clin Nutr 2000;71:1129–1137.

24. Bouthegourd JC, Roseau SM, Makarios-Lahham L, et al. A preexercise alpha-lactalbumin–enriched whey protein meal preserves lipid oxidation and decreases adiposity in rats. Am J Physiol Endocrinol Metab 2002;283: E565–E572.

25. Brandle E, Sieberth HG, Hautmann RE. Effect of chronic dietary protein intake on the renal function in healthy subjects. Eur J Clin Nutr 1996;50:734–740.

26. Burke DG, Chilibeck PD, Davidson KS, et al. The effect of whey protein supplementation with and without creatine monohydrate combined with resistance training on lean tissue mass and muscle strength. Int J Sport Nutr Exerc Metab 2001;11:349–364.

27. Burke LM. Energy needs of athletes. Can J Appl Physiol 2001;26(Suppl):S202–S219.

28. Burke LM, Kiens B, Ivy JL. Carbohydrates and fat for training and recovery. J Sports Sci 2004;22(1):15–30.

29. Butterfield GE, Calloway DH. Physical activity improves protein utilization in young men. Br J Nutr 1984;51: 171–184.

30. Campbell WW, Joseph LJ, Anderson RA, et al. Effects of resistive training and chromium picolinate on body composition and skeletal muscle size in older women. Int J Sport Nutr Exerc Metab 2002;12:125–135.

31. Campbell WW, Trappe TA, Wolfe RR, et al. The recommended dietary allowance for protein may not be adequate for older people to maintain skeletal muscle. J Gerontol Ser A Biol Sci Med Sci 2001;56: M373–M380.

32. Carter SL, Rennie C, Tarnopolsky MA. Substrate utilization during endurance exercise in men and women after endurance training. Am J Physiol Endocrinol Metab 2001;280:E898–E907.

33. Casey A, Mann R, Banister K, et al. Effect of carbohydrate ingestion on glycogen resynthesis in human liver and skeletal muscle, measured by (13)C MRS. Am J Physiol Endocrinol Metab 2000;278:E65–E75.

34. Castaneda C, Gordon PL, Fielding RA, et al. Marginal protein intake results in reduced plasma IGF–I levels and skeletal muscle fiber atrophy in elderly women. J Nutr Health Aging 2000;4:85–90.

35. Chesley A, MacDougall JD, Tarnopolsky MA, et al. Changes in human muscle protein synthesis after resistance exercise. J Appl Physiol 1992;73:1383–1388.

36. Cheuvront SN, Carter R III, Sawka MN. Fluid balance and endurance exercise performance. Curr Sports Med Rep 2003;2:202–208.

37. Cheuvront SN. The zone diet and athletic performance. Sports Med 1999;29(4):213–228.

38. Clarkson PM, Haymes EM. Exercise and mineral status of athletes: calcium, magnesium, phosphorus, and iron. Med Sci Sports Exerc 1995;27:831–843.

39. Convertino VA, et al. American College of Sports Medicine position stand. Exercise and fluid replacement. Med Sci Sports Exerc 1996; 1:i–vii.

40. Cordova A, Alvarez–Mon M. Behaviour of zinc in physical exercise: a special reference to immunity and fatigue. Neurosci Biobehav Rev 1995;19:439–445.

41. Coyle EF. Physiological determinants of endurance exercise performance. J Sci Med Sport 1999;2: 181–189.

42. Davis JM, Alderson NL, Welsh RS. Serotonin and central nervous system fatigue: nutritional considerations. Am J Clin Nutr 2000;72:573S–578S.

43. Delarue J, Couet C, Cohen R, et al. Effects of fish oil on metabolic responses to oral fructose and glucose loads in healthy humans. Am J Physiol 1996;270: E353–E362.

44. Demling RH, DeSanti L. Effect of a hypocaloric diet, increased protein intake and resistance training on lean mass gains and fat mass loss in overweight police officers. Ann Nutr Metab 2000;44:21–29.

45. Doi T, Matsuo T, Sugawara M, et al. New approach for weight reduction by a combination of diet, light resistance exercise and the timing of ingesting a protein supplement. Asia Pacific J Clin Nutr 2001;10:226–232.

46. Dorgan JF, Judd JT, Longcope C, et al. Effects of dietary fat and fiber on plasma and urine androgens and estrogens in men: a controlled feeding study. Am J Clin Nutr 1996;64(6):850–855.

47. Dorup I, Clausen T. Effects of magnesium and zinc deficiencies on growth and protein synthesis in skeletal muscle and the heart. Br J Nutr 1991;66:493–504.

48. Dreosti IE. Magnesium status and health. Nutr Rev 1995;53:S23–S27.

49. Esmarck B, Andersen JL, Olsen S, et al. Timing of post-exercise protein intake is important for muscle hypertrophy with resistance training in elderly humans. J Physiol 2001;535:301–311.

50. Flakoll PJ, Judy T, Flinn K, et al. Postexercise protein supplementation improves health and muscle soreness during basic military training in marine recruits. J Appl Physiol 2004;96:951–956.

51. Fleming J, Sharman MJ, Avery NG, et al. Endurance capacity and high-intensity exercise performance responses to a high fat diet. Int J Sport Nutr Exerc Metab2003; 13(4):466–478.

52. Fletcher RH, Fairfield KM. Vitamins for chronic disease prevention in adults: clinical applications. JAMA 2002; 287(23):3127–3129.

53. Ford F. Health benefits of omega–3s for the whole family. J Fam Health Care 2002;12:91–93.

54. Forslund AH, El Khoury AE, Olsson RM, et al. Effect of protein intake and physical activity on 24–h pattern and rate of macronutrient utilization. Am J Physiol 1999; 276:E964–E976.

55. Fournier PA, Brau L, Ferreira LD, et al. Glycogen resynthesis in the absence of food ingestion during recovery from moderate or high intensity physical activity: novel insights from rat and human studies. Comp Biochem Physiol A: Mol Integr Physiol 2002;133:755–763.

56. Garcia-Lorda P, Megias RI, Salas-Salvado J. Nut consumption, body weight and insulin resistance. Eur J Clin Nutr 2003;57(Suppl 1):S8–S11.

57. Graham TE. Caffeine and exercise: metabolism, endurance and performance. Sports Med 2001;31: 785–807.

58. Haff GG, Lehmkuhl MJ, McCoy LB, Stone MH. Carbohydrate supplementation and resistance training. J Strength Cond Res 2003;17:187–196.

59. Hawley JA. Effect of increased fat availability on metabolism and exercise capacity. Med Sci Sports Exerc 2002; 34:1485–1491.

60. Hawley JA, Schabort EJ, Noakes TD, et al. Carbohydrate-loading and exercise performance. An update. Sports Med 1997;24:73–81.

61. Ivy JL. Glycogen resynthesis after exercise: effect of carbohydrate intake. Int J Sports Med 1998;19(Suppl 2): S142–S145.

62. Ivy JL, Goforth HW, Jr., Damon BM, et al. Early post-exercise muscle glycogen recovery is enhanced with a carbohydrate–protein supplement. J Appl Physiol 2002; 93:1337–1344.

63. Ivy JL, Res PT, Sprague RC, et al. Effect of a carbohydrate–protein supplement on endurance performance during exercise of varying intensity. Int J Sport Nutr Exerc Metab 2003;13:382–395.

64. Jacobs KA, Sherman WM. The efficacy of carbohydrate supplementation and chronic high–carbohydrate diets for improving endurance performance. Int J Sport Nutr 1999;92–115.

65. Jakeman P, Maxwell S. Effect of antioxidant vitamin supplementation on muscle function after eccentric exercise. Eur J App Physiol 1993;67(5):426–430.

66. James MJ, Gibson RA, Cleland LG. Dietary polyunsaturated fatty acids and inflammatory mediator production. Am J Clin Nutr 2000;71(Suppl):343S–348S.

67. Jarvis M, Seddon A, McNaughton L, et al. The acute 1-weed effects of the zinc diet on body composition, Blood lipid levels, and performance in recreational endurance athletes. J Strength Cond Res 2002;16(1): 50–57.

68. Jentjens R, Jeukendrup A. Determinants of post–exercise glycogen synthesis during short–term recovery. Sports Med 2003;33:117–144.

69. Kay D, Marino FE. Fluid ingestion and exercise hyperthermia: implications for performance, thermoregulation, metabolism and the development of fatigue. J Sports Sci 2000;18:71–82.

70. Keith RE, Stone MH, Carson RE et al. Nutritional status and lipid profiles of trained steroid-using bodybuilders. Int J Sport Nutr 1996;6(3):247–254.

71. Koertge J, Weidner G, Elliott–Eller M, et al. Improvement in medical risk factors and quality of life in women and men with coronary artery disease in the Multicenter Lifestyle Demonstration Project. Am J Cardiol 2003; 91(11):1316–1322.

72. Kreider RB. Effects of creatine supplementation on performance and training adaptations. Mol Cell Biochem 2003;244:89–94.

73. Kriketos AD, Robertson RM, Sharp TA, et al. Role of weight loss and polyunsaturated fatty acids in improving metabolic fitness in moderately obese, moderately hypertensive subjects. J Hypertens 2001;19: 1745–1754.

74. Kuo CH, Hunt DG, Ding Z, et al. Effect of carbohydrate supplementation on postexercise GLUT-4 protein expression in skeletal muscle. J Appl Physiol 1999;87: 2290–2295.

75. Lambert EV, Goedecke JH. The role of dietary macronutrients in optimizing endurance performance. Curr Sports Med Rep 2003;2:194–201.

76. Lambert EV, Hawley JA, Goedecke J, et al. Nutritional strategies for promoting fat utilization and delaying the onset of fatigue during prolonged exercise. J Sports Sci 1997;15:315–324.

77. Layman DK. Role of leucine in protein metabolism during exercise and recovery. Can J Appl Physiol 2002; 27:646–663.

78. Layman DK, Boileau RA, Erickson DJ, et al. A reduced ratio of dietary carbohydrate to protein improves body composition and blood lipid profiles during weight loss in adult women. J Nutr 2003;133:411–417.

79. Layman DK, Shiue H, Sather C, et al. Increased dietary protein modifies glucose and insulin homeostasis in adult women during weight loss. J Nutr 2003;133: 405–410.

80. Lemon PW. Effects of exercise on dietary protein requirements. Int J Sports Nutr 1998;8:426–447.

81. Lemon PW, Berardi JM, Noreen EE. The role of protein and amino acid supplements in the athlete's diet: does type or timing of ingestion matter? Curr Sports Med Rep 2002;1:214–221.

82. Levenhagen DK, Carr C, Carlson MG, et al. Postexercise protein intake enhances whole-body and leg protein

accretion in humans. Med Sci Sports Exerc 2002; 34:828–837.

83. Levenhagen DK, Gresham JD, Carlson MG, et al. Post-exercise nutrient intake timing in humans is critical to recovery of leg glucose and protein homeostasis. Am J Physiol Endocrinol Metab 2001;280:E982–E993.

84. Lieberman HR. Nutrition, brain function and cognitive performance. Appetite 2003;40:245–254.

85. Long SJ, Jeffcoat AR, Millward DJ. Effect of habitual dietary-protein intake on appetite and satiety. Appetite 2000;35:79–88.

86. Lukaski HC. Magnesium, zinc, and chromium nutrition and athletic performance. Can J Appl Physiol 2001; 26(Suppl):S13–S22.

87. Lukaski HC. Magnesium, zinc, and chromium nutriture and physical activity. Am J Clin Nutr 2000;72:585S–593S.

88. Lukaski HC, Bolonchuk WW, Siders WA, et al. Chromium supplementation and resistance training: effects on body composition, strength, and trace element status of men. Am J Clin Nutr 1996;63(5):954–965.

89. Maughan RJ, Greenhaff PL, Leiper JB, et al. Diet composition and the performance of high–intensity exercise. J Sports Sci 1997;15:265–275.

90. McBride JM, Kraemer WJ, Triplett-McBride T, et al. Effect of resistance exercise on free radical production. Med Sci Sports Exerc 1998;30:67–72.

91. Miller SL, Wolfe RR. Physical exercise as a modulator of adaptation to low and high carbohydrate and low and high fat intakes. Eur J Clin Nutr 1999;53(Suppl 1): S112–S119.

92. Nieman DC. Exercise immunology: nutritional countermeasures. Can J App Physiol 2001;26(Suppl):S45–S55.

93. Niles, ES, Lachowetz T, Garfi, J, et al. Carbohydrate-protein drink improves time to exhaustion after recovery from endurance exercise. JEP online 2001;4.

94. Nindl BC, Kraemer WJ, Gotshalk LA, et al. Testosterone responses after resistance exercise in women: influence of regional fat distribution. Int J Sport Nutr Exerc Metab 2001;11(4):451–465.

95. Noakes TD. Fluid replacement during exercise. Exerc Sport Sci Rev 1993;21:297–330.

96. Parrish CC, Pathy DA, Parkes JG, et al. Dietary fish oils modify adipocyte structure and function. J Cell Physiol 1991;148:493–502.

97. Pascoe DD, Costill DL, Fink WJ, et al. Glycogen resynthesis in skeletal muscle following resistive exercise. Med Sci Sports Exerc 1993;25:349–354.

98. Pascoe DD, Gladden LB. Muscle glycogen resynthesis after short term, high intensity exercise and resistance exercise. Sports Med 1996;21:98–118.

99. Peters EM, Anderson R, Nieman DC, et al. Vitamin C supplementation attenuates the increases in circulating cortisol, adrenaline, and anti–inflammatory polypeptides following ultramarathon running. Int J Sports Med 2001;22(7):537–543.

100. Petibois C, Cazorla G, Poortmans JR, et al. Biochemical aspects of overtraining in endurance sports: a review. Sports Med 2002;32:867–878.

101. Petibois C, Cazorla G, Poortmans JR, et al. Biochemical aspects of overtraining in endurance sports: the metab-

olism alteration process syndrome. Sports Med 2003; 33:83–94.

102. Phillips SM, Tipton KD, Aarsland A, et al. Mixed muscle protein synthesis and breakdown after resistance exercise in humans. Am J Physiol 1997;273:E99–E107.

103. Poortmans JR, Dellalieux O. Do regular high protein diets have potential health risks on kidney function in athletes? Int J Sport Nutr Exerc Metab 2000;10:28–38.

104. Rampone AJ, Reynolds PJ. Obesity: thermodynamic principles in perspective. Life Sci 1988;43:93–110.

105. Rasmussen BB, Tipton KD, Miller SL, et al. An oral essential amino acid–carbohydrate supplement enhances muscle protein anabolism after resistance exercise. J Appl Physiol 2002;88:386–392.

106. Rauch LH, Rodger I, Wilson GR, et al. The effects of carbohydrate loading on muscle glycogen content and cycling performance. Int J Sport Nutr 1995;5: 25–36.

107. Reed MJ, Cheng RW, Simmonds M, et al. Dietary lipids: an additional regulator of plasma levels of sex hormone binding globulin. J Clin Endocrinol Metab 1987;64: 1083–1085.

108. Rennie MJ. Control of muscle protein synthesis as a result of contractile activity and amino acid availability: implications for protein requirements. Int J Sport Nutr Exerc Metab 2001;11(Suppl):S170–S176.

109. Rennie MJ, Bohe J and Wolfe RR. Latency, duration and dose response relationships of amino acid effects on human muscle protein synthesis. J Nutr 2002;132: 3225S–3227S.

110. Rennie MJ and Tipton KD. Protein and amino acid metabolism during and after exercise and the effects of nutrition. Annu Rev Nutr 2000;20:457–483.

111. Robinson SM, Jaccard C, Persaud C, et al. Protein turnover and thermogenesis in response to high–protein and high–carbohydrate feeding in men. Am J Clin Nutr 1990;52:72–80.

112. Rokitzki L, Sagredos, AN, Reuss F, et al. Assessment of vitamin B6 status of strength and speedpower athletes. J Am Coll Nutr 13(1):87–94.

113. Rosenthal MB, Barnard RJ, Rose DP, et al. Effects of a high-complex-carbohydrate, low-fat, low-cholesterol diet on levels of serum lipids and estradiol. Am J Med 1985;78(1):23–27.

114. Rotman S, Slotboom J, Kreis R, et al. Muscle glycogen recovery after exercise measured by 13C–magnetic resonance spectroscopy in humans: effect of nutritional solutions. Magn Res Mat Phys Biol Med 2000;11: 114–121.

115. Rowlands DS and Hopkins WG. Effect of high-fat, high-carbohydrate, and high-protein meals on metabolism and performance during endurance cycling. Int J Sport Nutr Exerc Metab 2002;12:318–335.

116. Roy BD, Luttmer K, Bosman MJ, et al. The influence of post-exercise macronutrient intake on energy balance and protein metabolism in active females participating in endurance training. Int J Sport Nutr Exerc Metab 2002;12:172–188.

117. Saris WH. The concept of energy homeostasis for optimal health during training. Can J Appl Physiol 2001; 26(Suppl):S167–S175.

118. Schutz Y, Bray G, Margen S. Postprandial thermogenesis at rest and during exercise in elderly men ingesting two levels of protein. J Am Coll Nutr 1987;6:497–506.

119. Sears B. The Zone. New York: Regan Books, 1995.

120. Shapiro S. Do trans fatty acids increase the risk of coronary artery disease? A critique of the epidemiologic evidence. Am J Clin Nutr 1997;66:1011S–1017S.

121. Skov AR, Toubro S, Bulow J, et al. Changes in renal function during weight loss induced by high- vs low-protein low-fat diets in overweight subjects. Int J Obes Rel Metab Disord 1999;23:1170–1177.

122. Stark AH and Madar Z. Olive oil as a functional food: epidemiology and nutritional approaches. Nutr Rev 2002;60:170–176.

123. Taubes G. What if it's all been a big fat lie? New York Times 2000;July 7.

124. Terpstra AH. Effect of conjugated linoleic acid on body composition and plasma lipids in humans: an overview of the literature. Am J Clin Nutr 2004;79:352–361.

125. Thompson D, Williams C, Garcia-Roves P, et al. Post-exercise vitamin C supplementation and recovery from demanding exercise. Eur J Appl Physiol 2003;89:393–400.

126. Thompson D, Williams C, Kingsley M, et al. Muscle soreness and damage parameters after prolonged intermittent shuttle–running following acute vitamin C supplementation. Int J Sports Med 2001;22(1):68–75.

127. Thompson D, Williams C, McGregor SJ, et al. Prolonged vitamin C supplementation and recovery from demanding exercise. Int J Sport Nutr Exerc Metab 2001;11(4):466–481.

128. Tipton KD, Borsheim E, Wolf SE, et al. Acute response of net muscle protein balance reflects 24-h balance after exercise and amino acid ingestion. Am J Physiol Endocrinol Metab 2003;284:E76–E89.

129. Tipton KD, Rasmussen BB, Miller SL, et al. Timing of amino acid–carbohydrate ingestion alters anabolic response of muscle to resistance exercise. Am J Physiol Endocrinol Metab 2001;281:E197–E206.

130. van Loon LJ, Greenhaff PL, Constantin–Teodosiu D, et al. The effects of increasing exercise intensity on muscle fuel utilisation in humans. J Physiol 2001;536:295–304.

131. van Loon LJ, Kruijshoop M, Verhagen H, et al. Ingestion of protein hydrolysate and amino acid–carbohydrate mixtures increases postexercise plasma insulin responses in men. J Nutr 2000;130:2508–2513.

132. van Loon LJ, Saris WH, Kruijshoop M, et al. Maximizing postexercise muscle glycogen synthesis: carbohydrate supplementation and the application of amino acid or protein hydrolysate mixtures. Am J Clin Nutr 2000;72:106–111.

133. Vogt M, Puntschart A, Howald H, et al. Effects of dietary fat on muscle substrates, metabolism, and performance in athletes. Med Sci Sports Exerc 2003;35(6):952–960.

134. Volek JS. Strength nutrition. Curr Sports Med Rep 2003;2:189–193.

135. Volek JS, Kraemer WJ, Bush JA, et al. Testosterone and cortisol in relationship to dietary nutrients and resistance exercise. J App Physiol 1997;82(1):49–54.

136. Webster S, et al. Physiological effects of a weight loss regimen practiced by college wrestlers. Med Sci Sports Exerc 1990;22(2):229–234.

137. Westman EC, Mavropoulos J, Yancy WS, et al. A review of low-carbohydrate ketogenic diets. Curr Atheroscler Rep 2003;5:476–483.

138. Willett WC and Leibel RL. Dietary fat is not a major determinant of body fat. Am J Med 2002;113(Suppl 9B):47S–59S.

139. Wong SH, Williams C, Adams N. Effects of ingesting a large volume of carbohydrate–electrolyte solution on rehydration during recovery and subsequent exercise capacity. Int J Sport Nutr Exerc Metab 2000;10:375–393.

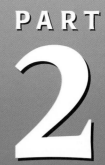

PART

2

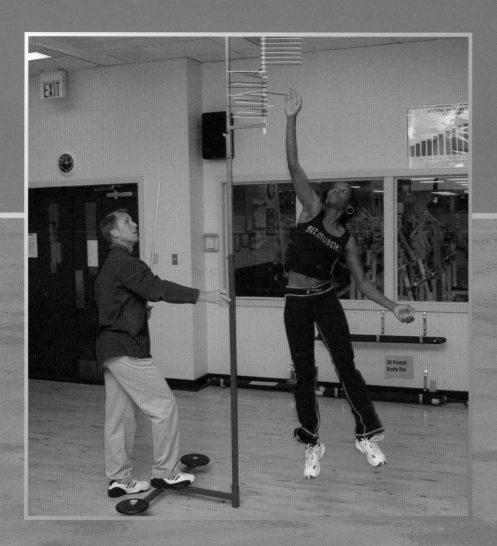

Organization and Administration

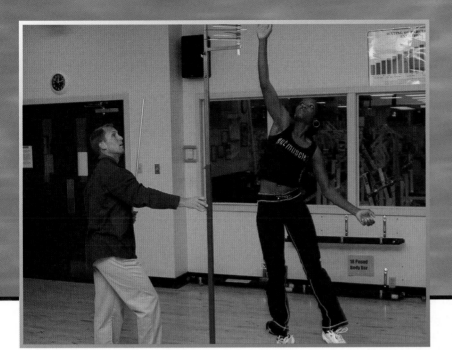

Test Administration and Interpretation

LEE E. BROWN
DANIEL MURRAY
PATRICK HAGERMAN

Introduction

Testing and measurement are at the heart of any resistance-training program. This is where initial decisions are made regarding the exercise prescription and such issues as frequency, intensity, and volume. Testing, however, is not a one-time task but rather an ongoing method of evaluation throughout the prescribed program. In this sense, it is the beginning, middle, and end of a truly individual periodized regime. The results can be used to evaluate performance and make decisions regarding the future of a program or individual. They may also be used to predict future performance in much the same way that college entrance exam scores are used to predict an individual's probability of graduating. Last, test scores may be used in a research environment as part of an in-depth analysis of an important question. Ultimately, the outcome of this entire process is the individualized exercise prescription that will best serve each athlete or client.

Physical testing is an ongoing task to assess the status of both the athlete and the program.

PURPOSE OF TESTING

The main reason testing and measurement are at the heart of resistance training is that they determine where an individual currently stands regarding his or her training status and, more importantly, where he or she is headed. The final outcome of any training program is to arrive at a peak level of performance or to achieve some predetermined goal (9). Therefore, having goals is of no consequence if neither the exerciser nor the strength and conditioning professional know the present state of the athlete. In short, before we can plan for a trip to go somewhere, we must first know where we currently are. In this way a cogent strategy can be designed and implemented based on the individual and the unique demands of the athlete, which have been determined through testing and measurement.

Using the results of a properly designed and implemented testing and measurement protocol will enable the tester or coach to make objective rather than subjective decisions regarding a client's or athlete's program. The ultimate assessment will be based on hard data collected through the judicious use of appropriate tests gathered under the scrutiny of a well-prepared tester. In this way individual bias can be reduced and the tester's prejudice eliminated in measuring an attribute on a test. There is, however, still a place for subjective reasoning during an evaluation process, but it is better utilized in the overall synergy of how the athlete's skills may be able to coordinate with the sport requirements rather than on the independent collection of raw data.

The purpose of this chapter is to lay the framework for a neat and concise assessment procedure in evaluating clients or athletes. Before proceeding, it is important to understand the nomenclature used during this process.

Population: An entire group of individuals sharing some common characteristic. This might be all third-graders in America or all NCAA Division I female pole vaulters. Such a group is nearly always too large in number to test every member, so a smaller sample is chosen as representative.

Subpopulation: The smaller sample mentioned above, containing a manageable number of people from whom to obtain performance measures. The results are then used to extrapolate data for the total population.

Test: A tool used to measure performance. This may take the form of a vertical jump test, a one-repetition-maximum (1-RM) strength test, or a timed muscular endurance test. The test is just a tool used to collect data in the course of the assessment procedure.

Measurement: The quantitative score derived from the test. It will be expressed in the form of the units described by the individual test, such as inches, feet, or pounds. Alone, it has very little meaning, since different tests have different scales, making comparisons difficult or impossible.

Evaluation: Placing a value on the measurement derived from the test. This is the point where the score must be compared to a scale and given worth. This part of the procedure requires a professional trained to choose the proper ranking scale and mindful of the intricacies involved in making decisions in the face of extraneous variables as well as individual differences associated with age, gender, and training status.

Assessment: Putting all three of the aforementioned events together. Choose a test, measure the score, and then make an evaluation based on a scale comparison.

Normative scale: A postmeasurement scale derived from the scores of a peer group. In making comparisons within a subpopulation, this scale is generally determined by placing the highest score at the top and then listing the descending scores in order of magnitude. In other words, if scores on a vertical jump test ranged between 28 and 12 in., then all the other scores would be ranked between them and some value placed on each performance. Breaks in the scale can be established according to statistical rules such as central tendency, standard deviation, or natural breaks.

Criterion: An a priori scale whereby the break points are known prior to testing and each person must meet an established level of performance to achieve that value level. It is important to understand that this scale is usually derived from many bouts of normative testing. When a considerable amount of data are collected on enough subpopulations to constitute a logical inference of the results to the total population, then a criterion scale can be established and used to evaluate subsequent scores. This scale requires participants to perform at a standard level of achievement. This may be reaching a specific height during the vertical jump for a basketball team, lifting a specific amount of weight as in a preemployment screening exam, or attaining a particular height before being allowed to enjoy an amusement park ride.

 Testing data can be useful in justifying a program or a training method.

TEST SELECTION

To accurately evaluate athletes, proper tests must be chosen that allow an in-depth view of an individual's performance level. This is best accomplished by choosing specific tests designed to measure only one aspect of human performance (10,12). Often many separate tests will be required to precisely measure an athlete's state of training, and each test should be chosen with risks and outcomes in mind. Sport coaches sometimes make choices based on anecdotal evidence or use insensitive tests that are incapable of discriminating variable human performance. The proper procedure is to first determine what the desired outcome is, then design a test and measurement protocol around that outcome (2).

 Tests chosen should be specific to the sport and to the population being tested.

Physical tests include measurements of cardiovascular and respiratory function, strength, power, endurance, and anthropometry, just to name a few. Each of these categories consists of a myriad of choices, every one of which is intended to measure a single factor of that performance characteristic within specific and detailed guidelines (8). Violation of these guidelines will result in spurious data, which are of no use whatsoever.

REAL-WORLD APPLICATION
Calculating Average Velocity During Sprint Running

The example is an athlete completing a 40-m sprint. We have electronic timing lights at 10, 20, and 30 m from the starting light gate. The average speed over the last 10 m might be used as an indication of maximum running speed. Let's assume that the times and distances are as follows:

Distance	10	20	30
Time	1.741	2.890	3.995

Velocity is change in distance over change in time. Therefore: velocity = (30–20)/(3.995–2.890) = 10/1.105 = 9.05 m/s.

Making decisions about an individual's physical state is not a trivial task and carries with it severe consequences for both the evaluator and client. The utilization of spurious data will ultimately lead to erroneous conclusions. The severe consequences of prescribing exercise for an individual that is beyond his or her capacity or returning athletes to play prior to their being able to participate without undue risk of danger cannot be overemphasized. Remember, bad data are worse than no data at all because they may constitute an unstable foundation on which to build further training.

Validity

Validity is the most important aspect of any assessment procedure. For a test to be valid, it must test what it purports to test (11). That is, if one wishes to measure leg strength, then a valid test might be the squat, leg press, or deadlift. Each test would result in different scores and care would need to be taken in choosing the proper test for a unique subpopulation, but each would be a valid test of leg strength. In contrast, the vertical jump test includes leg strength as a component but is a test of leg power. Therefore, the vertical jump test is not a valid test of leg strength because it measures an individual's ability to produce power. However related strength and power might be, they are still distinct mechanisms of physical performance. Again, this illustrates the sensitive nature of test selection.

Validity is historically been measured against a "gold standard" of performance. For instance, if someone has designed a new device to test leg strength, then the procedure would be to obtain measures using the new device and comparing those with the gold standard method (3). Using statistical techniques, it is possible to determine whether the two tests are conceptually similar and to what degree their results differ. A correlation analysis such as the Pearson product moment (r) may answer the conceptual question by determining the association of the two scores, while an analysis of variance (ANOVA) may answer the degree to which the tests scores differ. These techniques are beyond the scope of this chapter, but the concept should not be lost on the reader. The concept is that a test must measure what it has been designed to measure if the results are to be a valid quantification of that physical component.

The five major types of validity are:

1. **Face** validity states that the test is logical on the surface, as when having a person lift a weight to measure strength.
2. **Content** validity states that the test includes material that has been taught or covered; for instance, testing speed after training for speed.
3. **Predictive** validity states that test scores can accurately predict future performance. An example would be the National Football League measuring college football players prior to the draft to determine their potential.
4. **Concurrent** validity states that the test is a measure of the individual's current performance level. This happens when the test occurs shortly after training is completed.
5. **Construct** validity states that the test measures some part of the whole skill, such as measuring bench-press strength for football linemen.

Reliability

Reliability is loosely defined as repeatability. That is, the ability of a test to arrive at or near the same score upon repeated measurements in the absence of any intervention strategy. A reliable test should result in consistent scores. To accomplish this (using the new device scenario stated previously), the procedure would be to measure individuals using the new device, then allow a time delay of approximately 48 to 72 hours so no significant training effects could interfere with the results, and then measure each person a second time using the identical procedures as the first measurement. If reliability is high, then people scoring well on the first test should also score well on subsequent tests (4,5).

The rank order of participants should remain relatively constant, as in back-to-back days of handgrip strength testing. A perfect rank order between tests would mean that each person kept his or her spot in the ordinal sequence relative to all others.

REAL-WORLD APPLICATION
Reproducing Physical Test Results in Training and Conditioning

Reproducing the results of physical tests is important to maintain the test's validity and reliability. Testing athletes in the weight room or on the field presents special challenges in terms of reproducing test data.

Why is reproducibility important in training and conditioning? It is important for a number of reasons, even though the data may not be used for research purposes.

You will make a decision about the type of program you use based on the results you obtain. If your results are not accurate, then you may be making the wrong decision and choosing a program that is not producing the results you seek. Pre- and posttesting must use reproducible procedures so that you can accurately make your decision.

Conditioning programs should focus on specific areas of weakness in a particular athlete. Those areas must be monitored on a regular basis using reproducible tests. If the tests used are not reproducible, then, once again, an incorrect decision will be made.

Inconsistent test results may not motivate the athlete to improve. We know that hard work pays off with improved scores; but if the scoring is inconsistent, we are providing bad information.

Documenting improvement in the athletes you train is an indication that you, as a conditioning coach, are doing your job. Providing your administrators with accurate testing records obtained by using reproducible tests is an important step in justifying your position.

Are there steps that the conditioning professional can take to improve the reproducibility of the test results? Of course!

■ Standardize the testing procedures for every test. Have the procedures in writing and provide a copy to each data collector.
■ Train the data collectors to collect the test results accurately and consistently.
■ Use the same data collectors as much as possible.
■ Allow the same number of trials for each test.
■ Test in the same environmental conditions as much as possible. Environmental conditions are best controlled indoors, so test indoors as much as possible and practical.
■ Standardize the amount and type of external motivation provided to the athlete, and keep it consistent from one testing session to the next.
■ Test at the same time of day if possible.
■ Always test after a day of rest if possible. Strenuous training of specific muscle groups may decrease performance on some tests.
■ Maintain the same order of testing.

Control diet as much as possible. You may not be able to control diet to a great extent, but remember that it can have an effect on performance, both positive and negative.

This almost never occurs with human testing. Employing the statistical techniques of Pearson *r* would establish this rank order of the two measurements and establish reliability on a continuum ranging between 1.0 and −1.0. Reliability is not an either/or proposition but rather a floating scale of different levels.

Table 8.1 depicts one strategy to use to categorize the level of reliability between two measurements taken at two different times using the same population. Remember that a negative correlation still represents reliability but simply states that as one score increases, another score decreases, thereby inverting the rank order of participants. This may occur in comparing two different tests, such as vertical jump height and percent body fat. Figure 8.1 shows graphical representations of the scores as they appear when scatter-plotted. The trend line (sometimes referred to as the "line of best fit") has been added to illustrate positive, negative, and null relationships, respectively.

Although the Pearson *r* correlation can be used to determine the relationship between subsequent tests in our new-device scenario, it is no longer the gold standard in determining reliability. Instead, an **intraclass correlation coefficient (ICC)** can be used to better establish reliability. A Pearson *r* score close to 1 or −1 will denote that an individual has scored similarly with respect to his or her peers, but it does not take into account any changes in the mean test score. What would happen if the group of athletes we tested on our new device all finished in the same rank order on the second test but each scored several points higher? This would be a case in which Pearson *r* correlation would be high, because all of the athletes performed similarly with respect to their peers on both tests. The test would not be reliable, however, because the mean score was higher on the second test. Therefore,

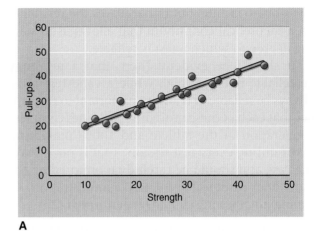

A

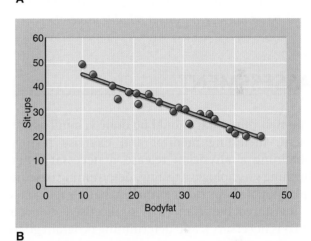

B

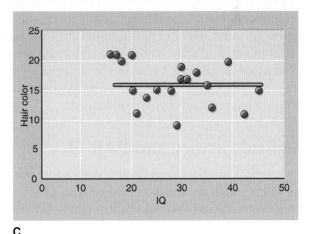

C

FIGURE 8.1 Graphical representation of scores when scatter-plotted. **A.** Positive relationship between strength and number of pull-ups. **B.** Negative relationship between body fat and number of sit-ups. **C.** No relationship between IQ and hair color.

the results are not repeatable. The ICC takes into account any difference that may be present, not only in the rank of each athlete but also in the overall difference in the value of the scores (7). It is important to remember that the ICC, like the Pearson *r*, does not determine the reliability of a test in

TABLE 8.1	CATEGORY SYSTEM TO DETERMINE LEVEL OF RELIABILITY
R VALUE	RELATIONSHIP
1.0–0.8	Very high
0.79–0.6	High
0.59–0.4	Moderate
0.39–0.2	Low
0.19–0	Very low

a yes-or-no fashion but rather places the reliability on a theoretical continuum that allows us to state the degree to which a test is reliable.

It should be evident, then, that a test may be reliable but not valid, while a valid test must always be reliable. It is always important to remember that each of these procedures assumes complete cooperation of the athlete and 100% maximum effort during every test session. That is not always the case and should be carefully monitored by the individual responsible for test administration, or submaximal testing should be performed (20).

 Tests chosen must be valid and reliable and must be administered using a reliable protocol.

ASSESSMENT

The first thing that should be done is a full assessment, including medical and exercise history, obtaining a physician release if necessary, performing physiological testing, determining baseline nutritional status [to determine whether referral to a registered dietician (RD) or licensed dietician (LD) is necessary], and determining program goals. The objective of the assessment is to provide a comprehensive view of the athlete, what he or she is capable of, what his or her limitations are, and any special needs that may have to be addressed. This initial assessment may be done the first time you meet, but will be an ongoing process as you work with and learn about the person's needs.

Medical History and PAR-Q

The medical history should begin with a few basic questions, such as those found on the Physical Activity Readiness–Questionnaire (PAR–Q). The PAR–Q is a limited tool that should not be considered to encompass all the information you will need. It is a quick and easy way to determine whether a potential client is at risk for any major complications during low to moderate but not vigorous exercise. In addition to the PAR–Q, it is appropriate to determine the following:

- Is the person diabetic? If so, is he or she able to control blood glucose levels, and how are these monitored? Additionally, has this person ever been on a regular exercise program as a diabetic?

- Does the person have asthma? If so, is his or her asthma exercise-induced, and at what levels? Does he or she use a fast-acting inhaler or other medication to control attacks?
- Is this person a smoker? If so, how much and how often?
- Is there a family history of heart attack, coronary artery bypass surgery, or sudden death before age 55 in men or age 65 in women?
- Does this individual have a history of hypertension (systolic pressure ≥ 140 or diastolic pressure ≥ 90), or is he or she on antihypertensive medications?
- Does this person have a total cholesterol level above 200 mg/dL?
- Is this individual obese, defined as a body mass index of ≥ 30, confirmed with a waist measurement of > 100 cm?

You will also need to know about any previous injuries that might interfere with your client's ability to perform certain exercises. Ask about such things as sprains and strains, arthritis, athletic injuries, unusual pain or swelling in any joint, and any tightness that might limits the ability to move with ease.

 Understanding an individual's medical and exercise history will help you make an informed decision regarding the best exercise prescription or whether referral to a medical professional for additional testing is indicated.

Physician Release

The words "Please consult with your physician before beginning an exercise program" are often found on the control panels of cardiovascular equipment. No matter how thorough a medical history you obtain, a physician will be better able to assess the medical ability of a person to begin an exercise program and may have information that can help you to determine the best course of action for that person. It is a good idea to have a medical release form that describes each of the exercise components, including the levels of intensity and duration.

Nutrition

It is important to get a basic understanding of the person's nutritional status. Nutritional programming should be performed only by a registered or licensed dietician. You can, however, obtain basic information—such as choice of foods, quantity, and timing of meals—from a simple 3-day recall. Having the client recall everything ingested for the past 3 days will allow you to decide whether more specific dietary interventions are necessary, in which case a referral to an RD/LD is necessary.

Needs Analysis

Two main concerns in choosing proper tests to be administered to athletes are the needs of the individual and the needs of the activity. Each of these brings specific requirements to the task of test selection and should be treated with equal diligence.

> *A needs analysis should be performed to evaluate the needs of the athlete and the demands of the sport.*

First, individual needs may be assessed through traditional physiological methods such as the assessment of body fat, cardiovascular fitness, muscular strength/power and flexibility. These tests are designed to evaluate the individual's present state of readiness to participate in the activity of choice. Not all tests will be required for each person, as not all physiological variables are equally required across sporting activities. Furthermore, each category may compel the investigator to pick appropriate ways to measure the individual.

Second, the needs of the particular sport or activity are unique and require different physiological performance levels of the athlete or client. Some sports, such as wrestling, require maximal isometric upper-body movements; others, such as cycling or running, require submaximal continuous lower-body movements. Once again, the specificity of a testing and measurement scheme is crucial to the success of the program.

In short, preparation for a comprehensive testing and measurement system requires time and diligence of the tester at the onset of the program to choose tests that measure the requisite needs of both the participant and the activity. These needs should consider all aspects of human performance, including but not limited to energy systems, duration of each repetition, duration of the entire event, muscle used, muscle actions used, range of motion involved, and speed of movement (16,17).

Table 8.2 displays a myriad of tests designed to measure strength and power, yet each is unique in that it requires different muscles, muscle actions, time limits, kinetic chain limitations, and energy systems. The tests presented in this chapter are by no means the only available methods of evaluating strength and power. Instead, they have been selected merely to represent the vast array of choices one has in assessing an athlete's training needs.

WINGATE ANAEROBIC CYCLE TEST

The Wingate anaerobic cycle test was designed as a means to measure overall anaerobic lower extremity power. The athlete is asked to cycle as fast as possible for 30 seconds with a predetermined resistance (Fig. 8.2). This resistance is derived by multiplying the athlete's body weight (kg) by the constant 0.075 (1,13).

Specialized cycle ergometers will record the athlete's peak and mean power during the 30-second test. This test is a good overall assessment of lower extremity power, as it requires contributions from all major muscle groups of the lower extremities. Also, it can be used to measure not only peak power, but also mean power over a 30-second period. For this reason it is a good test to include with sports that require maximal effort in bouts that last longer than just a few seconds. One negative aspect of this test is the need for a specialized cycle ergometer that will derive the athlete's peak and mean power. These ergometers are costly and are used primarily for research purposes.

MARGARIA-KALAMEN STAIR CLIMB TEST

This test of lower extremity power is easy and quick to perform. It is performed on a staircase and is a good measure of lower-body power and explosiveness, which is important to athletes requiring speed, agility, and quickness. First, measure the subject's body weight and calculate the height of each step. The test is performed by beginning in front of a flight of at least a dozen stairs. Each step height is approximately 17.5 cm (7 in.) high. Timing mats are placed on the third and ninth steps, which are connected to a timing device and are activated by the subject's body weight. The subject begins 6 m from the first step and then runs toward and up the steps, taking them three at a time (Fig. 8.3). The result (power) is the product of body weight and the steps' vertical distance and gravity divided by the total time from the third to the ninth step. Results of this test have shown a moderate correlation to the Wingate cycle test (15).

TABLE 8.2	VARIOUS STRENGTH AND POWER TESTS					
TESTS	**MUSCLE GROUPS AND JOINTS USED**	**MUSCLE ACTIONS**	**TIME LIMITS**	**KINETIC CHAIN**	**ENERGY SYSTEM**
Wingate anaerobic cycle	Hips, quads, ankles	Concentric	30 s	Closed	Anaerobic
Margaria-Kalamen stair climb	Hips, quads, ankles	Concentric and eccentric	2 s	Closed	ATP-PC
Isokinetic velocity spectrum	Each one individually	Concentric and eccentric	5 to 60 s	Open	ATP-PC and Anaerobic
Countermovement vertical jump	Hips and ankles	Concentric and eccentric	2 s	Closed	ATP-PC
1-RM power clean	Arms, shoulders, back, hips, quads, ankles	Isometric and Concentric and eccentric	5 s	Closed	ATP-PC
1-RM squat	Entire lower body	Isometric and Concentric and eccentric	5 s	Closed	ATP-PC
1-RM bench press	Entire upper body	Isometric and Concentric and eccentric	5 s	Closed	ATP-PC
Bench press body weight for total reps	Entire upper body	Isometric and Concentric and eccentric	30 to 60 s	Closed	Anaerobic
40-yd dash	Entire lower body	Concentric and eccentric	5 s	Closed	ATP-PC
Standing long jump	Entire lower body	Concentric and eccentric	2 s	Closed	ATP-PC

ISOKINETIC VELOCITY SPECTRUM

Isokinetic testing involves controlling the velocity of a given movement rather than the force or power with which it is performed. A computerized dynamometer is set to a specified velocity at which the lever arm of the machine can be moved. The athlete then attempts to move the lever arm as fast as he or she can through a preset range of motion. Torque (rotational force) and power produced during the movement are then recorded by the dynamometer. These measurements can be expressed as maximal values or averaged over several repetitions to derive mean torque and power values. This testing is often performed within a range, or spectrum, of velocities, so that the tester can get a better indication on whether potential deficits exist during slow- or fast-velocity movements.

Isokinetic dynamometers (Fig. 8.4) can be used to test a variety of joints in either seated or reclin-

ing positions. These machines can test each joint in only isolation and not as part of a dynamic movement. Therefore, they are limited in their application to the movement patterns specific to an individual sport. They do, however, provide precise, highly reliable data that can easily be compared between athletes, injured and uninjured limbs, or agonist and antagonist muscle groups (5,21,22).

COUNTERMOVEMENT VERTICAL JUMP

The vertical jump is performed primarily utilizing the hip extensor and ankle plantarflexor muscle groups. The athlete is instructed to jump as high as he or she can following a quick downward squatting movement. The athlete's jump height can be recorded simply by measuring the difference between chalk markings placed first on a wall while standing on the ground and reaching and then at the highest point that the athlete can reach while performing the countermovement jump. Commer-

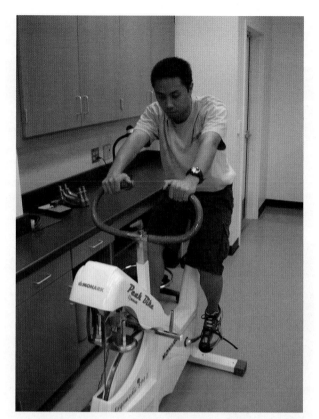

FIGURE 8.2 Wingate Anaerobic Cycle Test. This test is a good indicator of overall anaerobic lower extremity power.

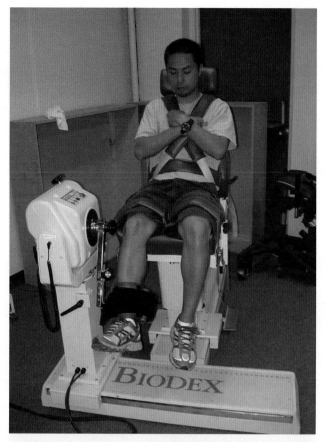

FIGURE 8.4 Isokinetic testing. Using a computerized dynamometer, this test measures torque and power at various velocities.

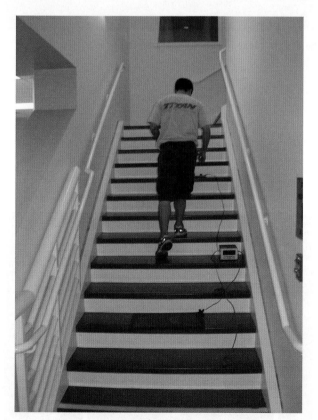

FIGURE 8.3 Margaria-Kalamen stair-climb test. This test is a good indicator of lower-extremity power.

cial products involving a series of plastic sticks that rotate about a vertical axis when touched are also available to measure vertical jump height (Fig. 8.5).

This test is often a good choice, as it is an essential skill in many sports. Therefore, the movement pattern and metabolic demands are similar to what the athlete might encounter in a game situation. Furthermore, improvement on a test such as this may have a direct effect on sport performance. One limitation of the countermovement vertical jump test is the fact that technique often differs among athletes. Thus, the examiner must be careful that differences in scores on subsequent tests are due to training and not variations in the athlete's jumping technique.

ONE-REPETITION-MAXIMUM POWER CLEAN

The power clean is an exercise performed using several upper extremity, lower extremity, and core muscle groups (Fig. 8.6). Because the exercise is designed for the athlete to lift the weight as quickly as possible, it is a good indication of ballistic strength. The 1-RM power clean is considered to

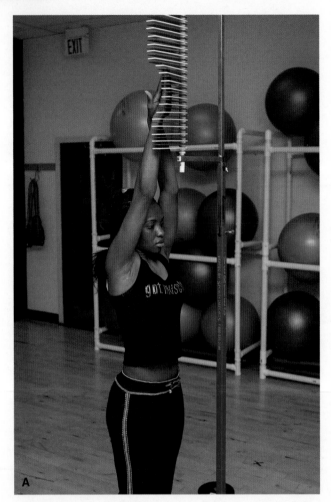

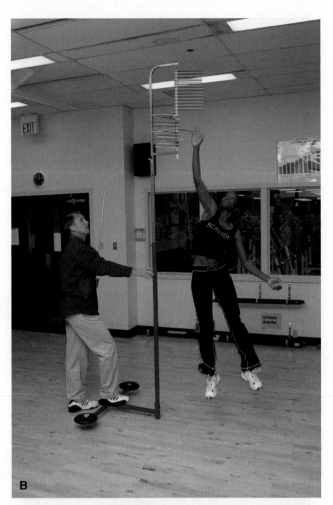

FIGURE 8.5 Countermovement vertical jump. **A.** First, determine the athlete's reach while standing on the floor. **B.** Then, have the athlete jump to determine maximum height.

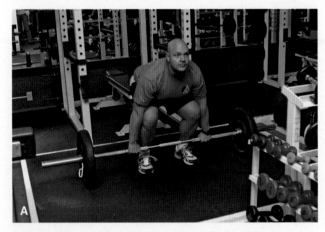

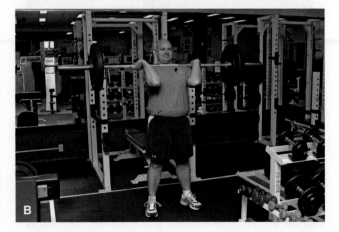

FIGURE 8.6 Power clean. **A.** Starting position. **B.** Catch.

be the greatest load with which the athlete can perform one repetition of the movement with proper form. This test is useful for power athletes who are required to move explosively for short durations.

ONE-REPETITION-MAXIMUM SQUAT

The 1-RM squat is considered the greatest load with which an athlete can perform the exercise in good form (Fig. 8.7). This test is a good indicator of overall lower body strength, as the movement requires contributions from all the major muscle groups of the lower body. It is an important test for athletes whose sports require a great deal of lower extremity strength, such as basketball and volleyball.

ONE-REPETITION-MAXIMUM BENCH PRESS

Like the squat test for the lower body, the 1-RM bench press is often used to estimate an athlete's overall upper-body strength (Fig. 8.8). Again, this value is obtained by determining the greatest load with which the athlete can perform the movement with good form. It is a particularly useful test for sports requiring upper-body strength, such as football. Since all athletes can benefit from improving their overall strength base, a general upper-body test such as this is good to include for all athletes.

Finding a true 1-RM may be both difficult and unnecessary in some cases. Like other RM tests, the bench-press test can be time-consuming to conduct (6). Long periods of rest are required between trials and several trials are necessary for each test. Therefore, RMs are often derived using prediction equations. Many prediction equations exist and are based on the mass lifted and the number of repetitions performed.

BENCH-PRESS BODY WEIGHT FOR TOTAL REPS

This test is another good indicator of general upper-body strength and muscular endurance. It may be a more valid measure than the 1-RM test because it takes into consideration individual differences in mass. Use of this test would allow the strength coach to compare an athlete to his or her peers more appropriately.

Although this test provides for variations in strength due to mass, it does not consider differences in training age. Athletes who have greater training ages may be able to bench press their body weight several times without much difficulty. Therefore, this test may provide a baseline of strength for some and muscular endurance for others. Deciding on an appropriate test for upper-body strength should take both differences in mass and training age into account.

40-YD SPRINT

The 40-yd sprint is another highly functional test to gauge total lower-body power. Sprinting at top speed is a skill required in many sports. Therefore, the 40-yd sprint is often a good test to include, as its performance may have direct application to many athletes' sports. Although many highly accurate timing devices are available, the test can easily be performed using a stopwatch.

One negative aspect of this test, however, is its potential to be overemphasized. In fact, such importance is placed on this test that highly competitive athletes often spend a great deal of time and effort practicing form drills in the hope of running a few tenths of a second faster. Although this is a very functional and useful test, its results should be used in conjunction with other tests to identify an ath-

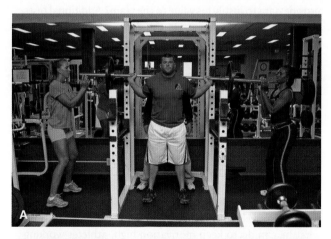
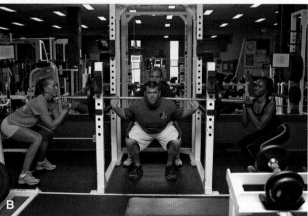

FIGURE 8.7 Squat. **A.** Starting position. **B.** Downward movement.

Q & A from the Field

The head strength and conditioning coach for the football team at our university only uses four tests for the players: the 40-yard dash, vertical jump, 1-RM squat, and 1-RM bench press. We had such a great season last year, when we won our conference championship, that the tests seem adequate, but should we be doing more?
—*graduate student intern*

Certainly we must take many things into consideration in designing a testing program. A mature, well-trained group of players might be able to continue to perform well with minimal testing. To determine the appropriate tests, we must review the basic rationale for testing athletes. Remember the primary reasons for testing:

1. To determine the fitness base of the athlete
2. To determine the performance characteristics of the better players in the sport
3. To motivate the athletes to continue to train hard

There are other possible reasons for testing. One reason might be that the S&C coach is in the process of justifying his position on the coaching staff. Good, solid data demonstrating improvement in a number of performance characteristics in the teams he trains would provide solid evidence that he is performing an important service for those athletes.

To get a total picture of the athlete's fitness base, you will probably need tests in a number of areas of performance. These areas might include the following:

1. upper-body strength
2. lower-body strength
3. upper-body endurance
4. lower-body endurance
5. upper-body power
6. lower-body power
7. aerobic capacity
8. speed
9. speed endurance
10. maximal anaerobic capacity.

You may choose some tests that overlap two of these characteristics, or you may determine that a test is not appropriate for a particular sport. Maximal anaerobic capacity tests that cause a dramatic rise in lactic acid production might not be appropriate for a golfer, for example. Do recall, however, that aerobic capacity is used in recovery,

even in anaerobic sports. Remember also that we base our decisions about the type of training program needed on the testing results. In a mature, highly performing group of athletes, it is possible that the training protocols are well established and the testing data will not greatly affect the program. Thus, a minimal testing program might work in some specific situations. Spending less time testing allows more time for conditioning or practice of the sport, which might be an advantage in some situations.

In summary, there are several reasons to consider adding tests to the testing program described above. It is also possible to spend too much time and energy on testing, taking away from training time and practice time. The correct answer to your question depends on the goals of your particular testing program. Do the athletes need more motivation to train hard? Additional tests may provide the additional motivation. Is it important for the S&C coach to provide data to justify his value to the team? Additional tests may prove his importance. Do the chosen tests adequately represent the physical requirements of the sport? If not, additional tests may provide the missing data. Are the tests position-specific? In football, the physical demands of different positions can vary. A 40-yard dash may be appropriate for backs, while a 10- or 20-yard dash may be more appropriate for linemen. Matching testing to position-specific physical requirements will provide useful information. The training program should provide position-specific benefits to the individual athlete.

Every group of athletes will differ to some extent, and the philosophy of conditioning programs will vary from school to school as well. An S&C coach is constantly thinking about what he can do to keep motivation high, athletes working hard, and maintain a positive attitude toward the training. The testing program should evaluate improvement in performance that is specific to the sport of football as well as to the athlete's position. A properly designed testing program can be a key component in achieving these goals!

lete's strengths and weaknesses. It should not be used as a direct predictor of how he or she will perform on the field.

STANDING LONG JUMP

The standing long jump is also a good functional test that measures total lower-body power (Fig. 8.9).

Although the vertical jump is used to measure vertical power, the long jump is used to measure horizontal power. As another test of lower-body power, it too is a good choice for athletes requiring speed, agility, and quickness. The test is very easy to conduct, since a tape measure is the only equipment needed. Although this is a valid measure of

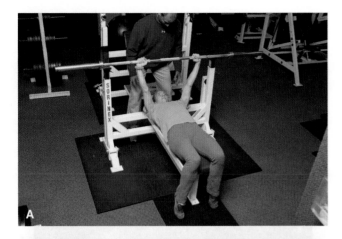

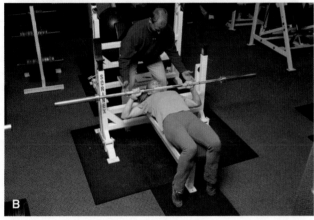

FIGURE 8.8 Bench press. **A.** Starting position. **B.** Downward movement.

lower-body power, the movement pattern of the standing long jump is not specific to many sports. Therefore, other field tests, such as the 40-yd sprint test and vertical jump, may have more specific applications for many athletes.

TEST INTERPRETATION

Administering a test and recording a measurement are the simple portions of any assessment routine. The final and most complicated portion is making an evaluation of those scores. This involves placing a value on the recorded score so it may be used to help design a program of training specific to the individual. To accomplish this, the scores must be put into a logical order and analyzed for practical significance. Once the scores have been collected, they must be compared to a proper criterion or normative scale based on the subpopulation (14,18,19). The scope of this book does not allow an in-depth discussion of statistical significance; therefore, this discourse focuses on the practical uses of test scores.

> *Once the test data are collected, they should be accurately interpreted to the coach and the athlete in terms of norms and expected improvement.*

Order Scales

Test scores fall into three main categories. **Nominal** scores are those that are coded for entry into a spreadsheet or statistical computer program. They represent the "real" item through the use of numbers. An example is coding gender as 1 for male and 2 for female, or vice versa. One might also use a code for positional differences on an athletic team, such as 1 for outside hitters, 2 for setters, and 3 for middle blockers on a volleyball team. This procedure allows the tester to add up the number of participants who possess similar characteristics but not to perform mathematical calculations on those values.

Interval scores are those that do not possess an absolute zero, meaning that zero does not represent the absence of that variable but that it sometimes contains negative scores and there is no standard unit of difference between scores. The most popular form of interval scoring is temperature expressed in Fahrenheit degrees. Freezing is expressed as 32 degrees: zero does not constitute no temperature, negative numbers are used to express colder temperatures, and 66 degrees is not twice as warm as 33 degrees.

Ratio scores possess all the traits not held by interval. They have an absolute zero, meaning a zero score is an absence of that variable, as in an elderly person's vertical jump score of zero inches. They contain no negative numbers and there is an absolute scale of measurement between scores, such that lifting 50 lb is scored at exactly half as much as lifting 100 lb. This is the most popular form of physiological measurement and is predominantly used in the literature on physical activity and testing.

Sometimes a fourth form of scoring order is expressed as **ordinal**, which is more accurately described as a ranking system rather than a scoring scale. An ordinal system ranks scores from top to bottom, highest to lowest, or greatest to least. All the other scales of measurement can be listed in ordinal rank, but it does not change them from their original scaling form.

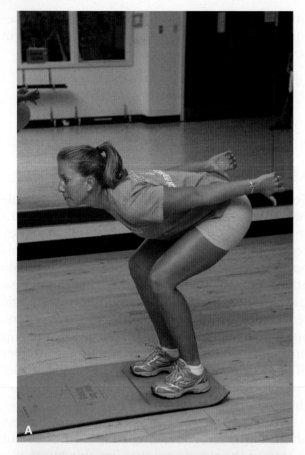

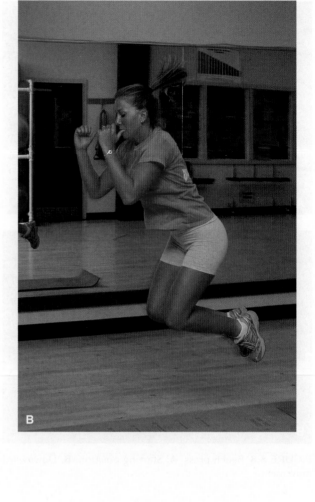

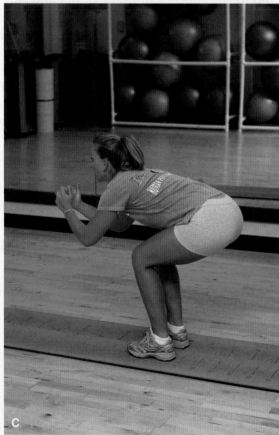

FIGURE 8.9 Standing long jump. **A.** Starting position. **B.** Jump. **C.** Landing.

Mathematical Measures

A few variables are associated with central tendency; these need to be discussed because they enable the investigator to draw conclusions from the collected data. These variables are fundamental in nature and require little mathematical skill but will provide the tester with valuable information regarding the data as a whole and each individual's relationship to the overall group.

Minimum and **maximum** refer to the least score and the greatest score, respectively.

The **range** is the difference between the minimum and maximum and represents the overall spread of scores as a whole number. The formula is max–min.

The **sum** is the total of all scores combined and added together. The formula is $X_1 + X_2 + X_3 + X_4$, etc.

N is the symbol used to denote the number of people in the test group and is used in conjunction with the sum to arrive at other important variables.

The **mean** is simply the arithmetic average derived from the sum divided by N. It is the most sensitive of all measures of central tendency and is also used most often. It considers every score in the group and is pulled away from the middle by extreme scores. The formula is sum/n.

The **median** is the exact middle of the total number of scores. It is not affected by outliers, shows a position only, and is rarely used for statistical calculations. To find the median, the scores should first be placed in an ordinal ranking; then, if there is an odd number of scores, the median will be the middle score (e.g., if there are 11 scores, then the median is score no. 6, since 5 scores are greater and 5 scores are less). If there is an even number of scores, then the median will be an average of the two middle scores (e.g., if there are 12 scores, then the median is the average of scores 6 and 7).

Mode is the score that occurs most frequently. There may be multiple modes or no mode at all. It too is not affected by extreme scores and is not often used in statistical calculations.

Distribution of Scores

Once all the scores have been collected, it is beneficial to determine their measures of central tendency. **Central tendency** is the measure of the middle of a distribution of scores. The measurement community relies on scores following a few basic rules, which causes them to take familiar shapes when presented graphically. The scores can then be analyzed using basic statistical assumptions. Figure 8.10 displays a normal bell curve, the basic element and starting point of many statistical techniques. The bell curve is a frequency histogram that plots the number of times a score occurs on the vertical, or Y axis, against the raw number itself on the horizontal, or X axis, where scores increase as they move from left to right. The conventional hump in the middle demonstrates that the greatest number of scores fall in the middle range with fewer and fewer scores out to either side. Most tests will produce a graph that is at least in part similar to a bell curve. In other words, there will be a few very low and very high scores, with the majority of scores being very similar. It is of paramount importance to remember that although many statistical calculations are based on the bell curve, *it almost never occurs in real-life data.* Therefore, a bit of error is built into all statistics, and statistics should always be read with this in mind. The only true bell curve occurs when the mean, median, and mode are exactly the same number.

The hump in the bell curve shows the likeness of scores. If many of the athletes scored similarly, then the hump will be tall and thin; whereas in a group with many varied scores, the hump will be short and flat. In some instances the curve does not follow such a symmetrical shape as that of the bell curve. Figure 8.11A displays a **positively skewed**

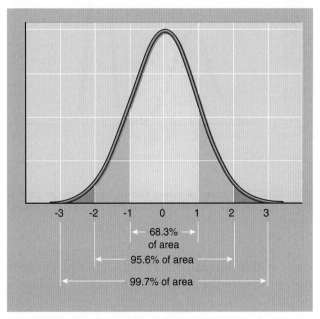

FIGURE 8.10 Normal bell curve. This commonly occurring frequency histogram demonstrates that the greatest number of scores falls in the middle range, with fewer scores at the extremes.

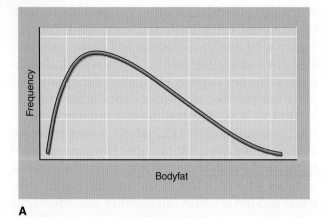

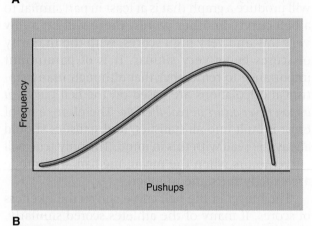

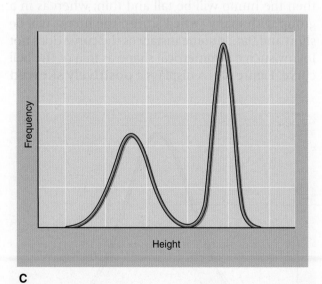

FIGURE 8.11 Likeness of scores shown by humps on graphs. **A.** Positively skewed curve. **B.** Negatively skewed curve. **C.** Bimodal curve.

curve with a long tail on the right and a hump near the left side of the graph. Figure 8.11B displays a **negatively skewed** curve with a long tail on the left and a hump near the right side of the graph. At times, a group of scores may even produce multiple humps. Figure 8.11C displays a **bimodal curve**

where the frequency of scores was greatest in two different portions of the final outcome. Since the hump exhibits similarity of scores, a bimodal curve may reveal that the group contains two like groups of people (e.g. two genders, two athletic teams, etc.).

Variability

The most commonly used measure of variability in scores is the **standard deviation (SD)**. It describes the scatter of scores about the mean and is used to show inclusion of scores for different percentages of the population and can be used as a measure of homogeneity when compared to the mean. It is derived through a few simple mathematical steps:

1. Calculate the deviation of each score from the mean by subtracting the mean from each raw score. Half of the deviation scores will be negative, since half the scores will fall below the mean. Do not let this concern you, as it will be remedied in the next step.
2. Square each deviation score by multiplying it by itself. This will convert all negative scores to positive scores.
3. Add all the squared deviations together to arrive at a sum.
4. Divide the sum of the squared deviations by $N - 1$ (e.g., if $N = 11$, then divide by 10); the answer is termed the **variance**. By eliminating one participant from the group, it will better assist the tester in using the resultant data to predict the performance of other similar groups that were not tested.
5. Take the square root of the variance to counterbalance the squaring process performed earlier in the second step. The answer is the SD.

Now the SD can be used to explain the variability of scores previously displayed in the bell curve. Figure 8.10 shows how the mean and SD can be used to calculate group inclusion numbers. Simply stated, the mean plus or minus 1-SD includes approximately 68% of the total group population. In other words if following a test the scores revealed a mean of 25 and an SD of 10 then it could be stated that approximately 68% of the group population had scores between 15 and 35 (e.g., 25–10 = 15 and 25 + 10 = 35). If $N = 75$, then 68% of that population would be 51 (e.g., 75 × 0.68). Likewise, the mean plus or minus 2 SD includes approximately

95% of the population while the mean plus or minus 3 SD includes approximately 99% or almost everyone in the test population. Remember that, since the bell curve almost never occurs (mean, median, and mode must be exactly the same number), there is always some error in the system. Therefore, the percentages rarely fall directly on those numbers but are most often close.

Standardized Scores

Another important use for the SD is to calculate **standardized scores**. These are scores that express each individual score as an SD, making it easier to determine each score's standard distance from the mean. This procedure allows tests with different units of measurement to be compared without confusion (e.g., vertical jump in inches versus 1 RM in pounds). They are therefore commonly used with standardized tests of knowledge or for large population groups following administration of a test battery.

Standardized scores are divided into two types. First, are **Z scores**, which range between −3 and +3 and are expressed out to two decimal places. They are calculated by subtracting the mean from the raw score and then dividing by the SD. If a raw score were 35 and the mean 25 with an SD of 10, then the equation would be (35 − 25) / 10 = 1. The resultant Z score of 1 means that the raw score of 35 is exactly 1 SD greater than the mean. Consequently the average Z score is zero and all positive Z scores are raw scores greater than the mean, while all negative Z scores are raw scores less than the mean.

Second, **T scores**, which range from 30 to 80, are almost identical to Z scores. They are the same because they are derived from Z scores. The procedure for T scores is to multiply the Z score by 10 then add 50. T scores are always positive whole numbers (i.e., no decimal places). Consequently the average T score is 50 and all T scores greater than 50 are raw scores greater than the mean, while all T scores less than 50 are raw scores less than the mean. T scores are used because the

resultant value is always positive and easy for the lay person to understand.

SUMMARY

A valid and reliable evaluation and assessment program begins with a careful needs analysis of both the client/athlete and the activity/sport. Appropriate tests are then chosen based on the individual needs of the situation, and the results are carefully analyzed using the basic mathematical calculations of central tendency and variability. By performing these simple calculations, assumptions can be made regarding the value of each score for each participant. Scores can then be compared to population-specific normative values or a criterion scale developed from those norms. In the final analysis, the well-prepared and knowledgeable tester will be able to evaluate each individual's needs and subsequently prescribe an appropriate training program to meet the derived client-specific goals.

MAXING OUT

1. A graduate student wanted to know something about the vertical jump of her classmates. She tested each one in the class and came up with the following data set: 19.5, 20, 21.5, 18, 17.5, 16, 22.5, 25, 24.5, 17.5. Find the mean, median, and mode of the data set and explain how to use these numbers to describe a team to a coach.
2. The basketball coach comes to you and wants an assessment of the team. You plan to do a "needs analysis" looking at both the individual player and the game of basketball. List the tests you will need to perform to answer the coach's query regarding the state of his team.
3. A colleague of yours has just developed a new assessment tool and has asked you to establish the validity and reliability of the new tool. What would you do to accomplish this? How are the two different?

CASE EXAMPLE
Designing a Performance Testing Program for an Elite Junior Tennis Athlete

BACKGROUND

You are employed in a major, well-equipped sports facility and have all testing equipment available to you. You are told to prepare for a complete fitness evaluation of a 16-year-old nationally ranked male tennis player preparing to turn pro. The player is the current national champion in the 16-and-under age group. He was first runner-up in the Junior U.S. Open this year.

The athlete is experienced in all areas of training and conditioning. He uses free-weight resistance training regularly in his program and performs a variety of multijoint and Olympic-style lifts. He participates in a variety of speed and agility training exercises.

The athlete does participate in clay court tournaments from time to time, but his primary surface, and the surface his game is expected to excel on is a hard court surface.

Using a needs analysis of the sport of tennis and a typical tennis athlete, design a complete fitness testing session to evaluate this athlete.

RECOMMENDATIONS/CONSIDERATIONS

Begin with a needs analysis of the sport of tennis. Professional tennis is an explosive, fast game, particularly on hard court surfaces. The tennis athlete is required to change direction rapidly several times in a point. The ability to generate ground reaction force and transfer that force to the upper body is a key component of success in tennis. The testing program for this athlete will likely include tests for the following: muscular endurance; lower extremity muscle strength; lower extremity power; upper extremity muscle strength; upper extremity power, speed, and agility; cardiorespiratory endurance; and joint range of motion. Injuries should be noted and the musculoskeletal adaptations to those injuries be considered.

IMPLEMENTATION

Maximal treadmill test with metabolic cart. Although tennis is primarily an anaerobic sport, recovery between points is aerobic. Moderate to moderately high levels of oxygen consumption are desirable in the tennis athlete. This test will provide information on the athlete's ability to work aerobically and to recover between points.

Bench press. Since the athlete trains using free weights, the bench press is a good measure of upper-body strength.

Squat. Again, since the athlete trains with free weights, the squat is a good choice for measuring overall lower extremity strength. The ability of a tennis player to generate ground reaction force is a key component of tennis performance.

Vertical jump. The vertical jump is an excellent choice to measure lower-body power. Performance on this test is relevant to tennis, as it is an indicator of the ability of the athlete to get a quick start and may also be an indicator of the athlete's ability to generate power in the service motion.

Seated medicine ball push. This test is a measure of general upper-body power.

20-yd dash. Speed in tennis is limited to short distances, and 20 yd would be the maximum a player would have to run all-out without stopping or changing direction.

Hexagon. This test is used to measure footwork and agility.

"T" test. This test measures lateral, backward, and forward movement over a short distance and the ability to transition between them.

Five-point agility run. This test measures the ability of the athlete to move in diagonal patterns, change direction, gain speed, decelerate, and stop.

Underwater weighing. This is an accurate way of determining body composition.

Push-ups in 60 s. In this athlete, pushups are a test of upper body muscular endurance. In the athlete who can perform only a few pushups, it becomes a test of muscular strength.

Sit-ups in 60 s. Sit-ups are a general measure of core body strength and endurance. The trunk is very important in tennis, as it transfers forces from the ground to the upper extremity.

RESULTS

Results are reported by percentile rank using a database of over 100 16-year-old male tennis athletes.

Maximal treadmill test with metabolic cart. 90th percentile.

Bench press. 96th percentile.

Squat. 91st percentile.

Vertical jump. 60th percentile.

Seated medicine ball push. 88th percentile.

20 yd dash. 88th percentile.

Hexagon. 85th percentile.

"T" test. 89th percentile.

Five-point agility run. 87th percentile.

Underwater weighing. 90th percentile.

These results should be reported to the athlete, the coach, and/or the player's parents. The one area of athletic fitness that obviously needs the most work is lower-body power. Remember, in conveying results to the player, to point needed areas of improvement and prescribe appropriate exercise regimens to correct the identified deficits.

REFERENCES

1. Bar-Or O. The Wingate test: An update on methodology, reliability and validity. Sports Med 1987;4:381–394.

2. Brown LE, Weir JP. ASEP procedures recommendations for the accurate assessment of muscular strength and power. J Exerc Physiol [serial online]. 2001;4(3):1–21. Available at: http://faculty.css.edu/tboone2/asep/August2001JEPonline.html. Accessed October 16, 2003.

3. Brown LE, Whitehurst M, Bryant JR. A comparison of the LIDO sliding cuff and the tibial control system in isokinetic strength parameters. Isokinet Exer Sci 1992;2(3):101–109.

4. Brown LE, Whitehurst M, Bryant JR. Reliability of the LIDO active isokinetic dynamometer concentric mode. Isokinet Exer Sci 1992;2(4):191–194.

5. Brown LE, Whitehurst M, Bryant JR, Buchalter DN. Reliability of the Biodex system 2 isokinetic dynamometer concentric mode. Isokinet Exer Sci 1993;3(3):160–163.

6. Chapman, PP, Whitehead JR, Binkert RH. The 225-lb reps-to-fatigue test as a submaximal estimate of 1-RM bench press performance in college football players. J Strength Cond Res 1998;12:258–261.

7. Chinn S, Burney PGJ. On measuring repeatability of data from self-administered questionnaires. Int J Epidemiol 1987;16:121–127.

8. Conway DP, Decker AS. Utilizing a computerized strength and conditioning testing index for assessment of collegiate football players. Natl Strength Cond Assoc J 1992;14(5):13–16.

9. Dolezal BA, Thompson CJ, Schroeder CA, et al. Laboratory testing to improve athletic performance. Strength Cond 1997;19(6):20–24.

10. Enoka RM. Neuromechanical Basis of Kinesiology. Champaign, IL: Human Kinetics, 1988.

11. Graham J. Guidelines for providing valid testing of athletes' fitness levels. Strength Cond 1994;16(6):7–14.

12. Magill RA. Motor Learning: Concepts and Applications. 5th ed. Madison, WI: Brown & Benchmark, 1998.

13. Maud PJ, Shultz BB. Norms for the Wingate anaerobic test with comparison to another similar test. Res Q Exerc Sport 1989;60:144–151.

14. Mayhew JL, Ware JR, Prinster JL. Using lift repetitions to predict muscular strength in adolescent males. Natl Strength Cond Assoc J 1993;15(6):35–38.

15. Patton JF, Duggan A. An evaluation of tests of anaerobic power. Aviat Space Environ Med 1987;58:237–142.

16. Plisk SS. Anaerobic metabolic conditioning: a brief review of theory, strategy and practical application. J Strength Cond Res 1991;5(1):22–34.

17. Plisk SS, Gambetta V. Tactical metabolic training: Part 1. Strength Cond 1997;19(2):44–53.

18. Schweigert D. Normative values for common preseason testing protocols: NCAA division II women's basketball. Strength Cond 1996;18(6):7–10.

19. Semenick D, Connors J, Carter M, et al. Rationale, protocols, testing/reporting forms and instructions for wrestling. Natl Strength Cond Assoc J 1992;14(3):54–59.

20. Swank AM, Adams K, Serapiglia L, et al. Submaximal testing for the strength and conditioning professional. Strength Cond J 1999;21(6):9–15.

21. Taylor NAS, Sanders RH, Howick EI, Stanley SN. Static and dynamic assessment of the Biodex dynamometer. Eur J Appl Physiol 1991;62:180–188.

22. Timm KE, Fyke D. The effect of test speed sequence on the concentric isokinetic performance of the knee extensor muscle group. Isok Exerc Sci 1993;3(2):123–128.

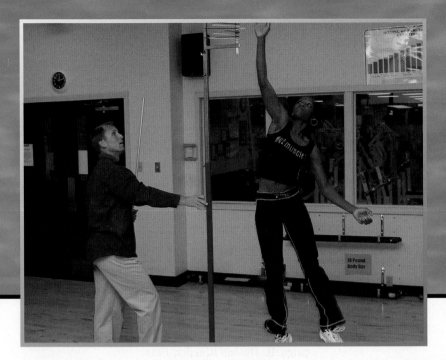

Warm-up and Flexibility

DUANE V. KNUDSON

Introduction

Athletes looking to improve sport performance or lengthen their athletic careers by modifying the risk of injury—as well as the exercising public—often focus on warm-up and flexibility routines in their training. Considerable research has been conducted on both of these issues and a surprising picture is emerging. The bulk of the current research is supportive of training and injury-prevention beliefs related to warm-up. Common beliefs about flexibility and stretching, however, are changing. This chapter summarizes what is known about the performance and injury-prevention benefits of warm-up and flexibility, since the two have complex relationships to performance and the risk of musculoskeletal injury. The chapter concludes with general recommendations for prescribing stretching exercises and programs.

WARM-UP

It is important to realize that warm-up and stretching are two different activities. Warm-up is designed to elevate core body temperature and stretching is primarily performed to increase the range of motion (ROM) at a joint or group of joints. It is well accepted that generalized warm-up movements are important to maximizing sport performance and reducing injury risk in physical activity. **Warm-up** consists of active or passive warming of body tissues in preparation for physical activity. **Active warm-up** consists of low-intensity movements that are effective in elevating body temperature, warming tissue, and producing a variety of improvements in physiological function. **Passive warm-up** includes external heat sources like heating pads, whirlpools, or ultrasound. Prior to vigorous exertion, athletes should perform several minutes of general body movements (**general warm-up**) of progressively increasing intensity. These movements should emulate the actual movements of the sport or exercise to follow. Low-intensity movement specific to the sport or activity of interest is called **specific warm-up**.

Warm-up benefits performance through thermal, neuromuscular, and psychological effects (9,10,22,46,87,89). In some people, warm-up may also decrease the occurrence of dangerous cardiac responses from sudden strenuous exercise (5). Active warm-up activities mobilize metabolic resources and increase tissue temperature. Much of the benefit of warm-up comes from the increased body temperature (22). Moderate-intensity active warm-up (general movements) and passive warm-up (e.g., diathermy, heating pads, whirlpool) can increase muscular performance between 3 and 9% (9,10). Large-muscle-group motor tasks benefit from warm-up more than fine motor tasks (22).

Another reason for warm-up is to prepare the tissues for the greater stresses of vigorous physical activity and thus to lower the risk of muscle-tendon injury. Biomechanical evidence supports this "injury-protective" hypothesis, since warmed-up muscle in animal models has been found to elongate more before failure (28,80,86,91). This, combined with prospective studies of warm-up (19), suggests that general warm-up prior to vigorous activity may decrease the risk of musculotendinous injury compared to no warm-up. More direct evidence of this relationship would be help-ful, but it is not possible to design studies that put subjects at risk of injury.

> *Warm-up activities are necessary to prepare the body for vigorous physical activity because they increase performance and decrease the risk of muscular injury.*

Athletes and other exercisers should therefore warm up prior to competition, practice, and physical conditioning. Recommendations for effective warm-up routines vary depending on the nature and duration of the exercise to be performed (10). In general, warm-up routines should use general, whole-body movements up to 40% to 60% of aerobic capacity for 5 to 10 minutes followed by 5 minutes of recovery (10). The American College of Sports Medicine recommends 5 to 10 minutes of calisthenic-type exercises and 5 to 10 minutes of progressive aerobic activity in warm-up (5). For example, tennis players may perform 5 minutes of light jogging, followed by the traditional 5-minute warm-up of ground strokes and serves prior to a match. Movement and muscular contractions commonly used in active warm-up also create decreases in passive tension (76,94) and increases in ROM as large as or larger than those due to passive stretching (40,77).

Most warm-up sessions should begin with general body movements of gradually increasing intensity, focusing on the muscles and joints to be used in training or competition. Static stretching currently is not recommended during warm-up routines (51). The reasons for this change from traditional practice are explored in the following sections on flexibility and stretching.

FLEXIBILITY

Flexibility is an important component of fitness and physical performance. Inconsistent use of terminology related to the term *flexibility* by a variety of health and exercise science professionals has led to confusion. There is a distinct difference between flexibility and joint laxity. **Flexibility** is "the intrinsic property of body tissues which determines the range of motion achievable without injury at a joint or series of joints" (37). The ability to move a joint without causing injury usually refers to the major anatomical rotations at joints rather than the joint laxity or accessory motion tests that orthopedists, physical therapists, and athletic trainers often evaluate to test joint and/or ligament integrity. Flexibility can be measured a variety of ways, and several variables of interest have emerged.

One variable is the common clinical measure of the limits of rotation through a ROM referred to as **static flexibility**. This is estimated by linear or angular measurements of the limits of motion in a joint or joint complex. For example, it might be of clinical interest to know the static flexibility of areas of the body that tend to lose ROM with inactivity, like the lower (lumbar region) back or hamstring muscle group. Many professionals employ a sit-and-reach test (Fig. 9.1), using a linear measurement that provides a good field measure of hamstring static flexibility (34). These tests are limited by the rise in passive tension as the muscle and connective tissue are stretched.

Tests of static flexibility, although easy to administer, have several limitations. A major weakness of these tests is that the measures obtained are subjective and largely related to the subject's stretch tolerance (28,32,68,70), as well as the way in which the endpoint of the ROM is determined. Accurate measurements also depend on testing methodology. Variations in instruments, body positioning, instructions, or the protocol used all heavily influence results. Another problem is the variety of conditions in which the measurements are made. For example, physical therapy uses both active ROM (unassisted) and passive ROM (therapist-assisted) tests (81). The ROM achievable with the assistance of the tester (passive) is usually greater than that obtained with unassisted ROM. A great deal of information must be known about testing conditions to interpret data on static flexibility.

In a research setting, we now have the ability to measure mechanical properties of the body in addition to the clinical measurements of ROM. Research laboratory measurements of flexibility using computerized dynamometers have allowed the measurement of new biomechanical variables related to the mechanical properties of muscle and tendon. Two of these variables that may be related to performance and injury risk are stiffness and hysteresis. These terms are used in physics to describe properties of materials. Since the human body is composed of materials that react to external forces in exactly the same as other materials, the terms are also applicable to the human body.

The term **stiffness**, sometimes also known as dynamic flexibility, refers to how quickly tissue resistance rises during a movement that requires the muscle-tendon unit to stretch. With passive stretching, the stiffness of the muscle-tendon unit measures how quickly the passive tension rises right before damage occurs. Studies show that dynamic flexibility accounts for only about 44% to 66% of the variance of static flexibility (70,74). Therefore, these variables are related but probably represent different functional properties of the musculature.

Figure 9.2 illustrates a schematic of a torque-angle curve of the elongation phase of repeated

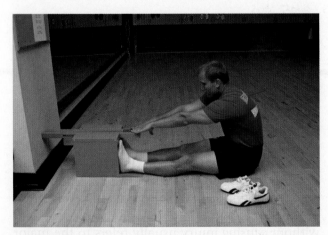

FIGURE 9.1 Since its development in the 1950s, the sit-and-reach test and several variations have become popular field tests of hamstring static flexibility.

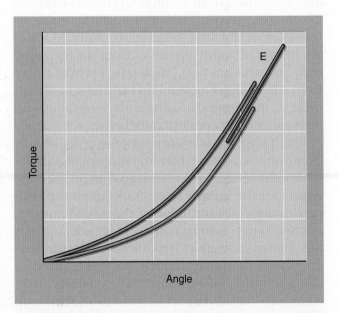

FIGURE 9.2 Schematic of a torque-joint angle plot during repeated passive stretches of a muscle group. Stress relaxation makes the passive torque at a given joint angle in subsequent stretches (blue line) less than in the first stretch (purple line). The stiffness (E) of the muscle group in these stretches, however, is not different.

passive stretches of a muscle group. These angular variables approximate well the load-deformation (linear) curve of the muscle (67) and provide an in vivo (in the living animal) functional estimate of the passive stiffness of muscle groups (25,70,74). Scientists normally use linear measurements of load and deformation to define the mechanical properties of materials. Note that in the graph, the torque (and also tension) in the muscle rises in a complex fashion, slowly and then rapidly as the muscle gets longer.

Biological tissues have other complex behaviors that influence their function. The muscle-tendon unit is considered to be **viscoelastic**. This means that the muscle-tendon unit can extend immediately when a tensile stress is applied and that it also continues to elongate with continued application of the stress. A faster stretch would have a similar shape but a higher stiffness because of this viscoelastic behavior. The tension developed during a stretch depends on the degree of elongation and the rate of the stretch. Also note in Figure 9.2 that the stiffness (E) of the muscle group does not change with repeated static stretching. Preliminary evidence suggests that although stretching does not affect muscle stiffness, passive motion does create significant reductions in muscle stiffness (76).

One problem in discussing the stiffness of muscles is the difference in the scientific and lay meaning of *stiffness* and *elasticity*. In biomechanics, stiffness and **elasticity** are synonymous, so a muscle with a quick rise in tension during stretch will tend to recover rapidly when the stretch is released. This conflicts with the colloquial meaning of the term *elasticity*, which refers to low resistance to elongation.

Although the application of materials science to the human body may seem complex, it is important to realize that the human body is a material that responds to stress in a predictable manner. Materials science defines stiffness as the slope of the stress-strain curve in the elastic (linear) region, which is how quickly the tension rises late in elongation before the elastic limit. The elastic limit is the point on the graph depicting the lengthening of the muscle-tendon unit just before the material begins to fail or the beginning of permanent damage. Beyond the elastic limit is the plastic region, so called because this is where the deformation is not immediately recoverable. Fortunately, small stretches beyond the elastic limit may be repaired by the body if it is given enough rest, but a very severe

elongation can cause rupture or complete failure of the tissue. Materials scientists call the maximum force or energy absorbed before complete failure the **mechanical strength** of the material.

When a muscle is stretched, but not beyond its elastic limit, it will return to resting length and recover some of the energy stored in it as it was stretched. Some of the energy, however, is lost as heat. The energy lost in the return to normal length from a deformed material is termed **hysteresis**. This represents the energy lost and can be visualized as the area (loop) between the loading (elongation) and unloading (restitution) phases in Figure 9.3. This figure illustrates a schematic of a torque-angle curve of the elongation phase (purple line) and the restitution phase (blue line) of a static stretch.

From Figure 9.3, note that in static stretching, 40% to 50% of the energy stored in the stretch is lost as the muscle returns to normal length (64). Much of this energy loss is in the contractile and connective tissue components within the muscle. To the contrary, studies of long tendons in normal activity show that they recover most (80% to 90%) of the energy stored in them in cyclic stretch-shortening actions (2,55).

Measuring energy may be better for examining the effect of stretching on muscle, as opposed to stiffness, because muscle tissue does not reach the elastic region of the stress/strain curve in typical

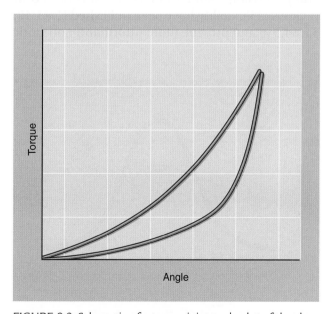

FIGURE 9.3 Schematic of a torque-joint angle plot of the elongation (purple) and restitution (blue) phases of a passive stretch of a muscle group. The energy lost (hysteresis) is the area of the loop between the loading and unloading phases.

hamstring stretches (67). Stretching has a greater effect on hysteresis than on the stiffness of muscle. This is important because it gives direction to where we should be performing research in the future if that research is going to be practical and meaningful in terms of improving performance.

> *The ability to move the joints of the body freely without injury is known as flexibility, and several mechanical properties can be used to document aspects of flexibility.*

Normal Static Flexibility

The wealth of research on static flexibility measurements provides a general picture of what is normal static flexibility for most joints and populations. Normal static flexibility is the typical joint movement allowed between two extremes (Fig. 9.4): ankylosis and hypermobility (85,93). **Ankylosis** is pathological loss of ROM, while **hypermobility** is excessive ROM. Static flexibility is not a whole-body characteristic but, like fitness, is specific to joints and directions of movement (33,39). People may tend to have low static flexibility in one part of the body and normal or high flexibility in another. It is also clear that females have greater static flexibility than males (33), and some of these differences are related to anthropometric differences (13).

Fitness professionals can access data on normal ranges of static flexibility for most joints from several professional sources (4–6,27). Several recent reviews of flexibility have been published (1,23,42, 51,64,59) and provide more information on static flexibility. It is unclear however, whether an "optimal" level of static flexibility for muscle groups or areas of the body exists. If this is the case, it is likely that different sports would require different optimal levels of static flexibility. Future research studies should be designed to focus on determining "normative" static ranges of motion at joints in athletes participating in specific sports, as well as documenting anomalies in athletes and active people who are outside of this normative range. It is too early to make a definitive statement, but it is possible that an athlete or active person whose muscles are too tight is more prone to *muscle* injuries and that one whose muscles are too loose is more prone to *joint* injuries as well as decreased performance in strength and power activities.

Common deviations from normal static flexibility are present in many joint(s). Some people lose ROM from physical inactivity. People may also lose static flexibility from workplace or sport-specific positions and/or repetitive movements. For example, the repetitive motion in several sports with overhead throwing patterns (baseball, tennis, etc.) without specific stretching intervention (47) can result in glenohumeral internal rotation deficit (GIRD). Persistent wearing of high heels can decrease ankle dorsiflexion ROM (Fig. 9.5).

> *Several resources provide normative data on the typical static flexibility of most major joints of the body, but current research does not identify an optimal level of static flexibility.*

Flexibility and Injury Risk

What appears to be desirable, based on data on the incidence of injury, is to avoid the extremes in static

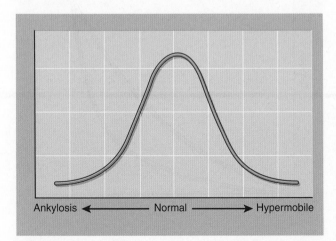

FIGURE 9.4 Schematic of a continuum of static flexibility. There is considerable research documenting the normal limits of static flexibility but little prospective research that links specific levels of static flexibility to increased risk of injury at either extreme.

Ankylosis ◄——— Normal ———► Hypermobile

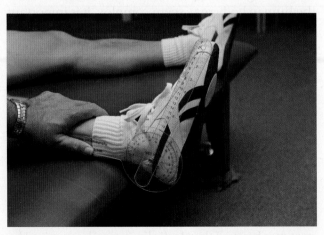

FIGURE 9.5 Repetitive work or body positions (like wearing high heels) can create tight muscles and decrease ankle static flexibility.

flexibility. Athletes and exercisers at both extremes of static flexibility may be at a higher risk for musculoskeletal injuries (45,48). The literature on clinical and basic science provides a very different view of the role of flexibility in injury risk and performance than what is commonly believed and practiced. This section focuses on the association between flexibility and injury risk: the sections on stretching, further on, discuss the association between stretching and changes in muscular performance and injury risk.

Low levels of hamstring flexibility have been related to a higher risk of muscular injury in soccer (103). The common belief that greater static flexibility will always decrease the risk of muscular injury, however, appears not to be valid. This may be explained by the stability-mobility paradox. The mechanical stability and ROM at a joint or joints are inversely related (14,59,93). It is possible that as static flexibility increases beyond the normal range, the potential benefits of greater motion and less tissue resistance are offset by the greater instability of the joint. More research is needed to begin to define the ranges of motion for various joints, so that the best compromise of stability and mobility may be provided, along with a lower risk of injury.

A good example of the lack of an association between high levels of static flexibility and lower injury risk is provided by low back fitness testing. Although it seems logical that less flexible back or hamstring muscles would be related to the incidence of low back pain, little evidence supports this association. A review of the literature found limited support (mixed results) for an association between lumbar/hamstring flexibility and the occurrence of low back pain (82). More recently, a large prospective study found no relationship between static flexibility and subsequent low back pain in adults (43). Therefore, the field tests of hamstring static flexibility commonly used in fitness test batteries may not be useful in predicting future low back injury.

People also commonly believe that less "stiff" muscles result in greater flexibility and a lower risk of injury. Unfortunately, little research is available on the association between dynamic flexibility and injury risk. Less stiff muscles may be less susceptible to muscle strain injury (102), but only one study has been conducted in this area (73). It appears that muscle with greater stiffness is more susceptible to eccentrically induced muscle damage. Currently, the evidence is insufficient to conclude that decreased dynamic flexibility will provide an injury-protective benefit. Combined with the unclear nature of the exact levels of static flexibility that decrease injury risk, this means that strength and conditioning professionals must educate athletes on the complexity of flexibility and injury risk.

A complex relationship exists between static flexibility and risk of muscular injury. Higher injury rates appear to be related to very flexible or very inflexible muscles.

Assessing Flexibility

Exercise prescriptions to modify flexibility should be based on valid measurements using standardized testing procedures. Static flexibility tests are based on both linear and angular measurements of the motion of a joint or group of joints. These tests can focus on single joints or compound movements of many body segments and joints.

Single-joint static flexibility tests are commonly used clinically in the medical professions (4,6,24,27,81); they often involve angular measurements (with goniometers or inclinometers) rather than linear measurements. Single-joint tests are considered better measurements of static flexibility than compound tests because they better isolate specific muscles and are less affected by anthropometric differences (15,58). The straight-leg-raise (30) and

REAL-WORLD APPLICATION
The Stability-Mobility Paradox

Static flexibility is like exercise in that more is not always better. Joint motion (mobility) is inversely proportional to the stability of the joint (93). Decreasing muscle passive tension around a joint increases the joint's ROM but also makes it easier for the joint to be pulled out of normal position. This presents the fitness professional with a paradox. What is the right amount of static flexibility? How much motion is necessary for normal and safe movement without adversely affecting the joint or ligaments? It is not possible to give easy answers to these questions. The amount of motion depends on the joint, the requirements of the sport/activity a person engages in, and other factors. Given that the lowest injury rates seem to correspond to normal flexibility and higher injury rates with the extremes in flexibility (inflexible and hypermobile), maintenance of normal or moderate amounts of static flexibility should be the goal for most people. Unless a person participates in an activity requiring extreme flexibility (dance, gymnastics, diving), most exercise prescriptions should focus on maintaining normal levels of static flexibility.

active-knee-extension (26) tests are the common hamstring flexibility tests used in physical therapy. The many variations of the sit-and-reach test (31, 36,38) are compound tests and are often validated with the straight leg raise or active knee extension.

Sit-and-reach scores are associated with hamstring flexibility but not with low back flexibility (72). Although the sit-and-reach test has been shown to be a moderately valid measure of hamstring flexibility which is only slightly affected by anthropometric variations (41,72), the prescriptive value of these measurements is limited. One study showed that 6% of children falsely passed and 12% falsely failed the sit-and-reach test relative to the straight-leg-raise test (15). If these data are consistent across all ages, people failing the sit-and-reach test should be retested with the straight-leg-raise or active-knee-extension test to make sure that they have limited hamstring static flexibility.

Current health-related norms for sit-and-reach or other static flexibility tests should be used only to identify individuals at the extremes who may be at higher risk for muscle injuries. Not enough data are available to provide specific static flexibility goals beyond the maintenance of normal flexibility. Fitness professionals must also remember that in measuring flexibility, exacting attention to testing details is necessary. Static flexibility scores are subjective and highly dependent on the subject's tolerance of the high muscle tension (discomfort) during testing. The clinical measurement of dynamic flexibility is not ordinarily practicable; it is limited to research settings because of problems related to expensive equipment, insufficient standardization, and the lack of normative data.

DEVELOPMENT OF FLEXIBILITY

Normal levels of flexibility can be maintained by regular physical activity and through specific programs of stretching and strengthening exercises. Kinesiology professionals should assess a client's flexibility, and based on these data and the client's history, develop a program to improve flexibility. Although poor flexibility can be treated with a combination of stretching and strengthening exercises (1), this section focuses on general recommendations for stretching in mass exercise prescription. Regular stretching exercises are usually

recommended for most people because of their often limited physical activity and also because regular participation in some activities is associated with sport-specific flexibility imbalances. In general, stretching recommendations should be limited to the maintenance of normal levels of static flexibility because of the complex nature of flexibility and the lack of data linking specific levels of flexibility to lower injury risk. This section concludes with recent evidence on the effect of stretching on muscular performance, which has implications for the placement of stretching in the training cycle.

Stretching exercises are usually classified into four types: passive, static, ballistic (dynamic), and **proprioceptive neuromuscular facilitation, or PNF** (8). **Passive stretching** uses an external force, usually another person, to stretch muscle groups (Fig. 9.6). **Static stretching** involves a slow increase in muscle group length and holding the stretched position at that length for a short time (usually 15 to 30 seconds). **Ballistic stretching** traditionally has meant fast, momentum-assisted, and bouncing stretching movements. These stretches are generally avoided because of the viscoelastic nature of muscle. For a given elongation, a fast stretch results in a higher force in the tissue and a greater risk of injury (61,88,95). Some refer to the active warm-up movements mentioned earlier as **dynamic stretching**. These stretches may be acceptable if they are performed in a relatively slow manner to create muscle elongation without imposing high levels of force on the tissue. This is probably how regular physical activity can maintain static flexibility.

The last group of stretching exercises focuses on PNF. PNF stretch routines use a specific series of

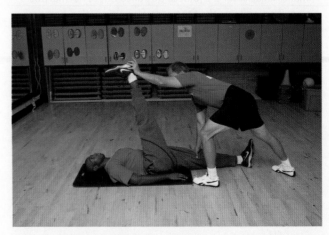

FIGURE 9.6 Passive stretching often uses external force from another person to produce a greater stretch of a muscle group.

movements and contractions to use neuromuscular reflexes to relax the muscles being stretched. PNF stretches can be performed with or without assistance. A simple PNF procedure is a "contract-relax" stretch where a person performs an isometric contraction of a muscle to be stretched, which is immediately followed by a static stretch of that muscle. This strategy takes advantage of the inhibitory effects of **Golgi tendon organs** as the muscle is slowly stretched. Assisted stretching procedures like PNF should be performed with care by trained subjects or sports medicine personnel. The practice of having athletes passively stretch partners should be used with caution until the athletes have been carefully trained in correct procedures and understand the risks of incorrect or high-force stretches.

The recommendations for stretching procedures are based on reviews of the basic science studies of the viscoelastic response of muscle to stretching (49,50). These recommendations (Table 9.1) are designed for group exercise prescription with normal subjects. Static or PNF stretching should be performed at least three times per week, preferably daily and after moderate or vigorous physical activity (in the cool-down phase of training). Exacting technique in stretching is recommended to safely focus tension on a muscle group or groups without systematic stress on other joint stability structures (ligaments, joint capsules, cartilage). Some experts have hypothesized, based on functional anatomy, that some stretching exercises are contraindicated because of potentially dangerous ligament and tissue loading (60,62,63).

Stretching programs should include up to four or five stretches for each major muscle group, with each stretch held for 15 to 30 seconds. The intensity (force) of each stretch should be minimized, slowly elongating and holding the stretched position just before the point of discomfort. The American College of Sports Medicine recommends holding static stretches "to a position of mild discomfort" (5). Slow elongation of muscles creates less reflex contraction through the action of **muscle spindles**. These sense muscle length and are responsible for the contraction of a stretched muscle (myotatic reflex). This reflex contraction is most sensitive to fast stretches, so slow muscle elongation in stretching exercises helps maintain relaxation in the muscle groups being stretched.

Static stretching will create a short-term increase in ROM and a decrease in passive tension in the muscle at a particular joint angle due to **stress relaxation**, which is the gradual decrease in stress (force per unit area) in a material stretched and held at a constant length. Most people can feel the decrease in passive tension in a muscle group held in a stretched position. This stress relaxation following stretching provides an immediate 10% to 30% decrease in passive tension (65,71,76), but the effect will have dissipated after about an hour (69). Holding stretches for 20 seconds is a good guideline, because most of the stress relaxation in passive stretches occurs in the first 20 seconds (64,75,95).

 Stretching to increase static flexibility in a muscle group should normally use four to five static stretches held for 15 to 30 seconds.

TABLE 9.1	STRETCHING RECOMMENDATIONS FOR GROUP EXERCISE PRESCRIPTION
FITNESS VARIABLE	**RECOMMENDATION**
Frequency	At least three times per week, preferable daily and after moderate or vigorous physical activity
Intensity	Slowly elongate muscle and hold with low level of force
Time	Up to four to five stretches held from 15 to 30 seconds. Stretch normally during the cool-down phase. Be sure to stretch only muscles that have been thoroughly warmed up from physical activity. Warning: Stretching in the warm-up prior to physical activity may weaken muscles and decrease performance
Type	Static or PNF stretches for all major muscle groups

Source: Reproduced with permission from Knudson D, Magnusson P, McHugh M. Current issues in flexibility fitness. PCPFS Res Digest 2000;3(10):1–8 (51).

Q & A from the Field

Our high school track-and-field athletes routinely stretch before, during, and after their events. I know that flexibility is an important component of performance, but I have heard rumblings in the running community for years that stretching before a sprint is a bad idea. Is it true that stretching prior to high-intensity track-and-field events is a bad idea?

—high school track coach

Athletes stretch in the warm-up for track events because they believe that it decreases their risk of injury and improves their performance. Unfortunately, research has shown that this practice is probably not justified for most athletes. Unless an athlete has a major deficit in ROM, stretching prior to vigorous exertion actually decreases most forms of maximal muscular performance for about an hour. Stretching prior to vigorous activity has also been shown to have no effect on the risk of muscular injury. The most important thing a coach can do is teach athletes that proper warm-up is essential for maximum performance and decreasing the risk of injury. Focus their precompetition routine around a progressive and specific warm-up. Most athletes with normal flexibility should perform their stretching routines after practice or competition.

Stretching should be performed during the cool-down period because of three important factors:

1. Warmed-up tissues are less likely to be injured.
2. The placement of stretching within the workout does not affect gains in static flexibility (16).
3. There can be performance decrements following stretching.

Programming static stretching during the cool-down period is also logical because stretching tends to relax or inhibit muscle activation (7,96). For example, static stretching is commonly used for the acute relief from muscle cramps or delayed-onset muscle soreness (DOMS). The former is indicated, but research on the latter indicates no effect of stretching before (44,99) or after activity (11,99) on the DOMS that occurs after unaccustomed exercise. Static stretching routines in the cool-down period primarily serve to help maintain normal levels of static flexibility.

Biomechanical Effects of Stretching

Stretching exercises are prescribed routinely to increase static flexibility. Research has shown that stretching can provide increases in static flexibility of 5% to 20%, but short-term and over the course of several weeks (50). Less well known are the facts that stretching has minimal effect on the stiffness of muscle (see Fig. 9.2), decreases muscular performance, and modifies the energy recovery of stretched muscle.

Passive stretching can create large tensile loads in the muscle, so it is possible to weaken and injure muscle with vigorous stretching programs. Stretching exercise is like any other training stimulus in that it results in temporary weakening before the body recovers and supercompensates for that activity. This decreased muscular performance following stretching has been documented by the growing consensus of many studies. Decreased performance of 4% to 30% has been observed in maximal strength tests (7,52,78,79) and jumping (12,17,35,104). Stretch-induced decrements in muscular performance appear to be equally related to neuromuscular inhibition and decreased contractile force (16) and can last up to an hour (21). This is why most stretching should be performed in the cool-down phase of training and avoided in the warm-up period for athletic competition. Only athletes who require extreme static flexibility for performance (dancers, gymnasts, divers) might need to stretch at the end of the warm-up phase.

Stretching should normally be performed in the cool-down phase of conditioning because stretching prior to activity decreases muscular performance.

We saw earlier that stretching does not create a short-term decrease in muscle stiffness, but several studies have also shown that stretch training *over time* does not decrease muscle stiffness (51). This is difficult for people to understand because they can feel the lower passive tension in the muscle group at a certain joint angle. Some researchers have also incorrectly defined stiffness as the change in tension over the change in angle from the beginning of the stretch, not as the true mechanical stiffness of the tissue (the slope in the linear region). Strength and conditioning professionals should instruct athletes and other exercisers that the primary benefits of stretching are maintenance of ROM and a decrease in the passive tension in the muscle. The stiffness or elasticity of muscle and tendon is a complex mechanical variable that is not easily understood or experienced.

Another performance-related mechanical variable of interest following stretching is hysteresis. Recall that hysteresis is the energy lost (see Fig. 9.3) when a viscoelastic material returns to its normal shape following a stretch. Only recently have studies begun to examine the effect of stretching on the hysteresis of muscle groups. Although stretching has minimal effect on the passive stiffness of muscle and tendon, it has a significant effect on hysteresis since the loss of recovery energy decreases from 17% to 37% after stretching (53,54,66). This appears to be a promising new area of research on the effects of stretching. Unfortunately, it is not clear whether short- or long-term stretching will increase muscular performance through reductions in hysteresis.

The relationship between muscle mechanical variables, like static and dynamic flexibility and performance, is quite complex. For example, lower levels of static flexibility have been associated with better running economy (18,29), but less stiff musculature is more effective in utilizing elastic energy in stretch-shortening cycle movements (56,57,97, 100,101). It is likely that the effects of stretching and flexibility on muscular performance are complex and activity-specific (28).

Prophylactic Effects of Stretching

The other traditional rationale for prescribing pre-activity stretching is a hypothesized reduction in the risk of injury. The logic was that if there were greater static flexibility from stretching, the chance that stretching the muscle beyond this point might lead to injury would be reduced. In the case of flexibility, this logic has not been supported by scientific evidence. Muscle strains (pulls) usually occur in eccentric muscle actions rather than passive elongation (87).

The larger and better-designed prospective studies have shown little or no effect of stretching on injury rate (3,83,84,98). The studies with larger samples and better controls (83,84) support the conclusion that flexibility and stretching may be unrelated to injury risk. Currently the data are insufficient to support the common prescription of stretching programs to modify flexibility based on the hypothesis of reducing the risk of muscle injury. Much more research on the effects of stretching and the associations between various flexibility levels and injury rates are needed before specific guidelines on stretching will be available.

 Research has not confirmed the belief that stretching decreases the risk of muscular injury, so general stretching prior to physical activity probably confers no protective effect.

SUMMARY

Both active and passive warm-up are common preparatory activities before exercise and athletic competition. Several lines of research have supported the beneficial effects of warm-up on improving performance and reducing injury risk. Typical warm-up should consist of general movements of gradually increasing intensity. The intensity of warm-up should be moderate (up to 40% to 60% of aerobic capacity) and sustained (5 to 10 minutes) to increase the tissue temperature. Flexibility is an important property of the musculoskeletal system that determines the ROM and resistance to motion at a joint or group of joints. This property can be examined by measuring the limits of the achievable motion (static flexibility) or the stiffness of passively stretched muscle group (dynamic flexibility). Normal ranges of static flexibility are well documented for most joints through a variety of tests. There is some evidence that extremes in static flexibility (top or bottom 20% of the distribution) may be associated with a higher incidence of muscle injury.

Sport science research and prospective studies of flexibility and stretching suggest that stretching should not be performed in warm-ups. Stretching prior to physical activity decreases muscular performance and does not reduce the risk of musculoskeletal injury. Currently, little scientific evidence is available on which to base precise, individualized prescriptions of stretching development beyond the maintenance of normal levels of static flexibility. Static or proprioceptive neuromuscular facilitation (PNF) stretching should normally be performed during the cool-down phase of physical activity. Stretches should slowly elongate and hold muscles with low levels of force for 15 to 30 seconds. Four to five stretches per muscle group or area of the body are usually recommended.

MAXING OUT

1. Dancer—A dancer/cheerleader requests your help in increasing hip flexion and abduction ROM to facilitate the split position for a variety of stunts. What stretching program would you recommend?
2. Personal training client—A manager seeks relief from neck and shoulder pain from long days on an office computer. What stretching and strengthening exercises would you recommend?
3. Athlete—An athlete who has undergone acute rehab wants to return to play and increase plantarflexion ROM following an ankle sprain. What assessments would you use to document progress and what stretching program would you employ?

CASE EXAMPLE
Postmatch Flexibility Routine in Tennis

BACKGROUND

You are a strength coach working with the university medical staff and a 20-year-old male collegiate tennis player. The player has limited internal shoulder rotation ROM in the dominant shoulder, which is common in repetitive overarm sports like tennis.

RECOMMENDATIONS/CONSIDERATIONS

Following matches, practice, and conditioning sessions, the cool-down phase will consist of a static stretching routine. This will be a typical whole-body routine but will focus extra stretching on sport-specific imbalances common in tennis players: reduced shoulder internal rotation and flexibility of the lower back and hamstrings.

IMPLEMENTATION

Three 20-second wrist flexor and extensor stretches

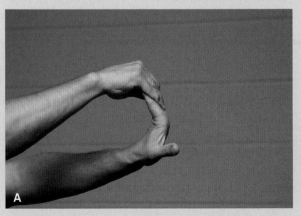
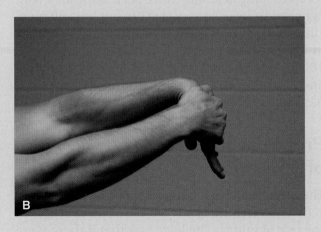

Wrist flexor and extensor stretches.

Four 20-second standing pectoralis major stretches

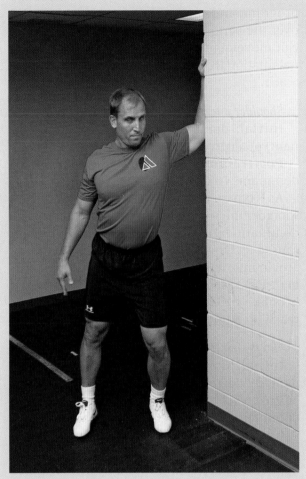

Standing pectoralis major stretch.

Four 20-second shoulder internal rotation stretches

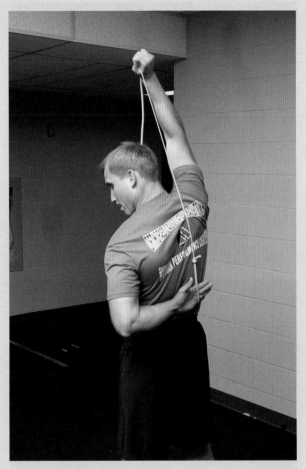

Shoulder internal rotation stretch.

Four 20-second knees to chest low back stretches

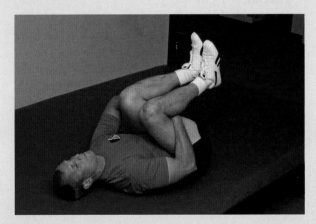

Knees to chest low back stretch.

Three 20-second trunk twists both directions
Three 20-second butterfly hip internal rotator stretches

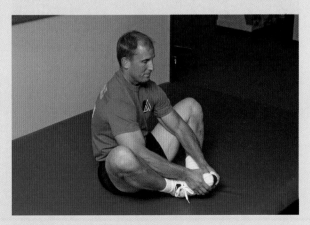

Butterfly hip internal rotators stretch.

(continued)

Four 20-second seated hamstring stretches

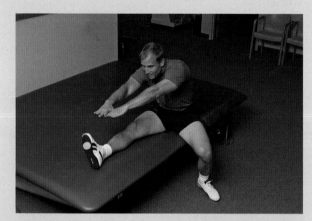

Seated hamstring stretch.

Three 20-second seated calf stretches

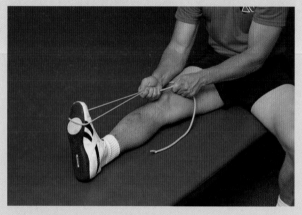

Seated calf stretch.

Three 20-second seated dorsiflexor stretches

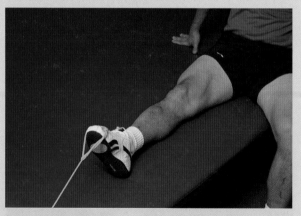

Seated dorsiflexor stretch.

RESULTS

Results before and after (a 10-week flexibility program) indicate an improvement in ROM over the period of the training program in specific movements. Tests included shoulder internal rotation ROM, hip flexion ROM, and sit and reach.

Shoulder internal rotation ROM

Initial: dominant, 33 degrees; nondominant, 66 degrees

Posttraining: dominant, 48 degrees; nondominant, 70 degrees.

As is typical with overhead throwing athletes, shoulder internal rotation was decreased in the dominant extremity. The prescribed program caused a change in the ROM of the dominant arm in internal rotation in the direction of normal. Because of the demands of the sport, it is unlikely that the dominant arm would ever reach the same ROM as the nondominant arm.

Hip flexion ROM with knee extended

Initial: dominant, 40 degrees; nondominant, 39 degrees

Posttraining: dominant, 49 degrees; nondominant 49 degrees

In hip flexion, a dominant-to-nondominant difference is not as pronounced as it is in the upper extremity. Both extremities demonstrated a small increase in ROM due to the prescribed flexibility program.

Sit-and-reach flexibility

Initial: + 1 cm

Posttraining: + 3 cm

The flexibility program resulted in a slight increase in ROM in trunk flexion.

Theoretically, these increases in ROM would indicate a reduction in injury risk to the shoulder, hamstrings, and lower back. The effect on performance (power, explosiveness) is undetermined at this time.

REFERENCES

1. Alter MJ. Science of Flexibility. 3rd ed. Champaign, IL: Human Kinetics, 2004.
2. Alexander RM. Tendon elasticity and muscle function. Comp Biochem Physiol Part A 2002; 133:1001–1011.
3. Amako M, Oda T, Masuoka K, et al. Effect of static stretching on prevention of injuries for military recruits. Mil Med 2003;168:442–446.
4. American Academy of Orthopaedic Surgeons. Joint motion: method of measuring and recording. Chicago, IL: AAOS, 1965.
5. American College of Sports Medicine. ACSM's Guidelines for Exercise Testing and Prescription, 7th ed. Philadelphia: Lippincott Williams & Wilkins, 2005.
6. American Medical Association. Guides to the Evaluation of Permanent Impairment. Chicago: AMA, 1988.
7. Avela J, Kyrolainen H, Komi PV. Altered reflex sensitivity after repeated and prolonged passive muscle stretching. J Appl Physiol 1999;86:1283–1291.
8. Beaulieu JE. Developing a stretching program. Phys Sportsmed 1981;9(11):59–66.
9. Bishop D. Warm up I: potential mechanisms and the effects of passive warm up on exercise performance. Sports Med 2003a;33:439–454.
10. Bishop D. Warm up II: performance changes following active warm up and how to structure the warm up. Sports Med 2003b;33:483–498.
11. Buroker KC, Schwane JA. Does postexercise static stretching alleviate delayed muscle soreness? Phys Sportsmed 1989;17 (6):65–83.
12. Church JB, Wiggins MS, Moode EM, et al. Effect of warm-up and flexibility treatments on vertical jump performance. J Strength Cond Res 2001;15:332–336.
13. Corbin CB. Flexibility. Clin Sports Med 1984;3:101–117.
14. Corbin CB, Noble L. Flexibility: a major component of physical fitness. J Phys Ed Rec 1980; 51(6),23–24,57–60.
15. Cornbleet SL, Woolsey NB. Assessment of hamstring muscle length in school-aged children using the sit-and-reach test and the inclinometer measure of hip joint angle. Phys Ther 1996;76:850–855.
16. Cornelius W, Hagemann RW, Jackson AW. A study on placement of stretching within a workout. J Sports Med Phys Fit 1988;28:234–236.
17. Cornwell A. Nelson AG, Heise GD, et al. Acute effects of passive muscle stretching on vertical jump performance. J Hum Mov Stud 2001;40:307–324.
18. Craib MW, Mitchell VA. The association between flexibility and running economy in sub-elite male distance runners. Med Sci Sports Exerc 1996;28:737–743.
19. Eckstrand J, Gillquist J, Liljedahl S. Prevention of soccer injuries: supervision by doctor and physiotherapist. Am J Sports Med 1983;11:116–120.
20. Fitness and Lifestyle Research Institute. Fitness and Lifestyle in Canada. Ottawa: Fitness and Lifestyle Research Institute, 1983.
21. Fowles JR, Sale DG, MacDougall JD. Reduced strength after passive stretch of the human plantar flexors. J Appl Physiol 2000;89:1179–1188.
22. Franks DB. Physical warm-up. In: Williams M H, ed. Ergogenic Aids in Sport. Champaign, IL: Human Kinetics, 1983:340–375.
23. Gajdosik RL. Passive extensibility of skeletal muscle: review of the literature with clinical implications. Clin Biomech 2001;16:87–101.
24. Gajdosik RL, Bohannon RW. Clinical measurement of range of motion: review of goniometry emphasizing reliability and validity. Phys Ther 1987;67:1867–1872.
25. Gajdosik RL, Guiliani CA, Bohannon RW. Passive compliance and length of the hamstring muscles of healthy men and women. Clin Biomech 1990;5:23–29.
26. Gajdosik R, Lusin G. Hamstring muscle tightness: reliability of an active-knee extension test. Phys Ther 1983;63: 1085–1088.
27. Gerhardt JJ, Russe OA. International SFTR Method of Measuring and Recording Joint Motion. Bern: Hans Huber, 1975.
28. Gleim GW, McHugh MP. Flexibility and its effects on sports injury and performance. Sports Med 1997;24: 289–299.
29. Gleim GW, Stachenfeld NS, Nicholas JA. The influence of flexibility on the economy of walking and jogging. J Orthop Res 1990;8:814–823.
30. Goeken LN, Holf AL. Instrumental straight-leg raising: results in healthy subjects. Arch Phys Med Rehabil 1993; 74:194–203.
31. Golding LA. Flexibility, stretching, and flexibility testing. ACSM Health Fit J 1997;1(2):17–20,37–38.
32. Halbertsma JPK, Goeken LNH. Stretching exercises: effect on passive extensibility and stiffness in short hamstrings of healthy subjects. Arch Phys Med Rehabil 1994;75:976–981.
33. Harris ML. Flexibility. Phys Ther 1969;49:591–601.
34. Hartman JG, Looney M. Norm-referenced and criterion-referenced reliability and validity of the back-saver sit-and-reach. Meas Phys Ed Exerc Sci 2003:7:71–87.
35. Hennig EM, Podzielny S. The effects of stretch and warming-up exercises on the vertical jump performance [German]. Dtsch Zeitschr Sportmed 1994;45:253–260.
36. Hoeger WW, Hopkins, DR. A comparison of the sit and reach and the modified sit and reach in the measurement of flexibility in women. Res Q Exerc Sport 1992; 63:191–195.
37. Holt J, Holt LE, Pelham TW. Flexibility redefined. In: Bauer T, ed. Biomechanics in Sports XIII. Thunder Bay, Ontario: Lakehead University, 1996:170–174.
38. Holt LE, Pelham TW, Burke DG. Modifications to the standard sit-and-reach flexibility protocol. J Athlet Train 1999;34:43–47.
39. Hoshizaki TB, Bell RD. Factor analysis of seventeen joint flexibility measures. J Sports Sci 1984;2:97–103.
40. Hubley CL, Kozey JW, Stanish WD. The effects of static stretching exercises and stationary cycling on range of motion at the hip joint. J Orthop Sports Phys Ther 1984; 6:104–109.
41. Hui SC, Yuen PY, Morrow JR, et al. Comparison of the criterion-related validity of sit-and-reach tests with and without limb length adjustment in Asian adults. Res Q Exerc Sport 1999;70:401–406.
42. Hutton RS. Neuromuscular basis of stretching exercise. In: Komi P, ed. Strength and Power in Sports. Oxford, UK: Blackwell, 1993:29–38.

43. Jackson AW, Morrow JR, Brill PA, et al. Relation of sit-up and sit-and-reach tests to lower back pain in adults. J Orthop Sports Phys Ther 1998;27:22–26.

44. Johansson PH, Lindstrom L, Sundelin G, et al. The effects of preexercise stretching on muscular soreness, tenderness and force loss following heavy eccentric exercise. Scand J Med Sci Sports 1999;9:219–225.

45. Jones BH, Knapik JJ. Physical training and exercise-related injuries. Sports Med 1999;27:111–125.

46. Karvonen J. Importance of warm-up and cool down on exercise performance. In: Karvonen, J, Lemon P, Iliev I, eds. Medicine in Sports Training and Coaching. Basel: Karger, 1992:189–214.

47. Kibler WB, Chandler TJ. Range of motion in junior tennis players participating in an injury risk modification program. J Sci Med Sport 2003:6:51–62.

48. Knapik JJ, Jones BH, Bauman CL, et al. Strength, flexibility, and athletic injuries. Sports Med 1992:14:277–288.

49. Knudson D. Stretching: science to practice. J Phys Ed Rec Dance 1998;69(3):38–42.

50. Knudson D. Stretching during warm-up: do we have enough evidence? J Phys Ed Rec Dance 1999;70 (7): 24–27,51.

51. Knudson D, Magnusson P, McHugh M. Current issues in flexibility fitness. PCPFS Res Dig 2000;3(10):1–8.

52. Kokkonen J, Nelson AG, Cornwell A. Acute muscle stretching inhibits maximal strength performance. Res Q Exerc Sport 1998;69:411–415.

53. Kubo K, Kanehisa H, Fukunaga T. Effect of stretching on the viscoelastic properties of human tendon structures in vivo. J Appl Physiol 2002a;92:595–601.

54. Kubo K, Kanehisa H, Fukunaga T. Effect of transient muscle contractions and stretching on the tendon structures in vivo. Acta Physiol Scand 2002b;175:157–164.

55. Kubo K, Kanehisa H, Fukunaga T. Gender differences in the viscoelastic properties of tendon structures. Eur J Appl Physiol 2003;88:520–526.

56. Kubo K, Kanehisa H, Kawakami Y, et al. Elastic properties of muscle-tendon complex in long-distance runners. Eur J Appl Physiol 2000;81:181–187.

57. Kubo K, Kawakami Y, Fukunaga T. Influence of elastic properties of tendon structures on jump performance in humans. J Appl Physiol 1999;87:2090–2096.

58. Leighton JR A simple objective and reliable measure of flexibility. Res Q 1942;13:205–216.

59. Liebesman J, Cafarelli E. Physiology of range of motion in human joints: a critical review. Crit Rev Phys Rehabil Med 1994;6:131–160.

60. Liemohn W, Haydu T, Phillips D. Questionable exercises. PCPFS Res Digest 1999;3(8):1–8.

61. Lin RM, Chang GL, Chang LT. Biomechanical properties of muscle-tendon unit under high-speed passive stretch. Clin Biomech 1999;14:412–417.

62. Lindsey R, Corbin C. Questionable exercises—some safer alternatives. J Phys Ed Rec Dance 1989;60(8):26–32.

63. Lubell A. Potentially dangerous exercises: are they harmful to all? Phys Sportsmed 1989;17(1):187–192.

64. Magnusson SP. Passive properties of human skeletal muscle during stretch maneuvers: a review. Scand J Med Sci Sports 1998;8:65–77.

65. Magnusson SP, Aagaard P, Nielson JJ. Passive energy return after repeated stretches of the hamstring muscle-tendon unit. Med Sci Sports Exerc 2000a;32:1160–1164.

66. Magnusson SP, Aagard P, Simonsen E, et al. A biomechanical evaluation of cyclic and static stretch in human skeletal muscle. Int J Sports Med 1998;19: 310–316.

67. Magnusson SP, Aagaard P, Simonsen EB, et al. Passive tensile stress and energy of the human hamstring muscles in vivo. Scand J Med Sci Sports 2000;10:351–359.

68. Magnusson SP, Simonsen EB, Aagaard P, et al. A mechanism for altered flexibility in human skeletal muscle. J Physiol 1996;487:291–298.

69. Magnusson SP, Simonsen EB, Aagaard P, et al. Biomechanical responses to repeated stretches in human hamstring muscle in vivo. Am J Sports Med 1996b;24: 622–628.

70. Magnusson SP, Simonsen EB, Aagaard P, et al. Determinants of musculoskeletal flexibility: viscoelastic properties, cross-sectional area, EMG and stretch tolerance. Scand J Med Sci Sports 1997;7:195–202.

71. Magnusson SP, Simonsen EB, Aagaard P, et al. Visoco-elastic response to repeated static stretching in human skeletal muscle. Scand J Med Sci Sport 1995;5:342–347.

72. Martin SB, Jackson AW, Morrow JR, et al. The rationale for the sit and reach test revisited. Meas Phys Ed Exerc Sci 1998;2:85–92.

73. McHugh MP, Connolly DAJ, Eston RG, et al. The role of passive muscle stiffness in symptoms of exercise-induced muscle damage. Am J Sports Med 1999;27: 594–599.

74. McHugh MP, Kremenic IJ, Fox MB, et al. The role of mechanical and neural restrains to joint range of motion during passive stretch. Med Sci Sports Exerc 1998;30: 928–932.

75. McHugh MP, Magnusson SP, Gleim GW, et al. Visco-elastic stress relaxation in human skeletal muscle. Med Sci Sports Exerc 1992;24:1375–1382.

76. McNair PJ, Dombroski EW, Hewson DJ, et al. Stretching at the ankle joint: viscoelastic responses to holds and continuous passive motion. Med Sci Sports Exerc 2000; 33:354–358.

77. Medeiros JM, Smidt GL, Burmeister LF, et al. The influence of isometric exercise and passive stretch on hip joint motion. Phys Ther 1977;57:518–523.

78. Nelson AG, Guillory IK, Cornwell A, et al. Inhibition of maximal voluntary isokinetic torque production following stretching is velocity specific. J Strength Cond Res 2001;15:241–246.

79. Nelson AG, Kokkonen J. Acute ballistic muscle stretching inhibits maximal strength performance. Res Q Exerc Sport 2001;72:415–419.

80. Noonan TJ, Best TM, Seaber AV, et al. Thermal effects on skeletal muscle tensile behavior. Am J Sports Med 1993;21:517–522.

81. Norkin CC, White DJ. Measurement of Joint Motion: A Guide to Goniometry. 3rd ed. Philadelphia: Davis, 2003.

82. Plowman SA. Physical activity, physical fitness, and low-back pain. Exerc Sport Sci Rev 1992;20:221–242.

83. Pope RP, Herbert RD, Kirwan JD. Effects of flexibility and stretching on injury risk in army recruits. Aust J Physiother 1998;44:165–172.

84. Pope RP, Herbert RD, Kirwan JD, et al. A randomized trial of preexercise stretching for prevention of lower-limb injury. Med Sci Sports Exerc 2000;32:271–277.

85. Russek LN. Hypermobility syndrome. Phys Ther 1999; 79:591–599.

86. Safran MR, Garrett WE, Seaber AV, et al. The role of warm-up in muscular injury prevention. Am J Sports Med 1988;16:123–129.

87. Safran MR, Seaber A, Garrett, WE Warm-up and muscular injury prevention: an update. Sports Med 1989;8: 239–249.

88. Sapega AA, Quedenfeld TC, Moyer R, et al. Biophysical factors in range-of-motion exercise. Phys Sportsmed 1981;12(9):57–65.

89. Shellock FG, Prentice WE. Warming-up and stretching for improved physical performance and prevention of sports-related injuries. Sports Med 1985;2:267–278.

90. Shephard RJ, Berrirdge M, Montelpare W. ON the generality of the "sit and reach" test: an analysis of flexibility data for an aging population. Res Q Exerc Sport 1990; 61:326–330.

91. Strickler T, Malone T, Garrett WE. The effects of passive warming on muscle injury. Am J Sports Med 1990;18: 141–145.

92. Suni JH, Miilunpalo SI, Asikainen A, et al. Safety and feasibility of a health-related fitness test battery for adults. Phys Ther 1998;78:134–148.

93. Surburg PR. Flexibility exercise re-examined. Athl Train 1983; 18:37–40.

94. Taylor DC, Brooks DE, Ryan JB. Viscoelastic characteristics of muscle: passive stretching versus muscular contractions. Med Sci Sports Exerc 1997;29:1619–1624.

95. Taylor DC, Dalton JD, Seaber AV, et al. Visoelastic properties of muscle-tendon units. Am J Sports Med 1990; 18:300–309.

96. Vujnovich AL, Dawson NJ. The effect of therapeutic muscle stretch on neural processing. J Orthop Sports Phys Ther 1994;20:145–153.

97. Walshe AD, Wilson GJ, Murphy AJ. The validity and reliability of a test of lower body musculotendinous stiffness. Eur J Appl Physiol 1996;73:332–339.

98. Weldon SM, Hill RH. The efficacy of stretching for prevention of exercise-related injury: a systematic review of the literature. Manual Ther 2003;8:141–150.

99. Wessel J. Wan A. Effect of stretching on the intensity of delayed-onset muscle soreness. Clin J Sports Med 1994; 4:83–87.

100. Wilson GJ, Elliott BC, Wood GA. Stretch shorten cycle performance enhancement through flexibility training. Med Sci Sports Exerc 1992;24:116–123.

101. Wilson GJ, Wood GA, Elliott BC. Optimal stiffness of series elastic component in a stretch-shorten cycle activity. J Appl Physiol 1991;70:825–833.

102. Wilson GJ, Wood GA, Elliott BC. The relationship between stiffness of the musculature and static flexibility: an alternative explanation for the occurrence of muscular injury. Int J Sports Med 1991;12:403–407.

103. Witvrouw E, Danneels L, Asselman P, et al. Muscle flexibility as a risk factor for developing muscle injuries in male professional soccer players: a prospective study. Am J Sports Med 2003;31:41–46.

104. Young W, Elliot S. Acute effects of static stretching, proprioceptive neuromuscular facilitation stretching, and maximum voluntary contractions on explosive force production and jumping performance. Res Q Exerc Sport 2001;72:273–279.

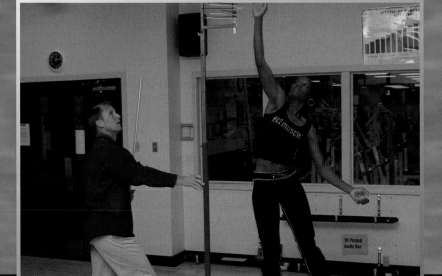

Resistance Exercise Techniques and Spotting

JOHN F. GRAHAM

Introduction

This chapter provides a description of the benefits and physiological aspects, safety, equipment, and techniques of resistance training. It also includes detailed descriptions of 22 free-weight, 8 machine-resistance-training, and 3 trunk exercises in the following classes: total-body (power/explosive), multijoint lower-body, single-joint lower-body, upper-body multijoint, and upper-body single-joint exercises. Total-body exercises emphasize loading the spine directly or indirectly in an explosive manner. Multijoint exercises involve two or more joints that change angles during the movement of a repetition. Single-joint exercises involve only one joint changing its angle during the completion of a repetition. Each exercise described in this chapter is accompanied by a detailed explanation of the type of exercise, muscles utilized, body and limb alignment, ascending and descending movement, safety points, and variations of exercise technique.

BENEFITS OF RESISTANCE TRAINING

Muscles adapt to resistance training by growing and developing. This process, called **hypertrophy** (3), involves an increase in the cross-sectional area of muscle fibers, not the splitting of the muscle into additional muscle fibers, which is called **hyperplasia**. Hypertrophy has been demonstrated to occur as a result of an increase in the thickness and number of myofibrils (8). It is believed to be the primary mechanism governing muscle growth. A number of factors generally are responsible for muscle hypertrophy:

- **Overload**. The resistance should be greater than the muscle's previous level of adaptation.
- **Muscle recruitment**. The maximal numbers of muscle fibers should be recruited.
- **Energy intake**. An adequate amount of carbohydrate and protein should be consumed (3).

Resistance training can enhance absolute and relative muscle strength (4,8). **Absolute muscular strength** is the strength an individual can develop regardless of body weight. **Relative muscular strength** is defined by absolute muscular strength divided by body weight in either kilograms or pounds. Increases in muscle and explosive strength are generally tied to inter- and intramuscular adaptations and muscle hypertrophy. The term **intermuscular adaptation** refers to the proper execution of exercise technique for exercises performed at both slow and explosive speeds. As an individual acquires the proper exercise technique, less energy is required to perform the exercise; therefore, the resistance utilized can be increased. **Intramuscular adaptation** refers to how many motor units are recruited during the effort, how quickly they are recruited, and whether antagonistic motor units interfere with the movement (4). By undergoing resistance training, individuals can expect an increased number of motor units to be recruited at an accelerated speed along with an increased inhibition of antagonistic muscle(s). As a muscle increases in cross-sectional area (hypertrophy), it will develop more force and power than will muscles with a smaller cross-sectional area.

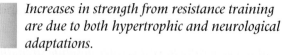

Increases in strength from resistance training are due to both hypertrophic and neurological adaptations.

Other benefits of resistance training include improvements in bone density and energy utilization and storage. The lack of weight-bearing activity with aging has often been linked to **osteopenia** (lowering of bone mineral mass to 1 standard deviation below young-normal levels) and **osteoporosis** (lowering of bone mineral mass to more than 2.5 standard deviations below young-normal levels). As discussed in Chapter 4, bone adapts to resistance training by increasing mineralization in a particular region of the bone to increase its strength and its ability to handle the stress due to resistance training (7). This may be accomplished through exercises using loads at greater than 75% of an individual's 3-RM (the maximum weight an individual can utilize for three repetitions) that are weight-bearing in nature (multijoint, closed-chain-kinetic exercises, such as leg presses, squats, and straight-leg dead lift). If the resistance training includes light to moderate loads (40% to 60% of 1 RM), higher repetitions (12 to 25), and shorter rest periods (30 to 60 seconds), moderate increases of 5% in $\dot{V}O_2$ (oxygen uptake) may be expected (2). With resistance training, individuals will utilize and store energy more efficiently. This will result in the muscle's ability to train at higher resistances and for longer periods of time. Resistance training performed with good technique through a full range of motion (ROM) can enhance muscle flexibility and reduce the likelihood of injury (2).

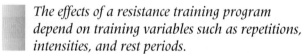

The effects of a resistance training program depend on training variables such as repetitions, intensities, and rest periods.

Although it is not surprising that males are typically stronger than females, the differences in muscle strength are not tied to the quality of the muscle tissue or its ability to produce force or power, since in these respects no difference exists between genders. A significant difference does exist, however, in the quantity of muscle tissue in the average male (40%) versus female (23%), which is largely responsible for the male strength advantage. It is this difference that also helps to explain why women are typically 43% to 63% weaker in upper-body strength and 25% to 30% weaker in lower-body strength (2). Conditioning programs for male and female athletes for the same sport should be essentially the same, as the physiological demands of the sport are the same.

 Males generally have a greater absolute strength than females, but males and females are very similar in relative strength.

Overtraining is characterized by a decline in performance over a time. This occurs when an individual's body is not given enough time to recuperate from training prior to the next training session (2). Symptoms of overtraining include but are not limited to the following:

- An increase in morning resting heart rate
- An unintentional decrease in body weight
- Inability to perform in a training session at the same level of strength, power, or endurance as had been achieved earlier
- An increase in muscle soreness from one training session to the next
- Extreme muscle soreness and stiffness on the day immediately following a training session
- A decrease in appetite

Once an individual becomes overtrained—that is, by exhibiting two or more of the warning signs listed above—the frequency, intensity, and duration of activity should be reduced until the symptoms dissipate. Obviously, it is more effective to prevent overtraining than to recover from it. Guidelines for preventing overtraining include increasing training intensity and duration gradually (< 5%), utilizing periodized training (gradual cycling of specificity, intensity, and volume of train-

---

 REAL-WORLD APPLICATION

Training Male and Female Athletes for the Same Sport

You are asked to evaluate the conditioning program for both the boys and girls on your high school's basketball teams. You are asked to make recommendations to the coaches as to changes that they could consider.

Observed: After observing the training program you note that the girls' team uses only body-weight exercises while the boys' team is using only machines.

Recommendations: The boys' and girls' teams should not be using separate programs, since they are training for the same sport. It is recommended that both teams use free-weight exercises that focus on lower-body power. Machines can be used to train areas of muscular weakness or imbalance.

---

ing to achieve peak levels of performance and/or fitness at a designated time), following sound nutritional guidelines, and devoting adequate time to sleep and recovery. The risk of overtraining may be increased in training the multisport athlete (see the case study further on).

 Proper planning using a periodized resistance training program will help prevent overtraining.

SAFETY

Training equipment and facilities can provide a safe environment for exercise as long as basic safety guidelines are utilized.

Spotting

Probably the most critical aspect of safe training once the facility and equipment utilized have been inspected is the use of a spotter or spotters, particularly with free-weight exercises. A **spotter** is a knowledgeable individual who assists in the proper execution of an exercise (5). His or her responsibility is to ensure that the exerciser completes all repetitions with good technique, to assist the exerciser with completion of a repetition when needed, and to summon help when necessary (5). This responsibility should be taken very seriously, as failure to do so may result in serious injury not only to the exerciser but to the spotter as well. Exercises that involve the use of free weights either over the head (standing barbell press), with the bar resting on the back (barbell lunge or back squat), racked at the front of the upper shoulders (barbell front squat), or over the face (barbell bench press or supine triceps extension) will require the use of one or more spotters who are skilled at safely spotting, since these maneuvers are the most potentially harmful to the athlete. Exercises involving raising the barbell or dumbbell to the side or front of the body below shoulder level and power exercises generally do not require a spotter.

Barbells should always be loaded evenly on both sides and the weights secured with collars.

Exercises performed overhead and with the barbell on the front or back of the shoulders should be performed inside a power rack with the safety bars placed at an appropriate height. Individuals who are not spotting or performing the exercise

Q & A from the Field

You notice that a particular athlete in your program looks fatigued. What questions might you ask him? What possible causes of the fatigue should you consider?

How much sleep he is getting? What are his eating habits? Is he getting enough recovery between training sessions? Is there enough variety in his exercises? You should consider

overtraining, drug use, disease, psychological problems, and normal emotional stresses as possible causes.

---

should remain at a safe distance from the power rack. Because the loads utilized in these exercises can be substantial, spotters ideally should be nearly as strong and as tall as the exerciser. All additional barbells, collars, plates, weight trees, and other equipment should be outside the area immediately surrounding the power rack. Collars should be utilized regardless of the level of the load being used so as to prevent weight plates from sliding off the barbell. For maximum safety, three spotters (one directly behind the exerciser and one on each side of the barbell) should be present. All three should assist with removing the load from the rack as well as returning the load to the rack on completion of the repetitions.

For exercises performed over the face, the spotter should hold the bar with an alternated grip inside the exerciser's grip to ensure that the barbell does not leave the exerciser's hands and land on the exerciser's face, neck, or chest. In the case of an exercise where the athlete's grip is narrow, the spotter may grasp the barbell immediately outside the exerciser's grip. Spotters should be conscious of body alignment (flat back, feet shoulder-width apart in a solid base, and a bent-knee position), as they may be called on quickly to help the exerciser by catching the barbell or by helping to lift the load. Dumbbell exercises may pose a different challenge to the spotter, as they require more skill to assist in exercises. For the safety of the exerciser, it is important for spotters to spot by standing as close to the dumbbells as possible and spotting near the wrists, so that the spotter can quickly support the exerciser if his or her elbows collapse, thus preventing the dumbbells from falling inward toward the exerciser's chest or face. For exercises in which one dumbbell is used, such as seated overhead triceps extension or supine dumbbell pull-over, it is impor-

tant to spot with the hands directly on or slightly below the dumbbell.

In selecting the number of spotters for a given exercise, an athlete should consider the load being lifted, the physical strength and height of the spotters, and the experience level of both the exerciser and spotters. The heavier the load, the greater the risk for injury and the severity of injury to both the exerciser and the spotter should the exerciser fail to complete a repetition and an inadequate spot be provided. For most exercises that involve overhead lifting with a barbell, a barbell on the back or shoulders with heavier loads, and over-the-face exercises with heavier loads, a lead spotter should be placed immediately behind the lifter to direct the other spotters placed on each side of the barbell. As the number of spotters increases, so does the potential for errors in timing. Prior to the first lift, the exerciser should tell the spotter(s) how the barbell will be lifted from the rack, how many repetitions will be performed, and how the barbell will be returned to the rack. This ensures the exercise can be performed safely and that the spotters do not disrupt the exercise.

Exercises that require explosive power should not utilize a spotter. Spotting these exercisers places both the exerciser and the spotter at increased risk for injury. Exercisers performing these explosive lifts should be taught the proper technique for missing a lift. To miss a lift when the barbell is in front of the body, the proper technique is to push the barbell forward and release it as the lifter moves backward. To miss a lift with the barbell behind the body, the lifter should release the barbell and jump forward. For the safety of not only the exerciser but also other exercisers in the surrounding area, power exercises should be performed on a segregated power platform clear of other exercisers and equipment.

Exercise Apparel

Proper clothing when exercising with resistance equipment is critical for two major reasons: safety and etiquette. It is important to wear a workout shirt that covers the chest, upper back, and shoulders to avoid losing control of a barbell on exercises where the barbell rests on the upper shoulders (e.g., barbell back squats). Without a shirt that covers those areas, a barbell may slip off the body, putting the exerciser, spotters, and other exercisers nearby at risk for injury. Covering the upper body with a T-shirt is also important on exercises that require the exerciser to lie prone or supine on a bench. Not doing so is poor etiquette and may also cause damage to the equipment's upholstery.

Footwear is also important in resistance training. Closed-toe training shoes that provide a solid, stable base should be used at all times. The proper shoes will ensure that the exerciser has a stable lifting base, which is critical for all explosive lower-body, squatting, overhead lift, or lifting from the floor exercises. Closed-toe shoes also provide some protection against dropped plates, barbells, and dumbbells. Sandals and bare feet should never be permitted in the resistance-training area for reasons of safety and hygiene.

 Safety is extremely important in a resistance-training program, and proper precautions should be taken at all times.

RESISTANCE TRAINING TECHNIQUE

If benefits are to be maximized, every resistance-training exercise will provide its own unique challenges. Many exercisers have similarities as well as differences. Understanding similarities and differences is essential for the proper selection of exercises in the design of a resistance-training prescription. The proper execution of a resistance training exercise has eight basic components:

1. Objective for exercise selection
2. Equipment alignment
3. Body alignment
4. Stabilization of body
5. Movement of body during exercise
6. Speed of movement
7. Breathing
8. Initiation and return of exercise equipment

In selecting an exercise, it is essential to ensure that the exercise matches the objective of the resistance-training program. For example, exercisers often perform numerous sets of chest exercises while not balancing them with an appropriate number of upper back exercises or failing to perform leg exercises. Spot enhancement or reduction of a given section of the body is not achievable (1). It is important for exercisers to recognize the importance of balance in a resistance-training exercise prescription. You are only as good as your weakest link.

 As a general rule, select exercises that work opposing muscle groups.

Equipment alignment means setting the equipment up properly so that the exercise can be performed safely and with maximum benefit. The proper resistance should be set on a machine exercise, the barbell should have equal resistance on each side, or dumbbells of identical resistance should be selected. Collars should be placed securely on each side of the barbell to make sure that weights do not slide or fall off the barbell, causing the barbell to tip. Hooks for barbell exercises in which the barbell is placed on the shoulder should be set 3 to 4 in. below shoulder level so that the exerciser can drop under the barbell to remove it from the rack to initiate the set and then return it to the rack above the hooks before sliding it back down on the hooks at the completion of the set. Safety bars on the power rack should be set slightly below the end ROM on squat or power exercises performed within the rack. Cams, seats, and arm and leg lengths on machines should be adjusted to the exerciser's optimal safe ROM.

In positioning the body during resistance training, the axial skeleton and its immediate attachments are of the highest priority (1). This means that particular attention should continuously be paid to the positioning of the pelvis, spinal column, and shoulder girdle before and during any resistance-training exercise. The spinal column is in its most stable and therefore strongest position when it and the pelvis are all in neutral positions with a slight thoracic kyphosis and lumbar lordosis. To place the torso in an ideal resistance-training position, the athlete should pull the shoulder blades back slightly and down, lift the sternum slightly out and up, and pull the chin slightly back and down, creating or maintaining the natural arch in the thoracic and lumbar regions of the spine (1). Once the body is positioned correctly, the positioning of the hands is important. The two primary handgrip positions are the **pronated grip** (palms down and knuckles up) and **supinated grip** (palms up and knuckles down). A variation of either grip is the **neutral grip** (knuckles point laterally). Other grips include the **alternated grip** (one hand supinated and the other pronated). In performing exercises that require a stronger grip (Olympic-style lifts), a **hook grip** (wrapping the index and middle fingers around the thumb, which is placed against the bar first, the ring and little fingers holding the bar rather loosely) designed to add at least 10% to any pulling motion is used (6). Along with the handgrip, grip width must be considered. The three grip widths are **common** (shoulder width), **wide** (outside of shoulder width), and **narrow** (inside shoulder width).

Prior to performing any exercise, it is important to know the correct grip and grip width.

Regardless of whether the exercise is performed utilizing a barbell, dumbbell, or machine, stabilization of the body is critical. A stable position enables an exerciser to maintain proper body alignment during an exercise, which in turn ensures that the appropriate stress is placed on the intended muscles and joints. Exercises that call for a standing position require the feet to be positioned shoulder width, with the feet securely in contact with the floor. Whether the exerciser is seated, prone (lying face down), or supine (lying face up), his or her head, shoulders (front or back), chest or upper back, lower back, and buttocks or pelvis should be in contact with the bench or machine. The feet must remain in contact with the floor unless the height of the machine does not permit or require the feet to be in contact with the floor or the exercise is a lower-body open-chain exercise.

The movement of the body during an exercise does not have a definitive set point. Although exercises generally have a maximum ROM, the ideal ROM will depend on variations in the exerciser's musculoskeletal, neurological, and biomechanical systems. Modern exercise machines are often designed with a range of controls for both the eccentric and concentric muscle actions. Additionally, power racks allow the exerciser to control ROM in barbell exercises when necessary owing to considerations of safety, injury reconditioning, or technique.

Speed of motion with exercises depends on the type of exercise being performed. With the exception of power or explosive lifts, exercises should be performed in a slow, controlled manner to increase the likelihood that a full ROM can be achieved. The eccentric muscle action should be performed over a 4-second period with a 1-second hold at completion before initiating the concentric movement. The concentric movement should be performed over a 2- to 4-second period with a 1-second hold at the completion before initiating the eccentric muscle action. When exercises are performed quickly, momentum will increase, negatively impacting body alignment, stabilization of the body, and movement.

In instructing exercisers on breathing during resistance training, the most important point to stress is to breathe at some point during every repetition. The most strenuous portion of a repetition, typically where the lifter is most likely to fail, is referred to as the **sticking point**. This is the point in the ROM of any joint where the mechanical advantage of the lever system is the lowest. The exact angle of the sticking point will depend on the mechanical properties of a specific joint. A general rule of thumb is for exercisers to inhale before initiating an exercise or at the less stressful phase of the repetition and to exhale upon passing the sticking point or the most stressful phase of a repetition. For more advanced exercisers, utilizing heavier resistances, such as those exercises that load the vertebral column and place stress on it, the use of the **Valsalva maneuver** (expiring against a closed glottis, which when combined with contracting the abdomen and rib cage muscles, creates rigid compartments of fluid in the lower torso and air in the upper torso) may be warranted in maintaining proper vertebral alignment and support (5). The Valsalva maneuver, however, should be utilized only through the sticking point of a lift. Periods that exceed 1 to 2 seconds of breath holding while working against a resistance may cause dizziness, disorientation, excessively high blood pressure, and blackouts.

As a final aspect of resistance-training technique, it is very important for exercisers to recognize the importance of properly lifting a resistance to initiate a set and returning the resistance to its starting position at the completion of a set. In using a barbell with a power rack or bench to perform exercises that require loading of the vertebral column or overhead or over-the-face exercises, at least one spotter should be used to guide the exerciser in removing the resistance from its starting position and then returning it at the completion of the set to ensure that the barbell is safely removed and returned. For the safety of the exerciser and others in the immediate area as well as for equipment maintenance, exercise should be initiated with the resistance being lifted from its resting position and returned to its starting position slowly.

Resistance-Training Exercises

Power Exercises
Power Clean
Power Snatch
Power Jerk

Hip/Thigh Exercises
Back Squat
Front Squat

Dead Lift
Barbell Lunge
Stiff-Leg Dead Lift
Leg Press
Leg Extension
Leg Curl
Standing Heel Raise

Chest Exercises
Bench Press, Dumbbell
Bench Press, Barbell
Incline Press, Dumbbell
Incline Press, Barbell
Dumbbell Fly

Upper Back Exercises
Dumbbell One-Arm
  Row
Lat Pull-Down
Seated Cable Row

Shoulder Exercises
Dumbbell Seated
  Shoulder Press
Machine Shoulder Press
Barbell Upright Row
Dumbbell Prone
  Posterior Raise

Triceps Exercises
Supine Triceps
  Extension
Triceps Pushdown

Biceps Exercises
Barbell Bicep Curl
Dumbbell Seated
  Alternate-Arm
  Bicep Curl

Forearm Exercises
Wrist Curl
Reverse Wrist Curl

**Abdominal and
Lower Back Exercises**
Abdominal Crunch
Back Extension

POWER EXERCISES

Power Clean

Type of Exercise

Total body/power (explosive) exercise

Muscles Used

Gluteus maximus, hamstrings (semimembranosus, semitendinosus, biceps femoris), quadriceps (vastus lateralis, vastus intermedius, vastus medialis, rectus femoris), soleus, gastrocnemius, trapezius, and deltoids (anterior, medial, and posterior)

Starting Position

Use a standard barbell. The lifting position is identical to that for the power snatch except for the hand position. The feet are between hip- and shoulder-width apart and pointing forward or just slightly outward. Squat and grasp the barbell with a shoulder-width or slightly wider pronated hand position using a closed or hook grip. Arms are outside the knees, elbows extended and pointing outward. Stand so that the barbell is over the balls of the feet and close to the shins. Back is rigid and flat or slightly arched. Head is up or slightly hyperextended.

Chest is held up and out. Shoulder blades should be squeezed together. Trapezius and upper back should be relaxed and in a slight state of stretch. With the heels always remaining in contact with the floor, the body weight should be balanced between the balls and middles of the feet. Shoulders are slightly in front of or over the barbell (Fig. 10.1A,B).

Upward Motion: First Pull

Initiate the power clean by taking in a deep breath and holding it. Lift the barbell off the floor through forceful hip and knee extension. Maintain a constant position of the torso in relation to the floor throughout the first pull. In other words, make sure that the hips do not rise faster or before the shoulders and keep the back flat or slightly arched. The head should remain in a neutral position in relation to the spine. The shoulders should remain slightly in front of or over the barbell. The elbows should still be fully extended. During the first pull, keep the barbell as close to the shins as possible. Continue to hold your breath (Fig. 10.1C,D).

Power Clean *(continued)*

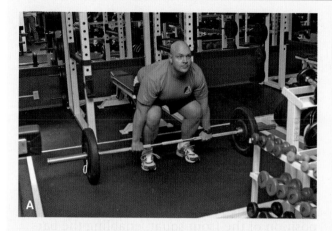

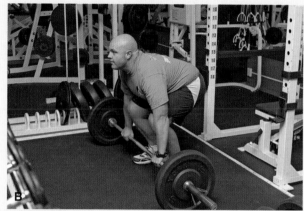

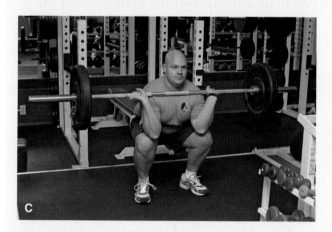

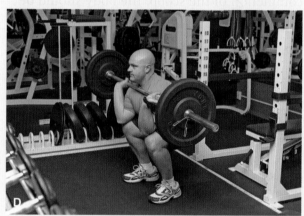

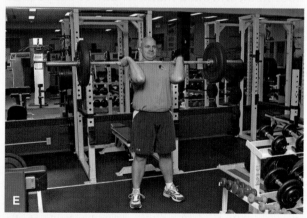

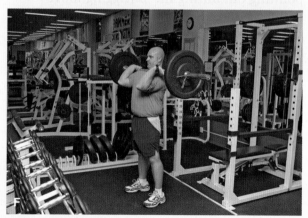

FIGURE 10.1 Power clean. **A.** Starting position, front view. **B.** Starting position, side view. **C.** First pull, front view. **D.** First pull, side view. **E.** Catch, front view. **F.** Catch, side view.

(continued)

Power Clean *(continued)*

Upward Motion: Transition (Scoop)

Explosively drive the hips forward and slightly increase the knee bend to enable the knees to move under and the thighs to move against the barbell. As the knee bend is increased, shift the body's weight forward toward the front half of the feet while still keeping the heels in contact with the floor. The back should remain slightly arched or flat. The shoulders should remain over or ahead of the barbell. The head should remain in line with the spine. Keep the elbows fully extended and pointing out. Continue holding the initial breath. At the completion of the scoop, the body should be in position for the initiation of the second pull.

Upward Motion: Second Pull (Power Phase)

With the barbell touching the body between the knees and midthigh, initiate the second pull by explosively extending the hips, knees, and ankles. Keep the shoulders over the barbell. Maintain a straight elbow position as long as possible while the hips, knees, and ankles are extending. Simultaneously fully extend the lower extremity joints and rapidly shrug the shoulders upward. The elbows should continue to remain extended and pointing out during the shrugging movement. Upon fully elevating the shoulders, rapidly flex the elbows to begin pulling the body under the barbell. With the elbows moving up and out to the sides, pull with the arms as high as possible. The powerful upward acceleration from the second pull will result in an erect torso and head. The feet will come off the floor.

Upward Motion: Catch

After the lower body has fully extended and the barbell reaches near maximal height, pull the body under the bar by rotating the arms and hands around then under the barbell. Rapidly bend the knees and hips to a half-squat position. The feet should return to the floor pointing straight ahead or slightly outward at a width slightly wider than that at the starting position. The barbell should be caught at the clavicles and anterior deltoids with the head facing forward; neck neutral; feet flat on the floor pointing straight ahead or slightly outward; body weight over the front half of the foot with the heels in contact with the floor; knees and hips should be flexed to a half-squat position to absorb the impact of the weight; back flat; upper arms parallel to the floor; elbows fully flexed; and the wrists extended. The barbell is caught with the torso almost fully erect and the shoulders slightly in front of the buttocks. The position is similar to the mid-position of the front squat, enabling the barbell to be directly over the body's center of gravity. If the torso is too erect, however, the momentum of the barbell will push the shoulders backward and possibly hyperextend the lower back, resulting in a potential risk of injury. Upon catching the barbell and establishing control and balance, complete the catch by standing to a fully erect position. Exhale and return to normal breathing pattern (Fig. 10.1E,F).

Downward Motion

Unless maximal or near maximal loads are used, the barbell should be returned to the floor in a controlled manner. Lower the barbell in two separate movements. While maintaining a flat back, slowly flex the hips and knees and lower the barbell to the thighs while keeping the barbell close to the body. Continue to maintain the flat back while continuing to flex the hips and knees as the barbell is lowered to the floor. Keep the barbell close to the thighs and shins during the descent. A rapid drop or release of the barbell should be avoided with any resistance below maximal or near maximal level. Once the barbell has reached the floor, reposition it and the body for the next repetition. In utilizing submaximal loads, the barbell should be lowered to the floor without relaxing or releasing tension; touch the plates to the floor, and then immediately (without a pause, provided that the body is in the correct starting position) and explosively lift the barbell for the next repetition.

Power Snatch

Type of Exercise

Total-body/power (explosive) exercise

Muscles Used

Gluteus maximus, hamstrings (semimembranosus, semitendinosus, biceps femoris), quadriceps (vastus lateralis, vastus intermedius, vastus medialis, rectus femoris), soleus, gastrocnemius, trapezius (upper portion), deltoids (anterior, medial, and posterior), and triceps brachii

Starting Position

Use a standard barbell. The lifting position is identical to the power clean except for the hand position. The feet are between hip- and shoulder-width apart and pointing forward or just slightly outward. Squat and grasp the barbell with a wider than shoulder-width grip (measured by measuring the distance from the knuckle edge of the clenched fist of an arm extended out to the side and parallel to the floor, across the back of the upper arm/upper back, to the outside edge of the opposite shoulder) and pronated hand position using a closed or hook grip. Arms are outside the knees, elbows extended and pointing outward. Stand so that the barbell is over the balls of the feet and close to the shins. Back is rigid and flat or slightly arched. Head is up or slightly hyperextended. Chest is held up and out. Shoulder blades should be squeezed together. Trapezius and upper back should be relaxed and in a slight state of stretch. With the heels always remaining in contact with the floor, the body weight should be balanced between the balls and middles of the feet. Shoulders are slightly in front of or over the barbell (Fig. 10.2A,B).

Upward Motion: First Pull

Initiate the power snatch by taking a deep breath and holding it. Lift the barbell off the floor through forceful hip, knee, and ankle extension. Maintain a constant position of the torso in relation to the floor throughout the first pull. Make sure that the hips do not rise faster or before the shoulders and keep the back flat or slightly arched. The head should

remain in a neutral position in relation to the spine. The shoulders should remain slightly in front of or over the barbell. The elbows should still be fully extended. During the first pull, keep the barbell as close to the shins as possible. Continue to hold your breath (Fig. 10.2C,D).

Upward Motion: Transition (Scoop)

Explosively drive the hips forward and slightly increase the knee bend to enable the knees to move under and the thighs against the barbell. As the knee bend is increased, shift the body's weight forward toward the front half of the feet while still keeping the heels in contact with the floor. The back should remain slightly arched or flat. The shoulders should remain over or ahead of the barbell. The head should remain in line with the spine. Keep the elbows fully extended and pointing out to the sides. At the completion of the scoop, the body should be in position for initiation of the second pull.

Upward Motion: Second Pull (Power Phase)

With the barbell touching the body between the knees and midthigh, initiate the second pull by explosively extending the hips, knees, and ankles. Keep the shoulders over the barbell. Maintain a straight elbow position as long as possible while the hips, knees, and ankles are extending. Simultaneously fully extend the lower extremity joints and rapidly shrug the shoulders upward. The elbows should continue to remain extended and pointing out during the shrugging movement. Upon fully elevating the shoulders, rapidly flex the elbows to begin pulling the body under the barbell. The upper-body movement resembles that of an elongated wide-grip upright row. While the elbows are moving up and out to the sides, pull with the arms as high as possible. The powerful upward acceleration from the second pull will result in an erect torso and head. The feet will come off the floor.

Upward Motion: Catch

After the lower body has fully extended and the barbell reaches near maximal height, pull the

(continued)

Power Snatch *(continued)*

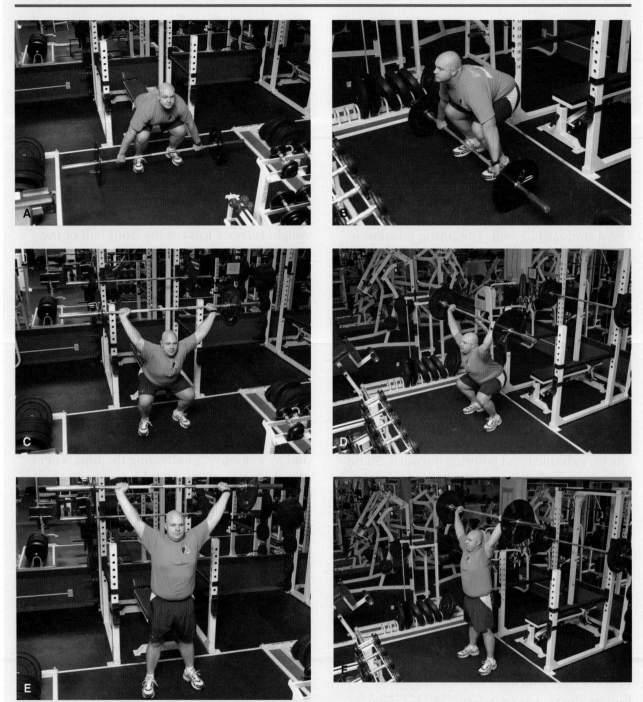

FIGURE 10.2 Power snatch. **A.** Starting position, front view. **B.** Starting position, side view. **C.** First pull, front view. **D.** First pull, side view. **E.** Catch, front view. **F.** Catch, side view.

body under the barbell by rotating the arms and hands around then under the barbell. Rapidly bend the knees and hips to a half-squat position. The feet should return to the floor pointing straight ahead or slightly outward at a width slightly wider than that of the starting position. As the arms reach a point under the barbell, the elbows extend rapidly to push the barbell up and the body downward under the barbell. The bar should be caught overhead with fully extended

Power Snatch *(continued)*

elbows, an erect/tight torso, the head in a neutral position in relation to the spine, knees flexed moderately, feet flat on the floor, the body weight over the center of gravity, and the barbell slightly behind or directly above the head. Upon catching the barbell and establishing control and balance, complete the catch by standing to a fully erect position. Exhale and return to a normal breathing pattern (Fig. 10.2E,F).

Downward Motion

If rubber bumper plates are used, the barbell may be returned to the floor by a controlled forward drop to the floor. The bounce of the bar should be controlled with the hands on or near the bar. Unless maximal or near maximal loads are used, however, the barbell should be returned to the floor in a controlled manner. Lower the barbell in two separate movements. While maintaining a flat back, slowly flex the

hips and knees while simultaneously reducing the tension of the upper body musculature and lower the bar to the thighs while keeping the barbell close to the body. Simultaneously, flex the knees and hips to cushion the impact of the barbell on the thighs. Continue to maintain the flat back while continuing to flex the hips and knees as the barbell is lowered to the floor. Keep the barbell close to the thighs and shins during the descent. A rapid drop or release of the barbell should be avoided, with any resistance below maximal or near maximal level. Once the barbell has reached the floor, reposition it and the body for the next repetition. In utilizing submaximal loads, the barbell should be lowered to the floor without relaxing or releasing tension. Touch the plates to the floor and then immediately (without a pause, providing the body is in the correct starting position) explosively lift the barbell for the next repetition.

Power Jerk

Type of Exercise

Total-body/power (explosive) exercise

Muscles Used

Gluteus maximus, hamstrings (semimembranosus, semitendinosus, biceps femoris), quadriceps (vastus lateralis, vastus intermedius, vastus medialis, rectus femoris), soleus, gastrocnemius, erector spinae, trapezius, and deltoids (anterior, medial, and posterior)

Starting Position

Position a standard barbell at chest level in a squat or power rack. Use a closed, pronated grip, slightly wider than the shoulders. Lift the barbell from its supports. If it is placed in front of the body, keep head slightly back with chin tucked in; shoulders elevated with elbows high/in front of barbell. If barbell is placed behind the head, keep head in neutral position or tilted forward slightly. Assume a natural stance (heels at shoulder width, toes pointing slightly outward). Feet should be firmly on training platform with weight distributed

between heel and forefoot. The torso is rigid and upright (Fig. 10.3A,B).

Upward Motion

Dip 6 to 8 inches (10% of body height) by flexing hips and knees, achieving a "power position" while maintaining complete foot contact with the platform. Immediately reverse direction with explosive extension of hips, knees, and ankles; weight may shift to forefoot. Jumping and pushing explosively enough to completely extend the body and lift the feet off the platform, complete upward drive. Drive barbell overhead with powerful leg action (not pressed with shoulders/arms) (Fig. 10.3C,D).

Downward Motion

Unless maximal or near maximal loads are used, the barbell should be lowered to the shoulders and then replaced on the rack (or platform) in a controlled manner (a rapid drop or release should be avoided with a submaximal resistance).

(continued)

Power Jerk *(continued)*

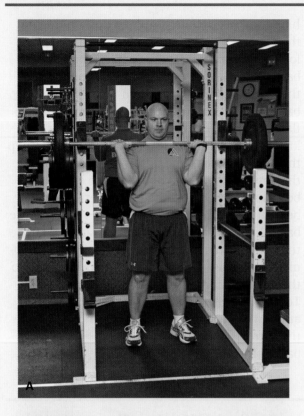
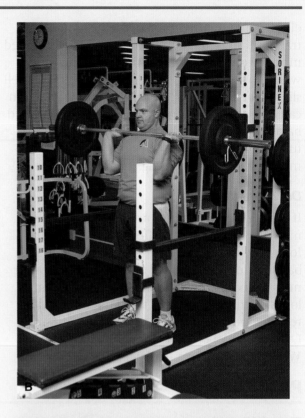
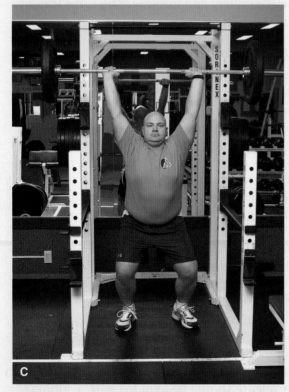
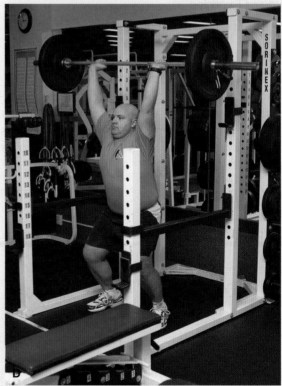

FIGURE 10.3 Power jerk. **A.** Starting position, front view. **B.** Starting position, side view. **C.** Upward motion, front view. **D.** Upward motion, side view.

Power Jerk *(continued)*

Variation in Upward Motion: Split Jerk

Athlete explosively splits legs front/back as barbell leaves torso and feet lift off platform. Key is dynamic placement of front-side foot one to two foot lengths ahead of hips (complete foot contact with platform is maintained). Shins are vertical. Back-side foot is placed two to three foot lengths behind hips; supported on forefoot (heel off platform); knee is slightly flexed. Hip-width stance should be maintained to maintain stable base. Athlete pushes himself or herself under the barbell, then straightens arms and locks barbell overhead. Head shifts to neutral position; barbell is caught directly above hips, shoulders, and elbows. Note: Once the basic mechanics of the lift are mastered, the split allows the athlete to receive the barbell in a lower overhead position. Athlete pushes off front leg first, bringing it back under hips. Rear leg is brought forward under hips. Final position (barbell, elbows, shoulders, hips, knees, and ankles) in same vertical plane. Assume a natural stance (heels at shoulder width, toes pointing slightly outward). Feet should be firmly on training platform with weight distributed between heel and forefoot. Hips and knees fully extended. The torso is rigid and upright. Shoulders elevated, arms fully extended and locked, supporting barbell overhead. Head in neutral position. Eyes focused straight ahead, not looking up at barbell. Barbell is under control.

Safety: Technique on How to Miss

If athlete loses control of the barbell or cannot complete a rep for any reason, he or she should quickly get out from underneath and let it drop (without trying to save it on the way down). Use the barbell's downward momentum to move out of the way (the athlete is told to "keep your grip and push yourself away from the barbell as it falls"). Stay between the plates (this does not mean that the athlete should remain under a falling barbell but rather should move backward or forward, not sideways, to escape).

HIP/THIGH EXERCISES

Back Squat

Type of Exercise

Lower-body/multijoint

Muscles Used

Gluteus maximus, quadriceps (vastus lateralis, vastus intermedius, vastus medialis, rectus femoris), hamstrings (semimembranosus, semitendinosus, biceps femoris)

Starting Position

Position a standard barbell at chest level in a squat or power rack. Step underneath the barbell and position the base of the neck/upper middle back and the hips and feet directly under the barbell. Grasp the barbell using a pronated grip slightly wider than shoulder width. Place the barbell evenly above the posterior deltoids at the base of the neck (high bar placement). Raise the elbows upward to provide a secure location for the barbell to rest on and prevent the bar from sliding down the back during the execution of the lift. To lift the barbell from the rack, extend the hips and knees and take a step backward. Feet are between hip- and shoulder-width apart and pointing forward or just slightly outward. Torso should remain erect. Keep chest out and up. Shoulders are back. Keep head and neck straight with eyes looking straight ahead. Before beginning the initial descent, take a breath and hold it (Fig. 10.4A,B).

(continued)

Back Squat *(continued)*

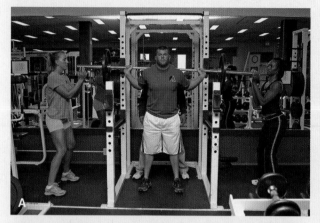
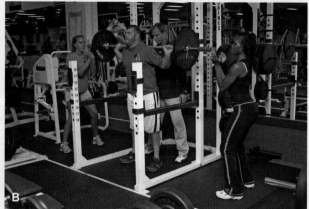
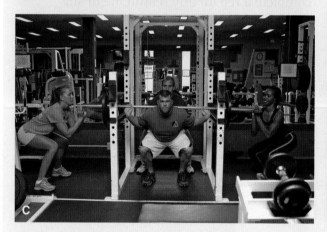
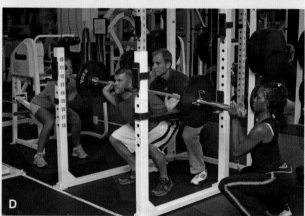

FIGURE 10.4 Back squat. **A.** Starting position, front view. **B.** Starting position, side view. **C.** Downward motion, front view. **D.** Downward motion, side view.

Downward Motion

Initiate the exercise by slowly flexing the knees and hips. Descend with control. Maintain a flat back with a high elbow position. Avoid leaning forward or rounding the upper back during the descent phase. Keep the eyes focused straight ahead with the head erect. Keep the body weight centered over the heels and midfoot portions of both feet. The heels of both feet should remain in contact with the floor at all times throughout the descent. Keep the knees above or slightly in front of the ankles. Do not allow the knees to move in front of the feet. Continue the descent until the backs of the thighs are parallel to the floor, heels begin to lift off the floor, or the trunk begins to round or flex in a forward direction. The flexibility of the lower body will determine the

actual depth of the descent. At the bottom position of the descent, avoid bouncing or increasing the rate of descent before beginning the ascent. Continue to hold your breath from the beginning of the descent (Fig. 10.4C,D).

Upward Motion

Lift the barbell forcefully and with control by extending the knees and hips. Keep the back flat. Do not round the upper back or lean forward during the ascent. Arms should remain tight and head erect with eyes looking straight ahead. Push through the entire foot on both feet with weight evenly distributed from the heels to the toes to make sure that the entire foot remains in contact with the floor. Keep the hips directly under the barbell. Avoid having the body weight move toward the toes. Keep the

Back Squat (continued)

Q & A from the Field

In observing an athlete in the squat, you note that she has too much forward trunk lean during the descent. Additionally, you notice that she has her heels on blocks of wood to raise them off of the floor. What advice would you consider for this athlete?

This athlete should lower the bar position and focus on keeping her head up during the lift. She should also work on gastrocnemius ROM so as to allow the heels to be flat during the lift.

---

knees positioned above to slightly in front of the ankles. Continue the ascent by extending the lower body joints at a consistent rate until the initial standing position is reached. Continue holding your breath from the beginning of the descent through the midpoint of the ascent, then exhale and breathe normally before beginning the descent of the next repetition.

Returning the Weight to the Rack

At the completion of the set, return the barbell to the rack by slowly walking forward and returning the bar to the support hooks of the rack.

Variation: Back Squat with Low Barbell Placement

Place the bar evenly on the posterior deltoids at the middle of the trapezius. Grasp the barbell with an overhand closed grip wider than shoulder-width grip. The handgrip is generally wider than in the high barbell position to adjust for the lower barbell position.

Front Squat

Type of Exercise

Lower-body/multijoint

Muscles Used

Gluteus maximus, quadriceps (vastus lateralis, vastus intermedius, vastus medialis, rectus femoris), hamstrings (semimembranosus, semitendinosus, biceps femoris)

Starting Position

Position a standard barbell at chest level in a squat or power rack. Grasp the barbell using a pronated grip slightly wider than shoulder width. Rotate the arms such that the barbell can be evenly placed across anterior deltoids/clavicles. The backs of the hands should be slightly outside the shoulders, located next to the barbell resting on the deltoids. Lift the elbows up and forward (upper arms should be parallel or as close as possible to the floor) to increase the stability of the barbell on the shoulders. Wrists should be hyperextended and elbows fully flexed. To lift the barbell from the rack, extend the hips and knees and take one to two steps backward. Feet are between hip- and shoulder-width apart and pointing forward or just slightly outward. The torso should remain erect. Keep chest out and up. Shoulders are back. Keep head and neck straight with eyes looking straight ahead. Before beginning the initial descent, inhale (Fig. 10.5A,B).

(continued)

Front Squat *(continued)*

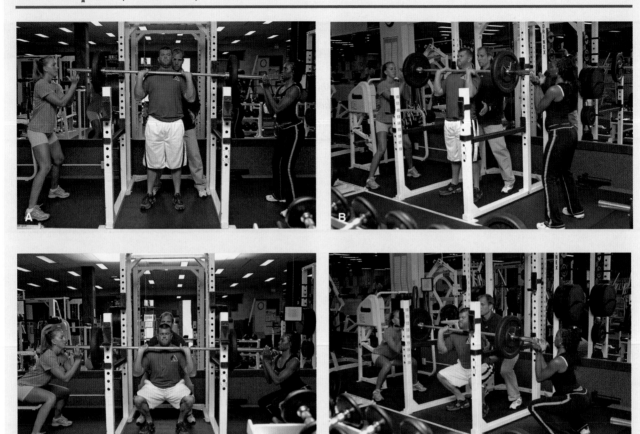

FIGURE 10.5 Front squat. **A.** Starting position, front view. **B.** Starting position, side view. **C.** Downward motion, front view. **D.** Downward motion, side view.

Downward Motion

Initiate the exercise by slowly flexing the knees and hips. Descend with control. Maintain a flat back with a high elbow position. Avoid leaning forward or rounding the upper back during the descent phase. Keep the eyes focused straight ahead with the head erect. Keep the body weight centered over the heel and midfoot portion of both feet. The heels of both feet should remain in contact with the floor at all times throughout the descent. Keep the knees above or slightly in front of the ankles during the descent. Do not allow the knees to move in front of the feet. Continue the descent until the backs of the thighs are parallel to the floor, heels begin to lift off the floor or the trunk begins to round or flex in a forward direction. The flexibility of the

lower body will determine the actual depth of the descent. At the bottom position of the descent, avoid bouncing or increasing the rate of descent before beginning the ascent (Fig. 10.5C,D).

Upward Motion

Lift the barbell forcefully and with control by extending the knees and hips. Keep the back flat. Do not round the upper back or lean forward during the descent. Arms should remain tight and head erect with eyes looking straight ahead. Push through the entire foot on both feet with weight evenly distributed from the heels to the toes to ensure the entire foot remains in contact with the floor. Keep the hips directly under the barbell. Avoid having the body weight move toward the toes. Keep

Front Squat *(continued)*

the knees positioned above to slightly in front of the ankles. Continue the ascent by extending the lower body joints at a consistent rate until the initial standing position is reached. Continue holding the breath from the beginning of the descent through the midpoint of the ascent, then exhale and breathe normally before beginning the descent of the next repetition.

Returning the Weight to the Rack

At the completion of the set, return the barbell to the rack by slowly walking forward and returning the bar to the support hooks of the rack.

Variation: Front Squat with Closed-Arm Grip

Flex the elbows and cross the forearms in front of the chest. Position the barbell evenly on the anterior deltoids without touching it with the hands. Once the barbell is correctly placed, put both hands on top of the barbell and utilize pressure from the fingers to keep it in position. This is an open grip, since the thumb will not be able to encircle the barbell because of the shoulders being in the way.

Dead Lift

Type of Exercise

Lower-body/multijoint

Muscles Used

Gluteus maximus, erector spinae, hamstrings (semimembranosus, semitendinosus, biceps femoris), quadriceps (vastus lateralis, vastus intermedius, vastus medialis, rectus femoris), trapezius, rhomboids, deltoids, and finger flexors

Starting Position

Use a standard barbell. The lifting position is identical to the power snatch and power clean except for the hand position. The feet are between hip- and shoulder-width apart and pointing forward or just slightly outward. Squat and grasp the barbell with an alternated grip [one palm supinated (facing forward) and one palm pronated (facing backward)] and hands slightly wider than shoulder-width apart. Arms are outside the knees, elbows extended and pointing outward. Stand so that the barbell is over the balls of the feet and close to the shins. Back is rigid and flat or slightly arched. Head is up or slightly hyperextended. Chest is held up and out. Shoulder blades should be squeezed together. Trapezius and upper back should be relaxed and in a slight state of stretch. With the heels always remaining in contact with the floor, the body weight should be balanced between the balls and middles of the feet. Shoulders are slightly in front of or over the barbell (Fig. 10.6A,B).

Upward Motion

Initiate the dead lift by extending the hips and knees at the same rate, maintaining a constant angle of the torso in relation to the floor. While keeping the body weight over the middle of the feet, ensure that the hips do not rise faster than the shoulders and keep the back rigid and flat or slightly arched. Shoulders should remain slightly in front of or over the barbell and elbows should be fully extended. Keep the barbell as close to the shins as possible during the ascent and slightly shift the body weight back toward the heels. As soon as the barbell reaches the knees, shift the body weight slightly forward toward the balls of the feet while keeping the heels on the floor. The back should remain rigid and flat or slightly arched, shoulders should remain slightly in front of or over the barbell, elbows should remain fully extended, and head is up or slightly hyperextended. Continue to simultaneously extend the hips and knees until the body reaches a fully erect torso position. The elbows should remain fully extended, like two steel rods, throughout the execution of the ascent. During the ascent the breath should be held until the barbell reaches the knees before exhaling and then breathing normally (Fig. 10.6C,D).

(continued)

Dead Lift *(continued)*

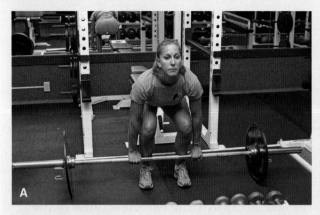
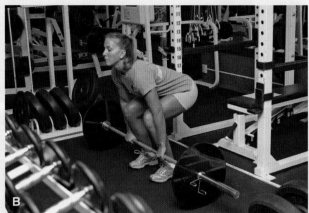
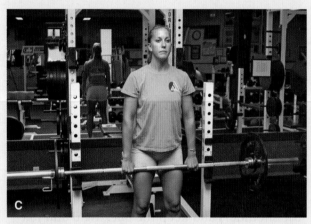
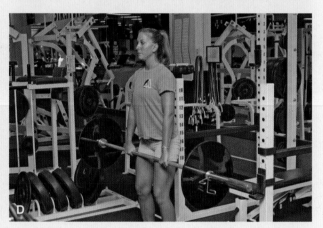

FIGURE 10.6 Dead lift. **A.** Starting position, front view. **B.** Starting position, side view. **C.** Upward motion, front view. **D.** Upward motion, side view.

Downward Motion

Keeping a rigid and flat or slightly arched back, flex the hips and knees and lower the barbell back to the floor with control. The barbell should remain close to the body (knees and shins) throughout descent. Lightly touch the plates on the barbell to the floor and come to stop without releasing the tension on the barbell. Inhale during descent. Begin the ascent for the next repetition.

Barbell Lunge

Type of Exercise

Lower-body/multijoint

Muscles Used

Gluteus maximus, iliopsoas, quadriceps (vastus lateralis, vastus intermedius, vastus medialis, rectus femoris), hamstrings (semimembra-

Variation

The dead lift may be performed with a shoulder-width grip, with both hands pronated to simulate the starting position utilized on a power clean. With this grip position, wrist straps may be utilized to improve grasp on the bar.

nosus, semitendinosus, biceps femoris), soleus, and gastrocnemius

Starting Position

Position a standard barbell at chest level in a squat or power rack. Load the barbell evenly on both sides and secure weights with collars.

Barbell Lunge (continued)

Step underneath the barbell and position the base of the neck/upper middle back and the hips and feet directly under the barbell. Grasp the barbell using a pronated grip slightly wider than shoulder width. Place the barbell evenly above the posterior deltoids at the base of the neck (high barbell placement). Raise the elbows upward to provide a secure location for the barbell to rest on and prevent the barbell from sliding down the back during the execution of the lift. To lift the barbell from the rack, extend the hips and knees to lift the barbell off the rack and take a few (two or three) steps backward to clear the rack and allow adequate room to lunge forward. Feet are between hip- and shoulder-width apart and pointing forward. Torso should remain erect. Keep chest out and up. Shoulders are back. Keep head and neck straight with eyes looking straight ahead. Before stepping forward, inhale (Fig. 10.7A).

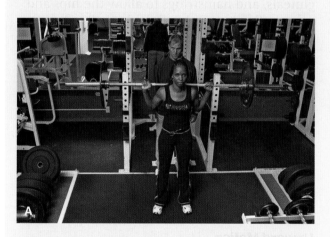

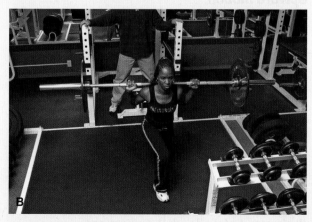

FIGURE 10.7 Barbell lunge. **A.** Starting position. **B.** Downward motion.

Downward Motion

Take an elongated step straight forward with one leg (lead leg). Keep the arms firm and the torso in an erect position as the lead foot goes forward and comes in contact with the floor. The rear leg (trail leg) remains constant in the starting position, but as the lead leg moves forward, balance should shift to the ball of the foot of the trail leg as the trail leg begins to flex. Place the lead foot flat on the floor with the foot pointing straight forward. To maintain balance, ensure that the lead leg moves directly forward from its original starting position and the lead ankle, knee, and hip remain in the same vertical plane. Avoid stepping to the right or left or allowing the knee to shift to one side or the other. Once balance is established on both feet, flex the lead knee to enable the trail leg to bend toward the floor. The trail leg should flex slightly less than the lead leg. The torso should remain erect with the shoulders kept directly above the hips and the head erect, facing forward. The lowest finish position of the ascent should occur when the trail leg is 1 to 2 in. from the floor, the lead leg is flexed to 90 degrees, and the knee is directly above or slightly in front of the ankle. To avoid potentially harmful shearing stress forces on the lead leg's knee joint, it is critical that the lead knee should not extend past the lead foot. At the completion of the descent, a concentrated effort to "sit back" on the trailing leg should be made, as if sitting on the front edge of a bench in the strength-training facility. The depth of the barbell lunge depends on the athlete's hip joint flexibility, particularly the iliopsoas muscles. The lead foot should remain flat on the floor as the toes of the trail foot are extended and the ankle is dorsiflexed (Fig. 10.7B).

Upward Motion

While maintaining an erect torso, shift the balance forward to the lead foot and forcefully push off the floor with the lead foot by plantarflexing it while extending the lead knee and hip joints. As the lead foot returns to the starting position, balance should shift to the trail foot, so that the trail foot regains full contact with the floor. The lead foot should be lifted

(continued)

Barbell Lunge *(continued)*

back to its original starting position with the feet between hip- and shoulder-width apart and pointing forward. Avoid touching the lead foot to the floor until it is returned to the finish position (unless balance is lost). Once the lead foot is returned to the starting position, divide the body weight equally over both feet. Torso should remain erect, as in the beginning position. Exhale at the completion of the ascent. Pause momentarily to fully gain balance, switch lead legs, and repeat the procedure.

Stiff-Leg Dead Lift

Type of Exercise

Lower-body/single-joint

Muscles Used

Gluteus maximus, erector spinae, hamstrings (semimembranosus, semitendinosus, and biceps femoris)

Starting Position

Use a standard barbell. The lifting position is identical to that used in the power clean. The feet are between hip- and shoulder-width apart and pointing forward or just slightly outward. Squat and grasp the barbell with a pronated closed grip and hands at or slightly wider than shoulder-width apart. Arms are outside the knees, elbows extended and pointing outward. Stand so that the barbell is over the balls of the feet and close to the shins. Back is rigid and flat or slightly arched. Head is up or slightly hyperextended. Chest is held up and out. Shoulder blades should be squeezed together. Trapezius and upper back should be relaxed and in a slight state of stretch. With heels always remaining in contact with the floor, the body weight should be balanced between the balls and middles of the feet. Shoulders are slightly in front of or over the barbell. Lift the barbell off the floor by performing a dead-lift exercise. The body alignment and barbell position at the completion of the dead-lift ascent (hips and knees extended, torso erect, barbell touching the front of the thighs, and elbows extended) is the starting position for the stiff-leg dead lift (Fig. 10.8A,B).

Returning the Weight to the Rack

At the completion of the set, return the barbell to the rack by slowly walking forward and returning the barbell to the support hooks of the rack.

Variation (Lunges with Dumbbells)

If balancing a barbell is too difficult for the exerciser, dumbbells held at the sides may be substituted as an alternative.

Downward Motion

Inhale before beginning the descent. Slightly flex the knees to reduce stress on the knee joint before initiating the descent. While keeping the back flat and the knees slightly flexed, gradually reduce the stress on the lower back, gluteals, and hamstrings to allow the hips and torso to flex forward and the barbell to be lowered slowly and with complete control toward the floor. Continue flexing the hips and torso until the trunk begins to round or the heels begin to lift off the floor (this is the endpoint of the descent). Keep the barbell close to the thighs and shins throughout the descent. Do not release or rapidly drop the barbell during the descent. Always lower the barbell without relaxing or releasing tension, keeping the knees in a slightly flexed position (Fig. 10.8C,D).

Upward Motion

Slowly extend the hips and torso and raise the barbell upward while keeping the knees stationary and slightly flexed. Maintain the flat back and extended elbow position. Do not flex the elbows to assist in the upward movement of the barbell. Once full hip extension has been reached, stand erect. Exhale at the completion of the ascent.

Variation

This movement may also be performed with a pair of dumbbells of equal weight or specially designated plate-loaded equipment.

Stiff-Leg Dead Lift *(continued)*

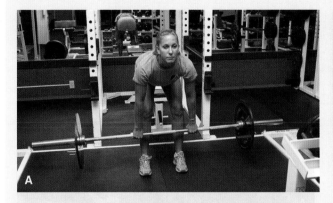
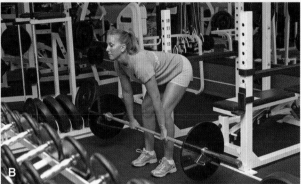
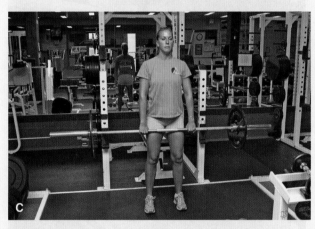
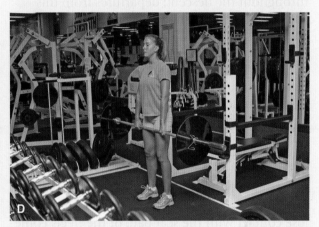

FIGURE 10.8 Stiff-legged dead lift. **A.** Starting position, front view. **B.** Starting position, side view. **C.** Upward motion, front view. **D.** Upward motion, side view.

Leg Press

Type of Exercise

Lower-body/multijoint

Muscles Used

Gluteus maximus, quadriceps (vastus lateralis, vastus intermedius, vastus medialis, rectus femoris), hamstrings (semimembranosus, semitendinosus, biceps femoris)

Starting Position

Load the machine with the appropriate weights. Set the machine seat and/or back pad at the appropriate position (hips and torso should form a 90-degree angle). Sit in the machine, positioning the lower back, with hips and buttocks pressed evenly and in the center of the pads. All body segments other than the legs must be firmly positioned and secured against any movement during the exercise so as to provide maximal support to the spine and lower back. Place the feet shoulder- and hip-width apart with the toes pointing straight up the footplate. It is important that both feet be in the same position vertically and horizontally on each side. Position both upper and lower legs parallel to each other. Grasp the handles on each side of the frame and extend the hips and knees to full extension without locking the knees. Keep the hips securely positioned on the seat and the back against the back pad as the platform is raised. Remove the support mechanism from the platform. The lower body should remain stationary as it absorbs the weight of the platform. When the platform is free of its sup-

(continued)

Leg Press *(continued)*

ports, regrasp the handles on each side of the machine frame to help keep the body firmly in place. All subsequent repetitions should be initiated from this position. Just prior to the descent, take a deep breath and hold it (Fig.10.9A).

Downward Motion

Begin the descent by flexing the knees and hips with control. Do not allow the platform to accelerate as it is lowered. Ensure that the upper and lower legs remain parallel to each other throughout the descent; departures from this position could place undue stress on the lower back, hips, or knees. The hips and buttocks should remain stationary against the seat pad while the back remains flat against the back pad. Avoid shifting the hips or allowing the buttocks to lose contact with the seat. Avoid releasing the handgrips during the descent. Maintaining a firm grip on the handles is essential to a stationary body position. Continue the descent by flexing the knees and hips until one of the following occurs: the thighs become parallel to the platform, the hips lift off the back pad, the buttocks lose contact with the seat pad, or the heels come off the footplate (Fig. 10.9B).

Note: The point where one of these four events occurs should be considered the end ROM or the completion of the descent. The extent of the exercise ROM is dependent upon the individual's magnitude of spinal, hip, knee, and ankle flexibility as well as the machine's individual setup and adjustment capabilities. At the completion of the descent, avoid bouncing the platform, releasing the handgrip, or relaxing the torso to initiate the ascent.

Upward Motion

Press the platform up forcefully under control through the heels by extending the knees

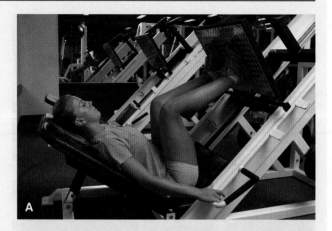

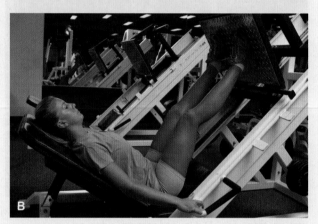

FIGURE 10.9 Leg press. **A.** Starting position. **B.** Ending position.

and hips. Keep the upper and lower legs parallel; do not allow the knees to move in or out. Avoid shifting the hips or allowing the buttocks to move off the seat pad. Continue pressing the platform upward until the knees are fully extended but not locked. Exhale as the platform passes the midpoint of the ROM. At the completion of the set, move the supports back into place and exit the machine.

Leg Extension

Type of Exercise

Lower-body/single-joint

Muscles Used

Quadriceps (vastus lateralis, vastus intermedius, vastus medialis, rectus femoris)

Starting Position

Adjust the seat so that the back of the knee touches the front of the seat pad and the knee joint lines up with the axis of the lever arm. Sit upright on the seat with the back and hips pressed evenly against their pads. Hook the

Leg Extension *(continued)*

feet under the ankle pad such that the insteps of the feet touch the pad when the ankles are dorsiflexed. The thighs, lower legs, and feet should be parallel to each other. Grasp either the side handles or the edges of the seating platform to steady the body throughout the movement. Inhale prior to beginning the exercise (Fig. 10.10A).

Upward Motion

Keeping the thighs, lower legs, and feet parallel to each other, extend the knees with control until the tops of the toes line up with knee height. Avoid rapidly lifting the resistance or accelerating the weight past the top position. To avoid upper and lower extremity movement, maintain contact with the machine pads

throughout the upward motion while keeping a firm grasp on the side handles or the edges of the seating platform during the upward motion. Exhale once the resistance has passed the sticking point (Fig. 10.10B).

Downward Motion

Slowly allow the knees to flex back to the initial starting position. Avoid lowering the resistance quickly during the descent. Keep the back and thighs in contact with their respective pads. Keep the thighs, lower legs, and feet parallel to each other throughout the descent. Stop the descent just before the resistance comes in contact with the remainder of the plates and begin the upward motion. Inhale as the resistance is lowered.

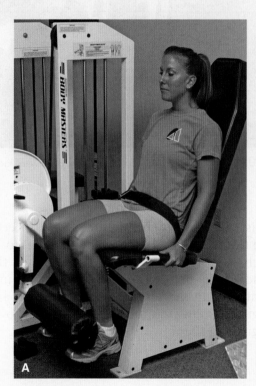
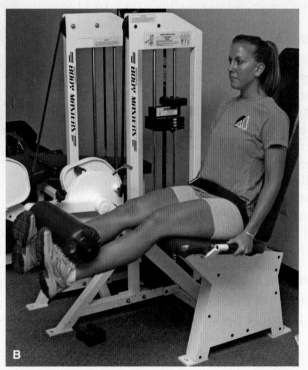

FIGURE 10.10 Leg extension. **A.** Starting position. **B.** Upward motion.

Leg Curl

Type of Exercise

Lower-body/single-joint

Muscles Used

Hamstrings (semimembranosus, semitendinosus, biceps femoris)

Starting Position

Lie prone on the machine with the hips, thighs, and torso resting on the padded surface. Place the tops of the kneecaps slightly over the edge of the padded surface of the machine with the knees lining up with axis of the lever arm. Adjust the position of the ankle pads such that the bottoms of the pads are 3 in. above the heels (just above the tops of the shoes). Position the feet, lower legs, and thighs parallel to each other. Grasp onto the side handles or padded surface of the machine (Fig. 10.11A).

Upward Motion

Inhale prior to initiating the ascent. Flex the knees with control and lift the resistance until the ankle pads nearly reach the buttocks, depending on the level of quadriceps flexibility and limb length. To minimize the use of hip and upper-body movement, maintain contact with the padded surface and keep a firm grip on the handles or torso pad throughout the upward motion. Avoid rapidly lifting the resistance or kicking with the legs to raise the resistance. Also avoid rapidly lifting the resistance through the sticking point before exhaling (Fig. 10.11B).

Downward Motion

Slowly allow the knees to extend back to the initial starting position. Avoid lowering the

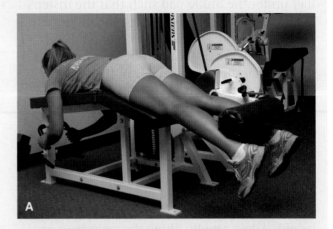

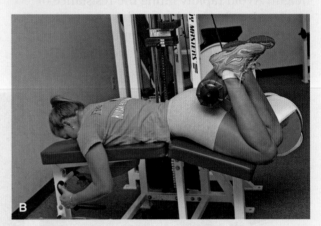

FIGURE 10.11 Leg curl. **A.** Starting position. **B.** Upward motion.

resistance quickly during the descent. Keep the thighs, lower legs, and feet parallel to each other throughout the descent. Stop the descent just before the resistance comes in contact with the remainder of the plates and begin the upward motion. Inhale prior to beginning the upward motion.

Standing Heel Raise

Type of Exercise

Lower-body/single-joint

Muscles Used

Gastrocnemius, soleus

Starting Position

The shoulder pads on the machine should be adjusted so that the exerciser is required to flex his or her knees to get under the pads. The body should be positioned evenly under the

Standing Heel Raise *(continued)*

shoulder pads. The feet should be positioned so that the heels hang over the back edge and slightly below the step with the arches and balls of the feet on the outside edge of the step. The legs and feet should be parallel to each other. The exerciser then stands erect, raising the resistance off the weight stack. The hips should be directly under the shoulders with the knees extended but not locked (Fig. 10.12A).

Upward Motion

Inhale prior to initiating the upward motion. Plantarflex the ankle through a full ROM while keeping the head up, torso erect, and legs and feet parallel to each other. Place equal pressure on the balls of both feet throughout the upward motion. Do not slightly invert or evert the ankles. Keep the legs straight but not locked throughout the upward motion. Avoid rapidly lifting the resistance through the sticking point before exhaling (Fig. 10.12B).

Downward Motion

Slowly allow the ankles to dorsiflex back to the initial starting position with the heels slightly below the step. Inhale as the heels lower back to the starting position. Stop at the bottom position before slowly reinitiating the upward motion for the next repetition.

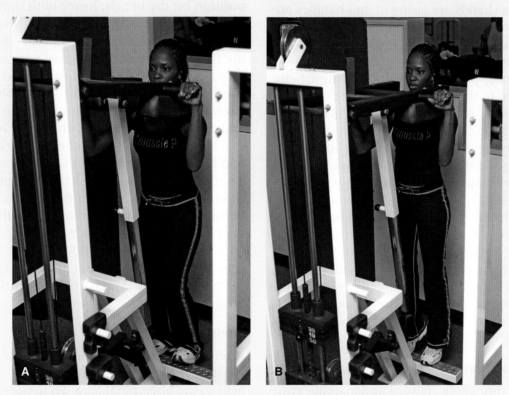

FIGURE 10.12 Standing heel raise. **A.** Starting position. **B.** Upward motion.

CHEST EXERCISES

Bench Press, Dumbbell

Type of Exercise

Upper-body/multijoint

Muscles Used

Pectoralis major, pectoralis minor, deltoid (anterior), serratus anterior, triceps brachii

Starting Position

Select two dumbbells of equal weight with a closed grip. Place the dumbbells on the floor next to the lower end of an adjustable bench. Lift the dumbbells up from the floor by using the legs. Align the dumbbells such that the end closest to the little finger is against the front of the thighs (hands are facing in and handles are parallel to each other) Sit down on the lower end of the adjustable bench with the dumbbells resting on the top of the thighs. Recline to the supine position such that the dumbbells are moved to the lateral aspect of the chest near the armpit even with the midchest level while reclining. Position the feet flat on the floor with the head, shoulders, and buttocks evenly and firmly on the bench. Dumbbells should be rotated to place the thumb side of the dumbbell against the lateral portion of the chest such that both handles are in line with one another, simulating a barbell running through both dumbbell handles. Another option is to perform the exercise with the dumbbell kept in the neutral position (with the handles of the dumbbells parallel to each other). Each repetition will begin from this same position (Fig. 10.13A,B).

Upward Motion

Press the dumbbells upward and together with control. Keep the head, body, and feet in their original position. Do not arch the lower back or lift the buttocks off the bench. The wrists should remain firm and straight, the forearms almost perpendicular to the floor and the hands aligned with each other. Do not allow the dumbbells to move out of control as they are being raised. Press the dumbbells upward until the elbows are fully extended but not locked. Bring the dumbbells together with control at the completion of the movement; do not bang the dumbbells together. Exhale as the dumbbells are lifted (Fig. 10.13C,D).

Downward Motion

Lower and separate the dumbbells with control toward the midchest. To maintain a stable position on the bench, lower both dumbbells at the same rate. Keep the wrists firm and straight, the forearms almost perpendicular to the floor and the hands aligned with each other. Avoid movements forward and backward or side to side. Lower the dumbbells to a lateral portion of the chest near the armpit at midchest level. Dumbbells should be lowered to a lateral portion of the chest such that both handles are in line with one another where a barbell would touch the chest. Dumbbells should not be bounced off the chest at the bottom position or arch the back to lift the chest upward. Maintain a stable position with the feet flat on the floor and the head, shoulders and buttocks evenly and firmly on the bench. Inhale as the dumbbells are lowered.

Completion of the Set

After lowering the dumbbells to the lateral chest on the last repetition, rotate the dumbbells to the abdominal area. Sit up slowly and return the dumbbells to the thigh before standing up and returning the dumbbells to the dumbbell rack or floor.

Bench Press, Dumbbell *(continued)*

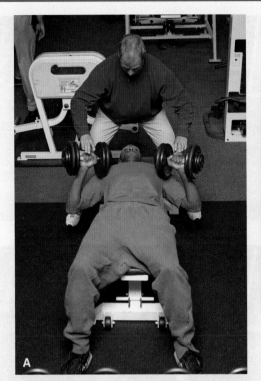

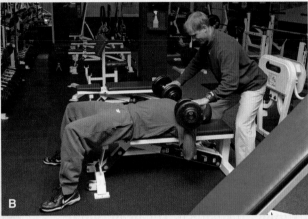

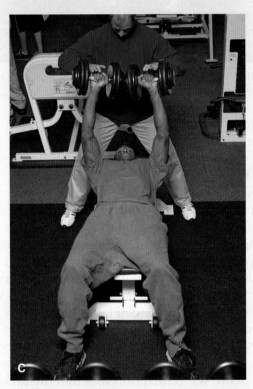

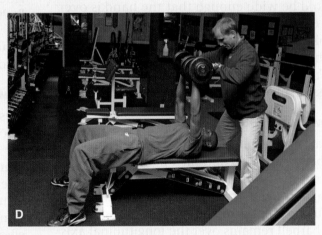

FIGURE 10.13 Bench press, dumbbell. **A.** Starting position, front view. **B.** Starting position, side view. **C.** Upward motion, front view. **D.** Upward motion, side view.

Bench Press, Barbell

Type of Exercise

Upper-body/multi-joint

Muscles Used

Pectoralis major, pectoralis minor, deltoid (anterior), serratus anterior, triceps brachii

Starting Position

Position a barbell on two equal standards of a bench or two equal hooks of a power rack with an adjustable bench. The two standards or hooks should be set such that the elbow is bent slightly (10 degrees) when grasping the barbell. Load barbell evenly on both sides and secure weights with collars. Lie supine on the bench and slide up or down until the eyes are directly under the barbell. The head, shoulders/upper back area, and buttocks should be firmly and evenly placed on the bench and both feet securely placed on the floor on either side of the bench. Both scapulas should be retracted and the pelvis should be tilted posteriorly. Once this position is established, it should be maintained throughout the set. Grasp the barbell with a closed pronated grip slightly wider than shoulder width. Grip should be wide enough that the hand is over the elbow. Lift the barbell off the standards or hooks to a position directly above the chest with the elbows fully extended. All subsequent repetitions begin from this position (Fig. 10.14A).

Downward Motion

Inhale and begin the descent by lowering the barbell in a slow, controlled manner toward the chest. The elbows will move down past the torso and slightly away from the body. Wrists should be kept firm and rigid, ensuring that the barbell remains over the longitudinal axis of the ulna and not in the distal portion of the hand. Forearms are parallel to each other and perpendicular to the floor. Lower the barbell to lightly touch the mid-chest; avoid bouncing the barbell off the chest or lifting the buttocks off the bench to raise the barbell. Keep the head, shoulders/upper back area, and buttocks in contact with the bench and both feet

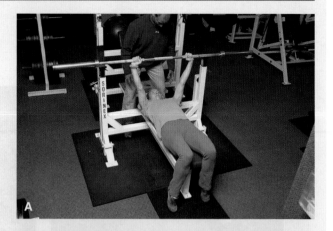

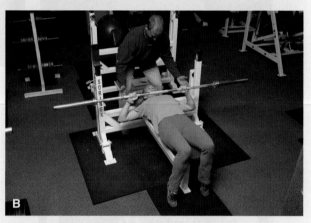

FIGURE 10.14 Bench press, barbell. **A.** Starting position. **B.** Downward motion.

securely on the floor. Keep the body rigid throughout the descent (Fig. 10.14B).

Upward Motion

Press the barbell up and slightly backward forcefully. Begin exhaling at the midpoint of the ascent. Avoid arching the lower back or lifting the feet or buttocks from their position. Keep the wrists rigid and the forearms perpendicular to the floor and parallel to each other. Continue pressing the barbell upward until the elbows are fully extended but not forcefully locked. At the completion of the lift, the barbell should be in line with the supporting joints (i.e., wrist, elbow, shoulder). At the completion of the set, return the barbell to the rack. Do not release the grip on the barbell until both ends of the barbell are securely on the standards or hooks. Keep the body rigid throughout the ascent.

Bench Press, Barbell *(continued)*

Q & A from the Field

An athlete states that she has reached a plateau in the bench press and is unable to increase in weight. What variations can you suggest to the program to help break this plateau?

Alternate exercises such as flies, incline press, or decline press can be used to add variety. Dumbbells can be used to require the athlete to balance the load, and lighter weights can be used explosively to increase power. The athlete may be overtraining, and some time off or a period of active rest may be necessary.

Incline Press, Dumbbell

Type of Exercise

Upper-body/multijoint

Muscles Used

Pectoralis major, pectoralis minor, deltoid (anterior), serratus anterior, triceps brachii

Starting Position

Select two dumbbells of equal weight and hold with a closed grip. Place the dumbbells on the floor next to the lower end of an adjustable bench. Adjust the bench such that the upper end of the bench is set at a 45-degree upward angle and the base of the bench is tilted upward to prevent lifter from sliding. Lift the dumbbells up from the floor by using the legs. Align the dumbbells such that the end closest to the little finger is against the front of the thighs (hands are facing in and handles are parallel to each other). Sit down on the lower end of the adjustable bench with the dumbbells resting on the top of the thighs. Lean back to the incline position such that the dumbbells are moved to the lateral aspect of the chest slightly above the armpit and midchest level while in the incline position. Position the feet flat on the floor with the head, shoulders, and buttocks evenly and firmly on the bench. Dumbbells should be rotated to place the thumb side of the dumbbell against the upper lateral portion of the chest such that both handles are in line

with one another, simulating a barbell running through both dumbbell handles. Another option is to perform the exercise with the dumbbells kept in the neutral position (parallel to each other). Each repetition will begin from this same position (Fig. 10.15A,B).

Upward Motion

Press the dumbbells upward and together with control. Keep the head, body, and feet in their original position. Do not arch the lower back. The wrists should remain firm and straight, the forearms almost perpendicular to the floor and the hands aligned with each other. Do not allow the dumbbells to move out of control as they are being raised. Press the dumbbells upward until the elbows are fully extended but not locked. Bring the dumbbells together with control at the completion of the movement directly above the eyes; do not bang the dumbbells together. Exhale as the dumbbells are lifted (Fig. 10.15C & D).

Downward Motion

Lower and separate the dumbbells with control toward the upper chest. To maintain a stable position on the incline bench, lower both dumbbells at the same rate. Keep the wrists firm and straight, the forearms almost perpendicular to the floor and the hands aligned with each other. Avoid movements

(continued)

Incline Press, Dumbbell *(continued)*

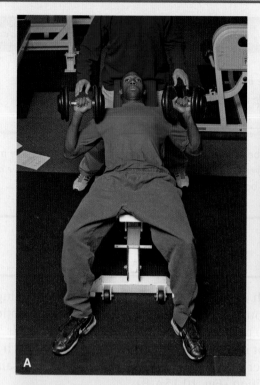

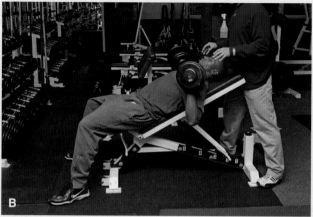

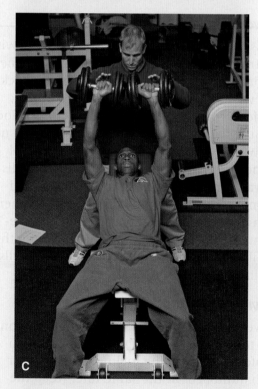

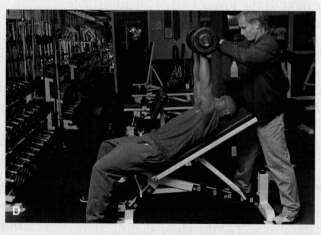

FIGURE 10.15 Incline press, dumbbell. **A.** Starting position, front view. **B.** Starting position, side view. **C.** Upward motion, front view. **D.** Upward motion, side view.

Incline Press, Dumbbell *(continued)*

forward and backward or side to side. Lower the dumbbells to a lateral portion of the chest slightly above the armpit and midchest level. Dumbbells should be lowered to a lateral portion of the chest such that both handles are in line with one another where a barbell would touch the upper chest. Dumbbells should not be bounced off the chest at the bottom position. Avoid arching the back to lift the chest upward. Maintain a stable position with the feet flat on the floor and the head, shoulders and buttocks evenly and firmly on the bench. Inhale as the dumbbells are lowered.

Completion of the Set

After lowering the dumbbells to the upper lateral chest on the last repetition, rotate the dumbbells toward the midline of the body and lower them to the thigh. Sit up completely and return the dumbbells to the dumbbell rack or floor.

Incline Press, Barbell

Type of Exercise

Upper-body/multijoint

Muscles Used

Pectoralis major, pectoralis minor, deltoid (anterior), serratus anterior, triceps brachii

Starting Position

Position a barbell on two equal standards of an incline bench or two equal hooks of a power rack with an adjustable bench. The two standards or hooks should be set such that the elbow is bent slightly (10 degrees) when grasping the barbell. Load barbell evenly on both sides and secure weights with collars. Lie supine on the bench and slide up or down until the eyes are directly under the barbell. The head, shoulders/upper back area, and buttocks should be firmly and evenly placed on the bench and both feet should be securely placed on the floor on either side of the bench. Once this position is established it should be maintained throughout the set. Grasp the barbell with a closed pronated grip, slightly wider than shoulder width. Grip should be wide enough that the hand is over the elbow. Lift the barbell off the standards or hooks to a position directly above the chest with the elbows fully extended. All subsequent repetitions begin from this position (Fig. 10.16A,B).

Downward Motion

Inhale and hold the breath throughout the descent and the change of direction. Begin the descent by lowering the barbell in a slow, controlled manner toward the chest. The elbows will move down past the torso and slightly away from the body. Wrists should be kept firm and rigid, making sure that the barbell remains over the longitudinal axis of the ulna and not in the distal portion of the hand. Forearms are parallel to each other and perpendicular to the floor. Lower the barbell to lightly touch the upper third of the chest, between the clavicles and the midchest; avoid bouncing the barbell off the chest or lifting the buttocks off the bench to raise the barbell. Keep the head, shoulders/upper back area, and buttocks in contact with the bench and both feet securely on the floor. Keep the body rigid throughout the descent (Fig. 10.16C,D).

Upward Motion

Press the barbell up and slightly backward forcefully. Begin exhaling at the midpoint of the ascent. Avoid arching the lower back or lifting the feet or buttocks from their position. Keep the wrists rigid and the forearms perpendicular to the floor and parallel to each other. Continue pressing the barbell upward until the elbows are fully extended but not forcefully locked. At the completion of the lift, the bar should be in line with the supporting joints (i.e., wrist, elbow, shoulder). At the completion of the set, return the barbell to the rack. Do not release the grip on the barbell until both ends of the barbell are securely on the standards or hooks. Keep the body rigid throughout the ascent.

(continued)

Incline Press, Barbell (continued)

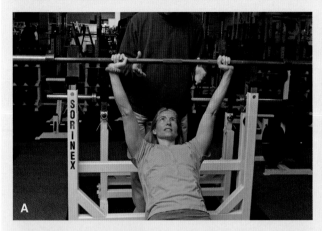
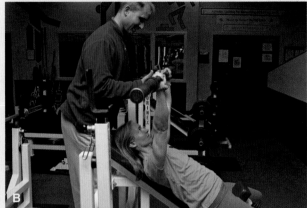
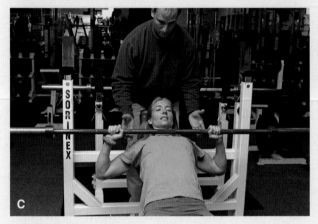
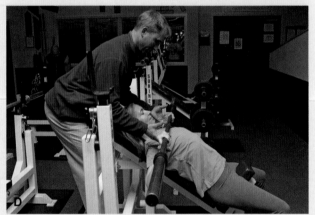

FIGURE 10.16 Incline press, barbell. **A.** Starting position, front view. **B.** Starting position, side view. **C.** Downward motion, front view. **D.** Downward motion, side view.

Dumbbell Fly

Type of Exercise
Upper-body/single-joint

Muscles Used
Pectoralis major, pectoralis minor, deltoid (anterior), serratus anterior

Starting Position
Select two dumbbells of equal weight and hold with a closed grip. Place the dumbbells on the floor next to the lower end of an adjustable bench. Lift the dumbbells up from the floor by using the legs. Align the dumbbells such that the end closest to the little finger is against the front of the thighs (hands are facing in and handles are parallel to each other). Sit down on the lower end of the adjustable bench with the dumbbells resting on the top of the thighs. Recline to the supine position such that the dumbbells are moved to the lateral aspect of the chest near the armpit even with the mid-chest level while reclining. Press the dumbbells up to an extended position of the elbows directly above the chest. Position the feet flat on the floor with the head, shoulders, and buttocks evenly and firmly on the bench. Dumbbells should be rotated to place them in a neutral position (parallel to each other) with the elbows rotating out. Flex the elbows slightly before beginning the downward motion. Each repetition will begin from this same position (Fig. 10.17A).

Dumbbell Fly *(continued)*

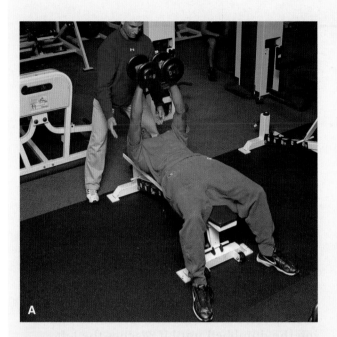

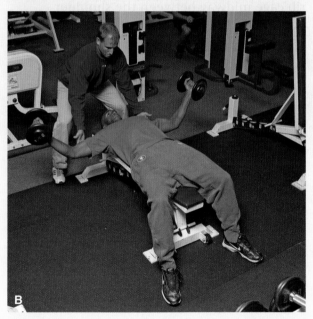

FIGURE 10.17 Dumbbell fly. **A.** Starting position. **B.** Downward motion.

Downward Motion

With a controlled motion, slowly lower the dumbbells with a wide arc. No movement should occur at the elbow joint, only at the shoulders. Inhale as the dumbbells are lowered. As the downward motion continues, the elbows will go from pointing out to the side to pointing toward the floor. Keep the shoulders, upper arm, elbow, lower arm, wrists, and hands in a nearly vertical plane parallel to the floor. The elbows and wrists should remain in a slightly flexed position throughout the downward motion. Continue the downward motion until they are level with the chest and parallel to each other. Avoid lifting the buttocks off the bench at the end of the downward motion (Fig. 10.17B).

Upward Motion

With a controlled motion raise the dumbbells in an arc, simulate hugging a large pillar with the arms. Keep the feet flat on the floor and the head, shoulders, and buttocks evenly and firmly on the bench; avoid arching the lower back or elevating the shoulders to assist with the upward motion. Keep the shoulders, upper arm, elbow, lower arm, wrists, and hands in a nearly vertical plane parallel to the floor as in the downward motion. The elbows and wrists should remain in a slightly flexed position throughout the upward motion. Exhale once the dumbbells pass the sticking point. Continue the slow, controlled, wide arc with the dumbbells until they are repositioned over the chest in the starting position.

Completion of the Set

After lowering the dumbbells to the lateral chest on the last repetition, rotate the dumbbells to the abdominal area. Sit up slowly and return the dumbbells to the thigh before standing up and returning the dumbbells to the dumbbell rack or floor.

UPPER BACK EXERCISES

Dumbbell One-Arm Row

Type of Exercise

Upper-body/multijoint

Muscles Used

Latissimus dorsi, middle trapezius, rhomboids, teres major, posterior deltoid, biceps brachii, brachialis, brachioradialis

Starting Position

Select a dumbbell of appropriate weight. Place the dumbbell on the floor next to the left upper end of an adjustable bench. Stand to the left of a bench that is elevated 30 degrees at the upper end of the bench. Kneel on the bench with the right leg on the bench and the left foot flat on the floor. Place the right hand at the upper end of the bench. Keep the body weight back toward the right heel with a minimum amount of stress placed on the right hand. Position the slightly flexed left leg on the left side of the bench behind the back end of the bench with the toes pointing forward. The left leg should remain in a slightly flexed position throughout the exercise. The upper extremity should remain parallel to the elevated bench. Reach down and grasp the dumbbell with a closed, neutral grip (palm of the hand facing in) of the left hand. Position both hips, left knee, and right elbow so that the torso is at a 30-degree angle to the floor (parallel to the bench). Hang the dumbbell (at a slightly upward angle) down at full elbow extension on the left side of the body while keeping the shoulders parallel. Keep the back flat and the eyes focused straight ahead.

Inhale just before raising the dumbbell (Fig. 10.18A,B).

Upward Motion

Begin by pulling the dumbbell up toward the torso. Keep the upper left arm and elbow next to the side of the body as the dumbbell is raised. Keep the wrist straight; do not curl the wrist upward. The left elbow should be pulled past the side to enable the dumbbell to be pulled to the rib cage midway between the shoulder and hip. Maintain the flat back at a 30-degree upward angle and stationary head, shoulder, elbow, hand, knee, and foot position throughout the ascent. Do not swing or jerk the upper body upward in an attempt to help raise the dumbbell. Continue pulling the dumbbell until it reaches the left rib cage midway between the shoulder and hip. Exhale as the dumbbell is lifted (Fig. 10.18C,D).

Downward Motion

Lower the dumbbell slowly and under control until the elbow is fully extended while keeping the shoulders parallel to each other. Maintain the flat back at a 30-degree upward angle and stationary head, shoulder, elbow, hand, knee, and foot position throughout the exercise. Keep the left knee slightly flexed and the left foot flat on the floor throughout the descent. Inhale as the dumbbell is returned to the starting position. After completing the set with the left arm, release the dumbbell, stand on the right side of the bench, and repeat the procedure using the right arm.

Dumbbell One-Arm Row *(continued)*

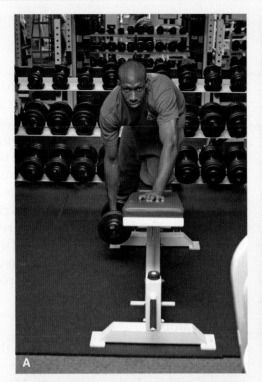
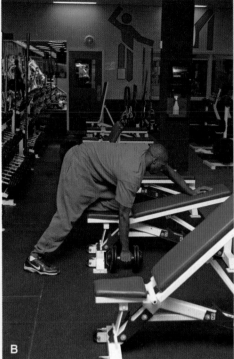
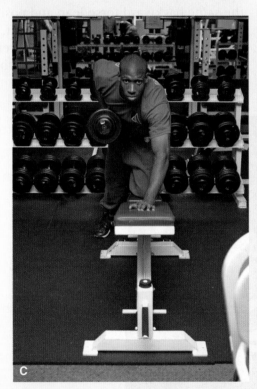
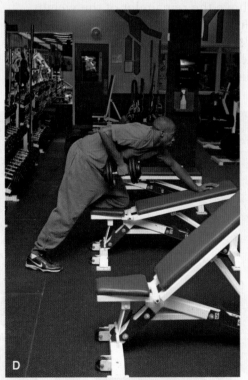

FIGURE 10.18 Dumbbell one-arm row. **A.** Starting position, front view. **B.** Starting position, side view. **C.** Upward motion, front view. **D.** Upward motion, side view.

Lat Pull-Down

Type of Exercise

Upper-body/multi-joint

Muscles Used

Latissimus dorsi, middle trapezius, rhomboids, teres major, posterior deltoid, biceps brachii, brachialis, brachioradialis

Starting Position

Place the pin at the desired training weight in the selectorized weight stack attached to the machine. Grasp the long bar with a closed, pronated grip. The grip width should be slightly wider than shoulder width on a straight bar or on the downward bend of a bent bar. Pull the bar downward and move into a seated position. If the seat is attached to the machine, sit down facing the weight stack with the legs under the thigh pads. The seat should be adjusted to enable the thighs to be parallel to the floor with the feet flat on the floor. The elbows should be fully extended with the selected load suspended above the remainder of the weight stack. Before initiating the descent, lean the torso back slightly and extend the neck to enable the bar to pass by the face as it is pulled down. This position will also decrease the

impingement stress on the shoulder joints (Fig. 10.19A).

Downward Motion

Inhale to initiate the descent. Begin the descent by adducting the scapulas and upper arms. The elbows should move down and back as the chest simultaneously moves up and out while the bar is lowered. Continue pulling the bar down and back until the bar lightly touches the upper chest near the clavicles. The torso should be leaning back slightly at the completion of the descent. The lower body should remain fixed throughout the descent. Avoid quickly leaning back farther or jerking the torso to help pull the bar down. Exhale at the completion of the descent (Fig. 10.19B).

Upward Motion

Return the bar back under control to the starting position. Avoid allowing the arms to return upward rapidly during the ascent. Maintain the same backward torso lean and position of the lower body throughout the ascent. Inhale as the bar rises to the start of the descent. The completion of the ascent is reached when the elbows reach full extension.

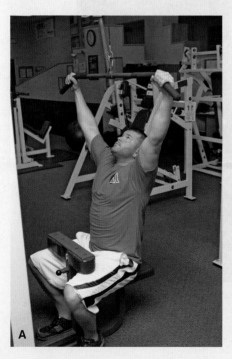 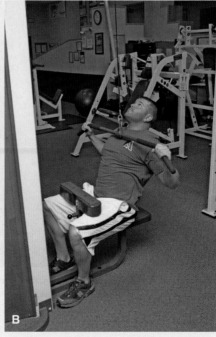

FIGURE 10.19 Lat pull-down. **A.** Starting position. **B.** Downward motion.

Seated Cable Row

Type of Exercise

Upper-body/multijoint

Muscles Used

Latissimus dorsi, middle trapezius, rhomboids, teres major, posterior deltoid, biceps brachii, brachialis, brachioradialis

Starting Position

Place the pin at the desired training weight in the selectorized weight stack attached to the machine. Sit erect with a flat back on the bench facing the handle and the pulley. Grasp the handles with a closed neutral grip (palms facing each other) and the elbows fully extended. Place the feet against the foot stops with a bent knee position. Keeping a flat back, slide back on the bench until the knees are bent slightly, keeping the elbows fully extended. Inhale prior to initiating the movement (Fig. 10.20A).

Backward Motion

Pull the handles toward the upper abdomen in a controlled motion. Maintain an erect torso throughout the backward motion. Keep the elbows close to the body as the handles are pulled back to the upper abdomen. Do not pull the handles quickly or arch the back to move the resistance. Exhale as the resistance is pulled through the sticking point (Fig. 10.20B).

Forward Motion

Keeping the torso erect and upright, elbows pointing down, allow the arms with control to fully extend back returning the resistance to the starting position. Inhale as the resistance is returned to the starting position.

Completion of the Set

Keeping a flat back slide forward on the bench allowing the knees to flex keeping the elbows fully extended until the resistance reaches the weight stack. Avoid rounding your back to return the resistance to the weight stack.

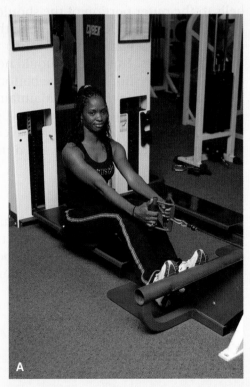 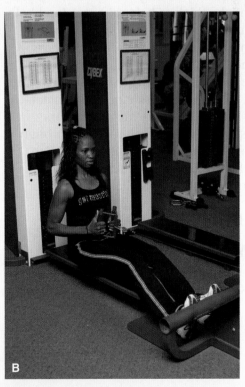

FIGURE 10.20 Seated cable row. **A.** Starting position. **B.** Backward motion.

SHOULDER EXERCISES

Dumbbell Seated Shoulder Press

Type of Exercise

Upper-body/multijoint

Muscles Used

Deltoid (anterior and medial), trapezius (upper portion), serratus anterior, triceps brachii

Starting Position

Select two dumbbells of equal weight using a closed grip. Place the dumbbells on the floor next to the lower end of an adjustable bench. Adjust the bench such that the upper end of the bench is set at a 90-degree upward angle and the base of the bench is parallel to the floor to prevent sliding. Lift the dumbbells up from the floor by using the legs. Align the dumbbells such that the end closest to the little finger is against the front of the thighs (hands are facing in and handles are parallel to each other). Sit down on the lower end of the adjustable bench with the dumbbells resting on the top of the thighs. Lift the dumbbells into their starting position by quickly flexing the hips one hip at a time, using the thigh to help raise the dumbbells to shoulder level. Position the feet flat on the floor with the head, shoulders, and buttocks evenly and firmly on the bench. Dumbbells should be rotated to place the thumb side of the dumbbell against the outside of the shoulder such that both handles are in line with one another, simulating a barbell running through both dumbbell handles. Another option is to perform the exercise with the dumbbells kept in the neutral position (parallel to each other). Each repetition will begin from this same position (Fig. 10.21A,B).

Upward Motion

Press the dumbbells upward and together with control. Keep the head, body, and feet in their original position. Do not arch the lower back. The wrists should remain firm and straight, the forearms almost perpendicular to the floor and the hands aligned with each other. Do not allow the dumbbells to move out of control as they are being raised. Press the dumbbells upward until the elbows are fully extended but not locked. Bring the dumbbells together with control at the completion of the movement directly above the middle of the head; do not bang the dumbbells together. Exhale as the dumbbells are lifted past the sticking point (Fig. 10.21C,D).

Downward Motion

Lower and separate the dumbbells with control toward the outer shoulder. To maintain a stable position on the bench, lower both dumbbells at the same rate. Keep the wrists firm and straight, the forearms almost perpendicular to the floor and the hands aligned with each other. Avoid movements forward and backward or side to side. Lower the dumbbells to the outer portion of the shoulder such that both handles are in line with one another where a barbell would touch the upper shoulders. Dumbbells should not be bounced off the shoulder at the bottom position. Avoid arching the back. Maintain a stable position with the feet flat on the floor and the head, shoulders, and buttocks evenly and firmly on the bench. Inhale as the dumbbells are lowered.

Completion of the Set

After lowering the dumbbells to the outer shoulder on the last repetition, rotate the dumbbells toward the midline of the body and lower them to the thigh. Return the dumbbells to the dumbbell rack or floor.

Dumbbell Seated Shoulder Press *(continued)*

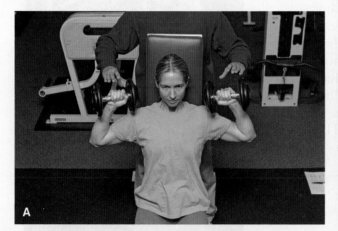

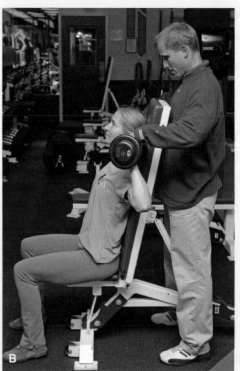

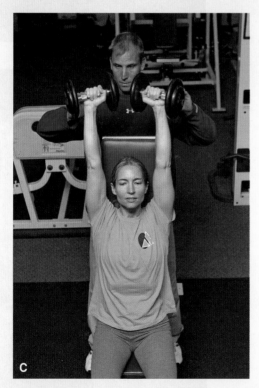

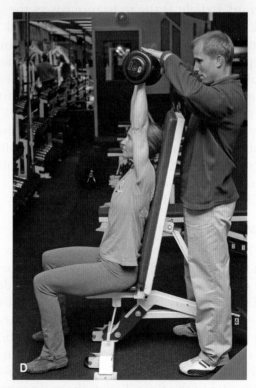

FIGURE 10.21 Dumbbell seated shoulder press. **A.** Starting position, front view. **B.** Starting position, side view. **C.** Upward motion, front view. **D.** Upward motion, side view.

Machine Shoulder Press

Type of Exercise
Upper-body/multijoint

Muscles Used
Deltoid (anterior and medial), trapezius (upper portion), serratus anterior, triceps brachii

Starting Position
Place the pin at the desired training weight in the selectorized weight stack attached to the machine. Adjust the seat height such that the handgrips are in line with the tops of the shoulders and the base of the neck. Position the feet flat on the floor with the head, shoulders, and buttocks evenly and firmly on the machine. The head shoulders, upper back and should be pressed against the vertical pad. Grasp both handles with a closed pronated or neutral (optional) grip (Fig. 10.22A).

Upward Motion
Begin the motion by pushing the handles upward. Exhale as the resistance passes the sticking point. Avoid arching the lower back or lifting the feet or buttocks from their position. Keep the wrists rigid and the forearms perpendicular to the floor and parallel to each other. Continue pressing the resistance upward until the elbows are fully extended but not forcefully locked. At the completion of the lift, the handles of the machine should be in line with the supporting joints (i.e., wrist, elbow, shoulder). Keep the body rigid throughout the ascent (Fig. 10.22B).

Downward Motion
Begin the descent by lowering the resistance in a slow, controlled manner toward the chest. The elbows will move down past the shoulder and slightly away from the body. Wrists should be kept firm and rigid, ensuring that the barbell remains over the longitudinal axis of the ulna and not in the distal portion of the hand. Forearms are parallel to each other and perpendicular to the floor. Lower the resistance to shoulder height; avoid bouncing the resistance off the weight stack, lifting the buttocks off the bench, or arching the back. Keep the head,

shoulders/upper back area, and buttocks in contact with the bench and both feet securely on the floor. Keep the body rigid throughout the descent.

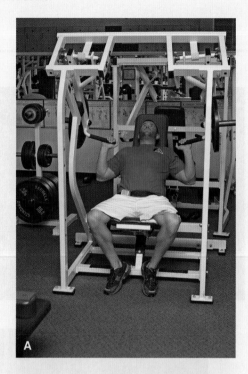

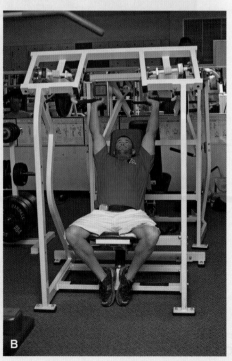

FIGURE 10.22 Machine shoulder press. **A.** Starting position. **B.** Upward motion.

Barbell Upright Row

Type of Exercise

Upper-body/multijoint

Muscles Used

Anterior, medial and posterior deltoid, trapezius, serratus anterior, brachialis, biceps brachii, brachioradialis

Starting Position

Load barbell evenly on both sides and secure weights with collars. Grasp the barbell evenly with a closed, pronated grip narrower than shoulder width but not closer than thumbs width apart from each other. Hold the barbell against the front of the thighs with the elbows fully extended. Position the feet flat on the floor shoulder width apart; knees flexed slightly, torso erect, shoulders back, and eyes looking straight ahead (Fig. 10.23A & B).

Upward Motion

Begin the upward motion by lifting the barbell vertically along the front of the body past the abdomen and chest by flexing the elbows and abducting the shoulders. Maintain an erect upper torso while keeping the knees still slightly flexed and feet flat on the floor. The barbell should not swing away from the body or upward in an uncontrolled manner. Avoid rising up on the toes, extending the knees, or shrugging the shoulders to assist in the ascent of the barbell. Keep the wrists rigid throughout the ascent. Continue with the upward pull of the barbell until the elbows are slightly higher than the shoulders and wrists (the barbell should be elevated to a point between the sternum and the chin depending upon the individual's arm length

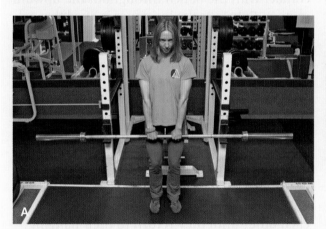
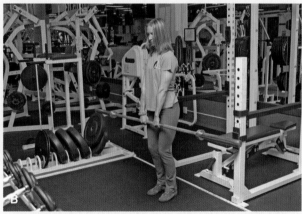
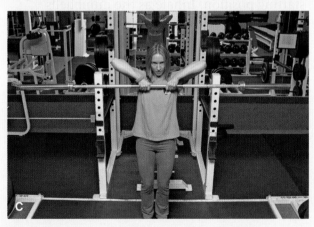
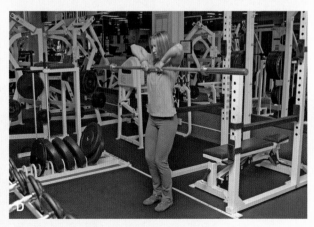

FIGURE 10.23 Barbell upright row. **A.** Starting position, front view. **B.** Starting position, side view. **C.** Upward motion, front view. **D.** Upward motion, side view.

(continued)

Barbell Upright Row *(continued)*

and shoulder flexibility). Exhale at the completion of the ascent (Fig. 10.23C,D).

Downward Motion

Slowly lower the barbell under control, keeping the barbell close to the body throughout the descent until the elbows are fully extended and the barbell is against the front of the thighs. Avoid bouncing the barbell against the thighs, rapidly extending the elbows, leaning forward with the torso, or shifting the body weight to the balls of the feet. Maintain an erect upper torso, knees slightly flexed and the feet flat on the floor shoulder width apart. Inhale as the barbell is lowered during the descent.

Dumbbell Prone Posterior Raise

Type of Exercise

Upper-body/single joint

Muscles Used

Infraspinatus, teres minor, trapezius, deltoids (anterior, medial, and posterior)

Starting Position

Select two dumbbells of equal weight. Place the dumbbells on the floor next to the upper end of a slightly elevated adjustable bench. Lie prone on the weight bench with the hips, thighs, and torso resting on the padded surface. Slide up the bench so that the chin rests over the top edge of the bench. Grasp the dumbbells with a closed grip and rotate them to a neutral hand position with the handles parallel to each other and with the elbows pointing out to the side. The arms extend straight down from the shoulders with a slight flex in the elbows (Fig. 10.24A,B).

Upward Motion

Inhale and raise the dumbbells with control simultaneously out to the sides while main-taining the slight bend in the elbows; movement should not occur at the elbow joints, only at the shoulders. Throughout the upward motion, the upper arms and elbows should rise together, before and slightly higher than the lower arm and hands. Avoid lifting the weight rapidly. Keep the head, neck, or upper torso in contact with the bench throughout the upward motion. Exhale as the resistance is lifted through the sticking point. Continue lifting the resistance until the arms are approximately parallel to the floor or nearly level with the shoulder height (Fig. 10.24C,D).

Downward Motion

Lower the dumbbells with control while keeping the head, neck, or upper torso in contact with the bench throughout the downward motion. Allow the dumbbells to continue to descend, keeping the dumbbells parallel to each other until they return to their hanging starting position. Inhale as the dumbbells return to the starting position.

Dumbbell Prone Posterior Raise *(continued)*

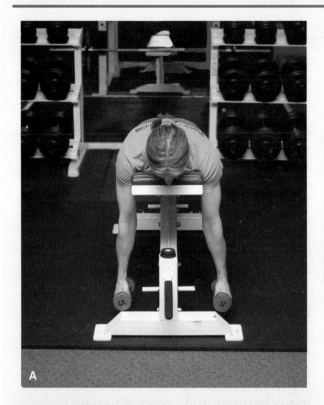

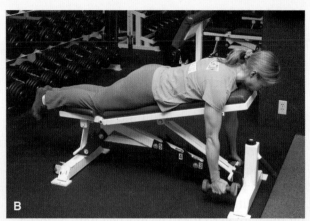

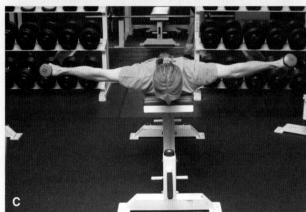

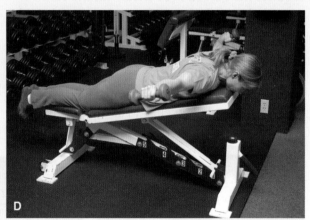

FIGURE 10.24 Dumbbell prone posterior raise. **A.** Starting position, front view. **B.** Starting position, side view. **C.** Upward motion, front view. **D.** Upward motion, side view.

TRICEPS EXERCISES

Supine Triceps Extension

Type of Exercise

Upper-body/single-joint

Muscles Used

Triceps brachii

Starting Position

Load an EZ curl barbell evenly on both sides and secure weights with collars. Sit at one end of an adjustable flat bench and then lie back so the head rests on the other end of the bench. The head, shoulders/upper back area, and buttocks should be firmly and evenly placed on the bench and both feet should be securely placed on the floor on either side of the bench. Have a spotter lift the barbell so it can be grasped with a closed, pronated grip at either the inside or outside hand position of the barbell. Move the barbell to a position where the arms are parallel to each other and perpendicular to the floor; this requires the barbell to be held with the elbows extended over the eyes. The upper arms should be externally rotated so that the elbows point toward the feet (Fig. 10.25A).

Downward Motion

Lower the barbell with control toward the top of the forehead. The elbows should point toward the feet as they begin to flex. The upper arms should remain parallel to each other and perpendicular to the floor. Keep the head, shoulders/upper back area, and buttocks firmly and evenly placed on the bench with both feet securely placed on the floor on either side of the bench. Avoid arching the back during the downward motion. The barbell should nearly touch the forehead at its lowest position. Caution should be taken to control the speed of the descent so that the barbell does not strike the face. Inhale during the downward motion (Fig. 10.25B).

Upward Motion

Lift the barbell upward with control by extending the elbows while keeping the elbow and upper arms stationary. Keep the head, shoulders/upper back area, and buttocks firmly and evenly placed on the bench with both feet securely placed on the floor on either side of the bench. Continue pressing the barbell until the elbows are fully extended with the barbell directly above the eyes. Exhale as the resistance is lifted through the sticking point.

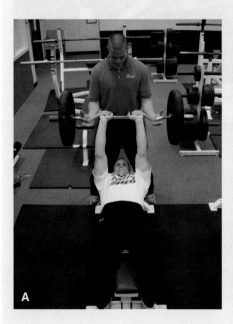
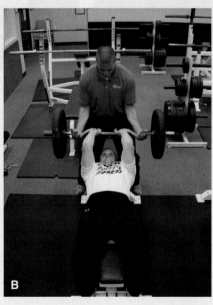

FIGURE 10.25 Supine triceps extension. **A.** Starting position. **B.** Downward motion.

Triceps Pushdown

Type of Exercise

Upper-body/single-joint

Muscles Used

Triceps brachii

Starting Position

Place the pin at the desired training weight in the selectorized weight stack attached to the machine. Grasp a Tri-V bar or rope with a closed pronated grip. Hands will be approximately 8 to 10 in. apart. Place the feet shoulder or hip width apart with the torso erect and the knees slightly flexed. Position the body so that the cable is positioned at a perpendicular angle in the starting position. Move the Tri-V bar down from its stationary position to a position where the elbows are next to the anterior portion of the torso touching the lower rib cage; the lower arm is straight out from the body with the wrists straight and hands even with chest level. Keep the head in a neutral position with the cable directly in front of the nose, with shoulders back and abdominal muscles slightly contracted. Avoid leaning forward or positioning the head to the side of the cable. Inhale prior to initiating the downward motion. All subsequent repetitions should begin from this position (Fig. 10.26A).

Downward Motion

While maintaining an erect posture, push the Tri-V bar down with control from the chest level toward the upper thigh. Keep the elbows tight to the anterior portion of the torso, touching the lower rib cage. Keep the body centered with the cable in front of the middle of the face. Maintain a slight flex in the knees throughout the downward motion. Exhale as the resistance is lifted through the sticking point. Avoid locking the elbows at the bottom position (Fig. 10.26B).

Upward Motion

Extend the elbows with control to allow the Tri-V bar to return to the initial starting position. The initial starting position is a position where the elbows are next to the anterior portion of the torso touching the lower rib cage; the lower arm is straight out from the body with the wrists straight and hands even with chest level. It is critical throughout the upward motion to ensure that the elbows are next to the anterior portion of the torso touching the lower rib cage. Inhale as the bar returns to the starting position.

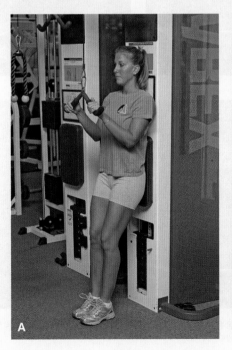
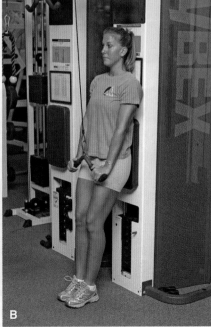

FIGURE 10.26 Triceps pushdown. **A.** Starting position. **B.** Downward motion.

BICEPS EXERCISES

Barbell Bicep Curl

Type of Exercise

Upper-body/single-joint

Muscles Used

Biceps brachii, brachialis, brachioradialis

Starting Position

Load barbell evenly on both sides and secure weights with collars. Grasp the barbell evenly with a closed, supinated grip shoulder width apart. Hold the bar against the front of the thighs with the elbows fully extended. Position the feet flat on the floor shoulder width apart; knees flexed slightly, torso erect, shoulders back and eyes looking straight ahead. Inhale prior to initiating the upward motion (Fig. 10.27A, B).

Upward Motion

Flex the arms at the elbows raising the barbell in an arc pattern with control. Keep the elbows tight to the anterior portion of the torso touching the lower rib cage as the barbell is raised. The movement should occur at the elbows, not at the shoulders. Keep the feet flat on the floor shoulder width apart; knees flexed slightly, torso erect, shoulders back and eyes looking straight ahead. Avoid swinging the barbell, arching the lower back, rising up on the toes or shrugging the shoulders to lift the resistance. Continue flexing the elbows until the barbell reaches a point above chest level approximately 2 to 3 in. from the body. Avoid moving the elbows forward at the completion of the upward motion. Exhale as the barbell passes the sticking point (Fig. 10.27C,D).

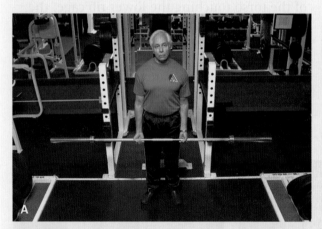
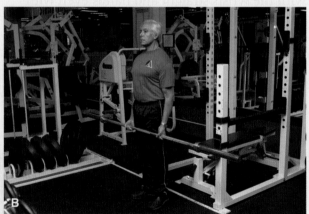
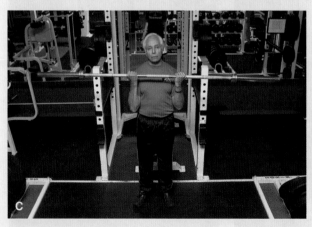
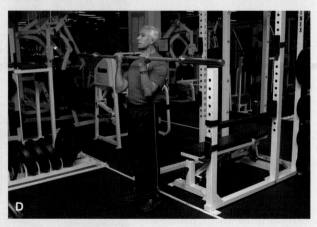

FIGURE 10.27 Barbell bicep curl. **A.** Starting position, front view. **B.** Starting position, side view. **C.** Upward motion, front view. **D.** Upward motion, side view.

Barbell Bicep Curl *(continued)*

Downward Motion

Lower the barbell with control until the elbows are fully extended. Avoid bouncing the barbell on the thighs at the bottom position. Flexing the torso forward, rise up on the toes or forcefully extend the elbows during the downward motion. Keep the elbows tight to the anterior portion of the torso touching the lower rib cage as the barbell is lowered. Maintain an erect upper body posture with the knees slightly flexed and the feet flat on the floor. Inhale during the downward motion.

Dumbbell Seated Alternate-Arm Bicep Curl

Type of Exercise

Upper-body/single-joint

Muscles Used

Biceps brachii, brachialis, brachioradialis

Starting Position

Select two dumbbells of equal weight with a closed grip. Place the dumbbells on the floor next to the lower end of an adjustable bench. Adjust the bench such that the upper end of the bench is set at a 75-degree upward angle and the base of the bench is parallel to the floor to prevent sliding. Lift the dumbbells up from the floor by using the legs. Sit down on the lower end of the adjustable bench with the dumbbells resting on the top of the thighs. Allow the dumbbells to hang at the side with the elbows fully extended and the hands supinated (palms facing forward). Inhale just before lifting the first dumbbell (Fig. 10.28A,B).

Upward Motion

Initiate the exercise by raising one dumbbell upward with control in an arc by flexing the arm at the elbow. Keep the elbows tight to the anterior portion of the torso, touching the lower rib cage as the barbell is raised. The movement should occur at the elbow, not at the shoulders. Keep the feet flat on the floor, torso erect, shoulders back, and eyes looking straight ahead. Avoid swinging the dumbbell, arching the lower back, rising up on the toes, or shrugging the shoulders to lift the dumbbell. Continue flexing the elbow until the dumbbell reaches a point above chest level approximately 2 to 3 in. from the body. Avoid moving the elbow forward at the completion of the upward motion. Exhale as the dumbbell passes the sticking point. Keep the opposite arm still at the side of the body (Fig. 10.28C,D).

Downward Motion

Lower the dumbbell with control until the elbow is fully extended. Avoid forcefully extending the elbow during the downward motion. Keep the elbow tight to the anterior portion of the torso, touching the lower rib cage as the dumbbell is lowered. Maintain an erect upper body posture with the feet flat on the floor. Inhale during the downward motion. Keep the opposite arm still at the side of the body until the repetition is completed and then repeat the upward and downward movements with the opposite arm.

Dumbbell Seated Alternate-Arm Bicep Curl *(continued)*

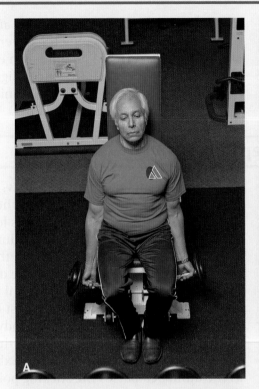
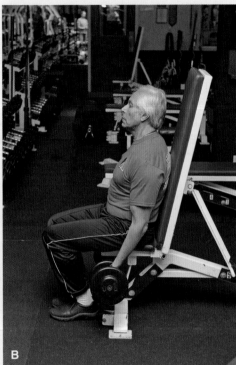
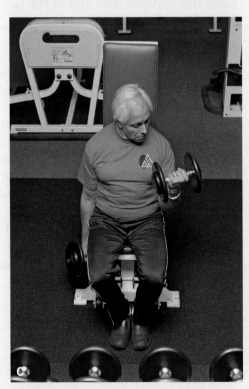
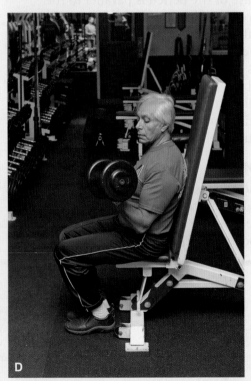

FIGURE 10.28 Dumbbell seated alternate arm bicep curl. **A.** Starting position, front view. **B.** Starting position, side view. **C.** Upward motion, front view. **D.** Upward motion, side view.

FOREARM EXERCISES

Wrist Curl

Type of Exercise

Upper-body/single-joint

Muscles Used

Flexor carpi radialis, flexor carpi ulnaris, palmaris longus, flexor digitorum superficialis, flexor digitorum profundus

Starting Position

Load barbell evenly on both sides and secure weights with collars. Grasp the barbell evenly with a closed, supinated grip shoulder width apart. Sit on the end of a bench. Grasp the barbell with a closed supinated grip 10 in. apart. Position the legs at a 90 degrees with the feet and legs parallel to each other and the toes pointing straight ahead. Place the forearms and elbows on top of the thighs and lean forward slightly. The wrists should extend slightly past the front of the knee. Extend the wrists with control toward the floor and open the fingers so that the barbell rests on the fingertips. Inhale before initiating the upward motion (Fig. 10.29A,B).

Upward Motion

Lift the barbell with control by flexing the fingers and then the wrists through a full ROM without moving the forearms or elbows. Do not jerk or rapidly move the barbell upward. Exhale as the barbell passes the sticking point (Fig. 10.29C,D).

Downward Motion

Return the barbell with control to the starting position by first extending the wrists and then the fingers. Avoid rapidly dropping the barbell during the downward motion. Inhale at the completion of the downward motion.

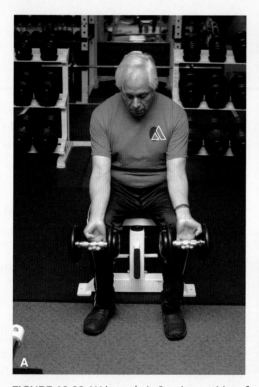
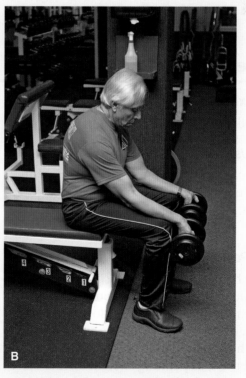

FIGURE 10.29 Wrist curl. **A.** Starting position, front view. **B.** Starting position, side view.

(continued)

Wrist Curl *(continued)*

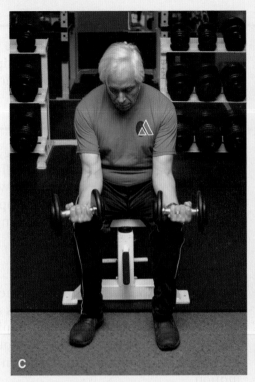
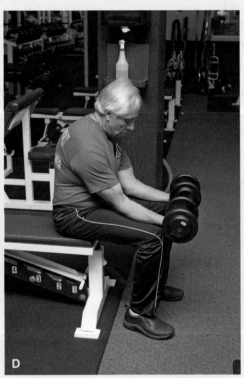

FIGURE 10.29 *(continued)* Wrist curl. **C.** Upward motion, front view. **D.** Upward motion, side view.

Reverse Wrist Curl

Type of Exercise

Upper-body/single-joint

Muscles Used

Extensor carpi radialis longus, extensor carpi radialis brevis, extensor carpi ulnaris, extensor digitorum, extensor digiti minimi, extensor indicis

Starting Position

Grasp the barbell evenly with a closed, pronated grip shoulder-width apart. Sit on the end of a bench. Grasp the barbell with a closed supinated grip 10 in. apart. Position the legs at a 90-degree angle with the feet and legs parallel to each other and the toes pointing straight ahead. Place the forearms and elbows on top of the thighs and lean forward slightly. The wrists should

extend slightly past the front of the knee. Extend the wrists with control toward the floor while keeping the fingers closed. Inhale before initiating the upward motion (Fig. 10.30A).

Downward Motion

Lower the barbell with control toward the floor by flexing the wrists. Avoid rapidly dropping the barbell during the downward motion. Inhale at the completion of the downward motion (Fig. 10.30B).

Upward Motion

Lift the barbell with control by extending the wrists through a full range of motion without moving the forearms or elbows. Do not jerk or rapidly move the barbell upward. Exhale as the barbell passes the sticking point.

Reverse Wrist Curl *(continued)*

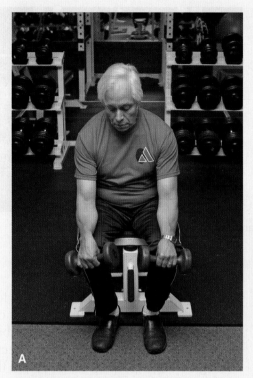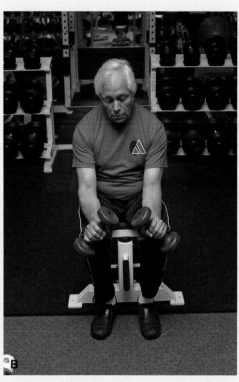

FIGURE 10.30 Reverse wrist curl. **A.** Starting position. **B.** Upward motion.

ABDOMINAL AND LOWER BACK EXERCISES

Abdominal Crunch

Type of Exercise

Trunk

Muscles Used

Rectus abdominis, obliquus externus abdominis, tensor fascia latae, rectus femoris

Starting Position

Lie supine on an exercise mat or padded floor. Place hands behind the head with fingers interlaced and elbows out to the side. Bend the knees to a 90-degree angle, and place the feet flat on the floor. Inhale prior to initiating the exercise (Fig. 10.31A).

Upward Motion

Keeping the neck straight cradled in the hands, the lower back and buttocks flat on the floor, and the knees at a 90-degree angle with feet on the floor, curl the torso upward with control until the upper back is lifted off the floor or exercise mat. Keep the fingers interlaced behind the head. Exhale as the sticking point is passed (Fig. 10.31B).

Downward Motion

With control, keeping the neck straight and cradled in the hands, the lower back and buttocks flat on the floor and the knees at a

(continued)

Abdominal Crunch *(continued)*

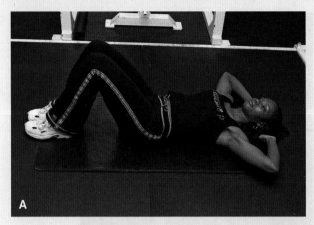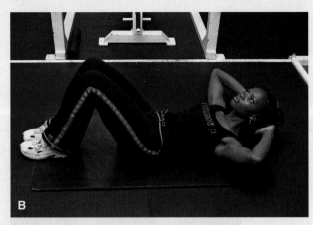

FIGURE 10.31 Abdominal crunch. **A.** Starting position. **B.** Upward motion.

90-degree angle with feet on the floor, allow the torso to uncurl back to the starting position when the upper back reaches the floor or exercise mat. Keep the fingers interlaced behind the head. Inhale at the completion of the downward motion.

Variation of the Exercise

For more experienced exercisers, the lower legs may be lifted parallel to the floor or placed on an exercise bench with the lower back and buttocks flat on the floor and the knees at a 90-degree angle perpendicular to the floor.

Back Extension

Type of Exercise

Trunk

Muscles Used

Longissimus thoracis, quadratus lumborum, iliocostalis lumborum, longissimus thoracis, iliocostalis thoracis, intertransversarii laterales lumborum, gluteus maximus, hamstrings (semimembranosus, semitendinosus, biceps femoris)

Starting Position

Sit on the machine in an upright posture with your feet on the footplate so your knees are slightly bent and the back of your legs are in

firm contact with the seat. Make sure the back pad is in contact with your shoulder blades, then place your hands, overlapped, across your chest (Fig. 10.32A).

Back Motion

Keep your head and neck in a neutral position and slowly begin to extend your torso backward until you reach a position that is straight from your feet to your head (Fig. 10.32B).

Forward Motion

Reverse your position while performing a slow trunk flexion movement until you return to the upright sitting posture.

Back Extension *(continued)*

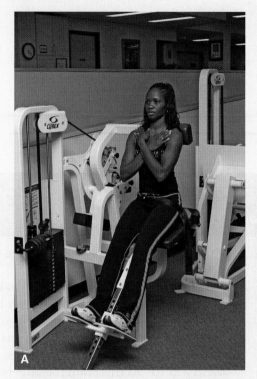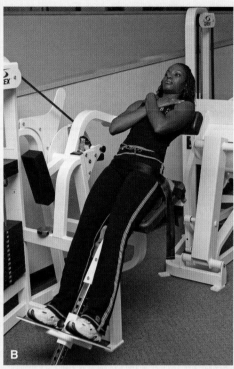

FIGURE 10.32 Back extension. **A.** Starting position. **B.** Downward motion.

SUMMARY

Resistance training has numerous benefits, including hypertrophy and increased bone mineral density. Prior to beginning a resistance training program, an athlete should be familiar with proper attire, spotting techniques, and breathing techniques. Prior to performing a specific exercise, an athlete should know the proper movement of the exercise as described in this chapter.

MAXING OUT

1. An experienced strength-training participant is performing a 3-RM exercise in the bench press. How many spotters are required? Where should they be positioned? What are their responsibilities?
2. Complete Table 10.1 for the listed upper-body exercises.
3. Complete Table 10.2 for the listed lower-body exercises.

TABLE 10.1	UPPER-BODY EXERCISES		
EXERCISE	**BENCH PRESS, BARBELL**	**BARBELL UPRIGHT ROW**	**SUPINE TRICEPS EXTENSION**
Type of exercise			
Muscles used			
Grip type			
Grip width			
Number of spotters			

TABLE 10.2	LOWER-BODY EXERCISES		
EXERCISE	POWER CLEAN	BACK SQUAT	DEAD LIFT
Type of exercise			
Muscles used			
Grip type			
Grip width			
Feet width			
Number of spotters			

CASE EXAMPLE

Designing a Resistance Training Program for a Young Multisport Athlete

BACKGROUND

You are a strength coach who is working with a 14-year-old male athlete who participates in multiple sports. He has been trained using weight machines for the past year. He wants to increase his sport-specific strength.

RECOMMENDATIONS/CONSIDERATIONS

After performing a needs analysis and on the basis of your client's potential, you decide to begin using free weights for squats and bench press. Free weights are chosen because of their increased specificity to sports.

IMPLEMENTATION

The free-weight squat and bench press are going to be implemented into the strength training program over a 10-week period.

Weeks 1 and 2. The first 2 weeks are used to introduce the free-weight exercises. Light weights are used and proper form is stressed. Half the sets performed will use the traditional machines and half will use the free-weight exercises.

Weeks 3 to 6. Once the athlete has learned proper form, moderate resistance can be used in weeks 3 to 6. Most of the sets are performed using free weights, but 1 to 2 sets a week may still be performed with machines.

Weeks 7 to 10. At this point the athlete should be comfortable with the free weights and be performing all of the sets with free weights using moderate resistance.

RESULTS

At the end of the 10-week period, the athlete was successfully incorporating the free-weight bench press and free-weight squat into his program. Testing after the program found the following results:

■ Increased body weight
■ No increase in percentage of body fat
■ Increased vertical jump
■ Increased push-ups in 1 minute

REFERENCES

1. Aaberg E. Resistance Training Instruction. Champaign, IL: Human Kinetics, 1999:35–48.
2. Baechle TR, Groves BR. Weight training: steps to success 2nd ed. Champaign, IL: Human Kinetics, 1998: 6–10.
3. Brooks GA, Fahey TD, White TP. Exercise Physiology: Human Bioenergetics and Its Applications. 2nd ed. Mountain View, CA: Mayfield, 1996.
4. Cissik JM. The Basics of Strength Training. New York: McGraw-Hill, 2001:17–21.
5. Fleck SR, Kraemer WJ. Designing Resistance Training Programs. 3rd ed. Champaign, IL: Human Kinetics, 2004.
6. Newton H. Explosive Lifting for Sports. Champaign, Il: Human Kinetics, 2002:49–51.
7. Nutter J. Physical activity increases bone density. NSCA J 1986;8:3;67–69.
8. Zatsiorsky VM. The Science and Practice of Strength Training. Champaign, IL: Human Kinetics, 1995.

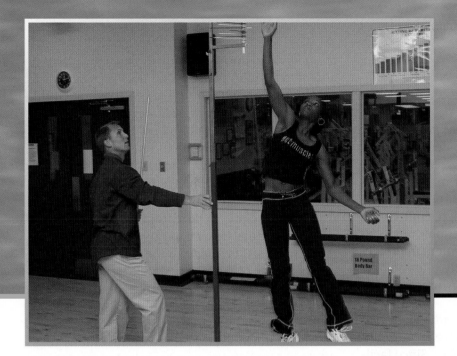

Facility Administration and Design

STEVEN PLISK

Introduction

The strength and conditioning profession involves the combined competencies of sport/exercise science, administration, management, teaching, and coaching. Practitioners must also comply with various laws and regulations. Collectively, this creates remarkable challenges in terms of facility administration and design, in turn requiring considerable experience, expertise, and resources. Practitioners and their employers are jointly responsible for addressing these challenges and, in turn, fulfilling the standard of care involved in providing safe and effective programs and services to athletes.

The major administrative issues include number of athletes and availability of competent coaches, equipment, space, and time (35). This chapter discusses these topics in the larger context of facilities and equipment, legal duties and concepts, liability exposure, and policies and procedures.

FACILITIES AND EQUIPMENT

Architects have an axiom: *Form follows function*—i.e., the design of a structure should be determined by its purpose. Although this concept seems straightforward enough, the reality is that many facilities were originally designed for another purpose. Furthermore, they often contain obsolete equipment. Even in state-of-the-art facilities, periodic upgrades may be desirable because the equipment manufacturing industry is dynamic, regularly offering new features and innovations based on practitioners' input.

Another axiom can be helpful: *Administer your programs in such a way that you would be proud to let a qualified visitor observe normal operations.* Since facility design and program administration are interrelated, this means that equipment content and arrangement should allow other practitioners with sound philosophies to implement their programs there without requiring significant changes. This concept also seems simple enough, but actually requires careful planning.

> *Administer your programs in such a way that you would be proud to let a qualified visitor observe your normal operations.*

Layout and Scheduling

The first step in planning and designing a new facility is to form a committee. This overall process can be subdivided into predesign, design, construction, and preoperation phases (21).

The practitioner should assess existing equipment based on the program needs of all athletic teams using the facility (21). This step should involve several issues, including number of athletes using the facility, specific types of training required by each group, age groups, and training experience (i.e., developmental needs) of athletes using the facility, when training fits into each team's schedule, as well as any repairs or adaptations that must be made to meet special needs.

The design of the facility should be considered in arranging existing equipment (21). Issues to consider include location, access, supervision location, ceiling height, flooring, environmental factors, electrical, mirrors, and other considerations (e.g., drinking fountains, rest rooms, telephones, signage, bulletin boards, storage, and repair areas).

In arranging equipment, safety is a key concern, along with the purpose and function of each individual piece (21). Issues to address include placement, spacing, and traffic flow. Figure 11.1 shows an example of a properly designed strength/power area. Specific concerns for particular areas (e.g., stretching/warm-up, circuit training, free weight, Olympic lifting, metabolic) should be considered in calculating space needs. For example (37):

■ For performing standing exercises from a rack, consider the bar length plus a double-wide (6-ft) safety space cushion, and multiply this by a suggested user space width of 8 to 10 ft [e.g., if using a 7-ft Olympic bar for

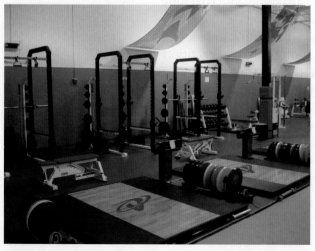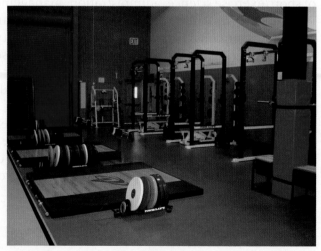

FIGURE 11.1 A strength/power area must be designed with regard to facility layout and arrangement as well as equipment safety and function.

the back squat exercise, (7 ft + 6 ft) × (10 ft) = 130 sq ft].

- For performing Olympic-style weightlifting exercises, consider the platform length plus a 4-ft perimeter walkway safety space and multiply this by the platform width plus another 4-ft perimeter walkway safety space [e.g., (8 ft + 4 ft) × (8 ft + 4 ft) = 144 sq ft].

In scheduling the facility, consider seasonal athletic priorities with regard to peak hours (specific recommendations are provided below under "Duties and Responsibilities: Liability Exposure"). Other issues to consider include staff-to-athlete ratios and equipment availability relative to group size.

Regardless of the training strategies used, a basic objective of facility design and layout is to optimize visibility and accessibility. In many cases, this must be achieved in spite of limited staff, high athlete volume, and time pressure. Depending on how various training methods and movements are prioritized, the challenge is to equip and arrange the facility for maximum capacity without compromising effectiveness, efficiency, or safety.

Although the specific content of each facility is a matter of discretion, some basic guidelines can be inferred from available evidence and practical experience. Practitioners should critically evaluate the pros and cons of various equipment choices rather than making decisions based on dogmatic beliefs about "free weights versus machines," "functional versus traditional training," and so on.

On one hand, training apparatus should be chosen according to transfer of training effect. This issue can be approached on several fronts, including mechanical specificity (also referred to as "dynamic correspondence"—i.e., the basic mechanics of training movements should be specific to the demands of competitive activity); metabolic effects (i.e., the influence of energy costs and endocrine responses on training adaptations); and coordination/skill acquisition. On the other hand, consideration should be given to practical issues, including the following:

- Versatility
- Coaching/teaching requirements (and corresponding staffing/spotting responsibilities)
- Safety
- Cost, space/time efficiency

In terms of strength/power training, the consensus emerging from the literature is that unguided-resistance equipment is superior in most regards, particularly when used with qualified instruction and supervision (43,45,57,59). There seem to be multiple reasons for this, which in turn provide useful criteria for selecting equipment. In general, the facility should be designed and equipped for a variety of training tasks consistent with the program's goals and objectives, enabling athletes to perform various multijoint, multiplane movements that challenge their coordinative abilities. Although certain stations are likely to get higher priority than others, most should be suitable for exercises where range of motion is an acceleration path involving high-power levels and rates of force development as well as different regimes of muscular work (concentric, eccentric, isometric, and stretch-shortening cycle where appropriate). Additional criteria are discussed below under "Duties and Responsibilities: Liability Exposure," but those outlined above can be used as a starting point in most settings.

Maintenance and Safety

The practitioner's primary responsibility is to provide a safe training environment for all athletes (20). Performance enhancement and injury prevention typically get high priority as well (20). Specialized activities and responsibilities can be delegated among staff members who, in turn, should work cooperatively as a team.

Practitioners have a responsibility to maintain and clean the facility and equipment (20). Establishing frequent maintenance and cleaning schedules—and keeping the required supplies, tools, and other items on hand—helps ensure safety, protect investments, and maintain appearance, cleanliness, and functionality.

Environmental factors are important for participants' health and safety. Some specific issues to consider include (20):

- Control of sound/video systems by the facility coordinator and qualified supervisors (e.g., volume low enough to allow clear communication between the spotter and lifter at all times)
- Air temperature kept constant at 72° to 78°F (22° to 26°C)
- Ventilation systems working properly (optimum 12 to 15 air exchanges/hr; minimum 8 to 10 air exchanges/hr); no detectable strong odors in the room

Q & A from the Field

I just accepted the position of strength and conditioning coordinator at a small university. The varsity weight room is filled with obsolete and nonfunctional equipment, and the budget is too small to afford all the items we'll need to reequip the facility this year. What should I do?

This is a common situation and can be a big challenge as well as an opportunity. Here are some suggestions:

Create a priority list of the equipment you plan to replace or upgrade. Be specific in terms of how many of each item you will need and how much they will cost, keeping in mind that many equipment vendors provide discount incentives for buying multiple pieces of equipment. Plan on upgrading in phases, being as objective as possible so your personal preferences don't influence your choices. Start with the "need to have" items, no matter how badly you want the "nice to have" ones. If it's ugly but functional, defer replacing it until later; for example, old/rusted barbells and plates may not be pretty but will be adequate temporarily. Spend the available money on high-priority equipment that cannot be donated or built on site.

Once you have compiled your upgrade plan, coordinate your efforts with your athletic director. Consider several issues here. Ask permission to approach local boosters or businesses for "gifts in kind." Most universities have a comprehensive incentive program for such donations, and many boosters are happy to exchange services and/or materials for tickets or other credits. The key is to be careful not to undermine your athletic director's fund-raising efforts—he or she may already be planning to approach some of the same people you have in mind. Many athletic directors set aside some

reserve budget money until late in the fiscal year in case there should be any unforeseen expenses. Ask him or her to consider directing some (or all) of that to the weight-room upgrade, being sure to emphasize how it can benefit every team's performance as well as recruiting!

If you have a particular vendor in mind for the majority of your upgrade, inquire about that company's computerized design capabilities. They may be able to offer floor plans, elevations, or other drawings that will help everyone involved in the project to visualize the end result.

Assuming that your athletic director gives his or her approval, approach the athletic department's fund-raising/development coordinator. Ask for referrals to specific boosters who can offer useful products or services—for example, building-supply centers that might donate lumber for platforms, welders who might fabricate equipment, etc. Do your homework before contacting them; boosters are usually gratified to know that you're giving them first consideration and have seen their advertisements in media guides, game-day programs, stadium signage, and so on.

One caveat: in recruiting the services of welders, carpenters, or other contractors, work with them to make sure that everything they build or modify meets industry specifications. If the equipment should fail at some point, the university will be liable for any resulting injuries or damages.

- Equipment and floor not slick due to humidity
- Facility well lighted and free of dark areas; bulbs changed regularly
- Exit sign well lit
- Extension cords large enough for electrical load; properly routed, secured, and grounded
- Safety, regulation, and policy signs posted in clear view

In keeping with these areas of responsibility, it is imperative to understand litigation issues (8,15, 22,23,28,37,49,51). In so doing, practitioners can effectively manage—but not totally eliminate—participants' risk of injury. It is also important to understand the concept of **product liability** [i.e., a manufacturer's and/or vendor's legal responsibilities if someone sustains injury or damage due

primarily to a defect or deficiency in design or production (8) as well as actions that can place one at risk for litigation.] These issues are discussed in detail in the following sections. Box 11.1 provides basic guidelines for planning and designing a new facility.

An important consideration relative to facility planning is to evaluating the needs of the athletes and teams who will be using the facility.

LEGAL DUTIES AND CONCEPTS

Practitioners and their employers share legal duties to provide an appropriate level of supervision and

11.1 FACILITIES AND EQUIPMENT

Form a committee of professionals to do the following:

■ Assess existing equipment based on the needs of all athletic teams using the facility.

■ Consider the design of the facility and arrange existing equipment. Safety and function are top priorities in determining equipment arrangement.

■ Consider seasonal athletic priorities, staff-to-athlete ratios, and equipment availability relative to group size.

■ Establish frequent maintenance and cleaning schedules to ensure safety, protect investments, and maintain the facility's appearance, cleanliness, and functionality.

instruction to do the following: meet a reasonable standard of care, provide and maintain a safe environment for athletes, inform users of the risks inherent in and related to their activities, and prevent unreasonable risk or harm resulting from negligent instruction or supervision (15,22,23,28). In fact, these legal duties and concepts define the organizational and administrative tasks of the profession.

> *The practitioner's primary responsibility is to provide a safe training environment for all athletes.*

A strength and conditioning professional should have an understanding of the following legal terms (21):

■ **Assumption of risk**. Voluntary participation in activity with knowledge of the inherent risk(s). Practitioners must thoroughly inform participants of the risks involved in athletic and conditioning activities. Ideally, athletes should be required to sign a statement indicating their understanding and acceptance of the risk.

■ **Liability**. A legal responsibility. Practitioners must take reasonable steps to ensure safe participation in conditioning activities, prevent injury, and act prudently when an injury occurs (8).

■ **Negligence**. Failure to exercise the care a prudent person would under similar circumstances. For a practitioner to be guilty of negligence, there must be duty, breach of duty, proximate cause, and damages (51). He or she is negligent if proven to have a duty to act

and to have failed to act with the appropriate standard of care, proximately causing injury or damages to another person.

■ **Standard of care**. What a prudent and reasonable person would do under similar circumstances. A practitioner is expected to act according to his or her education, training, and certification status.

> *Practitioners and their employers share a legal duty to provide an appropriate level of supervision and instruction.*

Types of Standards

In addition to standards for desired operational practices published by professional organizations such as the National Strength and Conditioning Association (NSCA), standards for technical/physical specifications have been published by independent organizations. In a negligence lawsuit, established standards of care can be used to gauge a practitioner's professional competence by comparing his or her actual conduct with written benchmarks of expected behavior. In addition to standards and guidelines established by allied organizations such as the American College of Sports Medicine (ACSM) (7,60), American Heart Association (AHA) (7,40), and National Athletic Trainers Association (NATA) (44), other associations have also delineated standards of practice (Aerobics and Fitness Association of America, American Physical Therapy Association, National Association for Sport and Physical Education). Moreover, relevant technical/physical specifications have been published by the U.S. Consumer Product Safety Commission (e.g., "Prevent Injuries to Children from Exercise Equipment"; CPSC Document #5028) and the American Society for Testing and Materials (2,3).

Applying Standards of Practice to Risk Management

Risk management is a proactive administrative process that helps minimize legal liability and also minimizes the frequency and severity of injuries and subsequent claims and lawsuits (14,15). It may not be possible to eliminate risk of injury and liability exposure, but these can be effectively minimized with risk-management strategies. Although the coordinator is ultimately responsible for risk management, all practitioners should be involved in various aspects of the process. Eickhoff-Shemek (16) proposes a four-step procedure [adapted from Head and Horn (25)] for applying standards of practice to the risk management process:

1. *Identify and select standards of practice as well as all applicable laws.* Because so many standards of practice are published by various organizations, it is challenging for the practitioner to be aware of all of them and to determine which ones are appropriate in implementing the risk-management plan. In terms of participant safety, the most conservative or stringent standards in a given industry should generally be used.
2. *Develop risk-management strategies reflecting standards of practice and all applicable laws.* This step involves writing procedures describing specific responsibilities and/or duties that staff would carry out in particular situations. The procedures should be written clearly, succinctly, and without excessive detail. Once the written procedures are finalized, they should be included in the staff policies and procedures manual.
3. *Implement the risk-management plan.* Implementation of the risk-management plan primarily involves staff training to ensure that the practitioner's daily conduct will be consistent with written policies and procedures and selected laws and standards of practice. The policies-and-procedures manual should be used in conjunction with initial training of new employees as well as during regular in-service training where all employees practice a particular procedure. From a legal perspective, it is also important to explain to

staff why it is essential to carry out such duties appropriately.
4. *Evaluate the risk-management plan.* Like the law, standards of practice are not static and need to be updated periodically to reflect change. The risk-management plan should be formally evaluated at least annually as well as after each incident of accident or injury to determine whether emergency procedures were performed correctly and what could be done to prevent a similar incident in the future.

> *Application of standards of practice to the risk-management process involves a four-step process: first, identify and select standards of practice as well as all applicable laws; second, develop risk-management strategies reflecting standards of practice and all applicable laws; third, implement the risk-management plan; and fourth, evaluate the risk-management plan.*

DUTIES AND RESPONSIBILITIES: LIABILITY EXPOSURE

Although every program and facility is unique, it is instructive to examine the practitioner's duties and responsibilities in terms of common areas of liability exposure (49). These are interrelated—for example, proper instruction and supervision are associated with personnel qualifications as well as facility layout and scheduling. Noncompliance in one area can affect others, thereby compounding

---

 REAL-WORLD APPLICATION

Policies and Procedures

Here is a sample policy for a strength and conditioning facility: "*Work with an attentive spotter—and use appropriate safety equipment (e.g., power racks)—for performing movements where free weights are supported on the trunk or moved over the head/face. Olympic lifts are an exception to the spotter rule and should be performed on an 8-ft by 8-ft platform that is clear of people and equipment.*"

Remember that when you write a policy, you have to think about how it can be enforced. To carry out this policy and to make sure it is enforced, several steps should be taken: (1) The staff must be trained on what is expected of them both in

terms of teaching spotting and dealing with athletes who fail to use a spotter. (2) The athletes must be trained in spotting, what lifts need a spotter, and the number of spotters needed. It is a necessity to train incoming athletes as they enter the program, and you may find that it is necessary to reinforce this training each year. (3) Decide in advance on the consequences for not following the policy. Be fair, but if you let some break the policy and not others, consider the legal implications if the athlete who has not followed the policy is injured.

Appendix B contains a sample policies-and-procedures document for a strength and conditioning facility.

the risk of negligence and potential litigation. Practitioners and their employers share the corresponding duties and responsibilities.

The NSCA's *Strength and Conditioning Professional Standards and Guidelines* (49) identifies nine areas of liability exposure: preparticipation screening and clearance; personnel qualifications; program supervision and instruction; facility and equipment setup, inspection, maintenance, repair, and signage; emergency planning and response; records and record keeping; equal opportunity and access; participation by children; and supplements, ergogenic aids, and drugs. Within these areas of liability exposure, a total of 11 standards ("must dos") and 13 guidelines ("should dos") are proposed (see Appendix C). These further define the tasks involved in facility organization and administration.

Preparticipation Screening and Clearance

A physical examination (preferably conducted by a licensed physician) is imperative for all athletes prior to participating in a program. This should include a comprehensive health and immunization history (as defined by current guidelines from the Centers for Disease Control and Prevention) as well as relevant physical exam, including an orthopedic evaluation. Cardiovascular screening, as discussed below, is also recommended. The practitioner does not need a copy of the results but must require a signed statement verifying proof of medical clearance to participate. Athletes who are returning from an injury or illness or have special needs must be required to show proof of medical clearance prior to beginning or returning to participation.

Currently, no universally accepted standards are available for screening athletes, nor are there approved certification procedures for health care professionals who perform such examinations. The joint Preparticipation Physical Evaluation Task Force of five organizations has published a widely accepted monograph, however, including detailed instructions on performing a preparticipation history and physical exam, determining clearance for participation, and a medical evaluation form to copy and use for each examination (50). The American Heart Association and American College of Sports Medicine have also published statements on preparticipation screening for those involved in fitness-related activities (7,40,41). Relevant issues can be summarized as follows:

Educational institutions have ethical, medical, and possible legal obligations to implement cost-efficient preparticipation screening strategies (including a complete medical history and physical examination), thereby ensuring that high school and college athletes are not subject to unacceptable risks. Support for such efforts—especially in large athletic populations—is mitigated by cost-efficiency considerations, practical limitations, and awareness that it is not possible to achieve zero risk in competitive sports.

A properly qualified health care provider (with requisite training, medical skills, and background to reliably perform a physical examination, obtain a detailed cardiovascular history, and recognize heart disease) should perform the preparticipation athletic screening. A licensed physician is preferable, but an appropriately trained registered nurse or physician assistant may be acceptable under certain circumstances in states where nonphysician health care workers are permitted to perform preparticipation screening. In the latter situation, a formal certification process should be established to demonstrate the examiner's expertise in performing cardiovascular examinations.

The best available and most practical approach to screening populations of competitive sports participants is a complete and careful personal and family medical history and physical examination designed to identify (or raise suspicion of) cardiovascular risk factors known to cause sudden death or disease progression. Such screening is an obtainable objective and should be mandatory for all athletes. Initially, a complete medical history and physical examination should be performed before participation in organized high school athletics (grades 9 to 12). An interim history should be obtained in intervening years. For collegiate athletes, a comprehensive personal/family history and physical examination should be performed by a qualified examiner initially upon entering the institution, before beginning training and competition. Screening should be repeated every 2 years thereafter unless more frequent examinations are indicated; an interim history and blood pressure measurement should be obtained each subsequent year to determine whether another physical examination, and possible further testing, is required (e.g., due to abnormalities or changes in medical status).

To initially classify participants by risk for triage and preliminary decision making, health appraisal questionnaires should be used before exercise testing and/or training. Participants can be further classified for exercise training on the basis of individual characteristics after the initial health appraisal (and medical consultation and/or supervised exercise test if indicated). Written and active communication between facility staff and the participant's personal physician or health care provider is strongly recommended when a medical evaluation/recommendation is advised or required. Participants should also be educated about the importance of the preparticipation health appraisal and medical evaluation/recommendation (if indicated) as well as potential risks incurred without them.

Personnel Qualifications

To properly supervise and instruct athletes utilizing facilities and equipment, qualified and knowledgeable personnel must be hired. A three-pronged approach is recommended:

1. *The practitioner should acquire expertise—and have a degree from a regionally accredited college/ university—in one or more of the topics comprising the "scientific foundations" domain identified in the Certified Strength and Conditioning Specialist (CSCS) Examination Content Description (46) or a relevant subject.* He or she should also make an ongoing effort to acquire knowledge and competence in the content areas outside his or her primary area of expertise.
2. *Professional organizations offer certifications with continuing education requirements as well as a code of ethics for practitioners interested in acquiring the necessary competencies.* Depending on one's specific duties, responsibilities, and interests, relevant certifications offered by other governing bodies may also be appropriate.
3. *The "performance team" model—i.e., aligning a staff composed of qualified professionals with interdependent expertise and shared leadership roles—can enhance practitioners' knowledge and skill development (see Appendix D)* (33,34). The profession's scope of practice has expanded and diversified to the point where it is very challenging—and often not possible—for one individual to acquire proficiency in all areas. The team model can also improve a hierarchical (single-leader) work group's productivity as well as each individual's learning and skill acquisition (33).

It is difficult to overemphasize the importance of qualified staffing in fulfilling the institution's and practitioner's shared legal duties for safety, supervision, and standard of care. Lack of qualified instruction and supervision can be identified—either directly or indirectly—as a causative factor in the available information on injuries and litigations associated with weight training. In some cases this is clearly documented (31,53,54), while in others it can be inferred. For example, despite the technical and athletic nature of Olympic-style weightlifting, the relatively high coach-to-athlete ratio and corresponding standard of care are likely reasons for its low incidence of injury (24,56).

Program Supervision and Instruction

About 80% of all court cases concerning athletic injuries deal with some aspect of supervision (8). Although serious accidents are rare in supervised exercise programs, the liability costs associated with inadequate or lax supervision are high; plaintiffs' recovery rate in such negligence lawsuits is almost 56% (42). Poor facility maintenance, defective equipment, and inadequate instruction or supervision are the main causes of these incidents. The importance of staffing is readily apparent in each circumstance. For example, in a review of 32 litigations arising from negligent weight-training supervision, three issues were raised by the plaintiff's attorneys in each case (52): poor instruction or instructor qualifications; lax/poor supervision; and failure to warn of inherent dangers in the equipment, facility, or exercise. The issue of professional instructors' qualifications, as discussed in the previous section, is a prevalent trend in such litigations.

Athletes must be properly supervised and instructed at all times to ensure maximum safety. Bucher and Krotee (9) recommend the following principles:

- Always be there.
- Be active and hands-on.
- Be prudent, careful, and prepared.
- Be qualified.
- Be vigilant.
- Inform athletes of safety and emergency procedures.
- Know athletes' health status.
- Monitor and enforce rules and regulations.
- Monitor and scrutinize the environment.

In addition to the physical presence of qualified practitioners, effective instruction and supervision involves several practical considerations (5,11,26, 28,42):

- A clear view of all areas of the facility—or at least the zone being supervised by each practitioner—and the athletes in it (this issue is related to facility design and layout; i.e., equipment placement with respect to visibility, versatility, and accessibility)
- A practitioner's proximity to the group of athletes under his or her care; i.e., the ability to see and communicate clearly with one another and quick access to athletes in need of immediate assistance or spotting
- Number and grouping of athletes; i.e., to make optimal use of available equipment, space, and time
- Athletes' age(s), experience level(s), and need(s)
- The type of program being conducted (i.e., skillful/explosive free-weight movements versus guided-resistance exercises) and corresponding need for coaching and spotting

In theory, practitioners should promote an optimal training environment by distributing activities throughout the day. Even with careful planning, however, most facilities have times of peak usage (e.g., as a result of team practices and athletes' class schedules). Beyond a certain point, it is impractical to simply schedule activities over a wider range of times in order to maintain an acceptable professional-to-athlete ratio. The central issue is to provide adequate facilities and qualified staff such that all athletes are properly instructed and supervised during peak usage times (30,39,60). Likewise, practitioners should emphasize proper techniques, movement mechanics, and safety—and utilize instructional methods, procedures, and progressions consistent with accepted professional practices—to minimize injury risk and liability exposure.

Even when reasonable steps are taken to make optimal use of facility and staff, a potential mismatch exists between available resources and demand for programs and services in many settings. The combined effects of explosive growth in collegiate/scholastic athlete participation (especially among females), corresponding liability exposures, and equal opportunity/access laws create a remarkable standard-of-care load and

liability challenge for practitioners and their employers. A two-pronged approach can thus be recommended:

1. *During peak usage times, activities should be planned—and required number of qualified staff should be present—such that recommended guidelines for minimum average floor space allowance per athlete (100 ft²)*, professional-to-athlete ratios (1:10 junior high school, 1:15 high school, 1:20 college), and number of athletes per barbell or training station (≤ 3) are achieved (5,30,32,37). Ideally, this corresponds to one practitioner per three to four training stations and/or 1,000 ft² area (junior high school); five training stations and/or 1,500 ft² area (high school); or six to seven training stations and/or 2,000 ft² area (college), respectively. Professional discretion can be used to adjust these guidelines with respect to the practical considerations discussed above.

2. *Practitioners and their employers should work together toward a long-term goal of matching the professional-to-athlete ratio in the facility to each sport's respective coach-to-athlete ratio.* This is relatively straightforward in collegiate settings, where the NCAA limits the number of coaches per sport and compiles sports participation data. In the absence of similar information in other settings, such determinations can be made on an individual-institution basis (or possibly according to trends within a district, division, or state).

Facility and Equipment Setup, Inspection, Maintenance, Repair, and Signage

In some cases, practitioners are involved in all phases of facility design and layout. Perhaps more commonly, they assume responsibility for an existing facility, in which case the opportunities to plan or modify it may be limited. In either case, the practitioner and his or her employer are jointly responsible for maximizing the facility's safety, effectiveness, and efficiency such that allotted space and time can be put to optimal use.

Practitioners should establish written policies and procedures for equipment/facility selection, purchase, installation, setup, inspection, maintenance, and repair. These should be included in the overall policies-and-procedures manual (as discussed in the next section). Safety audits and periodic inspections of equipment, maintenance, and repair should be conducted and status reports issued. Manufacturer-provided user's manuals, warranties, operating guides, and other relevant records regarding equipment operation and maintenance (e.g., selection, purchase, installation, setup, inspection, maintenance, and repair) should be kept on file and followed (9).

As mentioned previously, practitioners must understand the concept of **product liability**—i.e., a manufacturer's and/or vendor's legal responsibilities if someone sustains injury or damage due primarily to a defect or deficiency in design or production (6). Although this issue applies to manufacturers and vendors, certain actions and/or behaviors can increase the practitioner's responsibility, consequently putting him or her at risk for claims or lawsuits. The following steps can minimize equipment-related liability exposure (8,9,36):

- Buy equipment exclusively from reputable manufacturers and be certain that it meets existing standards and guidelines for professional/commercial (not home) use.
- Use equipment only for the purpose intended by the manufacturer; do not modify it from the condition in which it was originally sold unless such adaptations are clearly designated and instructions for doing so are included in the product information.
- Post any signage provided by the manufacturer on or in close proximity to the equipment.
- Do not allow unsupervised athletes to utilize equipment.
- Regularly inspect equipment for damage and wear that may place athletes at risk for injury.

Emergency Planning and Response

An emergency response plan is a written document delineating the proper procedures of caring for injuries that may occur to participants during activity (see Appendix E). All facilities should have such a document, but the document itself does not save lives. In fact, it may offer a false sense of security if not supported with appropriate training and preparedness by astute, professional staff. Therefore, practitioners must:

- Know the emergency response plan and the proper procedures for dealing with an emergency (i.e., location of phones, activating emergency medical services, designated personnel to care for injuries, ambulance access, and location of emergency supplies) (4,55).
- Regularly review and practice emergency policies and procedures (i.e., at least quarterly).
- Maintain current certification in guidelines for cardiopulmonary resuscitation (CPR) (1). First aid training and certification may also be necessary if sports medicine personnel [e.g., certified athletic trainer (ATC), physician] are not immediately available.
- Adhere to universal precautions for preventing exposure to and transmission of bloodborne pathogens (10,47).

Records and Record Keeping

Documentation is fundamental to program and facility management. A variety of records should be kept on file (9,13,17,29).

- Policies-and-procedures manual (as discussed in the next section).
- Manufacturer-provided user's manuals, warranties, and operating guides as well as equipment selection, purchase, installation, setup, inspection, maintenance, and repair records.
- Personnel credentials.
- Professional standards and guidelines (see Appendix C).
- Safety policies and procedures, including a written emergency response plan (see Appendix E).
- Training logs, progress entries, and/or activity instruction/supervision notes.
- Injury/incident reports, preparticipation medical clearance, and return to participation clearance documents (after the occurrence of an injury, illness, change in health status or an extended period of absence) for each participant under the practitioner's care.
- In collegiate and scholastic settings, athletes may already be required to sign protective legal documents (e.g., informed consent, agreement to participate, waiver; Appendix F) covering all athletically related activities; whereas in other settings, the practitioner should consider having participants sign such legal documents.

Legal and medical records should be kept on file as long as possible in the event of an injury claim or lawsuit. It is good practice to maintain files indefinitely or consult with a legal authority, because statutes of limitations vary from state to state (29). As is the case with other organizational and administrative tasks, adequate staff are necessary to properly keep and maintain such records.

Equal Opportunity and Access

In most organizations, institutions, and professions, discrimination or unequal treatment (e.g., according to race, creed, national origin, gender, religion, age, handicap/disability, or other such legal classifications) are prohibited by federal, state, and possibly local laws and regulations. For example, practitioners employed in federally funded educational settings must comply with civil rights statutes, including Title IX of the Education Amendments of 1972, which mandates gender equity in providing opportunity and access to athletic facilities, programs, and services. Practitioners must obey the letter and spirit of these laws when working with athletes and staff.

Participation in Strength and Conditioning Activities by Children

Resistance training can be an important component of youth fitness, health promotion, and injury prevention. When properly designed and supervised, such programs are safe and can increase children's strength, motor fitness skills, sports performance, psychosocial well-being, and overall health (18,19). Many of the benefits associated with adult activities are attainable by prepubescent and adolescent athletes who participate in age-specific training, but it is important for the practitioner to take certain precautions.

An alarming incidence of injuries to young children was observed in a 20-year retrospective review of weight-training injuries evaluated and/or treated in U.S. hospital emergency departments (31). Children under 7 years of age are almost six times more likely to be injured than those above 15 years of age, with most of such injuries (80%) resulting from playing with or around weight-training equipment in the home. According to the U.S. Consumer Product Safety Commission ("Prevent Injuries to Children from Exercise Equipment"; CPSC document #5028), about 8,700 children below 5 years of age are injured each year with exercise equipment, with an additional 16,500 injuries per year to children 5 to 14 years of age. This has clear implications regarding exposing children in these age groups to such equipment or facilities and the importance of supervision.

Supplements, Ergogenic Aids, and Drugs

The issue of nutritional supplement and drug use is complicated by several factors. According to the Dietary Supplement Health and Education Act of 1994, supplements are regulated as foods rather than drugs. This raises concerns about quality control/assurance and possible consequences for consumers.

Practitioners are often approached for advice on nutrition and supplementation and should be aware of the following: The Federal Trade Commission has primary responsibility for advertising claims. Simply stated, advertising for any product—including dietary supplements—must be truthful, substantiated, and not misleading. The U.S. Food and Drug Administration has primary responsibility for product labeling claims. The legislation enforced by this agency includes "Current Good Manufacturing Practices" and selected portions of the Federal Food, Drug and Cosmetic Act related to dietary supplements. Manufacturing practices for nutritional supplements established by the U.S. Pharmacopeia and National Formulary are cited as primary resources in this legislation.

The boundaries between dietary supplements, drugs, and conventional foods are not clear. This is especially challenging for competitive athletes and coaches, because such products may contain substances that are banned by one or more sport governing bodies, despite a manufacturer's or vendor's use of terms such as *herbal, legal, natural, organic, safe and effective,* and so on. Furthermore, supplement manufacturers are constantly developing new products with different combinations of ingredients, making it more challenging to identify those that may be problematic.

Banned-substance policies and procedures, testing protocols, and related rules and regulations differ among sport governing bodies. A compound that is legal according to one governing body may, therefore, be illegal according to another.

Standards and guidelines can be identified across nine areas of liability exposure: preparticipation screening and clearance; personnel qualifications; program supervision and instruction; facility and equipment setup, inspection, maintenance, repair, and signage; emergency planning and response; records and record keeping; equal opportunity and access; participation by children; and supplements, ergogenic aids and drugs.

POLICIES AND PROCEDURES

Strength and conditioning professionals must develop policies and procedures that allow them to provide safe and effective programs and services and to fulfill their standard of care for athletes. This requires a working understanding of facility and equipment considerations, legal concepts, and duties and responsibilities dictated by liability exposures, as described in previous sections.

It is important that the program have a well-defined mission along with identifiable goals and objectives (17). Safety, performance enhancement, and injury prevention are fundamental goals. These should be complemented with specific objectives as part of a holistic mission statement.

Clearly define and distinguish job titles, descriptions, and duties for various positions (17). These should be developed for the director, associate(s) and/or assistant(s), facility supervisor(s), and other staff members including interns, administrative assistants, and so on.

Understand pertinent staff policies and activities involved in achieving mission—that is, the goals and the specific objectives of the program (17). Staff members should be accountable for maintaining a professional code of conduct and working cooperatively as a team. This involves a wide range of issues—e.g., staff meetings, athlete orientation, annual planning, budgeting, staff facility use, relationships with athletes and other staff, professional goals, posted information, visitor tours, coaching and spotting procedures, testing, record keeping, athlete incentives, etc.

Understand the administrative decisions involved in the implementation of any strength and conditioning program to ensure safety and effectiveness (17). These issues are interdependent, as discussed throughout this chapter.

A written policies-and-procedures manual is essential to implementing a safe and effective program (17). In addition to the issues itemized above, the manual should address facility access, daily operation, telephone/music system use, rules and regulations, and emergency procedures as well as equipment/facility selection, purchase, installation, setup, inspection, and maintenance, and repair. This type of documentation may seem mundane, but is fundamental to managing programs or facilities involved in serving people.

Policies and procedures should be clearly delineated to all staff and athletes using the facility. They need not be rigid or static. On the contrary, they should be compiled with insight and discretion and revised periodically as circumstances dictate. Box 11.2 provides basic guidelines for writing policies and procedures.

Sound policies and procedures should be developed to ensure the safety of the athlete and guide administrative decisions.

SUMMARY

The issues of facility administration and design are fundamentally important in all aspects of strength and conditioning practice. Unfortunately, they often involve tasks in which the practitioner has little formal training.

Ample resources are available in some settings. In many others, however, they are not. Budgets,

---

REAL-WORLD APPLICATION
Mission Statement

Here is an example of a mission statement for a strength and conditioning program: "The strength and conditioning program will empower athletes and coaches to optimize their capabilities—and thereby achieve excellence—through learning and applying fundamentally sound principles."

Notice that it is broad, so it must be accompanied by goals and objectives to help professionals adhere to the mission statement. Mission statements will be different in different institutions and should be a product of the core beliefs of the administration and staff. From time to time, the mission statement should be reevaluated to make sure that it still reflects the core beliefs of the program.

Appendix A contains this mission statement and sample goals and objectives that support it.

11.2 GUIDELINES FOR POLICIES AND PROCEDURES

- Safety, performance enhancement, and injury prevention are fundamental goals in developing and clarifying the program's mission, goals, and objectives.
- Job titles, descriptions, and duties should be clearly defined and distinguished for respective positions.
- Practitioners should be accountable for maintaining a professional code of conduct and working cooperatively as a team.
- Understand the administrative decisions involved in safe and effective program implementation.
- Create a policies-and-procedures manual.

equipment, facilities, and staff are often limited or lacking altogether. This results in a mismatch between demand for—and provision of—safe and effective programs and services. Professionals and their employers share a legal duty to fulfill their standard of care for athletes. The individual practitioner is not solely responsible for fulfilling it (unless he or she is self-employed); the individual and his or her employer are jointly responsible for doing so.

The NSCA's *Strength and Conditioning Professional Standards and Guidelines* document is one of the main resources cited in this chapter. Its implementation will present significant challenges and involve ambitious changes in many programs. Resistance can probably be expected from some athletic directors/employers because it will prompt them to allocate more resources to their programs. Nonetheless, the employing institution or business has a legal responsibility to help practitioners provide or obtain the resources needed to fulfill their standard of care.

MAXING OUT

1. You are the strength and conditioning coordinator at a college program; a team coach approaches you with a program obtained from another university, asking you to implement it with her team in place of the one you have offered. Develop and explain your policy regarding such workouts, including how it will affect the team's programming and scheduling privileges in the varsity weight room.

2. You are the strength and conditioning coordinator at a college program, and your athletic director is expressing concern that the facility looks like a "football weight room" equipped with too many free weights. He feels that this is causing several problems (compromising the programs and services provided to other teams, discouraging other teams' recruits from attending the school, and placing the university at risk of a Title IX lawsuit). You are subsequently directed to put together a proposal on how to reequip the weight room with more machines and fewer free weights to make it more accommodating for all sports. Develop and explain your policy regarding equipment selection with respect to performance enhancement and injury prevention.

CASE EXAMPLE

Program Scheduling, Supervision, and Instruction

BACKGROUND

You coordinate a collegiate strength and conditioning program that is responsible for programming and servicing a total of 362 student-athletes in 16 sports:

SPORT	SQUAD SIZE (MEN)	SQUAD SIZE (WOMEN)
Baseball	31	—
Basketball	16	14
Cross country	13	13
Football	96	—
Golf	10	8
Soccer	26	23
Softball	—	18
Tennis	10	10
Track & field	32	28
Volleyball	—	14
Total athletes	234	128

(continued)

Including yourself, you have a three-person staff and 6,000 ft² weight room equipped with eight Olympic lifting platforms, eight self-contained power stations, four plyometric stations, and various (secondary) equipment. It is the first week of September; fall sport athletes have completed preseason camp and classes have begun. Your task is to schedule team workouts for the first 6 weeks of the fall semester such that in-season sports (cross country, football, soccer, volleyball) train 2 days per week, whereas off-season sports train 3 days per week. Your programs involve periodized multiset free-weight training, including explosive movements.

RECOMMENDATIONS AND CONSIDERATIONS

Begin by surveying team coaches regarding which days they prefer to train and whether their team is available in the morning (e.g., before 8 a.m.) or afternoon (usually after 3 p.m.). Make it clear to everyone in advance that in-season sports have scheduling priority in the weight room because their schedules are less flexible due to practices/meetings and games. Fall sport teams often compete twice weekly (e.g., Wednesdays and Saturdays), further limiting the number of days they're available to train.

The advantage of morning training sessions is that they reduce the demand for weight-room time during peak (afternoon) hours. The disadvantages are that they can conflict with athletes' sleep and/or meals and lengthen the staff's workday. The latter problem can be alleviated to an extent by allowing flex time for those staff working the early shift (e.g., leaving work after morning sessions are completed and returning in the afternoon).

Certain team coaches may allow some or all of their athletes to train during off-peak times individually or in small groups (e.g., between 8 a.m. and 3 p.m.; likewise, in any given week, there may be athletes on various teams who have academic commitments during their team workouts and need to use this option). Once

again, this reduces demand on the weight room during peak hours. And, of course, some coaches have no use for strength and conditioning programs and services at all, thus reducing the demand further.

Some coaches may also be willing to train varsity and junior varsity athletes on different schedules. This can be extremely useful with large teams in sports such as football.

Finally, it is helpful to recruit qualified interns to assist with program implementation, especially during busy times.

IMPLEMENTATION

With a 6,000-ft² facility and three-person staff, there may be opportunities to schedule two or three teams concurrently during peak usage times. With smaller teams, it may be feasible to start two sessions simultaneously; in larger-group situations, it may be advisable to stagger their starting times every 20 to 30 minutes. Since most of these sports have common demands in terms of total-body power and rate of force development (RFD) and can benefit from the same exercises/equipment, it is helpful to designate specific training stations for each group to minimize congestion. In any case, workouts should be planned to comply with the following recommended guidelines:

- 100-ft² average floor space allowance per athlete = maximum capacity of 60 athletes
- 1:20 professional-to-athlete ratio = up to three-group capacity, with each practitioner supervising one group and up to 6 or 7 training stations (or 2,000-ft² area)
- ≤ 3 athletes per barbell or training station = equipment capacity of 60 athletes (if distributed between platforms, power stations, and plyometric stations)

RESULTS

Here is an example schedule (**boldface** indicates in-season teams; shaded blocks are filled to capacity):

(continued)

DAY *Time*	MON	TUE	WED	THURS	FRI
7:00 am	**M. Soccer (26)** **W. Soccer (23)**			**M. Soccer (26)** **W. Soccer (23)**	M. Basketball (16) Softball (18) W. Tennis (10)
8:00	**V. Football (10)**	**J.V. Football (10)**	**V. Football (10)**	**J.V. Football (10)**	**J.V. Football (10)**
9:00	**V. Football (10)**	**J.V. Football (10)**	**V. Football (10)**	**J.V. Football (10)**	**J.V. Football (10)**
10:00	**V. Football (10)** M. Golf (3)	**J.V. Football (10)**	**V. Football (10)**	**J.V. Football (10)**	**J.V. Football (10)**
11:00	**V. Football (10)**	**J.V. Football (10)**	**V. Football (10)**	**J.V. Football (10)**	**J.V. Football (10)**
Noon	closed	closed	closed	closed	closed
1:00 p.m.	**V. Football (10)** M. Golf (5)	**J.V. Football (10)**	**V. Football (10)**	**J.V. Football (10)**	**J.V. Football (10)**
2:00	2:45 W. Basketball (14)		2:45 W. Basketball (14)		W. Basketball (14) 2:30 W. Golf (8)
3:00	3:30 Baseball (31)	W. Tennis (10)	3:30 Baseball (31)	M. Golf (10)	3:30 Baseball (31)
4:00	Softball (18)		Softball (18)		
5:00	Track and Field (60)	**M. X-Country (13)** **W. X-Country (13)**	Track and Field (60)	**M. X-Country (13)** **W. X-Country (13)**	Track and Field (60)
6:00	M. Basketball (16) **Volleyball (14)**	W. Golf (8) M. Tennis (10)	M. Basketball (16) **Volleyball (14)**	M. Tennis (10)	

Keep in mind that each time the fall, winter, or spring sports' in-season phases begin or end, you get to do it all over again. This means that you get to design six different versions of the schedule every academic year!

The author wishes to thank Tom Baechle, Mike Barnes, Roger Earle, Mike Greenwood, and Bob Jursnick.

REFERENCES

1. American Heart Association in collaboration with the International Liaison Committee on Resuscitation. Guidelines 2000 for cardiopulmonary resuscitation and emergency cardiovascular care: international consensus on science. Circulation 2000;102(Suppl 8).

2. American Society for Testing and Materials. ASTM Standard Consumer Safety Specification for Stationary Exer-cise Bicycles: Designation F1250-89. West Conshohocken, PA: ASTM, 1989.

3. American Society for Testing and Materials. ASTM Standard Specification for Fitness Equipment and Fitness Facility Safety Signage and Labels: Designation F1749-96. West Conshohocken, PA: ASTM, 1996.

4. Anderson JC, Courson RW, Kleiner DM, McLoda TA. National Athletic Trainers' Association Position Statement:

Emergency Planning in Athletics. J Athlet Training 2002; 37(1):99–104.

5. Armitage-Johnson S. Providing a safe training environment: part I. Strength Cond 1994;16(1):64–65.

6. Armitage-Johnson S. Providing a safe training environment: part II. Strength Cond 1994;16(2):34.

7. Balady GJ, Chaitman B, Driscoll D, et al. American Heart Association and American College of Sports Medicine. Recommendations for cardiovascular screening, staffing and emergency policies at health/fitness facilities. Circulation 1998;97(22):2283–2293; Med Sci Sports Exerc 1998; 30(6):1009–1018.

8. Baley JA, Matthews DL. Law and Liability in Athletics, Physical Education and Recreation. Boston: Allyn & Bacon, 1984.

9. Bucher CA, Krotee ML. Management of Physical Education and Sport. 11th ed. New York: McGraw-Hill, 1998.

10. Centers for Disease Control and Prevention/U.S. Department of Health and Human Services. Perspectives in disease prevention and health promotion update: universal precautions for prevention of transmission of human immunodeficiency virus, hepatitis B virus, and other bloodborne pathogens in health-care settings. MMWR 1988;37(24):377–388.

11. Clark M et al. Position Paper on the College Strength and Conditioning Professional. Colorado Springs CO: National Strength and Conditioning Association, 1998.

12. Coalition of Americans to Protect Sports. Sports Injury Risk Management. 2nd ed. North Palm Beach, FL: CAPS, 1998.

13. Cotten DJ, Cotten MB. Legal Aspects of Waivers in Sport, Recreation and Fitness Activities. Canton, OH: PRC Publishing, 1997.

14. Eickhoff-Shemek J. Distinguishing protective legal documents. ACSM Health Fit J 2001;5(3):27–29.

15. Eickhoff-Shemek J. Standards of practice. In: Cotten D, Wilde J, Wlohan J, eds. Law for Recreation and Sport Managers. 2nd ed. Dubuque, IA: Kendall/Hunt Publishing, 2001:293–302.

16. Eickhoff-Shemek J, Deja K. Four steps to minimize legal liability in exercise programs. ACSM Health Fit J 2000; 4(4):3–18.

17. Epley B. Developing a policies and procedures manual. In: Baechle TR, Earle RW, eds. National Strength and Conditioning Association. Essentials of Strength Training and Conditioning. 2nd ed. Champaign, IL: Human Kinetics, 2000:567–585.

18. Faigenbaum AD, Kraemer WJ, et al. National Strength and Conditioning Association. Youth resistance training: position statement paper and literature review. Strength Cond 1996;18(6):62–75.

19. Faigenbaum AD, Micheli LJ. Current Comment from the American College of Sports Medicine: Youth Strength Training. Indianapolis, IN: American College of Sports Medicine, 1998.

20. Greenwood M. Facility layout and scheduling. In: Baechle TR, Earle RW, eds. National Strength and Conditioning Association. Essentials of Strength Training and Conditioning. 2nd ed. Champaign, IL: Human Kinetics, 2000:549–566.

21. Greenwood M, Greenwood L. Facility maintenance and risk management. In: Baechle TR, Earle RW, eds.

National Strength and Conditioning Association. Essentials of Strength Training and Conditioning. 2nd ed. Champaign, IL: Human Kinetics, 2000:587–601.

22. Halling DH. Liability considerations of the strength and conditioning specialist. NSCA J 1990;12(5):57–60.

23. Halling DH. Legal terminology for the strength and conditioning specialist. NSCA J 1991;13(4):59–61.

24. Hamill BP. Relative safety of weightlifting and weight training. J Strength Cond Res 1994;8(1):53–57.

25. Head GL, Horn S. Essentials of Risk Management, vol I. 3rd ed. Malvern, PA: Insurance Institute of America, 1995.

26. Herbert DL, Herbert WG. Legal Aspects of Preventive, Rehabilitative and Recreational Exercise Programs. 3rd ed. Canton, OH: PRC Publishing, 1993.

27. Herbert D. L. Legal aspects of strength and conditioning. NSCA J 1993;15(4):79.

28. Herbert DL. Supervision for strength and conditioning activities. Strength Cond 1994;16(2):32–33.

29. Herbert DL. A good reason for keeping records. Strength Cond 1994;16(3):64.

30. Hillmann A, Pearson DR. Supervision: the key to strength training success. Strength Cond 1995;17(5):67–71.

31. Jones CS, Christensen C, Young M. Weight training injury trends: a 20-year survey. Phys Sportsmed 2000; 28(7):61–72.

32. Jones L. USWF Coaching Accreditation Course: Club Coach Manual. Colorado Springs, CO: U.S. Weightlifting Federation, 1991.

33. Katzenbach JR, Smith DK. The Wisdom of Teams. Boston: Harvard Business School, 1993.

34. Katzenbach JR, Beckett F, Dichter S, et al. Real Change Leaders. New York: Times Books/Random House, 1995: 217–224.

35. Kraemer WJ, Dziados J. Medical aspects and administrative concerns in strength training. In: Kraemer WJ, Häkkinen K, eds. Strength Training for Sport. Oxford, UK: Blackwell Science, 2002:163–175.

36. Kroll W. Selecting strength training equipment. NSCA J 1990;12(5):65–70.

37. Kroll B. Structural and functional considerations in designing the facility: part I. NSCA J 1991;13(1):51–58.

38. Kroll W. Structural and functional considerations in designing the facility: part II. NSCA J 1991;13(3): 51–57.

39. Kroll B. Liability considerations for strength training facilities. Strength Cond 1995;17(6): 16–17.

40. Maron BJ, Thompson PD, Puffer JC, et al. American Heart Association. Cardiovascular preparticipation screening of competitive athletes. Circulation 1996;94(4):850–856; Med Sci Sports Exerc 1996;28(12):1445–1452.

41. Maron BJ, Thompson PD, Puffer JC, et al. American Heart Association. Cardiovascular preparticipation screening of competitive athletes: addendum. Circulation 1998;97(22): 2294.

42. Morris GA. Supervision—an asset to the weight room? Strength Cond 1994;16(2):14–18.

43. Morrissey MC, Harman EA, Johnson MJ. Resistance training modes: specificity and effectiveness. Med Sci Sports Exerc 1995;27(5):648–660.

44. National Athletic Trainers' Association. Recommendations and Guidelines for Appropriate Medical Coverage of Intercollegiate Athletics. Dallas: NATA, 2003.

45. Nosse LJ, Hunter GR. Free weights: a review supporting their use in rehabilitation. Athlet Training 1985;20(4): 206–209.

46. NSCA Certification Commission. Certified Strength and Conditioning Specialist (CSCS) Examination Content Description. Lincoln, NE: NSCA Certification Commission, 2000.

47. Occupational Safety and Health Administration. U.S. Department of Labor. OSHA Regulations (Standards-29 CFR) 1910.1030: Blood-Borne Pathogens. Washington DC: OSHA, 1996.

48. Patton RW, Grantham WC, Gerson RF, Gettman LR. Developing and Managing Health/Fitness Facilities. Champaign, IL: Human Kinetics, 1989.

49. Plisk SS, Brass MS, Eickhoff-Shemek J, et al. Strength and Conditioning Professional Standards and Guidelines. Colorado Springs CO: National Strength and Conditioning Association, 2001.

50. Preparticipation Physical Evaluation Task Force. American Academy of Family Physicians, American Academy of Pediatrics, American Medical Society for Sports Medicine, American Orthopaedic Society for Sports Medicine and American Osteopathic Academy of Sports Medicine. Preparticipation Physical Evaluation. 2nd ed. New York: McGraw-Hill, 1996.

51. Rabinoff MA. Weight room litigation: what's it all about? Strength Cond 1994;16(2):10–12.

52. Rabinoff MA. 32 reasons for the strength, conditioning, and exercise professional to understand the litigation process. Strength Cond 1994;16(2):20–25.

53. Reeves RK, Laskowski ER, Smith J. Weight training injuries: part 1. Diagnosing and managing acute conditions. Phys Sportsmed 1998;26(2):67–96.

54. Reeves RK, Laskowski ER, Smith J. Weight training injuries: part 2. Diagnosing and managing chronic conditions. Phys Sportsmed 1998;26(3):54–63.

55. Schluep C, Klossner DA, eds. National Collegiate Athletic Association. 2003–04 NCAA Sports Medicine Handbook. 16th ed. Indianapolis, IN: NCAA, 2003.

56. Stone MH, Fry AC, Ritchie M, et al. Injury potential and safety aspects of weightlifting movements. Strength Cond 1994;16(3):15–21.

57. Stone MH, Borden RA. Modes and methods of resistance training. Strength Cond 1997;19(4):18–24.

58. Stone MH, Collins D, Plisk SS, et al. Training principles: evaluation of modes and methods of resistance training. Strength Cond J 2000;22(3):65–76.

59. Stone M, Plisk S, Collins D. Training principles: evaluation of modes and methods of resistance training—a coaching perspective. Sports Biomech 2002;1(1):79–103.

60. Tharrett SJ, Peterson JA, eds, for the American College of Sports Medicine. ACSM's Health/Fitness Facility Standards and Guidelines. 2nd ed. Champaign IL: Human Kinetics, 1997.

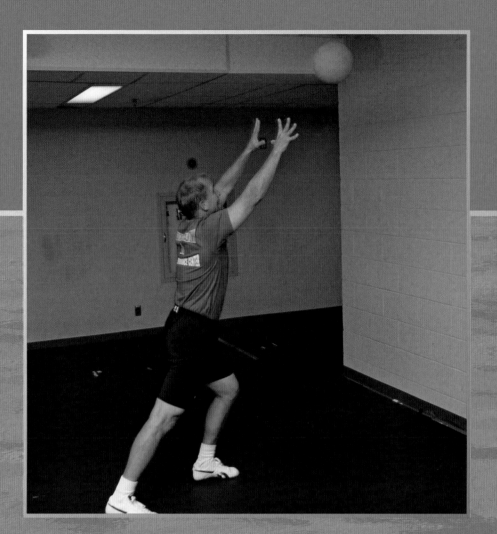

Exercise Prescription

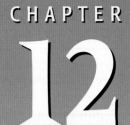

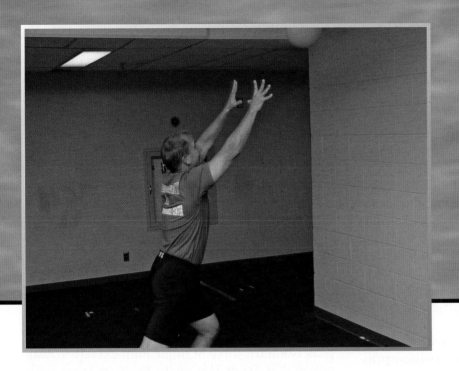

Strength and Conditioning for Sport

MICHAEL H. STONE
MEG E. STONE

Introduction

Until recently, most exercise and sports scientists focused their research on the physiological and performance effects of aerobic training. Many of the factors concerned with the intricacies of strength/power training and subsequent adaptations, particularly gender differences, are only just now beginning to emerge.

The purpose of this chapter is to briefly discuss performance adaptations to periodized resistance training as well as the periodization of training modes and methods that can enhance specific adaptations. This discussion includes both basic and traditional methods of programming for resistance training. For a more detailed discussion of advanced training methods, refer to Plisk and Stone (29).

BASIC TRAINING PRINCIPLES

Recent studies and reviews clearly indicate that the training method (reps and sets, velocity of movement, appropriate variation, etc.) can make a significant difference in the physiological and performance adaptations consequent to a resistance-training program (16,21,33). For example, high-volume programs generally have a greater influence on body composition and endurance factors than do low-volume programs (8,10,33,43). It is also probable that the choice of training mode (type of equipment) can influence the adaptations to a training program (42).

The three basic training principles are overload, variation, and specificity (43). If each of these principles is appropriately addressed through the exercise prescription, performance will be enhanced and the chance of overtraining will be reduced.

> *The three basic training principles are overload, variation, and specificity; to optimize the training adaptations, these principles must be appropriately integrated into the training plan.*

Overload involves providing an appropriate stimulus for attaining a desired level of physical, physiological, or performance adaptation. Overload can be conceptualized as an exercise and training stimulus that goes beyond normal levels of physical performance. An exercise prescription for overload could include range of motion, absolute and relative intensity levels, frequency, and duration factors. All overload stimuli will have some level of intensity, relative intensity (percentage of maximum), and volume. The quantification of overload stimuli for various modes (weights, variable resistance devices, semi-isokinetic devices, rubber bands, etc.) of resistance training can be challenging. Quantification of some forms of overload—elastic resistance, for example—is difficult. For this discussion, the quantification of overload stimuli deals with weight training.

Intensity is an often misunderstood component of an exercise prescription. There are several aspects to the intensity component. Intensity factors are associated with the rate of performing work and the rate at which energy is expended (43). Intensity factors can be separated into two aspects: training intensity and movement, or exercise, intensity (43).

Training intensity (TI) is concerned with the rate at which a training exercise or training session proceeds; it can be estimated by the average mass (weight) lifted per exercise, per day, per week, etc., and relates to the training density. For example, within a session, the average load lifted is directly related to the time taken to complete the exercise.

The **relative intensity** is a percent of the one-repetition maximum (1 RM). The 1 RM is stable only in advanced strength trainers. Thus, using relative intensity to plan training programs must be carried out with this aspect in mind.

Exercise intensity is the actual power output of a movement. Power is defined as a work rate or as the product of force and velocity. The product of force and velocity forms an inverted U, with peak power occurring at approximately 30% of the peak isometric force in single joint exercises. Peak power has been shown to be associated with approximately 30% to 80% of the 1 RM, depending upon the type of exercise and the trained state. The exact percentage of the 1 RM at which peak power occurs appears to depend on whether the exercise involves single or multiple joints, whether the body weight is also involved in the movement, and whether or not the movement is joint-range-limited or ballistic (27). Typically, for single-joint exercises, peak power occurs at about 30% to 40% of 1 RM; for whole-body movements, peak power occurs at approximately 30% to 50% for weighted jumps (39) and 70% to 85% for weightlifting movements (13,14).

The level of training may also influence the 1-RM percentage at which maximum power occurs, with stronger or more experienced strength athletes producing maximum power at slightly higher percentages than less trained or weaker athletes (2,27,39). Thus the relative intensity can be used to estimate (and to manipulate) the exercise intensity, with very heavy or very light weights producing lower power outputs than those in the middle range.

Training density deals with the frequency of training per session, per day, per week, etc. For example, day 1 might contain four training sessions, each of equal volume, and day 2 might contain two training sessions of similar volume. Day 1 would have a higher training density. One week could contain five training sessions while another could contain ten; the training density in week 2 would be higher.

Training volume is a measure or estimate of the total work performed and is strongly related

TABLE 12.1	DAY 1: GENERAL PREPARATION PHASE						
	SET	REPETITIONS	LOAD	VL	TI	TIME FOR SET EXECUTION (S)	KG/S
	1	10	60	600		40	15.0
	2	10	100	1,000		45	22.2
	3	10	140	1,400		47	29.8
	4	10	140	1,400		52	26.9
	5	10	140	1,400		55	25.5
TOTAL	5	50	580	5,800		239	119.4
Mean					116	47.8	24.3

Volume load (VL) = sum of load lifted (sets × mass); training intensity = VL/repetitions (or mean load/sets).

to total energy expenditure (6,25,47). Although training intensity (and relative intensity) can be estimated by the amount of weight lifted, the training volume is related to the number of repetitions and sets per exercise, the number and types of exercises used (large versus small muscle mass), and the frequency (i.e., number of times per day, week, month, etc.) with which these exercises are repeated.

Volume load (VL) is the best estimate of the amount of work accomplished during training and is commonly used in both research and practical settings. Volume load is calculated by summing the product of the load and the number of repetitions for each set. The application of training intensity and volume can be considered in terms of the train-

ing session (i.e., all of the exercises performed during a specified period) or in terms of single exercises. An understanding of overload factors can aid in the programming of training, including methods (i.e., sets and repetitions), velocity of exercise, and exercise selection.

The interaction/association of VL and TI can be illustrated by calculating these factors for two sample training sessions (using actual data from the squat as an example). Table 12.1 contains the data for day 1, the general preparation phase; Table 12.2 contains the data for day 2, the competition phase.

In this example, the VL for day 1 was larger than that for day 2 (5,800 kg versus 3,375 kg); however, the TI was larger for day 2 than for day 1 (135 versus 116). VL and TI are inversely related. Further-

TABLE 12.2	DAY 2: COMPETITION PHASE						
	SET	REPETITIONS	LOAD	VL	TI	TIME FOR SET EXECUTION (S)	KG/S
	1	5	60	300		15.0	20.0
	2	5	120	600		17.0	35.3
	3	5	165	825		25.0	33.0
	4	5	165	825		26.0	31.7
	5	5	165	825		28.0	29.4
TOTAL	5	25	525	3,375		111.0	149.4
Mean					135	22.2	30.4

Volume load (VL) = sum of load lifted (sets × mass); training intensity = VL/repetitions (or mean load/sets).

more, TI is directly related to the rate at which the load is lifted (kilograms per second) and is an indication of the rate of training. Calculation of the TI, while reflecting work rate (kilograms per second), is less time-consuming than measuring and calculating kilograms per second and thus has a practical advantage. The average VL and TI can be easily calculated per week, month, or phase of training. In this manner, using these variables, a reasonable record of training progress can be made.

Variation involves appropriate manipulation in training intensity, speed of movement, volume, and exercise selection. Appropriate variation is a primary consideration for continued adaptation over the course of long-term training programs (17,18). Appropriate sequencing of volume, intensity, and exercise selection, including speed-strength exercises in a periodized manner, can lead to superior enhancement of a variety of performance abilities (16).

> *Several different levels of variation are possible in a training program (i.e., long term, short-term, day-to-day, etc.) The level of variation in the training program is directly related to the level of the athlete.*

Specificity of exercise and training is the most important consideration in selecting both methods and modes for resistance training, especially if athletic performance enhancement is a primary goal. Specificity includes both bioenergetics and mechanics of training. This discussion is concerned with the mechanical aspects of specificity.

SPECIFICITY AND TRANSFER-OF-TRAINING EFFECT

As previously noted, *mechanical specificity* refers to the kinetic and kinematic associations between a training exercise and a physical performance. This includes movement patterns, peak force, rate of force development, acceleration, and velocity parameters. The greater similarity a training exercise has to the actual physical performance, the greater the probability of transfer (3,30,42,43). Mechanical specificity has been extensively studied as it affects strength-training exercise. Of particular importance is explosive strength and power.

> *Transfer-of-training effect deals with the degree to which a training exercise promotes adaptation in performance. To maximize the potential for "transfer-of-training effect," a training exercise must use reasonable levels of movement-pattern specificity and overload.*

Explosive Strength and Power

Among untrained and moderately trained subjects, heavy weight training can produce positive performance effects in the entire force velocity curve (15–21). Both observational and objective evidence indicates, however, that among advanced strength-trained subjects, considerable high-velocity training is necessary to make additional alterations in the high velocity end of the force velocity curve (15,16).

Although isometric training can result in an increased peak rate of force production and velocity of movement, especially in untrained subjects (3), the isometric training effect on dynamic explosive force production is relatively minor, particularly among well-trained athletes (15,23). Although several parameters can be affected, traditional heavy weight training primarily increases maximum strength, especially as measured by a 1 RM. In contrast, the primary effect of typical ballistic training is an increased rate of force production and velocity of movement, (15,16,21,23). Additionally, high-power training can alter a wide range of athletic performance variables to a greater extent than does traditional heavy weight training, especially in subjects with a reasonable initial level of maximum strength (16,49). Indeed, an initial high maximum strength level appears to potentiate the development of high power outputs and increased movement velocity (36,42,45).

> *The type of training program (i.e., high-volume, high-intensity) can make a marked difference in the type of adaptation (i.e., body composition, strength, power, etc.) to the program.*

It is also important to select modes of exercise that will have the greatest transfer-of-training effect. It is doubtful that single-joint exercises will have as much impact on performance, which is multi-joint in nature, as multijoint training exercises (42,50). In selecting training modes, a number of considerations and performance criteria can be used (32,42). These criteria can maximize the transfer-of-training effect.

Movement-pattern characteristics include the following (32,42):

1. The type of muscle action
2. Accentuated regions of force production
3. The complexity, amplitude, and direction of movement
4. Ballistic versus nonballistic movements

There also must be an overload application for successful performance adaptation. If there is no continued overload, then sport performance will not improve beyond adaptation to simple practice of the sport. Factors to be overloaded include force production, rate of force production, and power output. In choosing exercises for training explosive athletic performance, ballistic movements and rate of force production are especially important.

PROGRAM PLANNING

Program planning involves making decisions related to the number of sets, intensity of the exercise, volume, load, and rate of progression. In general, multiple-set periodized training programs will demonstrate greater gains in performance over the long term than single-set or nonperiodized programs.

Single Sets versus Multiple Sets

Although there has been controversy (7), the majority of studies and reviews that have carefully examined training with one set versus training with multiple sets, with both men and women, indicate that superior results can be obtained in a wide variety of performance and physiological variables by using multiple sets (4,19,31,43). Maximum strength, power, and positive adaptations in body composition are among the variables that can be altered to a greater extent by using multiple sets. The superior effects of multiple sets are particularly apparent among advanced weight trainers (17–19,43). Furthermore, these effects can be enhanced by the use of periodization/variation techniques along with the multiple set protocols.

Periodization

Periodization can be defined as a logical phasic method of manipulating training variables in order to increase the potential for achieving specific performance goals (40,41). Thus, a basic tenet of periodization is training nonlinearity. The primary goals of periodization are (1) reduction of overtraining potential and (2) peaking at the appropriate time or providing a maintenance program for sports with a specific season. The goals are met by appropriately manipulating volume and intensity factors and by appropriate exercise selection. It is important to understand that variation can take place at several different levels. A brief overview of periodization is provided in Box 12.1.

> *Periodization involves planned variation in volume and intensity of training to promote maximal performance at the desired time and to decrease the chance for overtraining.*

Traditional periodized training can be divided into three stages or levels: the **macrocycle** (long-length cycle), the **mesocycle** (middle-length cycle), and the **microcycle** (short-length cycle, or day-to-day variation). Each macro- and mesocycle

---

12.1 PERIODIZATION

Periodization is the manipulation of training variables to promote maximum performance at the appropriate time of the year while decreasing the chances of overtraining. Periodization principles can also be applied to seasonal sports such as rugby and American football.

In its simplest form, periodization is variation planning; both short- and long-term planning. As the competitive season approaches, training should progress from less specific to more specific. Less specific training is performed in the off season or during periods with less emphasis on competition and then progresses to sport-specific training as the competitive season approaches.

The decisions made in designing a periodized training program should be based on scientific evidence. The science of conditioning is a process of adaptation to new information, and conditioning programs should evolve with science. One potential limiting factor in the application of training principles and theory is that some sports or age groups have not been well studied. In this case, we must extrapolate from the research that is available to design the best possible training programs for these athletes.

Today, periodized training programs have been applied to a variety of individual and team sports. Some of these programs are based on direct scientific evidence and some are based on logical application of scientific principles based on similar sports or activities.

The application of periodization to training programs to improve athletic performance is an evolving science.

Q & A from the Field

I have heard the terms linear *and* undulating *periodization used lately. What do these terms mean?*

Linear periodization is used to describe periodized programs that increase load and intensity in a direct linear fashion over a specific time period. The term, however, is a misnomer, as all periodized programs should utilize variations in loading that include hard days followed by easier days or recovery days. *Undulating periodization* is a term used to describe periodized programs with wide variations in loads and intensities from day to day. Beginning athletes, for example, generally respond better to programs with less variation in load and intensity. Advanced athletes can generally maintain higher loads and intensities and greater variation from one day to the next. All periodized programs should vary the load and intensity of training; some programs contain more variation and some less.

generally begins with high-volume, low-intensity of training and ends with high-intensity, low-volume of training. The macro- and mesocycle can contain four phases: (1) preparation (general and special), (2) competition, (3) peaking, and (4) transition or active rest. Each of these phases typically has different goals and requires different degrees of variation in training variables. Figure 12.1 illustrates a traditional macrocycle for a novice athlete.

The **general preparation (GP)** is a high-volume phase, usually lasting a few weeks, designed to enhance sports-specific fitness and associated physiological parameters. **Special or specific preparation (SP)** deals with relatively high volume training in which the exercises are more specific to the activity in terms of movement pattern and velocity. It is used as a transition phase linking high-volume, less specific general preparation training to high-intensity, very specific training associated with competition. During the **competition phase (C)**, intensity factors are adjusted in keeping with the characteristics of the sport. For example, in a sport requiring high power outputs, more time is spent on using high exercise intensities; for a sport in which great strength is required, a greater emphasis can be placed on high training intensities. Volume during the competition phase is decreased. The competition phase can last several months.

> *The competition phase is generally characterized by a low volume of training and high intensity of training. The intensity of training should match the intensity required for participation in the sport.*

Peaking (P) is a phase lasting a short time (usually less than 4 weeks). During the early portion of peaking, volume is typically reduced as training intensity (or exercise intensity, depending on the sport or performance goals) is increased or maintained at relatively high levels. During the last few days before competition, intensity factors are also reduced to encourage adequate recovery. The later portion of a peaking phase, when volume is markedly reduced, is referred to as a "taper" (26).

> *Peaking is a short phase generally characterized by a low volume of training while maintaining sport-specific intensities. The last few days before competition, both the volume and intensity are reduced to promote recovery.*

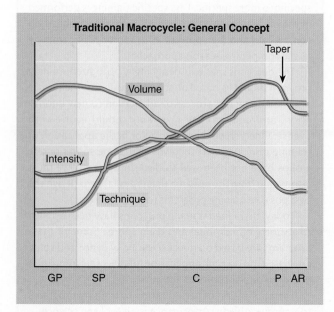

Traditional Macrocycle: General Concept

FIGURE 12.1 Traditional macrocycle for novices. GP = general preparation; SP = special preparation; C = competition; P = peaking; AR = active rest.

Active rest (AR) is a phase in which volume and intensity are decreased markedly to facilitate recovery from the training cycle. Recovery includes healing and rehabilitation of any injuries that may have occurred as well as recovery from the emotional rigors of competition. Complete rest allows sports-specific fitness to deteriorate to a degree from which it is difficult to recover without extensive training. Compared to complete rest, active rest allows for less deterioration of fitness and a faster return to peak fitness during the next cycle. Active rest usually lasts about 1 week. A modification of the typical scheme can be made for sports with a definite season in which winning all contests (games) is a goal, such as basketball. A typical general modification for seasonal sports is to prolong the competition phase and remove the peaking phase. For a more detailed discussion concerning periodization training, see Plisk and Stone (29), and Stone et al. (40,41,43).

Training Advanced Athletes

Most advanced and elite athletes use some form of periodization (Fig. 12.2). Advanced and elite athletes may require greater variation and more creative approaches to training compared to lower-level and beginning athletes. Greater variation is necessary as a result of several factors, including the facts that (1) advanced athletes train with greater volumes and intensities than beginners and novices, thus they may be closer to an overtraining threshold, and (2) as genetic limitations are approached, greater variation and novel approaches to training may be necessary to "provoke" additional adaptation. Several creative resistance-training approaches may stimulate further strength-power adaptations.

> *Advanced athletes may require greater variations in volume and intensity of training compared to beginning athletes to promote continued adaptations to the training stimulus.*

SEQUENCED TRAINING

As previously noted, prior exposure to strength training and increased maximum strength levels can potentiate gains in power resulting from power training. Examination of longitudinal and cross-sectional studies (15,43) suggests that sequenced training, heavy weight training over a few weeks followed by speed-strength training, or combination training (heavy training plus high-power or high-speed training), can produce superior results in speed and power gains compared to heavy weight training or speed-strength training alone. More importantly, evidence indicates that this type of sequenced training (a form of periodization) can beneficially alter a wide variety of athletic performance variables to a greater extent than either heavy weight training or speed-strength training

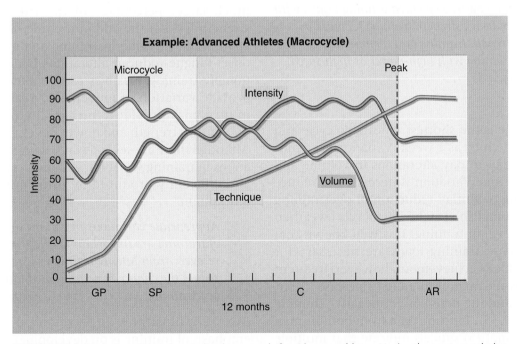

FIGURE 12.2 Typical traditional periodized approach for advance athletes. Notice the greater variation compared to Figure 12.1. GP = general preparation; SP = special preparation; C = competition; P = peaking; AR = active rest.

Q & A from the Field

I thought speed was one of those variables that really could not be improved. Can resistance training really improve the running speed of my athletes?

Yes, the appropriate resistance-training program can improve running speed assuming that the athlete has not reached his or her physiological peak. Running speed is a combination of several factors, some of which are genetic and not modifiable. Here are some components you can likely modify with resistance training: (1) One factor in running speed is generating ground reaction force; the more force you apply to the ground in the appropriate direction, the faster you will move. (2) Another factor is stride rate, which involves not only the force you apply to the ground but also the speed with which you can cycle your stride. A limiting factor here is bringing the trail leg forward rapidly. Resistance training of the hip flexors and integrating this training into running form can improve speed. (3) Speed of movement is partly a function of fast-twitch muscle fibers. Appropriately designed resistance-training programs facilitate speed and power development by training and improving the capacity of fast-twitch muscle fibers.

(16,24). To produce maximum gains in power, the following sequence would be reasonable (16):

Strength endurance → strength
→ power and speed

Each phase may last several weeks, depending on the needs of the athlete, type of sport, and placement in the overall macrocycle.

> *Evidence suggests that sequenced training may produce superior results in terms of improving speed and power. Sequenced training begins with a cycle of heavy strength training followed by speed-strength training or a combination of heavy training with high-power or high-speed training.*

MICROCYCLES

A microcycle is the shortest repeatable cycle and is typically defined as 1 week. Variation is accomplished by day-to-day alterations in volume and intensity factors. Variation is necessary to reduce overtraining potential; reduction of overtraining is better accomplished at the microcycle level then any other level of training. It is well known that heavy, intense training loads are necessary for ultimate athletic achievement; however, frequent heavy loads and training monotony increase "training strain" and the potential for negative training outcomes (9,35). Further, data from both human (9) and animal (5) models indicate that multiple "light" days within a microcycle can allow a given

training load to be accomplished with a greater potential for positive adaptations and fewer negative outcomes (9,40,41). Some of the negative side effects associated with training may be associated with changes in the maximum strength available in training (T_{max}). For example, observations by the authors indicate that T_{max} can decrease across a microcycle due to accumulated fatigue, thus the 1 RM representing T_{max} on Monday may not be T_{max} on Friday. If accumulative fatigue is not taken into consideration, loads based on a percentage of T_{max} (or a contest maximum) may actually represent a much larger percentage of the true maximum strength level at the end of the microcycle. Thus, appropriate variation in volume and intensity can offset fatigue-induced alterations in Tmax. Additionally training variables can be altered daily to provide variation in movement, a factor, which in turn, may provide a further stimulus for both maximum strength and power development (16). Although there are several ways of producing alterations in training variables, variation can be simply and efficiently produced by using a heavy/light day system.

> *Appropriate variations in volume and intensity of training are important to allow adequate recovery from intense training sessions and reduce the chance of accumulated fatigue and overtraining.*

Box 12.2 illustrates an example in which the emphasis of training is on development of leg and hip strength primarily using the squat.

REAL-WORLD APPLICATION
Fatigue and Decreased Performance

A weightlifter training for a competition is having trouble sustaining a reasonable level of training performance and is feeling quite fatigued. How would you examine her condition and what factors might you manipulate (as a coach) to remedy this problem?

Multiple factors may lead to decreased performance and fatigue in an athlete. Consider all possibilities, but focus on the factors that are most likely with the specific athlete you are working with.

1. The obvious factor to consider first is a potential imbalance between training and recovery. Evaluate the intensity of training.
2. Evaluate the nutritional habits of the lifter. Is the athlete eating properly? Is the athlete getting enough total calories? Carbohydrates? Protein?
3. What is the emotional/psychological status of the athlete? Maybe the athlete is burned out or is no longer enjoying the sport. Maybe there are personal problems with family members, friends, etc.
4. Are there any medical problems that could be causing fatigue? Perhaps a physical from a physician is needed to rule out specific medical conditions.

5. Is there a possibility the athlete is using or abusing drugs? Specific drugs are related to specific behaviors, and drug use and/or abuse can certainly be related to fatigue.

Obviously some of these problems need the assistance of other professionals: a medical doctor, a sport psychologist, etc. As the coach, you can do several things to help the athlete.

1. Make sure the training program is not too intense and that the athlete is getting adequate time for recovery. Hard days of training should be followed by lighter days or recovery days. There should be variation in intensity from one workout to the next. Adequate time should be allowed for recovery. Adequate sleep is critical to recovery. Make sure the athlete is not participating in additional physical activity that is detracting from the weightlifting performance.
2. Make sure the athlete is eating a balanced diet, eating enough calories, and adequately hydrated.
3. Monitor the athlete for common symptoms of overtraining.

In this example, several factors must be considered. First is the level of the athlete: this type of variation in intensity will not work well with beginners because of the instability of T_{max}. The second aspect is that intensity of training is altered through variations of relative intensity; the exact percentage used will change with individual athletes, the type of exercise, the set/repetitions scheme, and fatigue (37). Because of these factors, a percentage range should be used. So, in the above example, the athlete might squat 160 kg on Monday but only 140 kg on Friday for three sets of five repetitions. On both days maximum efforts would be made to enhance appropriate adaptations (22). Relative intensity can also be calculated based on set and repetition maximums rather than a 1 RM, as follows. Remember that relative intensity (RI) is the percent of maximum for the set and repetition protocol.

$$VH = 100\%$$
$$H = 90\% \text{ to } 95\%$$
$$MH = 85\% \text{ to } 90\%$$
$$M = 80\% \text{ to } 85\%$$
$$ML\ 75\% \text{ to } 80\%$$
$$L = 70\% \text{ to } 75\%$$

So, for example, if 100 kg were the maximum for 3 × 5 in the squat (i.e., 100% = VH) then on a moderate (M) lifting day only 80 to 85 kg would be used. This method works well with advanced athletes, for whom estimates of 100% for sets and reps can be predicted for various exercises with reason-

12.2 EXAMPLE OF SQUAT TRAINING PROGRAM

Squats: M and Th: 3 × 5 at target load
Pulls: W and S
Squat T_{max} = 200 kg

Day	M	T	W	TH	F	S	SU
RI	H	R	MH	M	R	M	R

Relative intensity (RI) = % of Tmax for 3 × 5.

H	80%–85%
MH	75%–80%
M	70%–75%
L	65%–70%
R	Rest

TABLE 12.3	ALTERATIONS IN VL RESULTING FROM CHANGES IN REPETITIONS						
	DAY 1: 3 × 10 REPETITIONS (TARGET LOAD)				DAY 2: 3 × 5 REPETITIONS (TARGET LOAD)		
	Set	*Repetitions*	*Load (kg)*	*VL (kg)*	*Set*	*Repetitions*	*Load (kg)*	*VL (kg)*
	1	10	60	600	1	5	60	300
	2	10	100	1,000	2	5	100	500
	3	10	140	1,400	3	5	140	700
	4–6	30	160	4,800	4–6	15	160	2,400
Total	6	60		7,800	6	30		3,900
Mean			130				130	

able accuracy, as their T_{max} and training loads are relatively stable over long periods.

In the creation of effective microcycle variation, the effects of other training activities must also be considered. If running or other conditioning activities are also included in the overall training program, then the additional energy demands and increased physical and emotional stress must be taken into account. In this context, planning and tracking alterations by volume load can be more valuable than tracking alterations in intensity. Volume load can change with the type of exercises, repetitions, and intensity. Table 12.3 illustrates alterations in VL resulting from changes in repetitions.

It can be noted that even when the load is constant, the addition or deletion of repetitions can alter the VL and therefore the total work accomplished. Importantly, the higher volume of work on day 1 will probably require more time and energy for recovery (25). On the other hand, higher inten-

sities of training would require greater recovery time and energy if the VL were equal.

Volume load (VL) can also be strongly effected by alterations in training intensity, as seen in Table 12.4.

In this example, using constant sets and repetitions, an increase in loading (training intensity) can produce a marked increase in VL, and therefore total work and total energy expenditure (exercise plus recovery). In actual practice, combinations of intensity and repetition changes accomplish alterations in VL. Often increases in load necessitate additional "warm-up" sets. The designation of heavy and light days based on VL must take into consideration the training intensity, relative intensity, number of sets, repetitions, and the trained state. Tables 12.5 and 12.6 illustrate actual data from heavy and light days within a microcycle on 2 days in which exercises were repeated.

From this example it can be observed that a reduction in target load by 20% (with appropriate

TABLE 12.4	ALTERATIONS IN VL RESULTING FROM CHANGES IN TRAINING INTENSITY						
	DAY 1: 3 × 5 REPETITIONS (TARGET LOAD)				DAY 2: 3 × 5 REPETITIONS (TARGET LOAD)		
	Set	*Repetitions*	*Load (kg)*	*VL (kg)*	*Set*	*Repetitions*	*Load (kg)*	*VL (kg)*
	1	5	60	300	1	5	60	300
	2	5	100	500	2	5	120	600
	3	5	140	700	3	5	160	800
	4–6	15	160	2,400	4–6	15	180	2,700
Total	6	30		3,900	6	30		4,400
Mean			130				147	

TABLE 12.5	DATA FROM A HEAVY DAY WITHIN A MACROCYCLE: MONDAY VL (HEAVY) SETS OF 5 (TARGET × 85)								
EXERCISE	SET	1	2	3	4	5	6	7	TOTAL
Squats	(1 RM = 200)	300	500	700	850	850	850	450*	4,500
Push press	(1 RM = 100)	250	300	400	400	400	250*		2,000
Bench press	(1 RM = 140)	300	500	600	600	600	325*		2,925
Total									9,425

*Reduced load sets for optimal power output.

alterations in warm-up sets) can result in a reduced volume load of approximately 22%.

Because total energy expenditure is related to the VL, care must be taken in "matching" the resistance-training program with the requirements for other aspects of conditioning. If one aspect is being emphasized—for example, strength adaptation—then a light day for training must remain a light day. It should be noted that increasing the amount of work performed in non-strength-training aspects, so that the day becomes a heavy-workload day, defeats the purpose of having a light day and can increase the probability of negative adaptation. So, for example, in a sport requiring strength/power training that also requires other conditioning aspects such as running and tactical training, it is imperative that the workloads for individual components complement each other and not interfere with the goals of the training period phase. Table 12.7 provides an example of a mesocycle in which improving maximum strength is the goal, where different aspects of training would be adjusted so that strength development is not reduced.

Or if tactical training were a priority, for example during football season, then a different schedule would be appropriate, as in Table 12.8.

Summated Microcycles

Microcycles can be grouped together or summated into "blocks," so that each block presents a specific pattern of volume and intensity loading. The blocks can then be repeated throughout a mesocycle such that specific stimuli are "re-presented" in a cyclical fashion. Generally, a block consists of 4 weeks. A typical block would be one in which volume and intensity is increased for 3 weeks followed by an "unload" week, creating a 3/1 block (12,20). The unload week can be used to reduce the potential for overtraining and to allow for adaptation and supercompensation (Fig. 12.3). Care should be taken in using this type of 3/1 approach because the heaviest loading takes place in the third week and the accumulation of fatigue from microcycles 1 to 3 may preclude adaptation to speed-strength work (therefore the need for an unload week). In advanced athletes, if improved maximum strength, power, and speed are the training goals, then other strategies may be more effective. One such strategy entails **planned overreaching**.

Summated microcycles consist of microcycles grouped into "blocks" so that each block presents a specific pattern of volume and intensity of

TABLE 12.6	DATA FROM A LIGHT DAY WITHIN A MACROCYCLE: THURSDAY VL (LIGHT) SETS OF 5—TARGET SETS REDUCED IN LOAD BY 20%								
EXERCISE	SET	1	2	3	4	5	6	7	TOTAL
Squats	(1 RM = 200)	300	500	700	700	700	450		3,350
Push press	(1 RM = 100)	250	300	325	325	325	250*		1,575
Bench press	(1 RM = 140)	300	400	475	475	475	325*		2,450
Total									7,375

*Reduced load sets for optimal power output.

TABLE 12.7	MESOCYCLE FOR IMPROVING MAXIMUM STRENGTH						
DAY	**M**	**T**	**W**	**TH**	**F**	**S**	**SU**
WTVL	H	R	MH	R	L	M	R
R/AV	L	M	R	M	R	M	R
TTV	L	L	R	L	R	L	R

WTVL = weight-training volume load; R/AV = running, agility training volume; TTV = tactical training volume.

loading. *The blocks can be repeated in a cyclical fashion with the desired result of maximizing training adaptation.*

Overreaching can occur as a result of a large increase in volume load. Overreaching can result in chronic fatigue and other symptoms similar to the initial stages of overtraining (35). Provided that the overreaching phase is not too extensive, a return to normal training volumes can result in a "super-compensation effect," promoting an increased performance. These supercompensation effects may be associated with the anabolic state and changes in the testosterone:cortisol ratio (11,34). By carefully planning the over-reaching phase (with subsequent return to normal training and adding a taper), performance may be enhanced (Fig. 12.4). It may also be possible to incorporate a short overreaching phase into a summated block scheme, so that the overreaching phase is periodically repeated and a cumulative effect is achieved. Figure 12.5 represents this type of approach. This approach of using planned overreaching with summated blocks can be used by intermediate and advanced athletes.

Planned overreaching is an intentional increase in volume and intensity that places the athlete in a state of overreaching. If the overreaching phase is not too extensive, recovery can result in a "supercompensation effect," promoting increased performance.

TABLE 12.8	MESOCYCLE FOR IMPROVING TACTICAL TRAINING						
DAY	**M**	**T**	**W**	**TH**	**F**	**S**	**SU**
WTVL	L	R	L	R	L	M	R
R/AV	L	M	R	M	R	M	R
TTV	H	L	M	MH	R	M	R

WTVL = weight-training volume load; R/AV = running, agility training volume; TTV = tactical training volume.

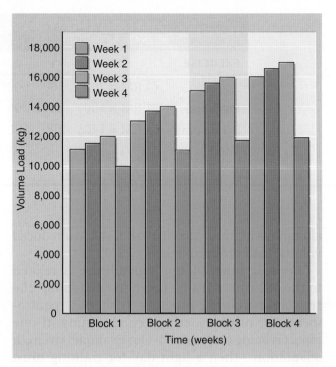

FIGURE 12.3 Summated microcycles. This graph represents a 3/1 cycle, or 3 weeks of increasing VL (volume load) followed by 1 unload week.

Fundamental conditioning addresses fitness parameters specifically associated with a sport. Fundamental conditioning usually emphasizes specific endurance aspects. For example, in strength-power sports, strength endurance would be a priority. It has been the observation of the authors that advanced athletes and their coaches often reduce or completely neglect fundamental condi-

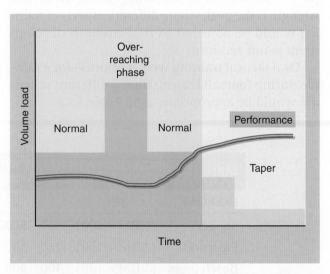

FIGURE 12.4 Planned overreaching (conceptual). Training volume is markedly increased for a short period. Performance may decline during overreaching. A return to "normal training" can result in a performance boost. A taper may further enhance the performance.

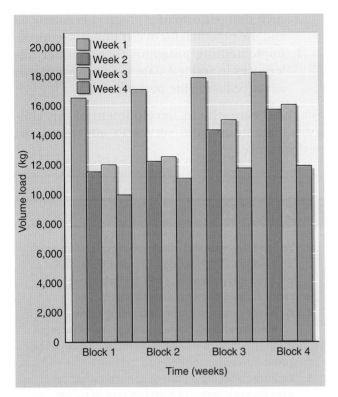

FIGURE 12.5 Planned overreaching (summated microcycles). Each block begins with an overreaching microcycle followed by a taper, producing a 1/2/1 block (1 week overreaching/2 weeks normal training/1 week taper). Taken from actual data among collegiate throwers using the squat.

tioning, believing that years of training obviate the need for more basic exercise or higher-volume work. However, there are several reasons why fundamental conditioning phases may be of benefit:

1. All training programs require occasional or periodic decreases in training volume and intensity or periods of rest. This decrease can result in a loss of sports-specific fitness, which can include negative alterations in body composition, endurance capabilities, and recoverability.
2. Periodically reintroducing this type of training variation offers a break (both physiologically and psychologically) from higher-intensity training.
3. Properly applied as a unidirectional concentrated load (46), fundamental training can enhance subsequent adaptation to higher-intensity exercise.

Figure 12.6 represents a mesocycle protocol in which concentrated loading (CL) lasting for 4 weeks is introduced as part of a general preparation phase. The advantages of an initial concentrated loading

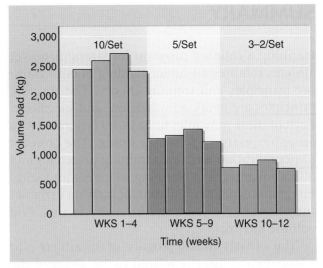

FIGURE 12.6 Strength training: model 1 (46). Concentrated loading (weeks 1 to 4), followed by normal training (weeks 5 to 9) and then a volume taper (weeks 10 to 12).

phase have been evaluated in both research (28,38, 48,51) and practical application/observation.

The concentrated loading phase can also be integrated with cyclically repeated overreaching phases to produce a training protocol, which can make use of the advantages of both phases (Fig. 12.7). Objective data using advanced strength trainers (44) as well as with national- and international-level athletes indicates that this approach can produce superior gains in maximum strength compared to other variation schemes or traditional training.

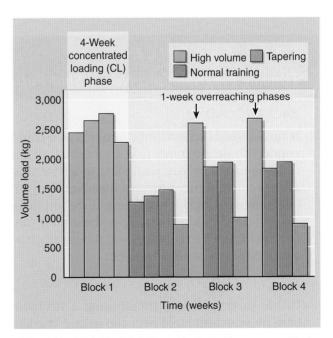

FIGURE 12.7 Strength/power training: model 2 (29). The combination of concentrated loading and short-term overreaching.

SUMMARY

Planning a training program for strength/power athletes requires an understanding of both training principles and training theory. The training principles are overload, variation, and specificity. Each of these principles must be incorporated into an appropriate system of training. The concept of periodization embraces training principles and offers advantages in planning, allowing for logical integration and manipulation of training variables such as exercise selection, intensity factors, and volume factors.

The adaptation and progress of the athlete is to a large extent directly related to the *ability* of the coach/athlete to create and carry out appropriate training plans. This ability includes:

1. An understating of how different types of exercises can affect strength and strength-related variables (i.e., maximum force, rate of force development, power, etc.).
2. An understanding of the characteristics of exercises necessary for maximizing transfer-of-training effect such that training exercises have the greatest potential for carryover to performance. This understanding includes both movement-pattern specificity as well as how to overload in specific manner.
3. Implementing programs with variations at appropriate levels (macro, meso, and micro)

such that performance progress is enhanced and the potential for overtraining is reduced.
4. Implementing programs that consider differences in trained state (i.e., novice versus advanced and elite performers).

For the coach/athlete, development of this ability is paramount and serves to advance sport performance.

MAXING OUT

1. You are strength and conditioning coach for track and field at a high school. Create a generalized plan for: (a) a thrower, (b) a sprinter, (c) a distance runner, (d) a basketball player.
2. A college distance runner is training toward the conference championships; what type of strength training program should be performed during the competitive season?
3. You are coaching a college sprinter; what type of resistance-training exercises would be performed in the general preparation and competition phases? Would there be differences based on gender?
4. You are coaching a high school American football team. How would you manipulate volume and intensity factors during various parts of the training program (summer versus fall versus in season)?

CASE EXAMPLE
Training Program for a Novice Shot-Putter

BACKGROUND

A novice (high school) shot-putter is in a competition phase. He comes to you for advice on his training program. Are you going to advise this athlete to work more toward speed and power or strength? Consider the long-term implications of the training program, as the athlete has the next 2 years to compete and potentially has a collegiate career ahead as well.

RECOMMENDATIONS/CONSIDERATIONS

In the novice athlete, establishing a strength base on which to build over the next 2 years is critical. Although the resistance-training pro-

gram will have variations within cycles and from one cycle to the next, a novice athlete should spend the bulk of his or her time establishing a strength base.

IMPLEMENTATION

For the first year, including the competition phase, the athlete could be advised to train throughout the year with training goals designed primarily toward strength. Cycles of speed and power or cycles that are a mixture of strength and power can be used on an occasional basis for variety. The second year, with an adequate strength base, the athlete can spend more time working toward speed, power, and explosiveness.

RESULTS

Maximum strength and power should be measured on a regular basis. Results in the first year should reflect rather large gains in basic strength, especially leg and hip strength. Although strength is being emphasized in the first years, some gain in power and speed should also be realized. It should be remembered that at this age (high school) the gains in performance will be a combination of matura-

tion and training adaptations. For an enthusiastic, well-motivated young athlete, the key may not be pushing him or her in the weight room but rather holding back. Although the coach does not want to dampen enthusiasm, care must be taken not to produce excessive fatigue or injuries. For example, over the first year for a 15-year-old 95-kg male novice shot-putter with good motivation, it would not be unusual to expect a 50-kg increase in the 1-RM squat, 25 kg in the bench press, and a 5- to 10-cm increase in the countermovement vertical jump.

REFERENCES

1. American College of Sports Medicine. Position stand (WJ Kraemer, chairperson): Progression models in resistance training for healthy adults. Med Sci Sports Exerc 2002; 34:364–382.
2. Baker D, Nance S, Moore M. The load that maximizes mechanical power output during jump squats in power-trained athletes. J Strength Cond Res 2001;15:92–97.
3. Behm DG. Neuromuscular implications and applications of resistance training. J Strength Cond Res 1995; 9:264–274.
4. Borst SE, De Hoyos DV, Garzarella L, et al. Effects of resistance training on insulin-like growth factor-I and IGF binding proteins. Med Sci Sports Exerc 2001;33:648–653.
5. Bruin G, Kuipers H, Keizer HA, Vander Vusse GJ. Adaptation and overtraining in horses subjected to increasing training loads. J Appl Physiol 1994;76:1908–1913.
6. Burleson MA, O'Bryant HS, Stone MH, et al. Effect of weight training exercise and treadmill exercise on post-exercise oxygen consumption. Med Sci Sports Exerc 1998;30:518–522.
7. Carpenelli RN, Otto RM. Strength training: single versus multiple sets. Sports Med 1998; 26:75–84.
8. Conley MS, Rozenek RR. Health aspects of resistance exercise and training. Strength Cond 2001;23:9–23.
9. Foster C. Monitoring training in athletes with reference to overtraining syndrome. Med Sci Sports Exerc 1998;30: 1164–1168.
10. Frobase I, Verdinck A, Duesberg F, Mucha C. Auswirkungen untersheidllicher belastungs-intensitaten im rahmen eines post-operativen stationaren aufbautrainings auf leistungsdefizite des m quadriceps femoris. Zeitshr Ortop 1993;131:164–167.
11. Fry AC, Kraemer WJ, Stone MH, et al. Relationships between serum testosterone, cortisol and weightlifting performance. J Strength Cond Res 2000;14(3):338–343.
12. Fry RW, Morton AR, Keast D. Periodisation of training stress: a review. Can J Sports Sci 1992;17:234–240.
13. Garhammer JJ. A comparison of maximal power outputs between elite male and female weightlifters in competition. Int J Sport Biomech 1991;7:3–11.

14. Garhammer JJ. A review of the power output studies of Olympic and powerlifting: methodology, performance prediction and evaluation tests. J Strength Cond Res 1993;7:76–89.
15. Hakkinen K. Neuromuscular adaptation during strength training, aging, detraining and immobilization. Crit Rev Phys Rehabil Med 1994;6:161–198.
16. Harris G, Stone MH, O'Bryant HS, et al. Short term performance effects of high speed, high force and combined weight training. J Strength Cond Res 2000;14:14–20.
17. Kraemer WJ. A series of studies: the physiological basis for strength training in American football: fact over philosophy. J Strength Cond Res 1997;11:131–142.
18. Kramer J, Stone MH, O'Bryant HS, et al. Effects of single versus multiple sets of weight training: impact of volume, intensity and variation. J Strength Cond Res 1997;11: 143–147.
19. Marx JO, Ratames NA, Nindl BC, et al. Low-volume circuit versus high-volume periodized resistance training in women. Med Sci Sports Exerc 2001;33:635–643.
20. Matveyev LP. Fundamentals of Sports Training. Moscow: Progress Publishers, 1981.
21. McBride JM, Triplett-McBride TT, Davie A, Newton RU. A comparison of strength and power characteristics between power lifters, Olympic lifters and sprinters. J Strength Cond Res 1999;13:58–66.
22. McBride JM, Triplett-McBride TT, Davie A, Newton RU. The effect of heavy- vs light-load jump squats on the development of strength, power, and speed. J Strength Cond Res 2002;16:75–82.
23. McDonagh MJN, Hayward CM, Davies CTM. Isometric training in human elbow flexor muscles. J Bone Joint Surg 1983;64:355–358.
24. Medvedev AS, Rodionov VF, Rogozkin VN, Gulyants AE. Training content of weightlifters during the preparation period. Yessis M (trans). Teoriya I Praktika Fizicheskoi Kultury 1981;12:5–7.
25. Melby C, Scholl C, Edwards G, Bullough R. Effect of acute resistance exercise on postexercise energy expenditure and resting metabolic rate. J Appl Physiol 1993; 75:1847–1853.

26. Mujika I, Padilla S. Scientific basis for precompetition tapering strategies. Med Sci Sports Exerc 2003;35: 1182–1187.

27. Newton RU, Kraemer WJ, Hakkinen K, et al. Kinematics, kinetics and muscle activation during explosive upper body movements. J Appl Biomech 1996;12:31–43.

28. O'Bryant HS, Byrd R, Stone MH. Cycle ergometer and maximum leg and hip strength adaptations to two different methods of weight training. J Appl Sports Sci Res 1988;2:27–30.

29. Plisk S, Stone MH. Periodization strategies. Strength Cond 2003;25:19–37.

30. Sale DG. Neural adaptations to strength training. In: Komi PV, ed. Strength and Power in Sport. London: Blackwell, 1992:249–265.

31. Rhea MR, Alvar BA, Ball SD, Burnett LN. Three sets of weight training superior to 1 set with equal intensity for eliciting strength. J Strength Cond Res 2002;16:525–529.

32. Siff M. Biomechanical foundations of strength and power training. In: Zatsiorsky V, ed. Biomechanics in Sport. London: Blackwell, 2001:103–139.

33. Stone MH, Fleck SJ, Triplett NT, Kraemer WJ. Health- and performance-related potential of resistance training. Sports Med 1998;11:210–231.

34. Stone MH, Fry AC. Increased Training Volume in Strength/Power Athletes. Overtraining in Sport. Champaign, IL: Human Kinetics, 1997:87–106.

35. Stone MH, Keith R, Kearney JT, et al. Overtraining: A review of the signs and symptoms of overtraining. J Appl Sports Sci Res 1991;5:35–50.

36. Stone MH, Moir G, Glaister M, Sanders R. How much strength is necessary? Phys Ther Sport 2002;3:88–96.

37. Stone MH, O'Bryant H. Weight Training: A Scientific Approach. 2nd ed. Minneapolis: Burgess Publishing, 1987.

38. Stone MH, O'Bryant H, Garhammer J, et al. theoretical model of strength training. NSCA J 1982;4:36–39.

39. Stone MH, O'Bryant HS, McCoy L, et al. Power and maximum strength relationships during performance of dynamic and static weighted jumps. J Strength Cond Res 2003;17:140–147.

40. Stone MH, O'Bryant HS, Pierce KC, et al. Periodization: Effects of manipulating volume and intensity. Part 1. Strength Cond 1999;21:56–62.

41. Stone MH, O'Bryant HS, Pierce KC, et al. Periodization: effects of manipulating volume and intensity. Part 2. Strength Cond 1999;21:54–60.

42. Stone MH, Plisk S, Collins D. Training principle: evaluation of modes and methods of resistance training—a coaching perspective. Sport Biomech 2002;1:79–104.

43. Stone MH, Plisk SS, Stone ME, et al. Athletic performance development: volume load—1 set versus multiple sets, training velocity and training variation. Strength Cond 1998;20:22–31.

44. Stone MH, Potteiger J, Proulx CM, et al. Comparison of the effects of three different weight training programs on the 1 RM squat. J Strength Cond Res 2000;14:332–337.

45. Stone MH, Sanborn K, O'Bryant HS, et al. Maximum strength-power-performance relationships in collegiate throwers. J Strength Cond 2003;17:739–745.

46. Verkhoshansky YV. Fundamentals of Special Strength Training in Sport. Moscow: Fizkultura i Spovt, 1977; [English version (trans Charniga A Jr)] Livonia, MI: Sportivny Press, 1986.

47. Williamson DL, Kirwan JP. A single bout of concentric resistance exercises increases BMR 48 hours after exercise in healthy 59–77 year old men. J Gerontol 1997;52A: M352–M355.

48. Willoughby DS. The effects of mesocycle-length weight training programs involving periodization and partially equated volumes on upper and lower body strength. J Strength Cond Res 1993;7:2–8.

49. Wilson GJ, Newton RU, Murphy AJ, Humphries BJ. The optimal training load for the development of dynamic athletic performance. Med Sci Sports Exerc 1993;25: 1279–1286.

50. Zajac FE, Gordon ME. Determining muscle's force and action in multi-articular movement. In: Pandolph K, ed. Exercise and Sport Sciences Reviews. Baltimore: Williams & Wilkins, 1989;17:187–230.

51. Zatsiorsky VM. Science and Practice of Strength Training. Champaign, IL: Human Kinetics, 1995.

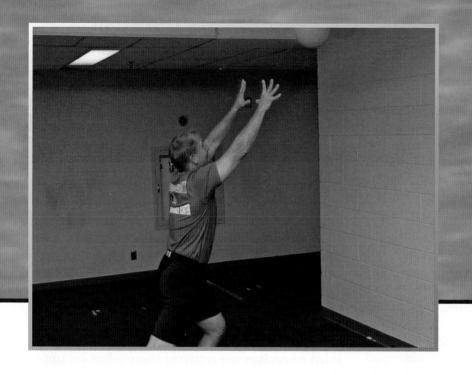

CHAPTER 13

Resistance Exercise Prescription

BARRY A. SPIERING
WILLIAM J. KRAEMER

Introduction

The prescription of a resistance exercise program presents a formidable challenge to the strength and conditioning professional. One must consider a multitude of variables (e.g., choice of exercises, number of repetitions) while attempting to design appropriate resistance-training programs that meet the needs of athletes involved in a variety of sports and activities. Fortunately, however, by following a sequential procedure based on scientific evidence and not on anecdotal recommendations, the practitioner can design a resistance-training program that is specific to the sport/activity, is individualized to the athlete's needs, allows for long-term progression, and provides the opportunity for athletic achievement.

NEEDS ANALYSIS

The first step in designing a resistance-training program is performing a needs analysis. To ensure optimal performance, it is imperative that the resistance-training program be individualized in accordance with the specific needs of the sport/activity and of the athlete. These needs can be ascertained by answering the following questions:

- What are the physiological needs of the sport (e.g., muscular strength, hypertrophy)?
- Which specific muscle groups are most important for the sport?
- What types of muscle actions are needed and used in the sport?
- What are the athlete's physical strengths and weaknesses? (These qualities are addressed in Chapter 8, "Test Administration and Interpretation.")
- What types of equipment are available?
- In which phase of the competitive season is the athlete?
- Does the athlete have any health/injury concerns?
- What are the common sites of injury for the sport/activity?

Answering these questions will provide the fundamental information necessary for designing the resistance-training regimen and set the stage for the implementation and manipulation of acute program variables.

Performing a needs analysis assists the strength and conditioning professional in designing a specific and individualized resistance exercise program.

ACUTE PROGRAM VARIABLES

Once the needs of the individual have been determined, the practitioner can begin to design a resistance-training program. Like any other professional, a strength and conditioning expert has specific "tools" with which to work, referred to as *acute program variables.* An appreciation of how to properly implement and manipulate acute program variables ensures that the program will meet the specific needs of the athlete, allow optimal pro-

gression over time, and prevent training plateaus. Therefore, this section introduces the acute program variables and their influence on the responses and adaptations to resistance exercise.

Exercise Selection

In general, exercises commonly used in resistance-training programs can be classified in terms of either single or multiple joints or either large or small muscle groups. **Single-joint exercises** stress one joint (or muscle group). For example, the arm curl stresses elbow flexion (biceps muscle group). These exercises are used to isolate and target specific muscle groups and are believed to pose less risk of injury due to the reduced level of skill and technique involved (66). Alternatively, **multiple-joint exercises** stress two or more joints (or muscle groups).

Multiple-joint exercises that stress large muscle groups invoke a greater metabolic and hormonal stimulus than single-joint exercises that stress small muscle groups.

For example, the back squat stresses hip and knee extension (gluteus, hamstrings, and quadriceps muscle groups). These exercises require more complex neural activation and coordination; however, it is believed that they are more effective for increasing muscular strength and power (66) (Box 13.1). Several forms of resistance training

---

13.1 FREE WEIGHTS AND MACHINES

Strength and conditioning professionals are often faced with the option of using free weights, machines, or both to train a specific movement or muscle group. Before making this decision, however, it is important that one be aware of the advantages and disadvantages of each. Weight machines are generally believed to be safer to use than free weights because they are easy to learn and allow the athlete to perform exercises that may be difficult with free weights (e.g., leg extensions, leg curls, pull-downs) (35,66). On the other hand, use of free weights may necessitate muscular coordination patterns that more closely mimic movement requirements of a specific task and thus are more beneficial for improving performance (66). Therefore, it is recommended that novice athletes use both free-weight and machine exercises, while free-weight exercises are emphasized for experienced athletes (66).

(Box 13.2) can be utilized in developing a sport-specific conditioning program.

Larger-muscle-group exercises (e.g., back squat) invoke significantly greater metabolic responses than smaller-muscle-group exercises (e.g., arm curl) (8). Furthermore, large-muscle-group exercises evoke greater acute anabolic hormonal responses (72). For example, exercises such as dead lifts (31), squat jumps (130), and Olympic lifts (72) produce greater testosterone and growth hormone responses than exercises such as bench press and seated shoulder press. Therefore, the amount of muscle mass involved has direct implications for metabolic and hormonal responses to resistance training.

An important concept to consider in designing a resistance-training program is the agonist/antagonist/stabilizer relationship. By performing physical activities and sport-specific resistance training, the prime movers undergo significant adaptations to increase performance. As the agonist increases its capabilities, however, the antagonist may become increasingly susceptible to injury. Therefore, it is recommended that all major muscle groups be trained during resistance exercise programs to ensure that appropriate attention is given to both agonist and antagonist muscle groups to prevent muscle imbalances and minimize the risk of injury.

> *All major muscle groups should be trained during a resistance exercise program.*

Exercise Order

Exercise order (the sequencing of specific exercises within a session) significantly affects force production and fatigue rate during a resistance exercise

---

13.2 FORMS OF RESISTANCE TRAINING

Although resistance training typically involves barbells, dumbbells, and machines, it should be pointed out that other forms of resistance training are available. For example, a strength and conditioning practitioner may also wish to include medicine balls, plyometrics, stretchable tubing, and partner-assisted exercises. These forms of resistance add diversity to the "choice of exercise" acute program variable. Moreover, since less resistance is applied during these exercises, high-velocity movements can be effectively trained in a sport-specific manner (e.g., plyometrics).

---

session (45). As already discussed, multiple-joint exercises are considered more effective in increasing muscular strength than single-joint exercises. Therefore, these exercises should be given priority within the training session (i.e., placed early in the training sessions when fatigue is minimal). The following recommendations regarding exercise order have been made (66). When all major muscle groups are being trained in a workout:

■ Perform large-muscle-group exercises before small-muscle-group exercises
■ Perform multiple-joint exercises before single-joint exercises
■ Rotate upper- and lower-body exercises
■ Also, for power training, perform total-body exercises (from most to least complex) before basic exercises. For example, perform power cleans before back squats (73). This is especially important when new exercises are being taught.

It is especially important to check for proper technique in an exercise anytime a change is made in the program design (e.g., changing the order of exercise, changing the rest period lengths) as this could have an impact on the skills of a particular lift, with the more complex multijoint exercises (e.g., power cleans) being more sensitive to such program alterations due to the higher technique demands. When training upper-body exercises on one day and lower-body exercises on a separate day:

■ Perform large-muscle-group exercises before small-muscle-group exercises.
■ Perform multiple-joint exercises before single-joint exercises.
■ Rotate opposing (agonist and antagonist) exercises.

When individual muscle groups are being trained:

■ Perform multiple-joint exercises before single-joint exercises.
■ Perform higher-intensity exercises (i.e., those that require a greater percentage of the exerciser's one repetition maximum) before lower-intensity exercises.

Loading

Load (i.e., intensity) is the amount of weight lifted or the resistance with which one exercises; it is highly dependent upon other acute program variables such as exercise order (114), muscle action

(62), and rest-interval length (64). Furthermore, there is an inverse relation between the load and the maximal number of repetitions performed: as the load increases the number of repetitions that can be performed decreases. Loading is typically prescribed as a percentage of the athlete's one-repetition maximum (1 RM) (e.g., 85% of 1 RM) (Box 13.3) or as a weight that allows a specific number of repetitions (e.g., 6 RM). Alterations in training load affect hormonal (67–69,72,103), neural (63,107), and metabolic (32,123) responses and adaptations to resistance training.

Certain muscular characteristics are best trained using specific RM loads (Fig. 13.1). For example, optimal gains in strength are obtained by training at loads heavier than 6 RM. This is not to say that improvements in hypertrophy or endurance will not occur at such loads; however, these characteristics will not be optimally trained.

Volume

Training **volume** is typically expressed as (66):

$$Volume = sets\,(number) \times repetitions\,(number)$$
$$\times resistance\,(weight)$$

Training volume can be manipulated by altering the number of exercises performed per ses-

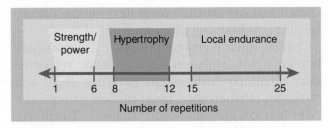

FIGURE 13.1 The repetition maximum (RM) continuum. Certain muscular characteristics are best trained using a specific RM load.

sion, the number of sets performed per exercise, or the number of repetitions performed per set. As with training intensity, changes in training volume influence neural (48), metabolic (132), and hormonal (23,39,65,67–69,95,129) responses and adaptations to resistance exercise.

Increased metabolic and hormonal responses are associated with high training volume.

Rest Intervals

Rest intervals between sets and exercises can have significant influence on the responses and adaptations to resistance exercise. Responses to short rest intervals include elevated heart rate and subjective ratings of perceived exertion (RPE) (71), increased lactate (21) and growth hormone (67–69) concentrations, and reduced performance during subsequent sets (64). Over the course of 4 weeks, short (30- to 40-second) rest intervals were shown to attenuate strength increases as compared to long (2- to 3-minute) rest intervals (102,105).

Short rest periods are associated with greater metabolic and hormonal responses; however, short rest periods may attenuate strength gains.

Frequency and Workout Structure

Training **frequency** is the number of training sessions performed during a specific period (e.g., 3 sessions per week) and is dependent on volume, intensity, exercise selection, level of conditioning and/or training status, recovery ability, nutritional intake, and training goals. Sessions using heavy loads, intense eccentric contractions, and/or large-muscle-group or multiple-joint exercises may

---

13.3 PROTOCOL FOR DETERMINING ONE-REPETITION-MAXIMUM (1-RM) STRENGTH

1. Ten repetitions at 50% of estimated 1 RM
   - One to two minutes rest
2. Three to five repetitions at 75% of estimated 1 RM
   - Two to four minutes rest
3. One repetition at 90% of estimated 1 RM
   - Two to four minutes rest
4. Increase the load by 5% to 10% and attempt another 1-RM lift
   - Two to four minutes rest
5. Continue process of increasing the load by 5% to 10% and attempting 1-RM lifts until the athlete can no longer lift the weight through the full range of motion using correct technique. 1 RM should be determined within five 1-RM attempts.

require increased recovery time before subsequent sessions. For example, it has been shown that untrained women of various ages recovered only 90% to 94% of their strength 2 days after a leg press routine of five sets of 10 repetitions using a 10-RM load (42), indicating that additional rest may be required for such populations before the next training bout.

Studies have shown that two to three sessions per week on alternating days is appropriate for untrained individuals (22,52); however, this does not imply that increased frequency is required for intermediate or advanced lifters. The primary advantage of increasing training frequency is that it allows for greater specialization (i.e., greater exercise selection and/or volume per muscle group in accordance with specific goals). For example, compare the two sample workouts in Table 13.1. Workout A uses a total-body exercise design with a frequency of two sessions per week. Alternatively, Workout B employs a **split-routine** design with a frequency of four sessions per week. If time restraints allow four exercises to be performed per workout, then using Workout B permits the athlete to perform twice as many exercises per muscle group per workout than Workout A while maintaining the number of times per week that each muscle group is trained; although, the total weekly time commitment is twice as much for Workout B.

With this in mind, the following recommendations have been made (66):

- For entire-body training, it is recommended that athletes train 2 to 3 days per week.
- For split-routine workouts, an overall frequency of 3 to 4 days per week is recommended, while ensuring that each muscle group is trained only 1 to 2 days per week.

The frequency of training is affected by the phase of the competitive season (Box 13.4). Table 13.2 provides recommendations on the frequency of resistance training based on the competitive season.

Muscle Action

Most resistance exercises include concentric (CON) and eccentric (ECC) muscle actions. CON means that the muscle is shortened as it is activated; ECC indicates that the muscle is lengthened as it is activated. For example, consider the arm curl exercise. As the weight is lifted, the biceps perform a CON action. Alternatively, as the weight is lowered, the biceps perform an ECC action. Although ECC actions result in more delayed onset muscle soreness (26) than CON actions, improvements in dynamic muscular strength are greatest when ECC actions are included in the repetition movement (as opposed to CON-only movements) (25). Considering that exercises typically used within resistance-training programs include CON and ECC muscle actions, that excluding CON movements reduces gains in strength, and that there is not much potential for variation in this acute program variable, it is

TABLE 13.1	EXAMPLE TRAINING FREQUENCIES AND WORKOUT STRUCTURES				
	MONDAY	TUESDAY	WEDNESDAY	THURSDAY	FRIDAY
Workout A	1. Back squat	Off	Off	1. Back squat	Off
Frequency:	2. Dead lift			2. Dead lift	
2 sessions · wk⁻¹	3. Bench press			3. Bench press	
Design: Total body	4. Lat pull			4. Lat pull	
Workout B	1. Back squat	1. Bench press	Off	1. Back squat	1. Bench press
Frequency:	2. Dead lift	2. Lat pull		2. Dead lift	2. Lat pull
4 sessions · wk⁻¹	3. Leg extension	3. Arm extension		3. Leg extension	3. Arm extension
Design: Split routine	4. Leg curl	4. Arm curl		4. Leg curl	4. Arm curl

13.4 TRAINING FREQUENCY AND THE COMPETITIVE SEASON

The prescription of resistance training frequency is affected by the phase of the competitive season (e.g., off season, in season). As greater emphasis is placed on sport skills and practice, the strength and conditioning professional must reduce the frequency of resistance training, which reduces the chance of overtraining the athlete and is necessary due to time constraints. See Table 13.2 for frequency recommendations based on competitive season.

recommended that CON and ECC muscle actions are included in all resistance-training programs.

Resistance-training exercises should include concentric and eccentric muscle actions.

Repetition Velocity

Force is equal to mass times acceleration; therefore significant reductions in force can occur when repetitions are moved slowly. Unintentionally and intentionally slow repetition velocity can occur during resistance exercises. Unintentionally slow velocities occur when individuals are attempting to exert maximal force but, due to high loading or fatigue, the weight travels at a slow velocity. This phenomenon was demonstrated in a study examining repetition velocity during a 5-repetition-maximum (5-RM) bench press set. It was shown that the first three repetitions were approximately 1.2 to 1.6 seconds in duration, while the last two were 2.5 and 3.3 seconds in duration, respectively (92).

Intentionally slow velocities are used with submaximal loads, which allow the individual greater control of the velocity. Research has shown that concentric force production was significantly lower for an intentionally slow velocity (5-second CON; 5-second ECC) compared to a voluntary velocity (771 versus 1,167 N, respectively) (61). Furthermore, over the course of 10 weeks, use of a very slow velocity (10-second CON; 5-second ECC) compared to a slow velocity (2-second CON; 4-second ECC) program led to significantly less strength gains (60). Compared to slow velocities, moderate and fast velocities have been shown to be more effective for increasing the number of repetitions performed, work and power output, and volume (77,94) and for increasing the rate of strength gains (51).

Athletes should intend to perform exercises with a fast lifting velocity, as intentionally slow lifting velocities diminish strength gains.

RESISTANCE-TRAINING PRESCRIPTION

After the needs analysis has been performed, the next step in designing a resistance-training program is to implement the acute program variables within an individualized regimen. One of the most critical principles for the strength and conditioning practitioner to keep in mind while designing a program is the **SAID principle: s**pecific **a**daptations to **i**mposed **d**emands. The essence of this principle is that the adaptations to resistance exercise, or any exercise for that matter, are specific to the demands of the program; the demands of the program, in turn, are determined by the acute program variables.

Specificity refers to the muscle groups being trained, the velocity of the movement, and the metabolic requirements of the exercise. For example, if an athlete requires increased muscular endurance of the lower-body extensors to be successful in his or her sport, then, to achieve the desired results, the strength and conditioning coach must implement a program that taxes the lower-body extensors and metabolic processes. Therefore, the following sections discuss the influence of the acute program variables on the trainable characteristics; specifically, strength, power, hypertrophy, and local muscular endurance.

TABLE 13.2	RESISTANCE TRAINING FREQUENCY RECOMMENDATIONS BASED ON COMPETITIVE SEASON (34,121,125)
PHASE OF COMPETITIVE SEASON	**TRAINING FREQUENCY (SESSIONS PER WEEK)**
Off season	4–6
Preseason	3–4
In season	1–2
Postseason	1–3

Muscular Strength

Muscular strength is the ability of the neuro-muscular system to generate force. The expression of muscular strength is dependent on the nervous system's ability to recruit motor units and the contractile capabilities of the muscle fibers. Resistance training is very commonly prescribed to increase muscular strength because it has been shown to enhance neural function (e.g., increased motor unit recruitment and frequency of stimulation) (78,90,107) and increase the muscle fibers' force-generating capacity via increased cross-sectional area (4,85,116).

EXERCISE SELECTION

Research has shown that single- (40,100) and multiple-joint exercises (46,47,64,120) are effective for increasing muscular strength. For optimal strength gains, however, it is recommended (66) that emphasis be placed on multiple-joint exercises (e.g., back squat, bench press). These exercises are regarded as most effective for increasing overall strength, since they enable a greater amount of weight to be lifted (122). Alternatively, single-joint exercises may be used to target specific muscle groups (e.g., arm curl). Single-joint exercises may also pose less risk of injury, since less skill and technique are involved.

For optimal gains in muscular strength, it is recommended that multiple-joint exercises be emphasized.

LOADING

Initial loading prescription depends heavily on the athlete's training status. For novices, loads as low as 45% to 50% of 1 RM have been shown to increase muscular strength (5,37,108,118,131). This initial phase of strength gain in untrained individuals is characterized by improved motor learning and coordination (106); therefore, heavy loads may not be required. Alternatively, for experienced lifters, greater loading is necessary for improvements in muscular strength. Studies (13,17,131) have shown that loads greater than approximately 80% to 85% of 1 RM (i.e., 1 to 6 RM) are most effective for increasing muscular strength.

Loading for strength gains is dependent on initial training status; novices may improve with loads as little as 45% to 50% of 1 RM, while experienced lifters may require loads of at least 80 to 85% of 1 RM.

VOLUME

Low-volume (i.e., high loads, low repetitions, and moderate to high number of sets) programs are characteristic of strength training (46). Research has shown that muscular strength can be improved using two (24,83), three (12,13,64,116,117), four to five (25,53,56,89), and six or more (54,108) sets per exercise. Much like training intensity, however, the optimal training volume seems to depend on training status.

Studies have compared a popular single-set training approach to multiple-set exercise programs. Some studies have reported that single-set training in untrained individuals was as effective as multiple-set programs in increasing muscular strength (20,115), although other studies have shown that multiple-set programs were superior (12,15,109,119,124). This is probably due to the fact that early training adaptations are a result of neural adaptations (e.g., improvements in muscle activation and coordination) (106). On the other hand, trained athletes seem to require a higher training volume than untrained athletes. Studies have shown that multiple-set programs are superior for improving strength in trained individuals (64,74,75,111), with one study showing equivocal findings (49).

Multiple-set programs are recommended for improving muscular strength in all athletes; however, single-set programs may be used during the initial weeks of training in untrained individuals.

REST INTERVALS

As previously stated, rest intervals affect physiological and performance responses and adaptations to resistance exercise. Since longitudinal studies (102,105) have shown greater strength increases with long rest intervals, it is recommended that rest periods of at least 2 to 3 minutes be used between sets for **fundamental exercises** (e.g., back squat). For **assistance exercises** (e.g., leg curls), 1 to 2 minutes of rest may suffice (66).

Programs aimed at improving muscular strength require long rest periods (i.e., > 2 to 3 minutes) between sets and exercises

REPETITION VELOCITY

Research has shown that muscular strength may be increased using repetition training velocities ranging from 30 to $300°·s^{-1}$ (22,54,30,58,76,91,

Q & A from the Field

The strength coach at a neighboring university trains his athletes using one set to failure for each exercise. I've noticed other strength coaches using a similar philosophy. Is it the best approach for improved athletic performance?

—*undergraduate exercise physiology major*

"One set to failure" programs are used in a few major university strength and conditioning programs; however, this does not mean that it is the best (or even a good) approach to training athletes.

In untrained athletes (e.g., college freshmen with little resistance training experience), one set *may* be as good as multiple sets for initial, short-term strength gains (20,115).

For athletes with significant resistance-training experience, however, it is clear that multiple-set routines are superior for strength gains (64,74,75,111). Therefore, although anecdotal reports may suggest that single-set programs are desirable for athletes, scientific evidence supports the use of multiple-set routines in experienced athletes for long-term gains in strength.

96,128). Strength increases are specific to the training repetition velocity, however, with some carryover above and below the training velocity (~30°·s⁻¹) (34). Training at a moderate velocity (180–240°·s⁻¹) appears to produce the greatest strength increases across all testing velocities (58).

 Moderate training velocities should be emphasized for increasing muscular strength.

Muscular Power

The expression of muscular power is important from a sport perspective, since athletes are typically required to produce a high level of force in a limited amount of time; for example, swinging a bat or jumping for a rebound. *Power* is defined as work divided by time. In a practical sense, power is increased by performing greater work in the same amount of time or by performing the same work in less time. Neuromuscular contributions to maximal muscle power include maximal rate of force development (43), muscular strength at slow and fast contraction velocities (59), stretch-shortening cycle performance (16), and coordination of movement pattern and skill (112,135). Maximal mechanical power appears to be best trained with resistances from 30% to 45% of 1 RM in exercises with minimum deceleration phases in the lift (e.g., hang pulls, squat jumps, etc.). Power output can be trained at higher percentages of the 1 RM, but translation to maximal mechanical power output must include higher-velocity exercise using lighter loadings. Thus, periodized training with a loading variety is essential for optimal training of power.

EXERCISE SELECTION

Multiple-joint total-body exercises (e.g., power clean, push press) have been used extensively for power training and have been shown to require rapid force production (36). The inherent problem with traditional resistance exercises is that the load is decelerated for a significant portion of the movement. Studies examining the bench press have shown that deceleration occurs during 24% to 40% of the concentric movement (27,99); the deceleration phase increases to 52% in performing the lift with a lower percentage (81%) of 1 RM (27), and it increases with attempts to move the bar rapidly to train at a high movement velocity (99). Ballistic resistance exercises (explosive movements that enable acceleration throughout the full range of motion) have been shown to limit this problem (97,98,134). For instance, loaded jump squats with 30% of 1-RM loads have been shown to increase vertical jump performance to a greater extent than traditional back squats (134).

 Multiple-joint ballistic exercises that minimize deceleration are recommended for improving muscular power.

LOADING

Several studies have shown improved power performance following a traditional resistance-training program (2,10,19,133,134). Traditional resistance training, however, typically improves power only at slow movement velocities (41). Programs utilizing relatively light loads have been shown to be more effective than traditional resistance training for improving vertical jump performance (43,44).

REAL-WORLD APPLICATION
Concentric Force-Velocity Curve

The concentric force-velocity curve is an important concept in training for power and maximal athletic performance. All exercises have a power output, some very low and some high. Highest power outputs are seen with heavy weights moved explosively. Power is a critical component of many competitive sports. "A" represents a high-force, low-velocity movement, such as a 1-RM max on a squat. "B" represents a low-force, high-velocity movement, such as throwing a baseball at maximal velocity. "C" represents training intentionally slowly, moving away from the force-velocity curve. To shift the force-velocity curve up and to the right (to improve power), training must be as close as possible to the curve. If sport-specific performance is at the high-force/low-velocity end of the force-velocity curve, as in the case of a powerlifter, for example, training should move to the high-force/low-velocity end of the continuum as the competitive season approaches. If sport-specific performance is at the high-velocity/low-force end of the force-velocity curve, as with a baseball pitcher, for example, training should move to the high-velocity/low-force end of the continuum as the competitive season approaches.

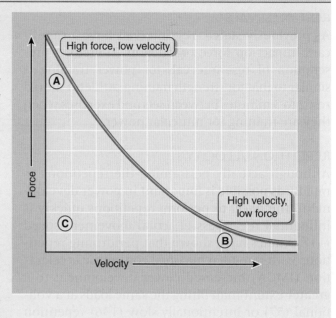

It appears that the use of light to moderate loads at high velocities increases force output at higher velocities (44).

The optimal load for maximal power output may vary between 30 and 60% of 1 RM, depending on the choice of exercise. Research using trained athletes has shown that loads of 30% of 1 RM maximized performance following ballistic jump-squat training (134), while loads of 45% to 60% of 1 RM maximized power output during single bouts of jump squats and bench-press throws (6,7). It is important to note, however, that simultaneously training for strength (i.e., heavy load training) and power (i.e., light load training) provides the basis for optimal power development and continued increases in power output by increasing the force and time components of the power equation. Figure 13.2 demonstrates that training at a variety of velocities and loads will cause positive adaptations along the entire force-velocity curve.

> *For optimal power development, a periodized program emphasizing strength development (i.e., 85% to 100% of 1 RM) with the integration of light-load, high-velocity movements (30% to 45% of 1 RM) is recommended. Training at a variety of loads and velocities will maximize power output through a continuum of velocities.*

VOLUME

Recommended volume for power training is similar to that for strength training. Multiple (three to six) sets of power exercises consisting of one to six repetitions integrated into a strength training

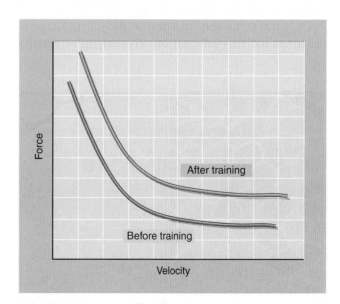

FIGURE 13.2 Impact of power training at fast, moderate, and slow velocities on the force-velocity curve. Training should be at a spectrum of velocities to see increases in power across all movement speeds.

program is recommended for maximizing power development.

REST INTERVALS

As previously stated, rest intervals have a significant impact on force production. Therefore, prescription of rest intervals for power training is similar to that for strength training. Athletes should rest 2 to 3 minutes between sets and exercises when they are training for muscular power.

REPETITION VELOCITY

Although actually performing the repetitions as rapidly as possible is important in power development, the *intent* to perform repetitions quickly is influential regardless of actual movement speed (11). Studies have shown that performing repetitions with intended maximal concentric acceleration (IMCA) increased power development to a greater extent than lifting the same loads at a volitional (57) or intentionally slow (136) repetition velocity.

 Regardless of the load used, in training for muscular power, repetitions should be performed with intended maximal concentric acceleration.

Muscular Hypertrophy

Resistance training promotes an increase in muscle cross-sectional area (CSA) (Fig. 13.3). Mechanical damage resulting from loaded eccentric muscle actions promotes hypertrophy (9,38,79,87); however, it has not been shown that muscle damage is required for this adaptation. Hypertrophy results

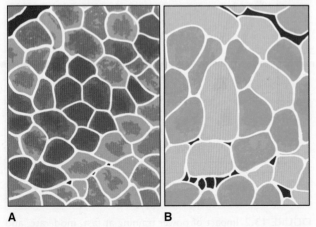

A   **B**

FIGURE 13.3 Micrographs of a muscle biopsy **A.** before and **B.** after 8 weeks of resistance training. It is easy to see that the fibers hypertrophied following the training program.

from an accumulation of proteins via increased rate of synthesis, decreased degradation, or both (14). Following a bout of resistance exercise, protein synthesis elevates at 2 to 3 hours, peaks at approximately 24 hours, and returns to baseline levels at around 36 to 48 hours after exercise (80). Fast-twitch muscle fibers typically increase in CSA to a greater extent than slow-twitch fibers (4,50, 85). The process of tissue remodeling is affected by concentrations of testosterone, growth hormones, cortisol, insulin, and insulin-like growth factor, which have been shown to increase during and following an acute bout of resistance exercise (1,65,68,69,72,86,103,116).

The time course of muscle hypertrophy has been examined during short-term training periods in previously untrained subjects. During the early weeks of training, it appears that the nervous system plays a primary role in the observed increments in strength (93). Muscle hypertrophy is evident by 6 to 7 weeks of training (101), although changes in the quality of proteins (116), fiber types (116), and rates of protein synthesis (101) take place much earlier. From this point onward, there appears to be an interplay between neural adaptations and hypertrophy in the expression of strength (107).

EXERCISE SELECTION

Single- and multiple-joint exercises have been shown to be effective for increasing muscular hypertrophy (21,64). Interestingly, the complexity of exercises may affect the time course of muscle hypertrophy. Multiple-joint exercises require a longer neural adaptive phase, which may delay the hypertrophic response (18). As previously stated, however, multiple-joint exercises induce a greater hormonal response, which is important for maximal gains in muscle size.

 Muscular hypertrophy can be induced by single- and multiple-joint exercises; however, multiple-joint exercises should be emphasized for maximal long-term gains in muscle size.

LOADING AND VOLUME

Various types of resistance-training programs have been shown to elicit muscular hypertrophy. Training programs aimed at maximizing hypertrophy, however, typically emphasize moderate to heavy loads (70% to 85% of 1 RM) and high volume (8 to 12 repetitions for multiple sets) (72). These programs stimulate greater acute increases in testosterone and growth hormone than high-load, low-volume regimens (i.e., programs that empha-size gains in muscular strength) (68,69). This has been supported in part by greater hypertrophy associated with high-volume, multiple-set pro-grams compared to low-volume, single-set pro-grams in resistance-trained individuals (64,74).

> *To optimize muscular hypertrophy, resistance-training programs should emphasize moderate to heavy loads (70% to 85% of 1 RM) and high volume (6 to 12 repetitions with multiple sets).*

REST INTERVALS

Short rest periods (of 1 to 2 minutes) used in accor-dance with moderate to high intensity and volume elicit greater acute anabolic hormone responses than programs utilizing very heavy loads and long rest periods (e.g., 3 minutes) (68,69). One study, however, reported no significant difference in mus-cle girth, skin folds, or body mass between proto-cols using 30, 90, and 180 seconds of rest between sets in recreationally trained men over 5 weeks (105). Therefore, to date, it is unclear whether the use of short rest periods to maximize the anabolic hormonal response to resistance exercise is impor-tant for maximizing muscular hypertrophy. Based on this information and the fact that rest periods significantly affect strength gains, we recommend rest periods of 2 to 3 minutes between sets in fun-damental exercises and 1 to 2 minutes between sets for assistance exercises.

REPETITION VELOCITY

Little is known about the effect of repetition veloc-ity on muscle hypertrophy. It has been suggested that higher velocities of movement pose less of a stimulus for hypertrophy than slow and moderate velocities (127); however, further research is nec-essary to substantiate this proposition. Therefore, in training for muscular hypertrophy, the prescription of repetition velocity is secondary to the load, rep-etition number, and goals of the particular exercise.

Local Muscular Endurance

Resistance exercise has been shown to improve local muscular endurance (5,55,81,88,123). Typ-ically, resistance training has been shown to increase absolute muscular endurance, which is the maximal number of repetitions performed with a specific pretraining load (e.g., 150 lb) (5,55,64); however, limited effects on relative muscular en-durance, which is the maximal number of repe-

titions performed at a specific relative intensity (e.g., 50% of 1 RM), have been found (84).

EXERCISE SELECTION

Exercises stressing multiple or large muscle groups are associated with the greatest acute metabolic responses (8,110,126). This is important, since high metabolic demand is a stimulus for adaptations leading to improved local muscular endurance (e.g., increased mitochondrial density and capillary number, fiber-type transitions, buffering capacity). Therefore, it is recommended that exercises for multiple or large muscle groups be emphasized in programs aimed at improving local muscular endurance.

LOADING AND VOLUME

Light loads used in accordance with high repeti-tions (20 or more) have been shown to be most effective for increasing local muscular endurance (5,118). Moderate to heavy loading is also effec-tive for increasing high-intensity and absolute muscular endurance when it is coupled with short rest periods (5,88). In general, high-volume pro-grams are optimal for endurance performance (64,82,118), especially when multiple sets per exercise are performed (64,82,88).

> *Light loads, high repetitions, and high overall volume should be emphasized for improving local muscular endurance.*

REST INTERVALS

Athletes who train using high volume and short rest periods (e.g., body builders) demonstrate a significantly lower fatigue rate in comparison with athletes who train with low to moderate volumes and long rest periods (e.g., power lifters) (71). This finding supports the use of short rest periods in training for local muscular endurance. Therefore, it has been recommended (66) that rest periods of 1 to 2 minutes be used for high-repetition sets (15 to 20 repetitions) and less than 1 minute for mod-erate-repetition sets (10 to 15 repetitions).

REPETITION VELOCITY

Studies examining isokinetic exercise perfor-mance have shown that a fast training velocity (i.e., $180° \cdot s^{-1}$) was more effective than a slow training velocity (i.e., $30° \cdot s^{-1}$) for improving local muscular endurance (3,34). Slow and fast veloc-ities, however, may be effective for improving local muscular endurance during constant external resistance training. Therefore, it has been recommended (66) that intentionally slow velocities be used when a moderate number of repetitions (10 to 15) are used and that moderate to fast velocities be used when a high number of repetitions (15 or more) are used.

PROGRESSION

Up to this point, we have discussed the manipulation of acute program variables to achieve a desired result. It should be noted, however, that these variables require continued alteration so that long-term progression can occur. **Progression** has been previously defined as "the act of moving forward or advancing toward a specific goal" (66). Although it is impossible to improve at the same rate over the course of a long-term resistance-training program, the proper manipulation of acute program variables can limit training plateaus and consequently enable achievement of a high level of muscular fitness. The three general principles of progression are progressive overload, variation, and specificity.

Progressive Overload

Progressive overload is the gradual increase of stress placed on the body during resistance-exercise training (66). As training duration proceeds, there is an increase in exercise tolerance. Continued gains in performance, however, will occur only if the body's adaptive processes are progressively taxed. Therefore, gradual increases in physiological demands are required for long-term improvements in physical performance.

Progressive overload may be induced by the following:

1. Increasing the load
2. Adding repetitions to the current load
3. Altering repetition speed according to program goals
4. Altering the length of rest periods according to program goals
5. Increasing volume within reasonable limits (2% to 5% until further adaptation has occurred) (34)

In some cases volume increases may be larger, depending on level of adaptation and starting loads; for example, extremely low starting loads may be rapidly outgrown in the early phases of a beginner program where technique is the limiting factor.

Variation

Variation (or *periodization*) is the alteration of acute program variables over time. Systematically varying volume and intensity is most effective for long-term progression (33,120). Therefore, to ensure long-term gains in performance, it is imperative to plan systematic changes in exercise choice, intensity, volume, and repetition velocity. Concepts of periodization are discussed in detail in Chapter 12.

Specificity

Training adaptations are specific to the muscle actions involved (25), speed of movement (58), range of motion (76), muscle groups trained (70), energy systems involved (71,113), and intensity and volume of training (17,104,111). These facts provide a valuable rationale for performing a needs analysis prior to prescribing a resistance-exercise program. Once the needs of the athlete have been identified, the strength and conditioning practitioner must keep these needs in mind in constructing a resistance-exercise regimen to ensure that the desired goals are being met.

Additionally, the progression of resistance exercise should follow a general-to-specific model (73). For example, if one's goal is to improve vertical jump performance, choice of exercise should progress from general lower-body strengthening exercises (e.g., dead lift, back squat) to explosive lower-body power exercises (e.g., power clean, jump squat). Box 13.5 provides key points in prescribing resistance training to improve athletic performance.

13.5 KEY POINTS IN PRESCRIBING RESISTANCE TRAINING TO IMPROVE ATHLETIC PERFORMANCE

1. The needs analysis determines the goals of the program.
2. The goals of the program determine the implementation of acute program variables.
3. The implementation of acute program variables determines the responses and adaptations to resistance exercise.
4. The responses and adaptations to resistance exercise influence athletic performance.

TABLE 13.3	SUMMARY OF RESISTANCE-TRAINING EXERCISE PRESCRIPTION				
	EXERCISE SELECTION	**LOADING**	**VOLUME**	**REST INTERVALS**	**REPETITION VELOCITY**
STRENGTH					
Novice	Single- and multiple-joint	45%–70% of 1 RM	Sets: 1–3 Reps: 8–12	2–3 min for fundamental 1–2 min for assistance	Slow, moderate
Experienced	Emphasize multiple-joint	> 80% of 1 RM	Sets: multiple Reps: 1–6	2–3 min for fundamental 1–2 min for assistance	Slow, moderate, fast
POWER					
Novice	Multiple-joint	Strength: > 80% of 1 RM Velocity: 30%–60% of 1 RM	Sets: 1–3 Reps: 3–6	2–3 min for fundamental 1–2 min for assistance	Intentionally fast
Experienced	Multiple-joint	Strength: > 80% of 1 RM Velocity: 30%–60% of 1 RM	Sets: multiple Reps: 1–6	2–3 min for fundamental 1–2 min for assistance	Intentionally fast
HYPERTROPHY					
Novice	Single- and multiple-joint	60%–70% of 1 RM	Sets: 1–3 sets Reps: 8–12	1–2 min	Slow, moderate
Experienced	Single- and multiple-joint	70%–85% of 1 RM	Sets: multiple Reps: 6–12	1–2 min	Slow, moderate
ENDURANCE					
Novice	Single- and multiple-joint	50%–70% of 1 RM	Sets: 1–3 sets Reps: 10–15	<1 min	Slow, moderate for MR Moderate, fast for HR
Experienced	Emphasize multiple-joint	30%–80% of 1 RM	Sets: multiple Reps: 10 or more	1–2 min for high rep ex. <1 min for moderate rep ex.	Slow, moderate for MR Moderate, fast for HR

HR = high repetitions; MR = moderate repetitions.

SUMMARY

The prescription of a resistance-exercise program is a sequential process that begins with a needs analysis to identify the specific needs of individual athletes. Identified needs can be met by manipulating the acute program variables in a precise manner to produce a desired outcome. Therefore, a sound resistance-training program can be developed via a thorough comprehension of the acute program variables and their respective impact on trainable characteristics. A detailed summary of the essential components of this chapter can be found in Table 13.3.

MAXING OUT

1. Before you design a resistance exercise program, you must first perform a needs analysis. Perform a needs analysis for a basketball team using the questions in the "Needs Analysis" section on page 274 as a guide.
2. You are a strength and conditioning coach for a high school football team. During the season, the head football coach instructs you to design an in-season workout that lasts no longer than 45 min-utes. You can choose resistance-training exercises. List the exercises you would choose and give a brief reason for your choices.
3. You are a strength and conditioning coach in a high school. The school is building a new weight room, and the athletic director wants to equip the weight room with various pieces of machine resis-tance equipment. You have a meeting with the athletic director to discuss your preference of free weights. Outline the major points you will make to the athletic director at this meeting.

CASE EXAMPLE

Designing a Resistance-Training Program for a College Football Player

BACKGROUND

You are a strength and conditioning profes-sional at a college and have been asked to design a resistance-training program for a football player. The player is a running back entering his junior season and has 5 years of resistance-training experience including multiple-joint and Olympic-style lifts. Perform a needs analysis and design an individualized resistance-training program.

CONSIDERATIONS

Football is a high-intensity sport with short peri-ods of play (approximately 5 seconds) inter-spersed with brief rest periods (approximately 30 seconds). Running backs require speed, strength, and power to be successful. This spe-cific athlete already possesses adequate muscle mass and minimal body fat; therefore hyper-trophy and/or changes in body mass are not desired. The athlete is beginning his summer break and is in a "preseason" training phase. The athlete has no injuries or health concerns.

IMPLEMENTATION

Exercise selection. Multiple-joint, large-muscle-mass exercises including power exercises should be emphasized.

Exercise order. (1) Power exercises; (2) multiple-joint large-muscle-mass exercises; (3) single-joint small-muscle-mass exercises

Loading. Power exercises: 30% to 50% of 1 RM
Strength exercises: >80% of 1 RM

Volume. Multiple sets, one to six repetitions per set

Rest intervals. Fundamental exercises: 2 to 3 minutes
Assistance exercises: 1 to 2 minutes

Frequency. Four sessions per week

Workout structure. Split routine

Muscle actions. Concentric and eccentric

Repetition velocity. Power exercises—the repeti-tions are to be performed as quickly as possible
Strength exercises: Volitional speed

RESULTS

Example of a week of training

MONDAY	TUESDAY	WEDNESDAY	THURSDAY	FRIDAY
Bench throws:	Hang pulls:	OFF	Incline press:	Squat jump:
4 sets	3 sets		3 sets	4 sets
3 reps	3 reps		6 reps	3 reps
30% of 1 RM (use medicine ball)	30% of 1 RM		6 RM	30% of 1 RM

MONDAY	TUESDAY	WEDNESDAY	THURSDAY	FRIDAY
Bench press:	Dead lift:		Lat pull-downs:	Back squat:
3 sets	3 sets		3 sets	3 sets
3 reps	6 reps		6 reps	3 reps
3 RM	6 RM		6 RM	3 RM
Bent-over rows:	Front squat:		Arm extension:	Leg press:
3 sets	3 sets		3 sets	3 sets
6 reps	6 reps		6 reps	6 reps
6 RM	6 RM		6 RM	6 RM
Shoulder press:	Leg extension:		Arm curl:	Calf raises:
3 sets	3 sets		3 sets	3 sets
6 reps	6 reps		6 reps	6 reps
6 RM	6 RM		6 RM	6 RM
Pull-ups:	Leg curls:			
3 sets	3 sets			
6 reps	6 reps			
6 RM	6 RM			

Note: This example is for 1 week of training. Follow fundamentals of progression to ensure long-term performance gains.

REFERENCES

1. Adams GR. Role of insulin-like growth factor-I in the regulation of skeletal muscle adaptation to increased loading. Exerc Sport Sci Rev 1998;26:31–60.

2. Adams KJ, O'Shea JP, O'Shea KL, et al. The effect of six weeks of squat, plyometric and squat-plyometric training on power production. J Appl Sport Sci Res 1992;6:36–41.

3. Adeyanju K, Crews TR, Meadors WJ. Effects of two speeds of isokinetic training on muscular strength, power and endurance. J Sports Med Phys Fit 1983;23:352–356.

4. Alway SE, Grumbt WH, Gonyea WJ, et al. Contrasts in muscle and myofibers of elite male and female body-builders. J Appl Physiol 1989;67:24–31.

5. Anderson T, Kearney JT. Effects of three resistance training programs on muscular strength and absolute and relative endurance. Res Q Exerc Sport 1982;53:1–7.

6. Baker D, Nance S, Moore M. The load that maximizes the average mechanical power output during explosive bench press throws in highly trained athletes. J Strength Cond Res 2001;15:20–24.

7. Baker D, Nance S, Moore M. The load that maximizes the average mechanical power output during jump squats in power-trained athletes. J Strength Cond Res 2001;15:92–97.

8. Ballor DL, Becque MD, Katch VL. Metabolic responses during hydraulic resistance exercise. Med Sci Sports Exerc 1987;19:363–367.

9. Barnett JG, Holly RG, Ashmore CR. Stretch-induced growth in chicken wing muscles: biochemical and morphological characterization. Am J Physiol 1980;239: C39–C46.

10. Bauer T, Thayer TE, Baras G. Comparison of training modalities for power development in the lower extremity. J Appl Sport Sci Res 1990;4:115–121.

11. Behm DG, Sale DG. Intended rather than actual movement velocity determines velocity-specific training response. J Appl Physiol 1993;74:359–368.

12. Berger RA. Effect of varied weight training programs on strength. Res Q 1962;33:168–181.

13. Berger RA. Optimum repetitions for the development of strength. Res Q 1962;33:334–338.

14. Booth FW, Thomason DB. Molecular and cellular adaptation of muscle in response to exercise: perspectives of various models. Physiol Rev 1991;71:541–585.

15. Borst SE, De Hoyos DV, Garzarella L, et al. Effects of resistance training on insulin-like growth factor-I and IGF binding proteins. Med Sci Sports Exerc 2001;33: 648–653.

16. Bosco C, Komi PV. Potentiation of the mechanical behavior of the human skeletal muscle through prestretching. Acta Physiol Scand 1979;106:467–472.

17. Campos GE, Luecke TJ, Wendeln HK, et al. Muscular adaptations in response to three different resistance-training regimens: specificity of repetition maximum training zones. Eur J Appl Physiol 2002;88:50–60.

18. Chilibeck PD, Calder AW, Sale DG, et al. A comparison of strength and muscle mass increases during resistance training in young women. Eur J Appl Physiol Occup Physiol 1998;77:170–175.

19. Clutch D, Wilton M, McGown C, et al. The effect of depth jumps and weight training on leg strength and vertical jump. Res Q 1983;54:5–10.

20. Coleman AE. Nautilus vs universal gym strength training in adult males. Am Correct Ther J 1977;31:103–107.

21. Colliander EB, Tesch PA. Effects of eccentric and concentric muscle actions in resistance training. Acta Physiol Scand 1990;140:31–39.

22. Coyle EF, Feiring DC, Rotkis TC, et al. Specificity of power improvements through slow and fast isokinetic training. J Appl Physiol 1981;51:1437–1442.

23. Craig BW, Kang H. Growth hormone release following single versus multiple sets of back squats: total work versus power. J Strength Cond Res 1994;8:270–275.

24. Dudley GA, Djamil R. Incompatibility of endurance- and strength-training modes of exercise. J Appl Physiol 1985;59:1446–1451.

25. Dudley GA, Tesch PA, Miller BJ, et al. Importance of eccentric actions in performance adaptations to resistance training. Aviat Space Environ Med 1991;62:543–550.

26. Ebbeling CB, Clarkson PM. Exercise-induced muscle damage and adaptation. Sports Med 1989;7:207–234.

27. Elliott BC, Wilson GJ, Kerr GK. A biomechanical analysis of the sticking region in the bench press. Med Sci Sports Exerc 1989;21:450–462.

28. Eloranta V, Komi PV. Function of the quadriceps femoris muscle under maximal concentric and eccentric contractions. Electromyogr Clin Neurophysiol 1980;20:159–154.

29. Evans WJ, Patton JF, Fisher EC, et al. Muscle metabolism during high intensity eccentric exercise. In: Biochemistry of Exercise. Champaign, IL: Human Kinetics, 1982.

30. Ewing JL Jr, Wolfe DR, Rogers MA, et al. Effects of velocity of isokinetic training on strength, power, and quadriceps muscle fibre characteristics. Eur J Appl Physiol Occup Physiol 1990;61:159–162.

31. Fahey TD, Rolph R, Moungmee P, et al. Serum testosterone, body composition, and strength of young adults. Med Sci Sports 1976;8:31–34.

32. Fleck SJ. Cardiovascular adaptations to resistance training. Med Sci Sports Exerc 1988;20:S146–151.

33. Fleck SJ. Periodized strength training: a critical review. J Strength Cond Res 1999;13:82–89.

34. Fleck SJ, Kraemer WJ. Designing Resistance Training Programs. 3rd ed. Champaign, IL: Human Kinetics, 2004.

35. Foran B. Advantages and disadvantages of isokinetics, variable resistance and free weights. NSCA J 1985;7:24–25.

36. Garhammer J, Gregor R. Propulsion forces as a function of intensity for weightlifting and vertical jumping. J Appl Sport Sci Res 1992;6:129–134.

37. Gettman LR, Ayres JJ, Pollock ML, et al. The effect of circuit weight training on strength, cardiorespiratory function, and body composition of adult men. Med Sci Sports 1978;10:171–176.

38. Gibala MJ, Interisano SA, Tarnopolsky MA, et al. Myofibrillar disruption following acute concentric and eccentric resistance exercise in strength-trained men. Can J Physiol Pharmacol 2000;78:656–661.

39. Gotshalk LA, Loebel CC, Nindl BC, et al. Hormonal responses of multiset versus single-set heavy-resistance exercise protocols. Can J Appl Physiol 1997;22:244–255.

40. Graves JE, Pollock ML, Jones AE, et al. Specificity of limited range of motion variable resistance training. Med Sci Sports Exerc 1989;21:84–89.

41. Häkkinen K. Neuromuscular and hormonal adaptations during strength and power training. J Sports Med 1989;29:9–26.

42. Häkkinen K. Neuromuscular fatigue and recovery in women at different ages during heavy resistance loading. Electromyogr Clin Neurophysiol 1995;35:403–413.

43. Häkkinen K, Komi PV. Changes in electrical and mechanical behavior of leg extensor muscles during heavy resistance strength training. Scand J Sports Sci 1985;7:55–64.

44. Häkkinen K, Komi PV. The effect of explosive type strength training on electromyographic and force production characteristics of leg extensor muscles during concentric and various stretch-shortening cycle exercises. Scand J Sports Sci 1985;7:65–76.

45. Haäkkinen K, Komi PV, Alen M. Effect of explosive type strength training on isometric force- and relaxation-time, electromyographic and muscle fibre characteristics of leg extensor muscles. Acta Physiol Scand 1985;125:587–600.

46. Häkkinen K, Komi PV, Alen M, et al. EMG, muscle fibre and force production characteristics during a 1 year training period in elite weight-lifters. Eur J Appl Physiol Occup Physiol 1987;56:419–427.

47. Häkkinen K, Pakarinen A, Alen M, et al. Neuromuscular and hormonal adaptations in athletes to strength training in two years. J Appl Physiol 1988;65:2406–2412.

48. Häkkinen K, Pakarinen A, Alen M, et al. Relationships between training volume, physical performance capacity, and serum hormone concentrations during prolonged training in elite weight lifters. Int J Sports Med 1987;8(Suppl 1):61–65.

49. Hass CJ, Garzarella L, de Hoyos D, et al. Single versus multiple sets in long-term recreational weightlifters. Med Sci Sports Exerc 2000;32:235–242.

50. Hather BM, Tesch PA, Buchanan P, et al. Influence of eccentric actions on skeletal muscle adaptations to resistance training. Acta Physiol Scand 1991;143:177–185.

51. Hay JG, Andrews JG, Vaughan CL. Effects of lifting rate on elbow torques exerted during arm curl exercises. Med Sci Sports Exerc 1983;15:63–71.

52. Hickson RC, Hidaka K, Foster C. Skeletal muscle fiber type, resistance training, and strength-related performance. Med Sci Sports Exerc 1994;26:593–598.

53. Hortobagyi T, Barrier J, Beard D, et al. Greater initial adaptations to submaximal muscle lengthening than maximal shortening. J Appl Physiol 1996;81:1677–1682.

54. Housh DJ, Housh TJ, Johnson GO, et al. Hypertrophic response to unilateral concentric isokinetic resistance training. J Appl Physiol 1992;73:65–70.

55. Huczel HA, Clarke DH. A comparison of strength and muscle endurance in strength-trained and untrained women. Eur J Appl Physiol Occup Physiol 1992;64:467–470.

56. Jones DA, Rutherford OM. Human muscle strength training: the effects of three different regimens and the nature of the resultant changes. J Physiol 1987;391:1–11.

57. Jones K, Hunter G, Fleisig G, et al. The effects of compensatory acceleration on upper-body strength and power in collegiate football players. J Strength Cond Res 1999;13:99–105.

58. Kanehisa H, Miyashita M. Specificity of velocity in strength training. Eur J Appl Physiol Occup Physiol 1983;52:104–106.

59. Kaneko M, Fuchimoto T, Toji H, et al. Training effect of different loads on the force-velocity relationship and mechanical power output in human muscle. Scand J Sports Sci 1983;5:50–55.

60. Keeler LK, Finkelstein LH, Miller W, et al. Early-phase adaptations of traditional-speed vs. superslow resistance training on strength and aerobic capacity in sedentary individuals. J Strength Cond Res 2001;15:309–314.

61. Keogh JWL, Wilson GJ, Weatherby RP. A cross-sectional comparison of different resistance training techniques in the bench press. J Strength Cond Res 1999;13:247–258.

62. Komi PV, Kaneko M, Aura O. EMG activity of the leg extensor muscles with special reference to mechanical efficiency in concentric and eccentric exercise. Int J Sports Med 1987;8(Suppl 1):22–29.

63. Komi PV, Vitasalo JH. Signal characteristics of EMG at different levels of muscle tension. Acta Physiol Scand 1976;96:267–276.

64. Kraemer WJ. A series of studies—the physiological basis for strength training in American football: fact over philosophy. J Strength Cond Res 1997;11:131–142.

65. Kraemer WJ. Endocrine responses to resistance exercise. Med Sci Sports Exerc 1988;20:S152–157.

66. Kraemer WJ, Adams K, Cafarelli E, et al. American College of Sports Medicine position stand. Progression models in resistance training for healthy adults. Med Sci Sports Exerc 2002;34:364–380.

67. Kraemer WJ, Fleck SJ, Dziados JE, et al. Changes in hormonal concentrations after different heavy-resistance exercise protocols in women. J Appl Physiol 1993;75:594–604.

68. Kraemer WJ, Gordon SE, Fleck SJ, et al. Endogenous anabolic hormonal and growth factor responses to heavy resistance exercise in males and females. Int J Sports Med 1991;12:228–235.

69. Kraemer WJ, Marchitelli L, Gordon SE, et al. Hormonal and growth factor responses to heavy resistance exercise protocols. J Appl Physiol 1990;69:1442–1450.

70. Kraemer WJ, Nindl BC, Ratamess NA, et al. Changes in muscle hypertrophy in women with periodized resistance training. Med Sci Sports Exerc 2004;36:697–708.

71. Kraemer WJ, Noble BJ, Clark MJ, et al. Physiologic responses to heavy-resistance exercise with very short rest periods. Int J Sports Med 1987;8:247–252.

72. Kraemer WJ, Ratamess NA. Endocrine responses and adaptations to strength and power training. In Komi PV, eds. Strength and Power in Sport. Malden, MA: Blackwell, 2003.

73. Kraemer WJ, Ratamess NA. Fundamentals of resistance training: progression and exercise prescription. Med Sci Sports Exerc 2004;36:674–688.

74. Kraemer WJ, Ratamess N, Fry AC, et al. Influence of resistance training volume and periodization on physiological and performance adaptations in collegiate women tennis players. Am J Sports Med 2000;28:626–633.

75. Kramer JB, Stone MH, O'Bryant H, et al. Effects of single vs. multiple sets of weight training: impact of volume, intensity, and variation. J Strength Cond Res 1997;11:143–147.

76. Knapik JJ, Mawdsley RH, Ramos MU. Angular specificity and test mode specificity of isometric and isokinetic strength training. J Orthop Sports Phys Ther 1983;5:58–65.

77. Lachance PF, Hortobagyi T. Influence of cadence on muscular performance during push-up and pull-up exercises. J Strength Cond Res 1994;8:76–79.

78. Leong B, Kamen G, Patten C, et al. Maximal motor unit discharge rates in the quadriceps muscles of older weight lifters. Med Sci Sports Exerc 1999;31:1638–1644.

79. MacDougall JD. Adaptability of muscle to strength training: a cellular approach. In: Biochemistry of Exercise, vol VI. Champaign, IL: Human Kinetics, 1986.

80. MacDougall JD, Gibala MJ, Tarnopolsky MA, et al. The time course for elevated muscle protein synthesis following heavy resistance exercise. Can J Appl Physiol 1995;20:480–486.

81. Marcinik EJ, Potts J, Schlabach G, et al. Effects of strength training on lactate threshold and endurance performance. Med Sci Sports Exerc 1991;23:739–743.

82. Marx JO, Ratamess NA, Nindl BC, et al. Low-volume circuit versus high-volume periodized resistance training in women. Med Sci Sports Exerc 2001;33:635–643.

83. Mayhew JL, Gross PM. Body composition changes in young women with high resistance weight training. Res Q 1974;45:433–440.

84. Mazzetti SA, Kraemer WJ, Volek JS, et al. The influence of direct supervision of resistance training on strength performance. Med Sci Sports Exerc 2000;32:1175–1184.

85. McCall GE, Byrnes WC, Dickinson A, et al. Muscle fiber hypertrophy, hyperplasia, and capillary density in college men after resistance training. J Appl Physiol 1996;81:2004–2012.

86. McCall GE, Byrnes WC, Fleck SJ, et al. Acute and chronic hormonal responses to resistance training designed to promote muscle hypertrophy. Can J Appl Physiol 1999;24:96–107.

87. McDonagh MJ, Davies CT. Adaptive response of mammalian skeletal muscle to exercise with high loads. Eur J Appl Physiol Occup Physiol 1984;52:139–155.

88. McGee D, Jessee TC, Stone MH, et al. Leg and hip endurance adaptations to three weight-training programs. J Appl Sport Sci Res 1992;6:92–95.

89. McMorris RO, Elkins EC. A study of production and evaluation of muscular hypertrophy. Arch Phys Med Rehabil 1954;35:420–426.

90. Milner-Brown HS, Stein RB, Lee RG. Synchronization of human motor units: possible roles of exercise and supraspinal reflexes. Electroencephalogr Clin Neurophysiol 1975;38:245–254.

91. Moffroid MT, Whipple RH. Specificity of speed of exercise. Phys Ther 1970;50:1692–1700.

92. Mookerjee S, Ratamess NA. Comparison of strength differences and joint action durations between full and partial range-of-motion bench press exercise. J Strength Cond Res 1999;13:76–81.

93. Moritani T, deVries HA. Neural factors versus hypertrophy in the time course of muscle strength gain. Am J Phys Med 1979;58:115–130.

94. Morrissey MC, Harman EA, Frykman PN, et al. Early phase differential effects of slow and fast barbell squat training. Am J Sports Med 1998;26:221–230.

95. Mulligan SE, Fleck SJ, Gordon SE, et al. Influence of resistance exercise volume on serum growth hormone and cortisol concentrations in women. J Strength Cond Res 1996;10:256–262.

96. Narici MV, Roi GS, Landoni L, et al. Changes in force, cross-sectional area and neural activation during strength training and detraining of the human quadriceps. Eur J Appl Physiol Occup Physiol 1989;59:310–319.

97. Newton RU, Kraemer WJ. Developing explosive muscular power: implications for a mixed methods training strategy. Strength Cond 1994;16:20–31.

98. Newton RU, Kraemer WJ, Hakkinen K. Effects of ballistic training on preseason preparation of elite volleyball players. Med Sci Sports Exerc 1999;31:323–330.

99. Newton RU, Kraemer WJ, Hakkinen K, et al. Kinematics, kinetics, and muscle activation during explosive upper body movements. J Appl Biomech 1996;12:31–43.

100. O'Hagan FT, Sale DG, MacDougall JD, et al. Comparative effectiveness of accommodating and weight resistance training modes. Med Sci Sports Exerc 1995;27:1210–1219.

101. Phillips SM. Short-term training: when do repeated bouts of resistance exercise become training? Can J Appl Physiol 2000;25:185–193.

102. Pincivero DM, Lephart SM, Karunakara RG. Effects of rest interval on isokinetic strength and functional performance after short-term high intensity training. Br J Sports Med 1997;31:229–234.

103. Raastad T, Bjoro T, Hallen J. Hormonal responses to high- and moderate-intensity strength exercise. Eur J Appl Physiol 2000;82:121–128.

104. Rhea MR, Alvar BA, Ball SD, et al. Three sets of weight training superior to 1 set with equal intensity for eliciting strength. J Strength Cond Res 2002;16:525–529.

105. Robinson JM, Stone MH, Johnson RL, et al. Effects of different weight training exercise/rest intervals on strength, power, and high intensity exercise endurance. J Strength Cond Res 1995;9:216–221.

106. Rutherford OM, Jones DA. The role of learning and coordination in strength training. Eur J Appl Physiol Occup Physiol 1986;55:100–105.

107. Sale DG. Neural adaptations to strength training. In Komi PV, eds. Strength and Power in Sport. Oxford, UK: Blackwell, 1992.

108. Sale DG, Jacobs I, MacDougall JD, et al. Comparison of two regimens of concurrent strength and endurance training. Med Sci Sports Exerc 1990;22:348–356.

109. Sanborn K, Boros R, Hruby J, et al. Short-term performance effects of weight training with multiple sets not to failure vs a single set to failure in women. J Strength Cond Res 2000;14:328–331.

110. Scala D, McMillan J, Blessing D, et al. Metabolic cost of a preparatory phase of training in weight lifting: a practical observation. J Appl Sport Sci Res 1987;1:48–52.

111. Schlumberger A, Stec J, Schmidtbleicher D. Single- vs multiple-set strength training in women. J Strength Cond Res 2001;15:284–289.

112. Schmidtbleicher D. Training for power events. In: Komi PV, ed. Strength and Power in Sport. Boston: Blackwell, 2001.

113. Schuenke MD, Mikat RP, McBride JM. Effect of an acute period of resistance exercise on excess post-exercise oxygen consumption: implications for body mass management. Eur J Appl Physiol 2002;86:411–417.

114. Sforzo FA, Touey PR. Manipulating exercise order affects muscular performance during a resistance exercise training session. J Strength Cond Res 1996;10:20–24.

115. Starkey DB, Pollock ML, Ishida Y, et al. Effect of resistance training volume on strength and muscle thickness. Med Sci Sports Exerc 1996;28:1311–1320.

116. Staron RS, Karapondo DL, Kraemer WJ, et al. Skeletal muscle adaptations during early phase of heavy-resistance training in men and women. J Appl Physiol 1994;76:1247–1255.

117. Staron RS, Malicky ES, Leonardi MJ, et al. Muscle hypertrophy and fast fiber type conversions in heavy resistance-trained women. Eur J Appl Physiol Occup Physiol 1990;60:71–79.

118. Stone MH, Coulter SP. Strength/endurance effects from three resistance training protocols with women. J Strength Cond Res 1994;8:231–234.

119. Stone MH, Johnson RL, Carter DR. A short term comparison of two different methods of resistance training on leg strength and power. Athlet Train 1979;14:158–161.

120. Stone MH, O'Bryant H, Garhammer J. A hypothetical model for strength training. J Sports Med Phys Fit 1981;21:342–351.

121. Stone MH, O'Bryant H, Garhammer J, et al. A theoretical model of strength training. NSCA J 1982;4:36–39.

122. Stone MH, Plisk SS, Stone ME, et al. Athletic performance development: volume load-1 set vs. multiple sets, training velocity and training variation. NSCA J 1998;20:22–23.

123. Stone MH, Wilson GD, Blessing D, et al. Cardiovascular responses to short-term olympic style weight-training in young men. Can J Appl Sport Sci 1983;8:134–139.

124. Stowers T, McMillian J, Scala D, et al. The short-term effects of three different strength-power training models. NSCA J 1983;5:24–27.

125. Tan B. Manipulating resistance training program variables to optimize maximum strength in men: a review. J Strength Cond Res 1999;13:289–304.

126. Tesch PA. Short- and long-term histochemical and biochemical adaptations in muscle. In: Komi PV, ed. Strength and Power in Sport. Boston, MA: Blackwell, 1992.

127. Tesch PA, Komi PV, Hakkinen K. Enzymatic adaptations consequent to long-term strength training. Int J Sports Med 1987;8(Suppl 1):66–69.

128. Tomberline JP, Besford JR, Schwen EE. Comparative study of isokinetic eccentric and concentric quadriceps training. J Orthop Sports Phys Ther 1991;14: 31–36.

129. Vanhelder WP, Radomski MW, Goode RC. Growth hormone responses during intermittent weight lifting exercise in men. Eur J Appl Physiol Occup Physiol 1984;53: 31–34.

130. Volek JS, Boetes M, Bush JA, et al. Response of testosterone and cortisol concentrations to high-intensity resistance exercise following creatine supplementations. J Strength Cond Res 1997;11:182–187.

131. Weiss LW, Coney HD, Clark FC. Differential functional adaptations to short-term low-, moderate-, and high-repetition weight training. J Strength Cond Res 1999; 13:236–241.

132. Willoughby DS, Chilek DR, Schiller DA, et al. The metabolic effects of three different free weight parallel squatting intensities. J Hum Mov Stud 1991;21:53–67.

133. Wilson GJ, Murphy AJ, Walshe AD. Performance benefits from weight and plyometric training: effects of initial strength level. Coach Sport Sci J 1997;2:3–8.

134. Wilson GJ, Newton RU, Murphy AJ, et al. The optimal training load for the development of dynamic athletic performance. Med Sci Sports Exerc 1993;25:1279–1286.

135. Young WA, Jenner A, Griffiths K. Acute enhancement of power performance from heavy squat loads. J Strength Cond Res 1998;12:82–84.

136. Young WB, Bilby GE. The effect of voluntary effort to influence speed of contraction on strength, muscular power, and hypertrophy development. J Strength Cond Res 1993;7:172–178.

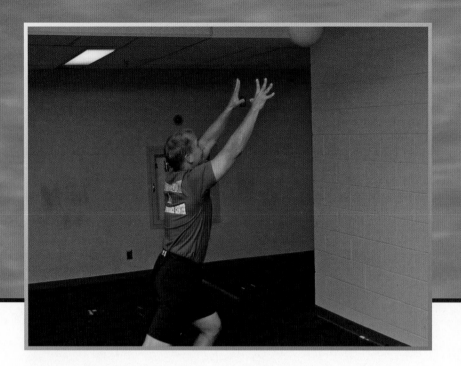

Improving Aerobic Performance

JOHN M. CISSIK

Introduction

Aerobic exercise is often used as a mode of training and conditioning for athletic and physical fitness. Clearly it is important to endurance athletes such as runners, cyclists, swimmers, triathletes, etc. It is unclear, however, to what extent aerobic exercise is necessary for athletes in nonendurance sports (i.e., football, baseball, basketball, etc.). With explosive nonendurance athletes where performance is measured over a matter of a few seconds or less, the case has been made that aerobic fitness is important for recovery from competition and training (since we use the oxidative system to recover from anaerobic training) and that aerobic energy pathways may contribute to anaerobic performance. As we refine our knowledge of specificity of training, the usefulness of aerobic exercise for nonendurance athletes is being called into question. Although traditional aerobic training may not be appropriate for explosively trained athletes, depending on the sport, sprint/interval training may be useful in maintaining or to some extent improving aerobic metabolism.

There seems to be no relationship between maximal oxygen consumption and recovery from anaerobic exercise in basketball players (10). Additionally, differences in aerobic power do not explain differences in performance during various phases of a 30-second all-out test (13). In this study, aerobic power provided only marginal contributions to anaerobic performance; therefore, it may not be worthwhile to devoting training time to it for specific types of athletes.

Although results like these are hardly conclusive, we should pause and reconsider the role of aerobic exercise in nonendurance athletes. Also remember that the aerobic/anaerobic requirements of athletic performance span a continuum. Some athletes need both anaerobic and aerobic training, and the way this is integrated into the athlete's overall program is important. That being the case, the remainder of this chapter examines aerobic exercise prescription from an endurance athlete's perspective and considers how these programs apply to the athlete needing both anaerobic and aerobic training programs. It is important for strength and conditioning professionals to understand this so that they also understand what endurance athletes are going through in their training before adding a strength and conditioning program.

Although we understand the importance of aerobic exercise in endurance athletes, we must reassess its role for nonendurance athletes.

FACTORS THAT INFLUENCE AEROBIC EXERCISE PERFORMANCE

Understanding those factors that influence aerobic exercise performance is important for helping both with athlete selection of and for planning endurance training programs. A number of factors influence aerobic performance. These include the following:

1. Maximal oxygen consumption
2. Lactate threshold
3. Fuel utilization
4. Fiber-type characteristics
5. Exercise economy

Maximal oxygen consumption refers to the maximum rate at which an individual can con-

sume oxygen. It is limited by cardiac output, pulmonary function, and cellular metabolism (3). Relative maximal oxygen consumption in elite female cyclists (i.e., milliliters per kilogram per minute) accounts for a significant part of bicycle racing performance (20). The results of studies like this should be interpreted with care, however, as they do not necessarily look at enough factors to determine whether other factors could make a more significant contribution to performance. For example, the only other variables studied were minute ventilation, heart rate, minute ventilation divided by maximal oxygen consumption, and heart rate divided by maximal oxygen consumption. As the next few paragraphs show, other factors may well have significant impacts on endurance performance.

Lactate threshold refers to the percentage of maximal oxygen consumption at which blood lactate increases above resting. This is sometimes referred to as the onset of blood lactate (OBLA). In one study, two groups of cyclists were compared (5). One group (group H) had an average maximal oxygen consumption of approximately 68 mL/kg per minute and 5 years of cycling experience. The second group (group L) had an average maximal oxygen consumption of approximately 66 mL/kg per minute and almost 3 years of cycling experience. Both groups exercised at 88% of maximal oxygen consumption and their time to fatigue and lactate accumulation was measured. Investigators found that group H could exercise for more than an hour (on average), while group L could exercise for an average of only about 30 minutes. Group L accumulated twice as much lactate as group H. In other words, since maximal oxygen consumption was nearly similar between the two groups, other factors, one of which may have been the accumulation of lactic acid, influenced endurance performance.

The ability to use fuel efficiently can have a huge impact on endurance performance. In the same study mentioned above (5), glycogen utilization was compared by having the subjects exercise at 80% of maximal oxygen consumption. Group L oxidized almost twice as many carbohydrates as group H, and group L used more than twice as much glycogen per kilogram. In other words, the group with the better performance (group H) was able to spare its glycogen stores during exercise, enabling it to exercise longer at a greater intensity.

Muscle fiber types will also have an influence on endurance performance. Theoretically, those individuals with a higher percentage of type I muscle fibers will perform better at endurance tasks. The higher-performing group (5) averaged approximately 66% type I fibers, while the lower-performing group averaged approximately 47%.

Finally, the economy with which one exercises will affect one's performance. This refers to the skill part of performing endurance exercise. One who can perform the exercises more efficiently may spare energy stores and move faster than one who cannot.

 Aerobic endurance is affected by maximal oxygen consumption, lactate threshold, fuel utilization, muscle fiber type, and exercise economy.

APPROACHES TO AEROBIC TRAINING

As with other modes of exercise (e.g., strength training, plyometrics, agility training, speed training, etc.) there are many opinions about how to train for aerobic endurance and what type of exercise to use. As with the other modes of exercise, this is made further confusing by a lack of standardization of terms, a lack of science to support some training approaches, and coaching prejudice. This chapter attempts to clear up some of the confusion by grouping the different approaches to endurance training into categories and explaining the advantages and disadvantages of each.

 Lack of standardization of terms, lack of scientific support, and coaching prejudice can make it difficult to understand the different approaches to aerobic training.

Several broad approaches to endurance training are considered in this chapter:

1. Continuous training
2. Fartlek training
3. Interval training
4. Repetitions

Continuous Training

Continuous training is designed to increase an athlete's endurance base, maximal oxygen consumption, and tissue respiration capacity (2,3). It is also known as long, slow distance (LSD) training, overdistance training, and aerobic threshold training (1,2). Typically, continuous training is done for lengths of between 30 minutes and 2 hours at a constant pace (lower intensity than race pace),

---

 REAL-WORLD APPLICATION
Strength Training and Endurance Athletes

Strength training, within reason, is important for endurance athletes. It can help to prevent injuries by targeting muscles and joints that are prone to injury. For example, it can help to improve strength imbalances in a runner's knee or a swimmer's shoulder. It can also help to improve an athlete's ability to apply force. Even though endurance athletes are taking many steps, strokes, or revolutions during a race, an athlete who can generate more force will still have the ability to get somewhere faster than one who cannot.

There are a number of guidelines for strength-training and endurance athletes:

1. Keep it in perspective. Endurance athletes are not strength and power athletes. They cannot tolerate high volumes and intensities of strength training combined with their endurance training; this can lead to overtraining or injury. Overly intense strength training can also be counterproductive in another way; putting on too much muscle mass on an endurance athlete will negatively affect his or her exercise economy, thereby detracting from event performance.

2. Resistance training does not have to mean weight training. Since the focus is not on drastically increasing maximal strength or hypertrophy, resistance training can be done in a number of ways, including in the weight room, through calisthenics, and with medicine balls or other implements.

3. Keep the stresses of the athlete's endurance training in mind. If the athlete's endurance training stresses a given joint (for example, the effect of pounding from running on the knee), then strength training should not further aggravate that.

4. Strength training is a terrible tool for training maximal oxygen consumption; it does not do a very good job of improving aerobic metabolism. However, it does an excellent job of improving one's anaerobic metabolism and one's tolerance to it. Adjusting the length of the sets and the recovery intervals can be a great way to further enhance these pathways.

generally between 60 and 70% of maximal oxygen capacity (1,8,19). Others recommend basing the training on competition distances. Overdistance training has been recommended to last between two and five times competition distances (17). This approach might be workable for an 800- to 5,000-m athlete, but it would be more difficult for a marathoner.

Some experts recommend a slightly different approach to continuous training (1). The method includes an approach similar to that for interval training but using longer work intervals (see below for more on interval training). Repetitions lasting between 10 minutes and 2 hours are recommended. Each repetition is performed between one and six times at approximately 60% of maximal oxygen consumption, with 1- to 2-minute recovery jogs between repetitions.

There is debate on the usefulness of continuous training for an endurance athlete. In one study, 7 weeks of steady-state pace training (21) improved maximal oxygen consumption in runners by an average of nearly 5 mL/kg per minute, improved 3.22-km-run performance by an average of just over a minute, improved by nearly 6 minutes the 10-km time, and improved anaerobic power by nearly 0.5 W/kg of body mass. Disadvantages include that this approach may lack specificity, in that it could teach the athlete to be slow, does not develop a sense of race pace, and may expose the athlete to overuse injuries (2,3).

Continuous training may lack specificity and may expose athletes to overuse injuries, but it does appear to improve maximal oxygen consumption and potentially performance for endurance athletes.

Continuous training is not the only type of training used to build up the athlete's endurance base and increase maximal oxygen consumption. Another popular approach is fartlek training.

Fartlek Training

Fartlek training, often referred to as "speed play," has been a mainstay of endurance training for decades. It refers to loosely structured training generally performed on cross-country trails. The runner alternates between fast, intense running and slower recovery jogs, often allowing the terrain to dictate the intensity. For example, a runner may jog to the first hill, sprint up it, jog down,

run at race pace for a few minutes, etc. Theoretically, fartlek provides the advantages of interval training without the boredom of performing laps on a track or the risks of intense work on hard surfaces (2,8). It also may be an event-specific way to develop running strength, especially in the ankle and shin, as the athlete must contend with the uneven surfaces found on cross-country terrain (8). One negative aspect of fartlek training is that it is more difficult to prescribe specific heart rates and/or exercise intensities with this approach.

Not everyone agrees that fartlek training should be loosely structured. One researcher derisively refers to the way fartlek is traditionally performed as "go as you feel and run as you like," pointing out that the way it is typically practiced may not allow it to be as effective as it might. He recommends that fartlek training should be hard, continuous, and structured (for example, run for 1 minute at race pace and then perform a recovery jog for 1 minute, repeat 25 times) (7).

Theoretically, fartlek training provides the benefits of interval training without some of the disadvantages. It may be too loosely structured, however, to maximize gains from training. As the body of knowledge in the field of training and conditioning grows, more evidence-based research will be available that can be used to prescribe sport-specific structured fartlek training programs.

Although fartlek and continuous training may be useful for improving an athlete's endurance base, they may not allow for a high enough exercise intensity to adequately address improving anaerobic metabolism, maximal oxygen consumption, and pace. Interval training may be a useful tool for addressing those components.

Interval Training

Interval training allows for a greater quantity of normally exhaustive exercise to be performed (17). An increase in total work in a given time period can be accomplished as a result of a properly structured interval training program. It has a number of benefits to an endurance athlete. First, it teaches race pace (3). Second, depending upon how the variables are manipulated, it can improve anaerobic metabolism (3,12,17,18). Finally, it can enhance maximal oxygen consumption (3,12,18).

Studies performed with highly trained cyclists show that interval training programs improve

40-km time-trial performance, maximal oxygen consumption, peak power output, time to exhaustion at 150% of peak power output, and buffering capacity (15,16,25). Interval training also improved the running velocity at maximal oxygen consumption, maximal oxygen consumption, and 3,000-m run time in middle-distance runners (23).

Several variables can be manipulated during interval training (17):

■ The intensity of the exercise
■ The duration of the exercise interval
■ The length of the recovery
■ The number of repetitions of the exercise-recovery interval

INTENSITY OF THE EXERCISE

Obviously, the intensity of the exercise interval will affect the workout's total volume. It will also affect the rest of the week's workouts (i.e., more intense exercise sessions will require more days of rest or light effort). Intense interval training can result in a dramatic reduction in muscle glycogen concentration, an increase in muscle lactate concentrations, and a decrease in pH. In one study, seven highly trained cyclists (mean maximal oxygen consumption of 5.14 L/minute) performed eight intervals on an ergometer (24). Each interval lasted 5 minutes, was performed at 86% of maximal oxygen consumption, and was followed by 60 seconds of active recovery. After the last interval, resting muscle glycogen concentrations had decreased by more than 50%. Muscle lactate had increased by nearly 500% and pH had dropped noticeably (24).

Recommendations for the intensity of an interval session vary. Some authors use maximal oxygen consumption as the determinant of exercise intensity. They recommend anywhere from 75% to close to 90% of maximal oxygen consumption (9,22). In addition to the wide variability of suggested exercise intensities, the other drawback to this approach is that one must know the maximal oxygen consumption (and the running, cycling, or swimming pace at which it occurs) for the athlete. Although useful, this may not be practical or possible in every athletic training situation.

The distance of the interval to be run and the athlete's best time for that interval distance represent another, perhaps more "field"-friendly way to determine interval intensity. For example, interval training guidelines are determined by one's best time running a given distance (17). If intervals are performed for 200 yd, one would add between 1.5 and 5 seconds to the best time at that distance and run the intervals with the new time. This may be a more practical way to determine interval intensities than basing them on maximal oxygen consumption.

DURATION OF THE EXERCISE INTERVAL

The duration of the exercise interval will be dictated by the goals of the training and sometimes by the distance to be covered in the race. Interval training can be organized around targeting specific energy systems (2,12,17). We know that up to about the first 6 seconds of exercise will be fueled primarily by ATP and CP. Up to about 2 minutes will be primarily fueled by glycogen, and if exercise is intense enough, lactic acid will be produced. After 2 to 3 minutes of exercise, oxygen will be used to break down glycogen and other energy stores for fuel.

In addition to guidelines about length of time, duration of the intervals can also be based on the distances to be run in the race. One recommendation is to perform intervals for one-quarter of the race distance, with the recovery based on the energy system that the athlete wishes to train (2). One must be careful with this guideline, as it would be useful for an 800-m runner but not for a long-distance endurance athlete.

LENGTH OF RECOVERY

If the duration of the interval can affect what energy system the interval trains, the length of the recovery can affect how that energy system is trained and how it adapts. For example, if one wants to increase an athlete's tolerance to lactic acid, then intervals would last up to 2 to 3 minutes and would not allow the athlete long to recover. This would result in the lactic acid accumulating in the muscles. If, however, the goal is to enhance the athlete's ability to remove lactic acid, intense intervals lasting up to 2 to 3 minutes would still be used, but complete recovery between intervals would be allowed.

Recovery times should also be driven by exercise intensity. Some recommendations more than double the amount of recovery time between intervals in moving from an intensity of 80% of maximal oxygen consumption to 90% (from 90 to 120 seconds to 120 to 300 seconds) (22). Unless the goal is to get the athlete used to functioning with high levels of lactic acid, recovery times must be increased as intensity increases.

Q & A from the Field

The university has had a successful cross-country team for the last several years. Recently I've been put in charge of designing their workouts. I understand how to incorporate the different types of endurance training, but I'm having trouble figuring out how to balance out the hard and easy days. How do I go about determining all that?

—*graduate assistant coach*

This can be a confusing topic for any strength and conditioning professional. First, determine when the competitions are; this will dictate the training calendar. The period around the competitions will be your competition phase. This period will see the most intense training. The remaining time will be divided between preparation and precompetition. The precompetition phase usually lasts 4 weeks and consists of training of increasing intensity. Preparation should ideally make up the bulk of the training, with low to moderate intensity (intensity should increase over time).

Once the rough calendar has been determined, break each phase into 4-week cycles. The easiest way to do this is to have a 3:1 approach (i.e., intensity increases for the first 3 weeks, then week 4 is a recovery week). This would mean that week 2 is more difficult than week 1, week 3 is more difficult than week 2, and week 4 is less difficult than week 2 (though slightly more difficult than week 1).

Within a 4-week cycle, decide on the intensity levels for each week. They may be high-intensity (i.e., three peaks), medium-intensity (i.e., two peaks), or low-intensity (i.e., one peak) work. Remember that a race always counts as a peak. In general the weeks in the competition phase will consist of high-intensity weeks; the rest of the training time (preparation and precompetition) will consist primarily of low- and medium-intensity weeks, with a few high-intensity weeks thrown in.

Once you've determined how many peaks a week will have, organize the training week around the peaks as described in Figure 14.1 (see p. 400).

In summary, to help determine how to balance our hard and easy days take several steps:

1. Determine when the competitions are.
2. Divide up the calendar into competition, precompetition, and preparation phases.
3. Break each phase into 4-week cycles.
4. Decide upon an intensity for each week within a 4-week cycle.

Distribute the peaks according to the guidelines laid out in this chapter.

NUMBER OF REPETITIONS

There are a number of approaches to calculating the number of repetitions (or total volume) of the interval training sessions. Workout volume can be based on the length of the athlete's competitive distance, with the workout's volume equaling between one and three times the competitive distance (2). For example, an 800-m runner would perform between 800 and 2,400 m of intervals in a workout. One must be careful with a guideline like this, as it will not serve a long-distance athlete such as a marathoner well.

A second method is to base volume on the intensity at which the intervals will be run. As intensity increases, total workout volume would decrease. For example, it has been recommended to cut the volume of 2,000-m intervals from 12,000 to −16,000 m to 6,000 to 12,000 m per workout when intensity increases from less than 85% to greater than 85% (22).

A final method is to determine volume by fatigue. Using this method, it is recommended that intervals be run until the athlete's heart rate is greater than 120 beats per minute after 2 minutes of recovery (9). This is a simple, "field-friendly" way to determine exercise volume, but it fails to take into account individual ages, heart rate responses to exercise, etc.

When it comes to interval training, remember that it is extremely demanding on the athlete and that the athlete is going to need a fitness base before engaging in it. Engaging in this type of training before the athlete's running form is consistent, endurance base is built up, and muscles/skeleton/connective tissue are ready is asking for an injury.

Interval training appears to be an effective way to target an athlete's deficiencies, but it is extremely demanding and requires a fitness base before this training activity is initiated.

As described, interval training may not be difficult enough to meet all of an endurance athlete's needs. When greater intensity is desired, repetitions are used.

Repetitions

Repetitions are a more intense version of interval training. Repetitions are performed at a faster pace with complete recovery between bouts (2). They are designed to increase speed as well as both the capacity for and the tolerance of anaerobic metabolism. Generally, repetitions are defined in the literature as being of high intensity, 90% of maximal oxygen consumption and above, with complete recovery between repetitions (2,22).

Repetitions are generally performed for 30- to 90-second bouts, with a work:rest ratio of around 1:5. For example, if an athlete performed a 30-second bout at 90% of maximal oxygen consumption, he or she would then perform low-intensity recovery work for 150 seconds. The workout approach just described would be ideal for cyclists, swimmers, recreational endurance athletes, and other athletes needing this type of work.

More concrete recommendations regarding repetitions and training for distance runners can be used (22). Middle-distance runners should perform repetitions with a total volume between $\frac{2}{3}$ and $1\frac{1}{2}$ times the length of the racing distance. For example, a 5-km runner should have a total volume of repetitions between 3,300 and 7,500 m per workout session. Long-distance runners should cover one-tenth, one-fifth, or one-third the total racing distance in each repetition workout. Recovery times would range from 5 to 30 minutes (22).

Now that we've reviewed the different approaches to training used with endurance athletes, we can consider how the different approaches fit together in an athlete's training.

ORGANIZING AEROBIC EXERCISE TRAINING

The rest of this chapter provides basic principles to help with the program design process. It then offers a sample training program to illustrate the application of these principles, such as the following:

1. Warm up properly (see Chapter 9). Warming up is important for decreasing the risk of injuries and for maximizing performance. In recent years, methods of warming up have been reassessed by conditioning professionals. In the past, an endurance athlete would start out slowly for 5 to 10 minutes, breaking a light sweat, then stretch for another 5 to 10 minutes, and finally would ease into the workout, gradually picking up speed and intensity. Although starting out slowly for the first 5 to 10 minutes is important (it moves blood into the muscles, warms joints to be trained, and raises heart rate gradually), today the thinking is that static stretching performed before a workout session is counterproductive (4,11). One option is to perform active activity-specific flexibility exercises (such as leg swings, high knee exercises, etc.) for 20 to 30 minutes prior to the actual workout. These train the muscles and joints in a way similar to their use in the workout, move more blood into the joints, raise temperature, etc. (4). Drills can become gradually faster and more intense as the athlete progresses through the warm-up, allowing them to begin the workout at full speed. An example of a warm-up for a runner is offered in Table 14.1.

2. Balance the hard and easy days. Most authors recommend alternating hard and easy days (2,3,6). Obviously this will be further complicated if there is a competition during the week. The 2 days before a competition should probably be low-intensity days (6). Low-intensity training days typically take the form of lower-intensity 30- to 40-minute efforts (9). Another possibility is to begin the training week with a less intense workout, using the following scheme, depending on the number of higher-intensity workouts (1) (samples are graphed in Fig. 14.1; note that these are weeks without competitions):
   a. One intense workout per week: This should be scheduled toward the middle of the week (i.e., Wednesday or Thursday).
   b. Two intense workouts per week: Separate the intense workouts with 1 or 2 less intense days in between (i.e., higher-intensity workouts on Tuesday and Friday, Wednesday and Saturday, etc.).
   c. Three intense workouts per week: Separate the intense workouts with low-intensity days (i.e., higher-intensity

TABLE 14.1	EXAMPLE OF A WARM-UP FOR A RUNNER		
EXERCISE	REPETITION/DURATION	SETS	REST
Jog	800 m	1	Walking recovery
Leg swings, front/back	10 each leg	2	jog 20 m after each set
Leg swings, side/side	10 each leg	2	jog 20 m after each set
Hip circles	10 each leg	2	jog 20 m after each set
Eagles*	10 each leg	2	jog 20 m after each set
Stomach eagles	10 each leg	2	jog 20 m after each set
Forward lunges	20 m	2	jog 20 m after each set
Backward lunges	20 m	2	sprint 20 m after each set
Inchworms†	20 m	2	sprint 20 m after each set
High knee walks	20 m	2	sprint 20 m after each set
High knee skips	20 m	2	sprint 20 m after each skip
Stride-length runs	sprint 20 m, set sticks up at 80% of stride length beginning at the 20-m mark, perform drill for 40–60 m	2	Walking recovery

*Eagles are performed with the athlete lying supine, arms stretched out to the sides. Keeping the right leg straight, the athlete attempts to lift the right leg across the body until it touches the left hand. This should be repeated with the left leg. Repeat for the desired number of repetitions.

†Inchworms start in the push-up position. Athlete will keep the legs as straight as possible while attempting to walk the feet up to the hands. When the feet reach the hands, the athlete should walk the hands out until he or she is again in the push-up position. Repeat for the desired distance.

workouts on Tuesday, Thursday, and Saturday, etc.).

3. Establish a fitness base first. Most endurance programs focus on continuous training and fartlek training for the first part of the training year. This is to give the athlete's muscles, joints, and skeleton a chance to adapt to training as well as to build up the athlete's cardiovascular system (1,3,6). Training volume should be increased by no more than 5% to 10% per week (6). Any more than such an increase could result in overuse injuries and burnout, and less might not promote maximal physiological development. For example, an athlete running a total weekly volume of 30 mi/week in the first week of training should move up to only 31.5 to 33 mi/week in the second week.

4. Determine weak points and deficiencies and train them. As with every other sport, once the fitness base has been established, it's important to determine what is limiting an athlete's performance and target it through training. For example, intervals can be used to get an athlete used to tolerating lactic acid or recovering from it. Continuous training can be modified to help push back the point at which lactic acid accumulation begins to exceed removal. To accomplish that, have the athlete train for 20 to 30 minutes at his or her lactate threshold. Sometimes this type of training is called "tempo training."

5. For purely endurance athletes, don't neglect resistance training. Resistance training is often overlooked by endurance athletes. Anecdotally, it's important for preventing injuries and for improving the ability to exert force. Resistance training does not have to be all weight-room training; it can take the form of calisthenics, cross-country running, hill running, etc.

In designing an aerobic exercise training program, keep the following factors in mind: warm up properly, balance the hard and easy days, establish a fitness base first, determine weak points and then train them, and don't neglect some type of resistance training.

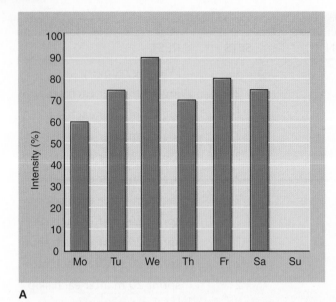

A

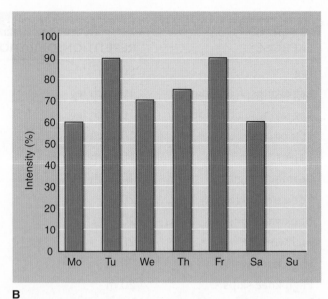

B

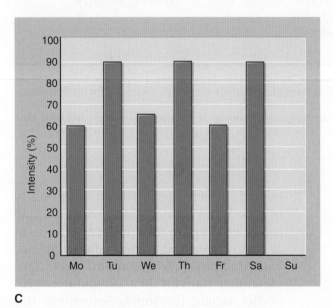

C

FIGURE 14.1 Examples of workouts with different numbers of peaks. **A.** Week with one peak. **B.** Week with two peaks. **C.** Week with three peaks.

Although there is research showing that each type of endurance training is effective, most of that is focused on one type of training. For example, the studies quoted above examining interval training (15,16,23,25) all demonstrate that interval training is effective. That, however, was the only type of training studied; i.e., it was not compared to other types of training. For example, is interval training more or less effective than continuous training at developing maximal oxygen consumption? This is a major limitation of the research on types of endurance training.

In addition to being unclear as to whether specific types of endurance training are more effective than others, there is little research looking into

how that training should be put together, balanced, or timed. This makes it difficult to put together endurance training programs scientifically.

The effect of different types of endurance training on performance in collegiate cross-country runners has been evaluated (14). The study surveyed the training of 14 division I cross-country teams that qualified for NCAA Cross-Country Nationals and 16 division I cross-country teams that did not qualify. Training was broken down into three phases; May to August (transition), August to October (competition), and November (peak). Nationals were in November.

Endurance training modes were divided into interval, tempo, repetition, hill, and fartlek. Note that the modes had slightly different definitions than those given in this chapter (14).

In the transition phase, those teams that qualified for the Nationals had more days of rest and used cross-training more than nonqualifiers. On average, the longest run of the week was 2 mi longer for nonqualifiers than for qualifiers. They also found a positive correlation between performing tempo runs, repetitions, intervals, fartlek, and twice-per-day training and team performance (i.e., the more those training modes were used, the slower the team's mean 10-km time was) (14).

During the competition phase, the qualifying teams ran more speed work and had higher mileage than the nonqualifying teams. A positive correlation was found between mean team time with running intervals and mean team time with fartlek training during the competition phase. The more interval running and fartlek training were used, the slower the team's mean 10-km time was (14).

During the peak phase, the more intervals a team used, the higher its placing was (14). These results may be limited because they were based on the self-reporting of the various coaches. This self-reporting may or may not have accurately reflected what was actually done in training.

This study suggests a number of interesting possibilities for a collegiate cross-country team preparing for November NCAA Nationals. First, the extensive use of intervals during transition and competition phases may be too intense. Second, fartlek training may not be structured and difficult enough to produce training adaptations. Finally, twice-daily training, or at least excessive amounts of training, can result in overtraining, which could have a negative impact on performance.

The above study has interesting implications for a college cross-country coach, but its applications to other situations is limited at best. However, the study does demonstrate that this type of research is possible and could be done in other athletic situations.

The rest of this chapter covers a sample cross-country training program, using the guidelines and recommendations from this chapter, for a 10-km runner. The cross-country season can be broken down into the following phases:

1. General preparation: June (4 weeks)
2. Special preparation: July (4 weeks)
3. Precompetition: August (4 weeks)
4. Competition: September to November (10 weeks)

General Preparation Phase

During this phase, as the athlete should be developing his or her fitness base, the focus will be on continuous training. For the sake of this chapter, the general preparation phase will consist of weeks with a single peak (Wednesday). During this phase, the peak will be the longest run of the week, which will be twice the competition distance on the first week of training. Friday will consist of a "structured" fartlek training session. Strength-training work will be performed on Tuesdays and Saturdays. Training volumes will increase by 5% from the first week to the second, then 7.5% from the second to the third. Table 14.2 provides a sample week of workouts from the general preparation phase of training.

Figure 14.2 shows an example of how this program would look over a 4-week period. Note that volume increases during the first 3 weeks and then backs off during the fourth week to give the athlete a chance to recover.

Special Preparation Phase

The special preparation phase will continue increasing the volume. More specialized work will begin to be integrated into the training. Training

TABLE 14.2	SAMPLE GENERAL PREPARATION TRAINING WEEK
DAY OF THE WEEK	**WORKOUT**
Monday	10,000-m (6.2-mi) run, 60% effort
Tuesday	Morning: 5,000-m (3.1-mi) run, 70% effort
	Afternoon: Weight training
Wednesday	20,000-m (12.4-mi) run, 60% effort
Thursday	Morning: 5,000-m (3.1-mi) run, 60% effort
	Afternoon: Hill training, ten 30-second efforts, 1-minute recovery
Friday	Structured fartlek: fifteen 400-m runs at race pace, 200-m jog recoveries
Saturday	Calisthenics/medicine ball circuit
Sunday	Off

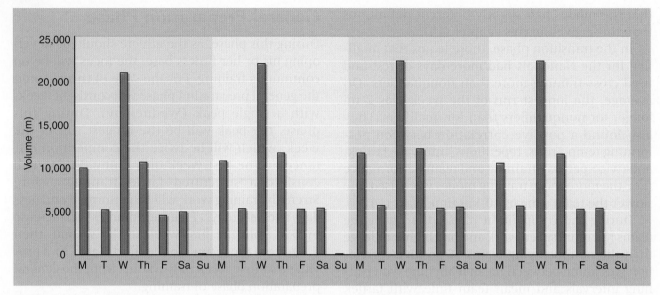

FIGURE 14.2 General preparation phase. Running volume in meters over 4 weeks.

will be reorganized slightly around two peaks per week; Tuesday will be the longest distance day (though the volume will not increase beyond the 22,600-m peak reached in the general prep phase). Monday and Saturday will be lower-intensity training days. Friday will include an interval training session (Friday is the second peak). Note that the intensities of the continuous workouts will be increased compared to the general preparation phase. Table 14.3 shows a sample special preparation training week.

Special preparation workouts will continue to follow the 5% to 10% rule for increasing volume. Between the first and second weeks, volume will increase by 5%. Between weeks 2 and 3, volume will increase by 7.5%. The fourth week will once again serve as a recovery week. Note that the distance of the Tuesday run will never exceed 22,600 m.

Precompetition Phase

Now that the athlete's base has been established, precompetition training will be used to correct deficiencies. Interval training may be utilized more extensively, while continuous training is used for recovery and to maintain endurance. More specialized continuous training (for example, at the point where lactate accumulation begins to exceed removal) may be performed depending upon need.

Workouts in this phase will revolve around three peaks: Tuesday (intervals), Thursday (inter-vals), and Saturday (specialized continuous training). Monday, Wednesday, and Friday will be days of less intense effort. Table 14.4 shows the sample workouts for this phase.

As with the other phases, this phase will increase volume from week 1 through week 3. The fourth week will serve as a back-off week to allow for recovery.

TABLE 14.3	SAMPLE WEEK OF SPECIAL PREPARATION WORKOUTS
DAY OF THE WEEK	**WORKOUT**
Monday	10,500-m (6.52-mi) run at 65% effort
Tuesday	21,000-m (13-mi) run at 60% effort
Wednesday	Morning: 5,250-m (3.3-mi) run at 60% effort
	Afternoon: Resistance training
Thursday	Structured fartlek training: 15×500 m at race pace (with 250-m jog recoveries)
Friday	Intervals: 2×4×600 m run (with 2-minute jog recoveries)
Saturday	Morning: 5,000-m (3.1-mi) run at 60% effort
	Afternoon: Calisthenic/medicine ball resistance training
Sunday	Off

TABLE 14.4	SAMPLE WEEK OF PRECOMPETITION WORKOUTS
DAY OF THE WEEK	**WORKOUT**
Monday	15,000-m (9.3-mi) run at 65% effort
Tuesday	Intervals: 2×6×600-m runs at 80% effort (with 200-m-jog recoveries)
Wednesday	Morning: 5,500-m (3.4-mi) run at 60% effort
	Afternoon: Resistance training
Thursday	Intervals: 2×4×400 m runs at 85% effort (with 150-m-jog recoveries)
Friday	5000-m (3.1-mi) run at 60% effort
Saturday	10,000-m (6.2-mi) run at threshold
Sunday	Off

TABLE 14.5	SAMPLE WEEK OF COMPETITION WORKOUTS
DAY OF THE WEEK	**WORKOUT**
Monday	Repetitions: six 1,000-m runs at 90% effort with 5-minute jog recovery
Tuesday	Morning: 15,000-m (9.3-mi) run at 60% effort
	Afternoon: Calisthenic/medicine ball resistance training
Wednesday	Intervals: ten 1,000-m runs at 80% effort with 2 minutes recovery
Thursday	7500-m (4.7-mi) run at 60% effort
Friday	Off
Saturday	Race
Sunday	Off

Competition Phase

The competition phase is designed to make sure that the athlete is at his or her best during the important competitions. The process of determining the athlete's deficiencies and correcting them will continue. All types of training will be included as needed, although this phase will see the greatest amount of interval and repetition training. For this example, this phase will also have three peaks. Because competitions are on the weekend, however, the competition will be one of the peaks. The other peaks will be on Monday and Wednesday, so that Thursday and Friday can serve as recovery days. Table 14.5 lists the workouts for the competition phase.

SUMMARY

Performance in aerobic exercise depends on the interaction of a number of factors, including maximal oxygen consumption, lactate threshold, fuel utilization, muscle-fiber types, and exercise economy. There are many approaches to training to improve aerobic performance, each of which seeks to develop one or more of the factors that limit performance. Each of these approaches has advantages and limitations that must be carefully

thought out during the planning of an athlete's training. The jury is still out on precisely how those exercise modes should be organized, balanced, and timed in a training program, although research is being done in this area.

MAXING OUT

1. A track coach comes to you and wants to determine the distances for continuous training sessions for 800-m runners. If you were to base those distances on the length of the race, how long should the continuous runs be?
2. A high school cross-country coach is trying to determine the duration, recovery time, and number of intervals for her high school athletes. What are the different ways presented in this chapter for determining this information? Which one would be the most appropriate for the coach's situation?
3. A recreational 5-km runner is having trouble with her warm-ups. She complains of feeling sluggish and has been having hamstring trouble during her runs. Her warm-ups currently consist of stretching for 5 minutes and then beginning her run, gradually increasing her pace over the first mile. List some things that can be modified in her warm-up to improve its effectiveness.

CASE EXAMPLE

Designing Continuous, Interval, and Repetition Training Programs for a Recreational Cyclist

BACKGROUND

You are employed as a personal trainer and hired by a recreational cyclist who wants to compete in a 20-mi race in 16 weeks' time. This individual has been cycling for 3 years recreationally and can easily complete the 20 mi; however, she would like to improve her speed and does not know how to go about doing so. Apply the guidelines presented in this chapter to design a 16-week-long workout program, training three times per week, to improve her performance in a 20-mi race.

RECOMMENDATIONS/CONSIDERATIONS

We have 16 weeks. Starting backwards from the competition, the 4 weeks prior (which we'll designate weeks 1 through 4, week 1 being the week of competition) will be our competition phase and will consist of the most intense workouts (intervals and repetitions, some continuous work). Weeks 5 through 8 will be a peaking phase and will see the gradual integration of high-intensity workouts (continuous work and intervals). Weeks 9 through 16 will be our preparation phase and will primarily consist of low-and medium-intensity workouts, mostly continuous work.

IMPLEMENTATION

Preparation Phase. Our athlete will train three times per week; Tuesdays, Thursdays, and Saturdays. Bowing to reality, the longest ride of the week will occur on Saturday (i.e., Saturdays will be the peak). On Tuesdays there will be a shorter ride at approximately 60% effort. On Thursdays there will be a moderate ride at 60% to 70% effort. On week 16 (i.e., the first week of training), the longest training session will be performed at the race distance (i.e., 20 mi); Tuesday's workout will be conducted at 50% of Saturday's distance (i.e. 10 mi); Thursday's workout will be conducted at 75% of Saturday's distance (i.e. 15 mi). Volume will be increased for the following weeks: 15, 14, 12,

11, and 10. Volume will be increased by 5% ion each of these weeks. Weeks 13 and 9 will serve as recovery weeks, volume for these weeks will be equal to that for weeks 15 and 11. This means that by week 10, the distances for each day will be:

Tuesday: 12.1 mi
Thursday: 18.15 mi
Saturday: 24.2 mi

Peaking Phase. Our athlete will continue training three times per week. Beginning with this phase, Thursday will become the peak and will consist of interval training. Saturday will remain the long day, with Tuesday as a recovery ride. Saturday's distances will never increase over 24.2 mi. Interval training will be designed initially to improve our athlete's ability to recover from lactic acid. As she is not an elite athlete, intensity will be 75%. Intervals will last 3 minutes. Since we're targeting recovery, she will achieve close to full recovery between intervals (i.e., 2 minutes of slow riding between each interval).

Week 8 will see long-ride volumes equal to that of week 12; this step back is being taken because of the addition of the intervals. In week 8, our athlete will perform only four intervals. The number of intervals, like the distance of the other rides, will increase over weeks 7 and 6, with week 5 being a recovery week. With this in mind, week 6 (the most difficult week) will look like this:

Tuesday: 12.1 mi
Thursday: six 3-minute intervals
    (with 2-minute recovery rides)
Saturday: 24.2 mi

Competition Phase. With this phase, repetitions will be used on Tuesday's workouts, Thursday will remain interval training, and Saturday will remain a continuous training session. Repetitions will consist of 90 seconds of near-maximal activity, followed by 450 seconds of recovery riding (i.e., 1:5 work:rest ratio).

Intervals will now focus on training her to tolerate large levels of lactic acid; they will remain 3 minutes in length but recovery will be cut in half to 1 minute. Continuous training will continue to be capped at 24.2 mi.

Week 4 will see continuous training distances equivalent to those of week 7 and the performance of only four intervals on Thursday's workout. This step back is being taken because of the addition of repetitions on Tuesday. Tuesday's workout will consist of four repetitions during week 4. Weeks 3 and 2 will

see an increase in the number of repetitions, intervals, and continuous training distance (to 24.2 mi). Week 1 will be a recovery week, with the race being at the end of that week.

Week 2 (the most difficult week) will look like this:

Tuesday: six 90-second repetitions
  (450-second recovery rides)
Thursday: six 3-minute intervals
  (1-minute recovery ride)
Saturday: 24.2 mi

REFERENCES

1. Bompa TO. Periodization: Theory and Methodology of Training. 4th ed. Champaign, IL: Human Kinetics, 1999.
2. Bowerman WJ, Freeman WH. High-Performance Training for Track and Field. 2nd ed. Champaign, IL: Leisure Press, 1991.
3. Brooks GA, Fahey TD, White TP. Exercise Physiology: Human Bioenergetics and Its Applications. 2nd ed. Mountain View, CA: Mayfield, 1996.
4. Cissik JM, Barnes M. Sport Speed and Agility. Monterey, CA: Coaches Choice, 2004.
5. Coyle EF, Coggan AR, Hopper MK, Walters TJ. Determinants of endurance in well-trained cyclists. J Appl Physiol 1988;64(6):2622–2630.
6. Daniels J. Designing periodized training programs: Distance running. In: Foran B, ed. High-Performance Sports Conditioning. Champaign, IL: Human Kinetics, 2001.
7. de Swardt A. Cross-country methods for year 2000. Mod Athl Coach 2000;28(4):38–40.
8. Dick FW. Sports Training Principles. 4th ed. London: A & C Black, 2002.
9. Freeman W. Peak When It Counts. 3rd ed. Mountain View, CA: Tafnews Press, 1996.
10. Hoffman JR, Epstein S, Einbinder M, Weinstein Y. The influence of aerobic capacity on anaerobic performance and recovery indices in basketball players. J Strength Cond Res 1999;13(4):407–411.
11. Holdeman J. Minimizing injury and maximizing performance in fast running: warming up and warming down. Track Coach 2004;167:5336–5341, 5346.
12. Karp JR. Interval training for fitness professionals. Strength Cond J 2000;22(4):64–69.
13. Koziris LP, Kramer WJ, Patton JF, et al. Relationship of aerobic power to anaerobic performance indices. J Strength Cond Res 1996;10(1):35–39.
14. Kurz MJ, Berg K, Latin R, DeGraw W. The relationship of training methods in NCAA division I cross country

runners and 10,000 meter performance. Strength Cond J 2000;14(2):196–201.
15. Laursen, PB, Shing CM, Peake JM, et al. Interval training program optimization in highly trained endurance cyclists. Med Sci Sports Exerc 2002;34(11):1801–1807.
16. Lindsay FH, Hawley JA, Myburgh KH, et al. Improved athletic performance in highly trained cyclists after interval training. Med Sci Sports Exerc 1996;28(11):1427–1434.
17. McArdle WD, Katch FI, Katch VL. Exercise Physiology: Energy, Nutrition, and Human Performance. 6th ed. Baltimore: Lippincott William & Wilkins, 2006.
18. McNeely E. Adding precision to aerobic exercise prescription. 26th Annual National Strength and Conditioning Association National Conference and Exhibition Conference Proceedings. Colorado Springs, CO: NSCA, 2003.
19. Pfeifer H, Harre D. Fundamentals and methods of endurance training. In: Harre D, ed. Principles of Sports Training. Berlin: Sportverlag, 1982.
20. Pfeiffer RP, Harder BP, Landis D, et al. Correlation indices of aerobic capacity with performance in elite women road cyclists. J Strength Cond Res 1993;7(4):201–205.
21. Priest JW, Hagan RD. The effects of maximum steady state pace training on running performance. Br J Sports Med 1987:21(1):18–21.
22. Schmolinsky G. Track and Field: The East German Textbook of Athletics. Toronto, Ontario: Sports Books Publishers, 1996.
23. Smith TP, McNaughton LR, Coombes JS. Effects of a 4-week interval training program using Vo₂max and Tmax on performance in middle distance athletes. Med Sci Sports Exerc 1999;31(5 Suppl):S282.
24. Stepto NK, Martin DT, Fallon KE, Hawley JA. Metabolic demands of intense aerobic interval training in competitive cyclists. Med Sci Sports Exerc 2001;33(2):303–310.
25. Weston AR, Myburgh KH, Lindsay FH, et al. Skeletal muscle buffering capacity and endurance performance after high-intensity interval training by well-trained cyclists. Eur J Appl Physiol 1997;75(1):7–13.

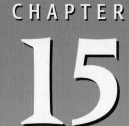

CHAPTER

15

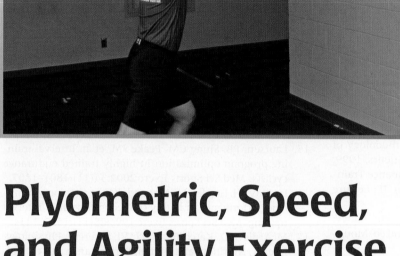

Plyometric, Speed, and Agility Exercise Prescription

JASON D. VESCOVI

Introduction

Participation in most individual and team sports requires athletes to perform short (5- to 20-yd) or long (20- to 40-yd) sprints, change direction rapidly, or jump for maximal height or distance. In other words, linear acceleration and speed, agility, and vertical, horizontal, and lateral jumping actions are essential elements of successful athletic performance. These locomotor skills are learned at relatively young ages as children participate in playful activities. Maturation and experience will help refine the movement patters associated with these skills; however, instruction on the mechanical aspects of locomotion is still required. Once the global and segmental mechanical aspects of a skill have been mastered, training can focus on improving and ultimately maximizing performance. The types of exercises or drills prescribed to an athlete will be based on identified mechanical flaws or muscular weaknesses. To date the manipulation of acute training variables for speed, agility, and plyometric training is unclear but will certainly depend on the developmental stage of an athlete as well as chronological and training age.

To design a training regimen for an athlete, sport performance professionals need to consider aspects from several domains. First, a clear understanding of the sequence of motor development from childhood to adulthood for running, jumping, and changing direction is important. This will help guide the selection of appropriate drills or exercises for inexperienced, mature, and advanced athletes. Second, sports performance professionals should clearly recognize mature movement patterns associated with global and segmental mechanics and understand the specific muscular actions involved. This will help them to identify movement flaws, instruct athletes on appropriate changes, and assist skill improvement during childhood and through adolescence. Finally, understanding how to manipulate acute training program variables (e.g., sets, reps, frequency, volume) will prove to be the most challenging aspect of improving and maximizing performance, since research is scarce regarding sprint, agility, and plyometric training. Nevertheless, appropriate training principles are applied to ensure sufficient stimulation to improve performance while minimizing excessive overload.

This chapter begins with an overview of the stretch shortening cycle (SSC) and briefly describes factors that impact SSC efficiency. Next, the developmental sequence of sprinting, jumping, and changing direction is illustrated, which includes characteristics for mature motor skill performance. Then a brief list of exercises and drills is provided to help develop and improve sprinting, jumping, and agility skills. Finally, general guidelines for program design are recommended.

THE STRETCH SHORTENING CYCLE

The common thread that links sprinting, jumping, and changing direction is the **stretch shortening cycle (SSC)**, which can simply be described as the coupling of an eccentric action with a concentric action. In other words, when a muscle or muscle group is eccentrically loaded (i.e., stretched) and is immediately followed by a shortening action, then a SSC has occurred. Although SSCs are common in everyday tasks (e.g., walking), their use in athletics is often intended to enhance performance. By rapidly coupling eccentric-concentric actions,

the muscular force and power output during the concentric phase are enhanced (83). This, in turn, allows athletes to run faster, jump higher, and change direction more rapidly.

Although the SSC has been studied in great detail, the mechanisms responsible for greater power production are still debated (12,13,29, 31,83). Two models may contribute to a complex mechanism, which results in enhanced power production during the concentric portion of the SSC. The mechanical model, first illustrated by A. V. Hill (40), describes contractile and noncontractile elements (discussed in Chapter 3).

Contractile elements are contained within the sarcomere of a muscle and consist of actin and myosin. **Noncontractile elements** consist of the series elastic component (SEC), also known as the muscle-tendon unit (31), and the parallel elastic component (PEC), which consists of the connective tissues surrounding individual fibers, muscle bundles, and the entire muscle (i.e., endomysium, perimysium, and epimysium). The mechanical model states that muscle force is increased due to the reutilization of elastic energy by the SEC (31). In other words, when a muscle is eccentrically loaded (i.e., stretched) and immediately followed by a concentric action, energy will be produced, stored, and ultimately released from the muscle-tendon unit and increase force and power output.

On the other hand, the neuromuscular model suggests that preactivation of a muscle or muscle group is partially responsible for the force and power potentiation during the concentric phase of a SSC (13,83). A comparison of jumps initiated from either a static squat position or by beginning with a countermovement shows that there is a greater amount of time to develop force and muscular activation prior to shortening by the con-

REAL-WORLD APPLICATION
Muscle Elasticity

Releasing a rubber band from a stretched position will allow it to snap back into its original shape. Similarly, stored elastic energy will provide additional force when muscle shortening is preceded immediately by a stretch. During the stretch, energy is stored in the muscle, just as it is stored in the stretched rubber band. The stored elastic energy of muscle is one reason plyometric exercises increase power output.

tractile element during the countermovement jump (13). In addition, sprinting and agility skills have shown preactivation of a majority of the leg muscles prior to the support phase (7,49,84), suggesting that movement speed would be dramatically reduced otherwise.

In all likelihood both models contribute to the enhancement of force and mechanical power output during SSC. In fact, during the early extension phase of a static squat jump, it has been shown that the SEC is stretched only slightly (48). This is most likely due to the large amount of shortening of the contractile element. Just prior to toe-off (about 100 milliseconds), there is a reversal in roles where the contractile element does not change in length and the SEC rapidly shortens and releases prestored energy (48). Therefore, each model may provide a stimulus during different portions of a given SSC.

> *The SSC is an important physiological reflex that enhances muscular power output. Both mechanical and neural factors contribute to power potentiation.*

Neural control and reflexes of skeletal muscle are governed by two receptors: namely, muscle spindles and the Golgi tendon organ. Each has a distinct purpose of facilitation and inhibition, respectively (32,79). **Muscle spindles** contain several intrafusal fibers that are arranged in parallel with extrafusal fibers. They provide information via **sensory neurons** regarding muscle length. Specifically, spindles detect the rate of change in length (velocity) and report the information to the central nervous system (CNS). In response to a rapid muscle stretch, **alpha motor neurons** are stimulated, causing a contraction of the agonist muscle. It is for this reason that instructions for SSC exercises focus on performing a rapid eccentric action (stretch) to maximally stimulate the stretch reflex (71); the jury is still out, however, regarding the rate of stretch and SSC performance (13).

The other muscle receptor is the Golgi tendon organ. **Golgi tendon organs (GTOs)** are located in the muscle-tendon complex and monitor tension, which in turn provides an inhibitory reflex on motor neurons of the agonist muscle (32,63). GTO stimulation may be overridden however, by voluntary impulses and under certain circumstances could provide an excitatory stimulus (70). There-

fore, in regards to SSC activities, the net effect of GTO stimulation remains in question.

> *Muscle spindles and GTOs are responsible for the enhancement or inhibition of muscular actions by monitoring the rate of stretch and detecting tension in muscle.*

Impacting Factors

In performing exercises that involve SSC, there are several factors that can impact the enhancement of force or power output of the movement. For example, fiber-type distribution may significantly affect SSC (80). An athlete with predominantly slow-twitch fibers should take advantage of the neuromuscular model and slow movement speeds slightly to allow more time to build up muscular force. This may not be a realistic option, however, when one is concerned with sprinting, changing direction, or jumping for maximal performance. Conversely, an individual with predominantly fast-twitch fibers should focus on increasing movement speeds to maximize power output.

As an example, let's consider a 100-m sprinter and compare him to a distance runner (2 to 3 mi). We will assume that both athletes have mastered the technique of their respective activities. On one hand, to make sure that power will be improved for the sprinter, speed drills and plyometric exercises should focus on maximizing movement velocity, especially during the eccentric action. On the other hand, because the support phase during running can be 60% to 70% greater compared to sprinting (57), movements could be performed at slightly slower speeds, maintaining specificity to the particular activity. Keep in mind that these suggestions may differentiate only what is necessary for the eccentric portion of the SSC and should be applied only to certain types of SSC movements (i.e., jumping) (13). Therefore, stretching velocity may need to be altered so that the appropriate deceleration rates favor the greatest return in performance (78), but all movements should be performed to maximize concentric shortening velocity, acting to potentiate the contractile element and SEC activity.

Another factor affecting SSC, especially during jumping, is the use of the upper extremities. Swinging the arms while performing a countermovement jump creates more downward vertical ground reaction force; consequently a greater amount of upward vertical force is generated (Newton's law of action-reaction), propelling the body higher or further during flight (36). Arm swing also contributes to takeoff velocity during vertical and horizontal jumping actions (2,36) and is important for maximizing momentum of the lead leg during high jumping (50). Swinging the arms during sprinting increases velocity compared to sprinting without arm actions (84). So, choosing whether or not to swing the arms can significantly contribute to the execution of SSC drills and consequently affect athletic performance.

Studies have reported gender differences in SSC ability by using indirect measurements such as countermovement jump height or sprinting ability. Typically boys and men exhibit greater absolute power than girls or women. In addition, larger increases are observed in maximal power for boys compared to girls during growth and maturation (59). Greater amounts of lean body tissue (i.e., muscle mass) are believed to be responsible for these differences; however, when normalized for body weight, the differences between boys and girls are often minimized (46,81). Reports have shown higher peak velocity during countermovement jumps for men as compared to women (20,37). In fact, one study concluded that the difference in peak power between men and women was solely due to movement velocity (20). Other factors such as fiber-type composition, anaerobic metabolism, and neuromuscular aspects may also contribute to gender differences (59). Although these differences exist, there is no evidence to suggest that men and women respond to SSC training differently; therefore, program design should reflect developmental stage, training experience, and the particular sport rather than gender.

Sprinting, jumping, and changing direction require complex multijoint movements, which must have specific coordination between agonists and antagonists to ensure movement efficiency. It would be extremely ineffective, for example, if during sprinting the hip flexors were stimulated in the late swing phase, when maximal hip extension activity is necessary. There are reflexes that stimulate agonists while simultaneously inhibiting antagonists. This is termed **reciprocal innervation** (32,63). Alterations in this relationship can be impacted by increased strength or fatigue (3,43,44). For example, strengthening agonists

will increase acceleration of the movement, while strengthening antagonists will allow deceleration to occur over a shorter time (44). The overall effect would be a heightened capacity to perform explosive SSC actions.

Fatigue, on the other hand, reduces the effectiveness of the SSC through a host of mechanisms, the effects of which may persist for several days (6,41). It has been shown that a decrease in muscle spindle sensitivity occurs, which impairs elastic energy utilization, in turn reducing SSC potential (3–5). The mechanisms responsible for altered SSC function may be influenced by whether the fatigue was generated during submaximal or maximal exercise (75,76). Therefore, the duration of recovery from previous training sessions may be heavily dependent on the type and intensity of SSC drills performed.

This brief overview of SSC identifies several aspects that must be considered in designing a training regimen or exercise session. First, the use of arm swing is an integral component of locomotion and should be considered in selecting drills or exercises. For example, proper arm actions should always be implemented for younger, inexperienced athletes who are still learning the fundamental locomotor skills. For advanced athletes, limiting arm action may be implemented into certain training phases for specific training outcomes. Second, improving overall strength should be regarded as a priority for improving locomotor skills that require SSC. Children will become stronger through growth and development, but they may still benefit from playful activities or body-weight exercises that can increase strength. Mature athletes can include resistance training to enhance force capacity. Although gender will play a role in the difference of force and power production following puberty, variations between boys and girls at younger ages are minimal. Therefore, children should be taught proper movement mechanics regardless of gender; however, beyond puberty, training regimens should target performance limitations of the individual athlete and may be designed toward particular gender differences. Finally, unless there are specific needs that require an athlete to perform sprints, jumps, or changes in direction in a fatigued state, SSC exercises should be performed early within a training session and appropriate rest given between subsequent training sessions.

Q & A from the Field

I work with many youth soccer teams (12- to 14-year-olds) and continually find the need to work on fundamental movement skills, such as sprinting and agility. What are appropriate drills and progressions to use with this age group?

—*high school strength and conditioning coach*

The ability to perform stopping and starting tasks in sports such as soccer is important. Coupling deceleration with reacceleration, however, may be one of the most challenging motor skills to teach younger athletes, since other things like balance, orientation, rhythm, and anticipation will set the foundation for more advanced skills. Nevertheless, an appropriate progression is an important consideration in selecting drills for your athletes.

First, teach your athletes how to accelerate properly. Next, develop their ability to stop or decelerate. Then begin to combine these skills in a linear acceleration, deceleration, and reacceleration sequence. Finally, couple linear stopping with reacceleration in different directions. Each of these steps must start at slow speeds and progress to faster movements, ultimately producing athletes who can start, stop, and restart in a variety of directions at maximal speed. Below are two drills to include in your training plan.

Linear Walk to Stride: Instruct the athletes to transition from walking to a jog and then slow back down again over short distances (5 to 10 yd). Once slower speeds are per-

fected, have your athletes increase the speed of acceleration. Be sure they use a multiple-step stopping technique when slowing down and avoid using one large step. You can also specify a distance for your athletes to stop within (e.g., 2 to 4 yd) and thereby heighten the intensity.

Jog-Stop-Turn-Jog: Once your athletes can perform linear stopping and starting drills at higher speeds, you can introduce slight changes in direction by having the athletes move between cones. Initially instruct your athletes to completely stop when they reach a cone, plant their outside foot, simultaneously rotate their torso toward the new direction, and finally resume jogging. You should begin with shallow angles (130 to 160 degrees) and progressively make them more challenging (90, 60, and 45 degrees). When your athletes can perform changes in direction at slower speeds with minimal flaws, gradually increase the speed.

Be sure to progress slowly; it may take several months or longer to develop appropriate movement skills. Provide ample practice time when athletes are fresh (at the beginning of practice) and continually give feedback.

 Many factors can contribute to SSC function, such as fiber-type distribution, gender, age, muscle activation patterns, fatigue, and arm actions.

PLYOMETRICS

Plyometric exercises are specifically designed to utilize the SSC. Many upper- and lower-body exercises exist; it is beyond the scope of this chapter to include an all-inclusive list, but several examples are provided at the end of the chapter. This section provides a discussion on intended uses, the importance of instructions, complex training outcomes, and proper exercise terminology for plyometric training.

Plyometric exercises should include activities such as jumping, landing, hopping, leaping, bounding, galloping, and skipping. By performing these activities explosively, we train the body first to utilize the nervous system to help us move faster and second to utilize the energy stored in muscles when

we stretch them rapidly. The activities demonstrated in these figures should be performed explosively for the exercise to be considered plyometric.

Terminology

The plyometric literature has yet to clearly define movement skills using the lower extremities to propel the body off the ground. In an effort to clarify the language used by sports performance professionals, terminology from physical education is used in this chapter to describe plyometric motor skills. There are three main movement skills; a few of their derivatives are listed below. First, a **jump** involves a takeoff from one or both feet and a landing on both feet simultaneously. Second, a **leap** (sometimes called a bound) occurs from taking off on one foot and landing on the other. Finally, a **hop** is when the takeoff and landing occur on the same single foot. Other common fundamental skills are the gallop, shuffle, and skip. **Galloping** and **shuffling** are a combination of a step and leap, whereas **skipping** requires combining a step with a hop. It becomes somewhat more difficult to distinguish types of upper-body actions. One distinction that can be used is throwing and tossing. **Throwing** actions will be considered when an overhand movement is used to propel an object, while a **toss** occurs when an underhand action is employed. Plyometric exercises also exist for the core. Core exercises can be classified as stability, anterior-posterior flexion and extension, rotation, and lateral flexion and extension.

Developmental Sequence

Jumping, leaping, and hopping are the three primary fundamental motor skills to project the body off the ground. All individuals will develop these skills based on experiences throughout childhood, and some will perfect them later in life due to coaching from more knowledgeable instructors. It is important to understand some of the key movement characteristics as well as to be able to identify the developmental difficulties associated with these motor skills. With that said, it is beyond the scope of this chapter to provide all of the criteria to evaluate the different stages of all jumping skills; therefore a brief overview follows for vertical jumping and horizontal leaping. More detailed information can be found in the references (33,38).

Vertical jumping is common to many sports, and its initiation can begin as early as 2 years of age (33). Many steps are involved in the developmental transition from inefficient jumping actions to proficient movement skills. In younger or inexperienced jumpers, there is only a small preparatory countermovement action. In addition, full extension of the hips, knees, and ankles does not occur. Often the legs are tucked (knee flexion)

under during the flight phase, so the center of mass is not elevated. Another characteristic is that there is difficulty jumping and landing on both feet. A small step can usually be observed when a one-footed takeoff and landing occurs. Arm action is also asymmetrical and is not necessarily coordinated with the body or legs. Mature jumping patterns differ dramatically, and changes will occur quickly. For example, there is an appropriate preparatory countermovement action of the legs that is followed by a more forceful extension of the hips, knees, and ankles (33). The movement patterns of the legs are now also coordinated with those of the arms, so that there is an increase in ground reaction forces (preparatory countermovement phase) as well as an improvement in peak vertical velocity (extension phase). During the flight phase, the trunk remains upright; and upon landing, there is appropriate flexion of the hips, knees, and ankles to reduce the forces on impact.

Horizontal leaping (or bounding) is another common jumping skill that is similar to running in that there is an air phase when body weight is transferred from one leg to the other. Unlike running, leaping requires a prolonged air phase with greater vertical height and more horizontal distance covered. Early attempts at leaping typically resemble modestly exaggerated running movements. There is an inability to propel the body upward or for greater horizontal distances (33). There is a high degree of conscious effort to perform this movement; therefore, the entire motion is ineffective and often appears stiff. The arms are not used for generating force but rather for maintaining balance. Mature leaping includes forceful extension of the support leg to maximize horizontal and vertical distances, and the arms are now coordinated and assist in force development.

REAL-WORLD APPLICATION
Angular Motion and Human Movement

The human body is designed for angular motion around joints, which causes linear motion of the center of gravity of the body. Think about rowing a boat: the blade of an oar enters the water, the oar itself is relatively inflexible, and there is an oarlock providing a pivot point. This lever system works to provide the propulsion that moves the boat forward. Foot contact during the support phase, muscle activation providing stiffness, and motion around the hip joint all ultimately allow horizontal motion.

REAL-WORLD APPLICATION
Absorption of Energy

An egg that has been thrown at you will break when you catch it unless you "give" with it and catch it softly. Similarly, in landing from a jump, or similar movement, the athlete can learn to land softly. Instead of all of the energy dissipating on impact, it is spread out over a larger period. Landing softly decreases the chance of impact-related injuries. The transition from eccentric to concentric muscle action, however, must occur rapidly to utilize the stored elastic energy in the muscle.

Interestingly, chronological age does not guarantee mature jumping or leaping patterns, as adolescents and adults have been found to display immature or ineffective mechanical characteristics. These can range from preparatory, takeoff, and landing inefficiencies. Therefore, sports performance professionals should not assume that movement skills have been mastered simply due to chronological age. A critical examination of these motor skills is important to identify performance deficiencies. Only when proper takeoff and landing characteristics are evident should a training program focus on improving and maximizing performance.

Intended Purpose

Plyometric exercises are used in a variety of settings (e.g., athletic training, strength and conditioning, physical therapy); although no formal classification system has been developed, it is important to understand the purpose and expected outcomes of any plyometric exercises chosen for a training program. For simplicity, the following section describes the instructions used for two very distinct areas of motor development: injury prevention and performance enhancement, both of which are important for any athlete.

INJURY PREVENTION

Some approaches to injury prevention have used plyometric exercises in an attempt to improve neuromuscular control, alter biomechanical risk factors, and provide instructions on general proprioceptive and stability development (19,35,39,73). This requires specific instructions that typically focus on reducing landing forces to minimize risk potential. These types of instructions can be effective in a short time (e.g., one to three sessions) (62,66), but they must be used regularly, because adaptations appear temporary (69).

A common mechanism of injury occurs on landing from a jump. This is often due to improper mechanics, where landing forces are not appropriately dissipated because the hips, knees, or ankles are extended and/or rotated. As an example, these mechanical flaws are associated with noncontact injuries to the anterior cruciate ligament (ACL). By instructing athletes to land with greater hip, knee, and ankle flexion, the landing forces can be significantly reduced (39,55). Although programs using these types of instructions have shown success

in reducing landing forces and noncontact ACL injury rates, the effect on performance enhancement is extremely questionable, because no attention is given to maximizing concentric movement velocity. Therefore, these types of instructions for plyometric exercises may be reserved for younger athletes who require proprioceptive and motor development or kept within the context of clinical rehabilitation. Healthy or more advanced athletes might also benefit from this type of work if fundamental motor skills are not fully developed; however, if performance improvement is the intended outcome, other instructions may be necessary.

IMPROVING POWER

Plyometric drills are most often incorporated into a strength and conditioning program with the intention of improving SSC capability, power, and ultimately performance (e.g., vertical jump, linear sprint speed). Since power is related to both force and velocity, the question regarding which is more responsible for power improvements is often asked.

It has been reported that the use of plyometric exercises alone can improve jumping ability (17,30, 53,85). Peak velocity during the concentric phase, however, appears to be the key component for countermovement jump performance (2,36,50). Research has shown that improvements of 12.7% in takeoff velocity accounted for 71% of the observed improvement in jumping performance (2). In addition, the use of light (30% of 1 RM) compared to heavy (80% of 1 RM) squat jump loads has been shown to provide greater velocity specificity and improvements in jumping and acceleration (61). This underscores the importance of instruction for takeoff technique and the ability to take off with maximal velocity. Therefore, landing and jumping mechanics should be viewed as separate motor skills and trained independently.

> *Plyometric drills used for injury prevention, rehabilitation, or motor skill development should focus on proper jumping and landing mechanics. Training with the intention to improve performance (maximal takeoff velocity) should be the focus.*

The performance of SSC drills in isolation during training is not common, and the combination of resistance training and plyometric exercises is often integrated into training regimens. One classic study demonstrated that the combination of resistance and plyometric training caused greater improvements in vertical jump ability than either training modality alone (1). Other research has provided indirect support for this notion by reporting that neither resistance training nor plyometric exercises alone can provide a stimulus any greater than the other when targeting performance enhancement (85). It therefore appears that one cannot increase power simply by becoming stronger and that utilizing any increase in strength at appropriate speeds is the key factor for performance enhancement (14). These data, however, do support the fact that increasing agonist strength will enhance SSC capacity and performance.

The implementation of plyometric exercises at appropriate times to maximize performance for a particular competition requires careful program design. The duration for a given mesocycle may be as short as several weeks and as long as several months. Shorter-duration programs (6 weeks) do not provide adequate stimulation or enough time for adaptation to occur (89), but interventions implemented over 8 to 12 weeks can improve vertical jump height and power production (30,34). Therefore, a minimum of 8 weeks should be used in designing a training program that includes plyometrics to improve athletic performance.

> *The combination of resistance and plyometric training provides a significant stimulus for improving performance. The use of high-intensity drills for a minimum of 8 weeks seems necessary.*

Acute Training Variables

The acute training variables—volume, frequency, and intensity—must be planned on a daily basis and are key components of the exercise, which relate strongly to the potential effectiveness of the training program.

VOLUME

Foot contacts or distance covered are the most common methods for determining plyometric volume. Often volume is prescribed based on classifying the individual as a beginner, intermediate, or advanced athlete (71); however, there is no scientific support for this approach. In fact, studies examining the effects of plyometrics on performance have used between 30 and 200 jumps per day (1,17,21,24,34,68,85,89), which is well outside the range frequently cited. The volume of work should be based on the intent of the session

(i.e., performance versus learning), the intensity of the drills (i.e., high versus low), the training age of the athlete (i.e., inexperienced versus advanced), and other variables, such as the sport itself and the particular goals of the training cycle.

FREQUENCY

The number of plyometric training sessions performed weekly will be governed by many factors. In general, one or two sessions during the season and three to four sessions during the off season may be sufficient; however, available evidence suggests that 2 to 3 days per week may be optimal for improving performance (1,17,21,24,34,68,85,89). The frequency of plyometric sessions will be dictated by the need for recovery from other training or practice sessions. It may also be affected by the demands of the sport. For example, volleyball and basketball require a large volume of jumps to be performed on a daily basis. Therefore, it may be unreasonable to include in-season plyometric sessions. If plyometric exercises are implemented with the intent to teach proper motor skill development and the demands are small, then more frequent (4 to 5 days per week) sessions could be prescribed.

INTENSITY

The intensity of plyometric drills is often qualified with terms such as *high, moderate,* or *low intensity.* Unfortunately no research has quantitatively identified intensity of plyometric exercises by measuring landing forces for a particular exercise. Even if such information existed, there are several factors that will affect the intensity of a plyometric exercise. An athlete with a greater body mass will have greater landing forces. A heavier athlete who lands with greater hip, knee, and ankle flexion, however, might have less landing forces than a lighter athlete who lands with less flexion in those joints. Therefore, landing mechanics will also affect the intensity of plyometric drills. Adding complexity to a drill will alter the intensity. For example, a single-leg hop with rotation will be more intense than a countermovement jump.

The intensity of the exercises used may impact the outcome in targeting performance enhancement. For example, one study compared depth jump training to countermovement jump training; even though both groups significantly improved jump height, the range of improvement was larger for the individuals performing depth jumps (34).

On the other hand, if injury prevention is the primary focus, it will be helpful to implement a variety of less challenging exercises. Much more research is necessary in this area prior to drawing any definitive conclusions regarding an intensity classification system for plyometrics.

LINEAR SPRINTING

Linear sprint speed is a key component for successful athletic performance in most sports. Linear sprinting can typically be divided into three distinct phases: **acceleration** (0 to 10 yd), **attainment** (10 to 35 yd), and **maintenance** (above 35 yd). These distances will certainly differ between individuals and should be used only as a temporal guide to the various phases. An understanding of the movements involved and specific muscular actions responsible for creating movement will allow sports performance professionals to design drills and develop training regimens that are appropriate for improving linear sprinting performance. Several key sprint mechanics drills are displayed at the end of this chapter.

Developmental Sequence

The main difference between walking and running is the absence of a double support phase and the presence of a flight phase, respectively. The earliest attempts to run occur around 2 to 3 years of age or approximately 6 to 7 months after a child learns how to walk (33,38). By observing these movements in young children, one often notes a brief flight phase with a limited range of motion in the legs. This will result in shortened stride length. In addition, the thighs and arms swing away from the body, most likely acting to help stabilize and balance the body during the flight and support phases (38). Also to aid in balance, the stance is often wide. As children mature, they develop movement patterns that are more efficient and powerful. For example, maturity will bring about an increase in muscle mass and strength, which will provide more ground force and increase stride length. Other changes in sprint mechanics include full leg extension, keeping the actions of the extremities in the anterior-posterior plane, and maintaining bent elbows (38). The development of motor skill patterns will impact energy expenditure, fatigue rates, injury risk, and ultimately linear sprint performance.

Sprinting Gait

Sprinting is a complex motor skill for which specific kinetic and kinematic patterns emerge. Box 15.1 shows a basic breakdown of leg actions for sprinting. In addition, Figure 15.1 shows the average moments around the hip, knee, and ankle joints during a complete stride. The following discussion briefly outlines the two phases of a sprint: the **swing phase** and **support phase**. This overview describes factors associated with mature movement patterns and should provide a context from which to design drills and develop a training program targeted at improving or maximizing sprinting speed in advanced athletes.

SWING PHASE

At toe-off, maximum extension (about 185 degrees) of the hip occurs (74), while knee extension is approximately 145 degrees (47). During early follow-through, both hip flexor and knee extensor muscle activity greatly increases, as they are eccentrically loaded. This acts to decelerate leg rotation (58) and helps with quick leg recovery (Fig. 15.2). The transition from follow-through to forward swing is the first SSC observed in the sprint cycle. This is caused by concentric hip flexor action, which rotates the upper leg anteriorly (57). Maximum hip flexion occurs two-thirds of the way through the swing phase and corresponds with

---

15.1 SPRINTING GAIT (57)

1. **Swing phase.** The time the foot is in midair and not in contact with the ground
2. **Follow-through.** From toe off to maximal hip extension
3. **Forward swing.** From the beginning of hip flexion to maximum hip flexion
4. **Foot descent.** From maximum hip flexion to foot contact
5. **Support phase.** The time the foot is touching the ground
6. **Foot contact.** Time of initial foot contact until the acceptance of full body weight
7. **Midsupport.** From full weight acceptance until plantarflexion of ankle joint begins
8. **Toe-off.** From the onset of plantarflexion to toe-off

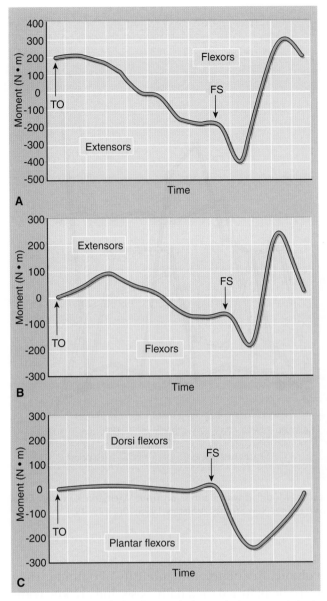

FIGURE 15.1 Muscle dominance during sprinting around the **A.** hip, **B.** knee, and **C.** ankle. TO = toe off; FS = foot strike. (Modified with permission from Mann RV. A kinetic analysis of sprinting. Med Sci Sports Exerc 1981;13:325–328.)

The adductors are active during early follow-through (just after toe-off) and early foot descent, stabilizing the knee by counterbalancing the external rotation and abduction action of the gluteus group (84) (see Fig. 15.2). Tibialis activity begins at toe-off and remains throughout the entire swing phase, whereas gastrocnemius activity is minimal during most of this phase and does not increase until immediately prior to foot contact (25). This preactivity is thought to help prepare the joint to assist in decreasing the vertical forces at foot contact as well as creating a more efficient SSC of the gastrocnemius.

SUPPORT PHASE

Once the foot has made contact with the ground, hip extensor muscles (e.g., hamstrings and gluteus) act concentrically until midsupport (49). The gluteus maximus is continuously active (42), extending the hip but also stabilizing it (see Fig. 15.2). The hamstrings are responsible for providing the necessary force to propel the body forward and are the key to linear sprint speed (84). Higher-level sprinters have shown the ability to decrease horizontal braking by creating larger forces and generating more power in the hip extensors and knee flexors during early support (58). This extremely brief subphase should be recognized as the most important time of the sprinting cycle, realizing that hip extension is the main action responsible for linear sprinting speed. Therefore, to maximize speed, power must be created as early in the support phase as possible.

A transition of muscle action occurs between midsupport and toe-off when the hip flexors begin to act eccentrically and decelerate leg rotation (58). It appears the main function of the knee joint during the support phase is to transfer power in a proximal-to-distal direction (i.e., hip to ankle). There is a large amount of knee extensor muscle activity up through midsupport to stabilize the knee, transfer forces from the hip to the ankle, and keep the height of the center of mass constant. Lending support to this notion, one study reported negligible power from the knee during midsupport (45). Therefore, during the attainment and maintenance phases of a sprint, the knee extensors should not be considered a muscle group that produces forward propulsion. In fact, if the knee extensors activated maximally during support, it would produce a disproportionate upward force rather than forward propulsion. This would lead to a higher

contralateral toe-off. About this time there is a switch from knee flexion to knee extension. Figure 15.2 shows relatively little muscle activation of the quadriceps during this time in the swing cycle (84), indicating that knee extension is mainly brought about by momentum from hip flexion, which provides a whip-like action of the lower leg during the swing phase. The hamstrings now act eccentrically, halting knee extension while simultaneously beginning hip extension during foot descent (56). This is the second SSC observed during the swing phase of the sprinting cycle.

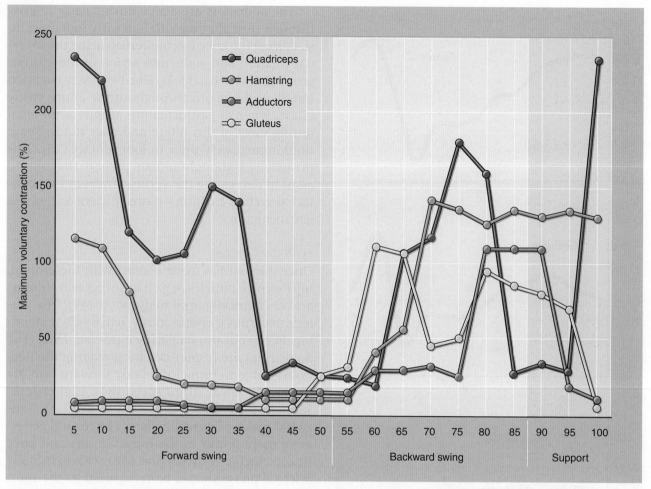

FIGURE 15.2 Relative muscle activation patterns during a sprint stride. [Modified with permission from Wiemann K, Tidow GN. Relative activity of hip and knee extensors in sprinting: implications for training. New Studies Athletics 1995;10(1):29–49.]

and subsequently longer flight phase (84), in turn reducing linear sprinting performance. The primary role of the muscles surrounding the ankle joint is to assist in maintaining the height of the center of mass at foot contact and to provide some thrust, albeit minimal, of the body in the anterior-posterior plane (25,56).

> *Sprinting requires horizontal power production from the hip extensors and knee flexors to propel the body forward during the early portion of the support phase. Maintaining a stable center of gravity occurs through eccentric actions of the gluteus, quadriceps, and gastrocnemius muscle groups.*

Acute Training Variables

The acute training variables are the specific variables that are manipulated to produce variation in volume, frequency, and intensity of training. They must be planned on a daily basis and are key components of the exercise, which relate strongly to the potential effectiveness of the training program.

VOLUME

The volume of linear sprint work will be characterized by the total distance covered during a given training session. It might be beneficial to consider sprint drills (e.g., A-steps, B-skips, etc.) and sprint capacity exercises separately. Sprint drills may be included daily during the warm-up routine with a focus on perfecting mechanical technique. On the other hand, the volume of work dedicated to improving sprint capacity will be governed by the characteristics of a given sport and possibly by requirements of a specific position. This includes the metabolic and linear sprint characteristics (i.e., average frequency and distance). Sprinting short distances (< 60 yd) depends heavily on anaer-obic metabolism. Therefore, the set and repetition scheme should ultimately target improving the enzymes associated with this particular energy system. Although abundant research has examined the impact of sprint interval training on metabolic adaptations (22,27,54,65), there is a great deal of variability in program design, so definitive guidelines on linear sprint volume are limited.

FREQUENCY

Performing high-intensity sprint training is physically demanding; therefore the number of weekly sessions will depend on recovery from other training and practice sessions. It may be sufficient to schedule two to three sessions per week, depending on additional demands placed on the athlete.

INTENSITY

Training to improve sprint capacity will typically involve maximal efforts; however, submaximal bouts of work can be used with inexperienced athletes to induce metabolic adaptations. It will be necessary to have the majority of training be of high intensity, so it should be prescribed only to athletes who have mastered sprinting mechanics. With that in mind, younger athletes should focus on drills that will enhance mechanics, while more advanced athletes can be prescribed maximal-effort bouts of work, targeting specific linear sprint distances.

Two additional methods often used in sprint training are assisted and resisted sprints. Both of these methods are considered to be of high-intensity and should not be prescribed to any athlete who has not mastered linear sprint mechanics. Extreme caution is warranted even for those athletes who have mature movement patterns, since resisted and assisted sprints can have negative consequences.

Assisted running (e.g., high-speed treadmill exercises, towing, or downhill running) will permit an athlete to run faster than his or her natural pace and is typically prescribed to help increase stride frequency (i.e., improve turnover). In spite of the anecdotal evidence, research clearly shows that running at supramaximal speeds will increase stride length and decrease stride frequency compared with maximal running (16,23,67). These alterations will consequently cause an increase in the horizontal distance from the foot to the center of mass at ground contact, resulting in greater braking forces during the support phase and increasing the likeli-

hood of injury (23). In addition, high-speed treadmills set below 80% or above 90% of maximal running velocity will cause a breakdown in sprint mechanics (47). Therefore, this type of training should be limited to elite athletes and completely avoided by younger inexperienced athletes.

Resisted running includes dragging a sled or running uphill and is often prescribed to increase force production and consequently stride length during unresisted sprinting. Several mechanical alterations occur with resisted sprints. For example, greater hip, knee, and ankle flexion occurs, which indicates less stiffness in the entire kinetic chain and less potential to maximize sprint velocity. In addition, overall posture is altered when running up slight grades (3 degrees) or pulling minimal weight (12% of body mass) (52,67). During resisted sprints, a larger amount of the leg cycle is spent in the support phase and there is a decrease in stride length (52,67,77,90). These changes in sprint mechanics may be detrimental to linear speed; therefore extreme caution is warranted in prescribing resisted sprint drills.

Clearly additional research is necessary to determine whether acute changes in sprint mechanics can be permanent if resisted and assisted training methods are chronically integrated into an athlete's regimen. Based on the available information, it would seem prudent to avoid any type of resisted or assisted method with younger and inexperienced athletes.

AGILITY

Changes in direction occur often during many athletic activities and include deceleration followed immediately by reacceleration of the entire body or individual body segment(s). This ability, termed **agility**, has been described as an efficient, coordinated movement in multiple planes performed at multiple velocities (26,82). A fighter dodging a punch or kick, a ballroom dancer performing the mambo, or a wrestler finishing a take-down are all examples of agility. Individuals involved in the development and improvement of sport performance, however, often regard agility as a locomotor skill where an athlete changes direction by decelerating the body and reaccelerating in a new direction (26,82). Although agility has been shown to be an independent athletic attribute (51), additional qualities are considered important, including dynamic balance, spatial awareness, rhythm, and visual processing (28). A high degree of complexity is present within this fundamental athletic motor skill.

Developmental Sequence

Learning to become agile requires the development of appropriate movement patterns and, more importantly, the ability to integrate locomotor skills efficiently (e.g., running, jumping) with proprioceptive awareness. As children learn to walk fast and run (at 1.5 to 3 years of age), they make attempts to be elusive and change direction when being chased. Their movement efficiency is often poor, however, and associated with awkward arm motion, overall unbalanced posture, and a general lack of timing and coordination. These are all characteristics described earlier in the section on the developmental sequence of sprinting. Because a variety of aspects are included in the ability to change direction, it is difficult to precisely identify a specific developmental sequence, as found in other locomotor skills.

Nevertheless, at particular windows of time, or critical periods, either general or specific drills can be implemented to develop agility appropriately. For instance, children aged 5 to 8 years should perform a large variety of general movement patterns in an effort to develop a foundation of motor skills. This could include arm and leg movements in a stationary position, rhythmic jumps in place, or locomotor drills that incorporate spatial orientation. Learning the temporal characteristics of general movements is extremely beneficial, especially prior to initiating more specific drills or activities. Closed agility drills, where the initiation, execution, and termination of a drill are clearly established, should dominate during this period. Children involved with athletics should be able to perform general drills with minimal flaws prior to advancing to more demanding exercises.

Young athletes between the ages of 9 and 13 years will be able to move more quickly as they mature. For reasons of safety and injury prevention, however, they should initially perform drills at submaximal speeds. In addition, drills should not yet include sharp changes in direction but rather involve rounded patterns. Weaving within a set of linear cones, running a figure-eight pattern, or learning how to integrate several locomotor skills

into one exercise are all acceptable drills during this stage of development. Drills that include sharp changes in direction performed at high running speeds are unlikely to benefit agility development, especially when mastery has not yet been achieved (10,72). Closed drills should still predominate in this window of time; however, some open drills can be included sparingly to add a reactive component with visual or audio stimuli.

Alterations in body size, structure, and body mass will influence a young athlete's coordination and proprioception. During this stage, take the time to perfect locomotor skills that are already developed, allowing the athlete to become more comfortable with his or her "new" body (26). Greater difficulty and more challenging drills can certainly be added to the training regimen, but throughout this stage sport-specificity should be avoided, as it may hinder overall athletic development.

More complexity and specificity are the focus of agility training during later teenage years (17 years and beyond) and can now be regularly implemented within the training plan (26). The same drill can be made more difficult simply by using different field conditions, including a partner, or implementing an area or time restriction. These are all acceptable methods to increasingly challenge an athlete's ability to change direction effectively (26). Athletes should perform nearly all of the drills at high speeds, as slower movements have been shown to alter muscle activation patterns (64). A shift toward open and away from closed drills is often typical; however, understand that performing open reactive exercises at high speeds can increase rotational loads placed on the joints with little change in the magnitude or pattern of muscle activation. This suggests that greater stresses will be placed on the joints, with a potentially increased risk of injury (9,10).

Critical periods of development do exist and generally correspond to a range of chronological ages. These critical periods can certainly guide appropriate athletic development, but in selecting drills or exercises, it is also important to consider an athlete's developmental stage and training age. In other words, it might be appropriate to use a large variety of closed drills with a 16-year-old who has had less than a year of training experience. On the other hand, it may be appropriate to include a greater proportion of open drills with a 13-year-old has had 4 years of consistent training experience and has mature locomotor skills. Do not depend solely on chronological age, but take the time to understand the limitations of each individual athlete. This will provide the strongest rationale for exercise prescription.

Impacting Factors

The ability to coordinate a smooth and rapid transition between stopping and starting is a distinct advantage for athletes performing changes in direction. Inefficient transitions caused by poor deceleration mechanics or an elongated support phase might allow a defender to maintain close proximity, not allowing an offensive player to become open to receive a pass (e.g., football, soccer, lacrosse). Enhanced agility must be developed in concert with many other proprioceptive and kinesthetic skills, such as balance, orientation, reactiveness, rhythm, visual processing, timing, and anticipation (28). With that in mind, several variables will impact how drills and exercises are performed, namely movement velocity, the angle of direction change, and whether a movement is planned (closed skill) or unplanned (open skill).

Effects of Movement Velocity

Agility drills can be performed at slow or fast running speeds. Slower running speeds are associated with greater ground-contact time during the deceleration phase compared to faster running speeds (300 versus 170 milliseconds, respectively) (8,64,72). As in linear sprinting, preactivation of knee flexors and extensors occurs immediately prior to ground contact, which serves to prepare the joints for eccentric loading during deceleration. An increase in muscle preactivation at higher running speeds has led some to suggest that a neural feed-forward mechanism exists to protect the hip and knee joints from the increased eccentric and rotational loads. A neural **feed-forward mechanism** indicates that the protective musculature would preactivate as a protective mechanism to decrease the chance of injury through neural control. It may also stimulate an increase in SSC ability and enhance the transition from eccentric to concentric muscle actions.

During the support phase, the adductors and gluteus medius are constantly active and are primarily responsible for stabilizing the hip. A highly integrated agonist-antagonist relationship between the quadriceps and hamstrings provides the ability

to change direction (64). More specifically, the knee extensors work to decelerate the body upon ground contact, while hip extensor activity predominates during the late support phase. Hip extension provides the necessary horizontal propulsion of the body in the new direction. Recall from the section on linear sprinting that hip extension is important during the early portion of the support phase. This apparent difference from linear sprinting should be considered in developing drills or exercises focused on improving agility performance.

Effects of Angles

Changes in direction can be considered shallow (less than 45 degrees) or sharp (more than 45 degrees). When athletes are observed in the laboratory and asked to perform sharp changes in direction, there is a large reduction in approaching velocity. Often there is an inability to appropriately execute the drill even with the reduction in approaching velocity (10,72). The fact that these movements are preplanned further highlights the difficulty of performing such maneuvers. It also indicates the need for incorporating drills into training regimens for elite athletes with mature movement skills. Drills that focus on the ability to make drastic changes in movement while maintaining speed will provide the necessary stimulus for adaptation and transfer to competition. On the other hand, inexperienced athletes should focus on more rounded patterns performed at slightly slower speeds and avoid demanding drills.

Changes in direction can be performed with an open or a crossover step. During the early stages of development, it might be beneficial to teach young athletes both movement skills. These steps should be performed at slow speeds, with specific attention given to proper mechanics. An analysis of open-step changes in direction shows internal rotation, whereas crossover steps produce external rotation on the knee. These loads can be up to five times greater than in linear running (10,11). In addition, crossover steps produce varus loads, while open steps show a mixture of varus and valgus loading at the knee (10,11). Changes in direction using an open step increase the activity of the vastus medialis and gluteus medius (9,72). This acts to (a) create stability around the hip joint during stance and (b) to counter the valgus loads associated with this movement. Closely observe your athletes as they perform agility drills to ensure proper mechanics, and include resistance training exercises that target the quadriceps and gluteus muscles, which will help stabilize the knee.

Effects of Anticipation

Whether a skill is preplanned (closed) or unplanned (open) will also impact movement patterns and joint loads. For example, an offensive lacrosse player may attempt several preplanned cutting maneuvers to elude a defensive player. On the other hand, the defensive player must continually adjust to the visual stimulus and anticipate the movements of the offensive player, making changes of direction reactive, or unplanned. The difference between preplanned and unplanned changes in direction has effects on external varus/valgus and internal/external rotational loading (9,10), muscle activation patterns (9), and body preparation (72).

Compared to an unplanned change in direction, a preplanned open step change in direction shows a slight crossover with the step prior to the pivot foot being planted, an earlier rotation of the pivot foot in the new direction, and a greater body lean (72). Flexion/extension loads are similar in planned and unplanned cutting actions, but there is greater knee flexion when movements are unplanned (11). In addition, a reduction in the whole movement angle occurs during an unplanned change of direction (10,72). These are all protective mechanisms that provide additional time for appropriate muscle activation, proper joint stabilization, and decreased internal joint forces.

Performing an unplanned cutting maneuver increases the valgus and internal rotation loads by 70% and 90%, respectively. Interestingly, muscle activation only increases by 10% to 20% (9,10). Furthermore, general muscle activation patterns emerge during unplanned changes in direction, indicating nonspecific coordination between anterior/posterior and medial/lateral synergistic muscle pairs (10). On the other hand, preplanned actions produce specific activation patterns of the vastus medialis and biceps femoris to counter the external valgus and internal rotation loads, respectively (10). The inability of the neuromuscular system to initiate the appropriate adjustments during unplanned changes in direction reduces the efficiency and velocity of the movement. Therefore, to enhance the ability to decelerate, include exercises that increase the eccentric ability of muscles (e.g., resis-

tance training) as well as drills that focus on improving reactive ability (e.g., plyometrics).

> *Factors such as velocity of movement, angle of change, or anticipation will impact muscular activation patterns, kinematics, and joint forces. Exercises that develop muscular stability, eccentric muscle strength, and reactive ability should be included for maximal athletic development.*

Acute Training Variables

Limited information exists on how to improve agility; however, training for linear speed will not improve the ability to change direction and vice versa (87,88). In fact, linear sprint speed, power, and agility are independent performance characteristics, where ability in one variable is not associated with the others (60). This means that agility training should be an integral component of an athlete's training regimen. Differences should exist, however, between inexperienced and advanced athletes.

VOLUME

Specific training sessions dedicated to the development or improvement of agility can utilize guidelines similar to those of linear sprint training, where volume is the total distance covered. Inexperienced athletes may require more time to learn proper mechanics and perform general movement patterns. On the other hand, advanced athletes can perform a greater volume of work. Understanding the relative contribution of changing direction to the sport or position will help to guide the sports performance professional in determining the appropriate volume appropriate for high-level athletes.

There are numerous agility drills; the conditioning specialist is limited only by the imagination when designing these drills. Agility drills should focus on changing direction quickly and using multiple footwork patterns. These drills should also be sport-specific in terms of movement patterns, footwork patterns, distances, work intervals, rest intervals, and intensities. Although it would be impossible to make a comprehensive list of agility drills, sample drills are described in Figures 15.19 to 15.22. These drills can be easily changed from one workout to the next for variety.

FREQUENCY

Inexperienced athletes can include agility daily as a part of a warm-up routine. Regular attention to proper mechanics is vital for the development of appropriate movement skills. Program design for advanced athletes will depend on the time of the year, sport specific requirements, and other training demands. The intent or focus of exercises can be adjusted to incorporate them more or less frequently.

INTENSITY

The intensity of agility drills will depend on factors such as running velocity, preplanned (closed) versus unplanned (open) drills, and sharpness of the angles. Young, inexperienced athletes need to perfect general, preplanned motor patterns before performing sport-specific drills. The drills should include rounded patterns performed at slow to moderate speeds. Body-weight resistance exercises and less demanding plyometric drills will also benefit the ability to change direction. As an athlete becomes more advanced, specific movement patterns can be included. The drills can be increasingly reactive and may include a wide variety of angles.

INTEGRATION OF SPEED AND AGILITY DRILLS

Depending on the sport and the time of the training cycle, the focus may be on either speed or agility or possibly both. If the focus is on maximizing forward running speed, three to four training sessions per week may be devoted to speed. Agility training may be performed occasionally for variety. The opposite will be true if the focus is on agility.

Some sports—soccer, for example—require both speed and agility. If speed and agility are both training goals, one to two sessions per week can be devoted to speed, and one to two to agility. Well-conditioned athletes may be able to benefit from combined sessions, using both speed and agility exercises. These exercises should be performed early in a training session so that the athlete is fresh. Performing speed and agility exercises while the athlete is fatigued on a regular basis may not be as effective in improving performance.

Speed and Agility Exercises

PLYOMETRIC EXERCISES

Countermovement Jump

Starting Position

The athlete stands with feet shoulder width apart, the body in an upright posture and looking straight ahead (Fig. 15.3A).

Movement Sequence

Begin with a preparatory countermovement by flexing the hips and knees. Maintain an upright body posture (Fig. 15.3B). Once at the bottom position, immediately jump vertically (Fig. 15.3C). Land in same spot from where the jump was initiated and flex the hips and knees to reduce landing forces.

Variations

Manipulate the depth of the preparatory countermovement. Keep the hands placed on the hips to eliminate arm swing. Add degrees of rotation so that the athlete will land facing a different direction.

(continued)

Countermovement Jump (continued)

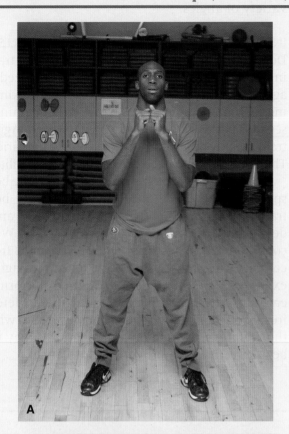

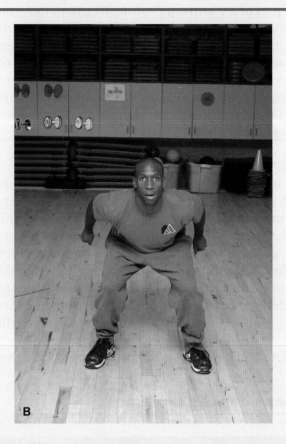

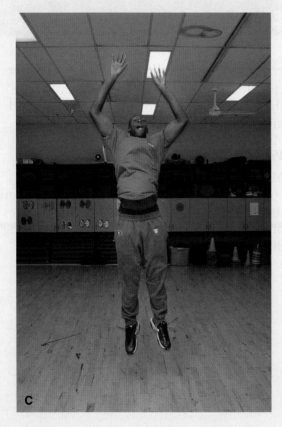

FIGURE 15.3 Countermovement jump. **A.** Starting position. **B.** Countermovement. **C.** Jump.

Scissor Jump

Starting Position

The athlete stands with the feet a shoulder width apart, the body in an upright posture, looking straight ahead. Take a half step forward with the right foot and a half step backward with the left.

Movement Sequence

Begin with a preparatory countermovement by flexing the hips and knees. Maintain an upright body posture (Fig. 15.4A). Once at the bottom position, immediately jump vertically

(Fig. 15.4B). While in the air, switch the positions of the legs so that the landing will occur with the left leg forward and the right leg behind. Be sure that the knees remain pointed forward and avoid caving inward (Fig. 15.4C).

Variations

Keep the hands placed on the hips to eliminate arm swing. Attempt to perform a double switch of the legs while in the air, so that landing occurs in the same position as the takeoff.

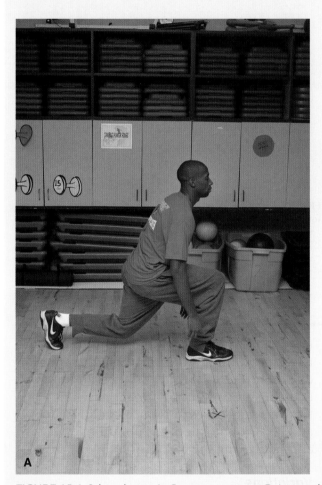

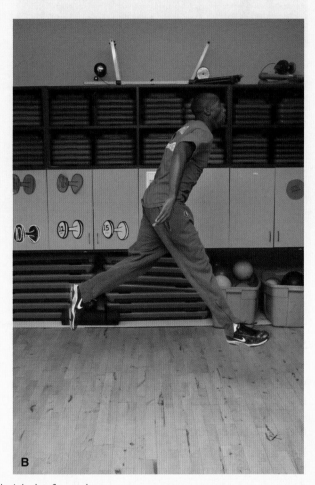

FIGURE 15.4 Scissor jump. **A.** Countermovement. **B.** Jump, with right leg forward.

(continued)

Scissor Jump *(continued)*

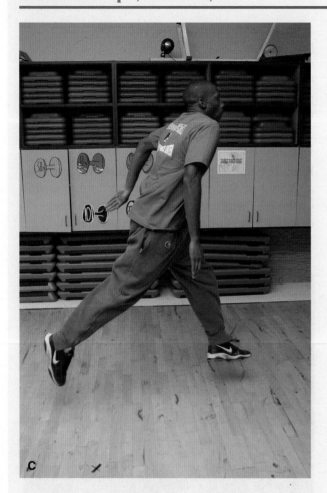

FIGURE 15.4 *(continued)* Scissor jump. **C.** Landing, with left leg forward.

Broad Jump

Starting Position

The athlete stands with the feet a shoulder width apart, the body in an upright posture, looking straight ahead.

Movement Sequence

Begin with a preparatory countermovement by flexing the hips and knees. During the downward movement, the body will lean slightly forward and the arms should be coordinated with a posterior swing

(Fig. 15.5A). At the bottom of the counter-movement, jump horizontally in the anterior direction (Fig. 15.5B). Land with an upright body posture and head looking forward. Flex the hips and knees to reduce landing forces and be sure the knees are pointing forward and not caving inward (Fig. 15.5C).

Variations

Eliminate arm swing. Take off from two feet and land on one foot.

Broad Jump (continued)

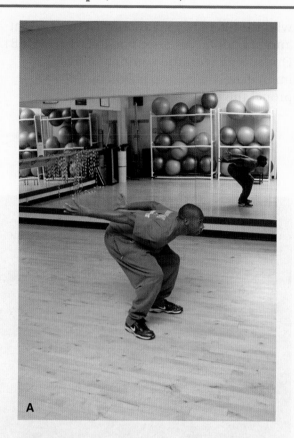

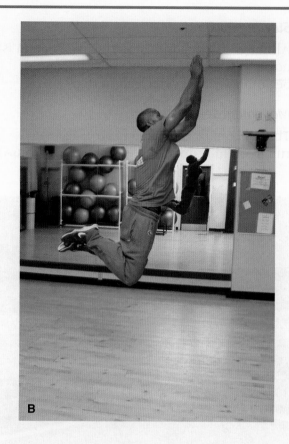

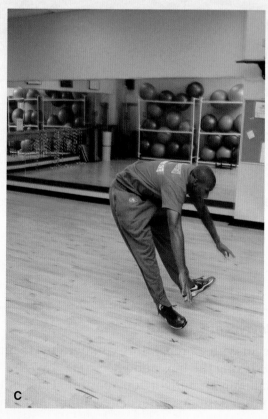

FIGURE 15.5 Broad jump. **A.** Countermovement. **B.** Jump. **C.** Landing.

Linear Bounds

Starting Position

Although starting from a stationary position is possible, it may be more comfortable by beginning with several lead-in steps.

Movement Sequence

This drill can be compared to an exaggerated run. Forcefully drive off the rear leg (Fig. 15.6A)

with the intent to gain as much vertical height and horizontal distance possible (Fig. 15.6B). On landing with the contralateral leg, immediately generate maximal force to propel the body again.

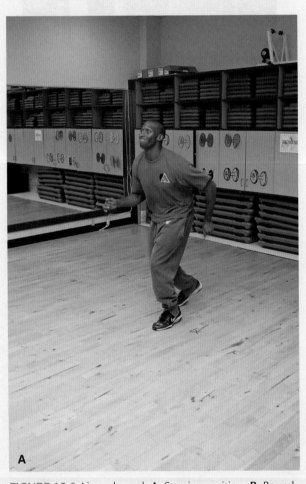

A

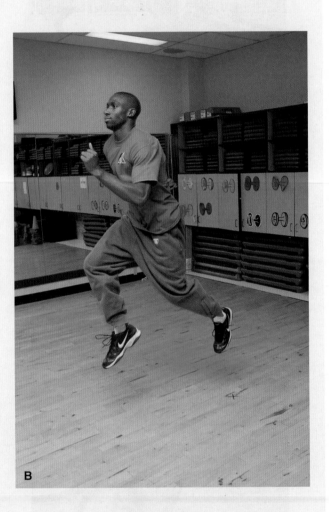

B

FIGURE 15.6 Linear bound. **A.** Starting position. **B.** Bound.

Lateral Cone Jump

Starting Position

The athlete stands with the feet a shoulder width apart, the body in an upright posture, looking straight ahead, with a cone placed directly to the side.

Movement Sequence

Begin with a preparatory countermovement by flexing the hips and knees (Fig. 15.7A). Maintain an upright body posture. Once at the bottom position, immediately jump, propelling

Lateral Cone Jump *(continued)*

the body vertically as well as laterally (Fig. 15.7B). Land on the opposite side of the cone and flex the hips and knees to reduce landing forces (Fig. 15.7C).

Variations

Keep the hands placed on the hips to eliminate arm swing. Add degrees of rotation so as to land facing in a different direction.

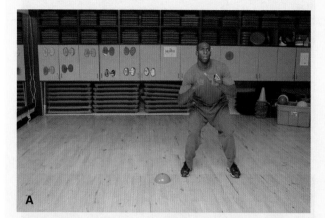

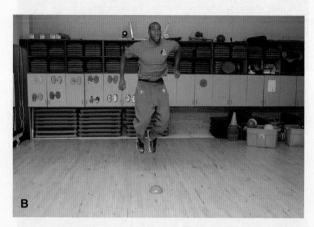

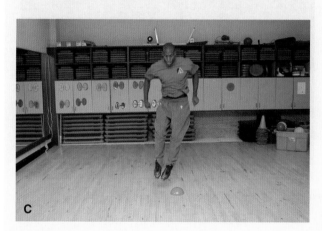

FIGURE 15.7 Lateral cone Jump. **A.** Countermovement. **B.** Lateral jump. **C.** Landing.

Lateral Bounds

Starting Position

The athlete stands with the feet a shoulder width apart, the body in an upright posture, looking straight ahead.

Movement Sequence

Begin with a preparatory countermovement by flexing the hips and knees. Maintain an upright body posture. During the downward phase, begin to shift the body weight to the left leg (Fig. 15.8A). Once at the bottom

position, propel the body laterally with the left leg (Fig. 15.8B) and land on the right (Fig. 15.8C). Be sure to flex the hips and knees on landing while also keeping the body inside the vertical plane of the knee (Fig. 15.8D).

Variation

Add anterior movement to this drill where the athlete will follow a zig-zag or diagonal pattern with each bound.

(continued)

Lateral Bounds *(continued)*

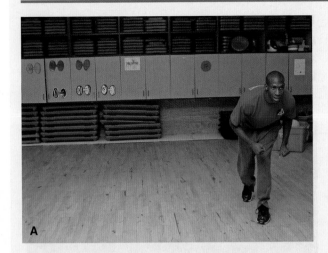
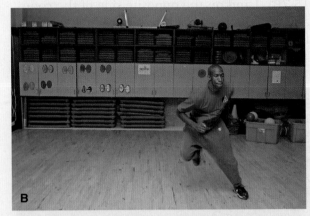
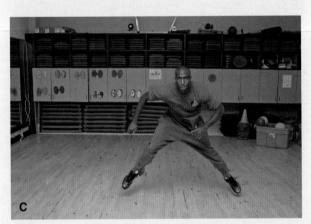
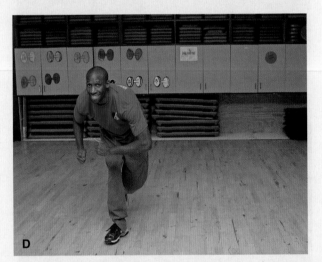

FIGURE 15.8 Lateral bound. **A.** Countermovement. **B.** Lateral movement. **C.** Downward movement. **D.** Landing.

Chest Throw

Starting Position

The athlete stands with the feet a shoulder width apart, holding a medicine ball in the center of the chest.

Movement Sequence

Begin with a preparatory countermovement by flexing the hips and knees. Maintain an upright body posture (Fig. 15.9A). During the upward phase, begin to simultaneously extend the arms with the legs. As the legs reach peak extension, the medicine ball is released with the intent of obtaining maximal horizontal distance (Fig. 15.9B).

Variation

Perform this exercise from your knees or with a partner.

Chest Throw *(continued)*

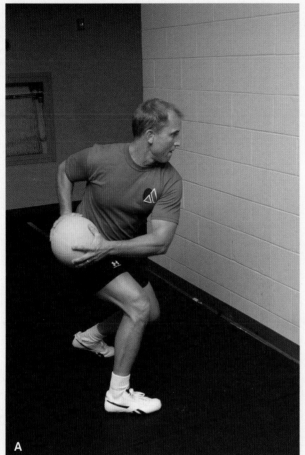 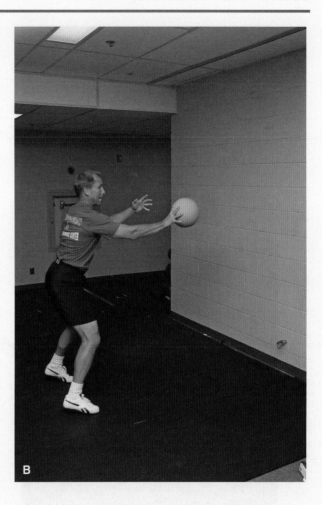

FIGURE 15.9 Chest throw. **A.** Countermovement. **B.** Release.

Scoop Toss

Starting Position

The athlete stands with the feet a shoulder width apart, holding a medicine ball by the hips with the arms fully extended.

Movement Sequence

Begin with a preparatory countermovement by flexing the hips and knees. Maintain an upright body posture and extended arm position (Fig. 15.10A). During the upward phase, while the legs are extending, begin to flex at the shoulders, keeping the elbows extended (Fig. 15.10B). As full leg extension is reached (Fig. 15.10C), release the medicine ball with the intent of obtaining maximal vertical height (Fig. 15.10D).

Variation

Perform this drill will a partner.

(continued)

Scoop Toss *(continued)*

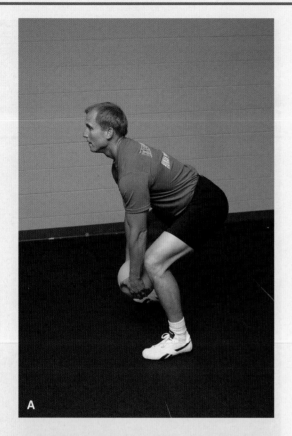

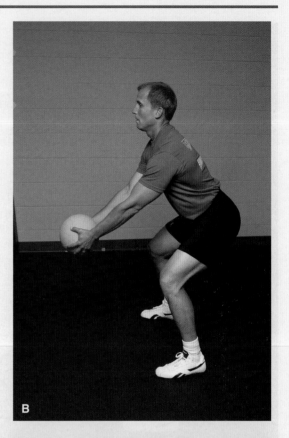

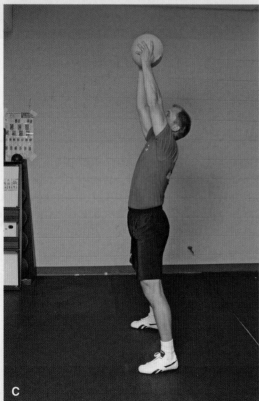

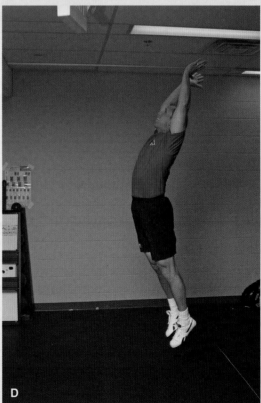

FIGURE 15.10 Scoop toss. **A.** Countermovement. **B.** Upward phase. **C.** Full leg extension. **D.** Release.

Overhead Throw

Starting Position

The athlete stands in a staggered stance, with an upright posture, holding a medicine ball directly overhead with the elbows extended.

Movement Sequence

Begin with a preparatory flexion of the elbows so that the medicine ball is behind the head (Fig. 15.11A). Immediately extend the elbows (Fig. 15.11B) and release the ball toward the wall (Fig. 15.11C). Attempt to hit the wall so that the ball rebounds directly into your hands with your elbows still extended.

Variation

Perform this drill by maintaining extended elbows, moving only from the shoulder.

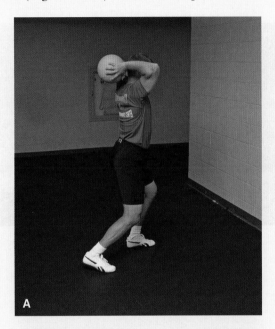

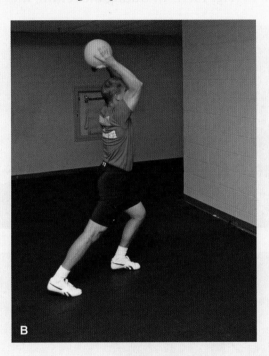

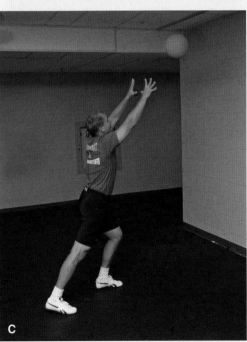

FIGURE 15.11 Overhead throw. **A.** Starting position with elbows flexed. **B.** Extension of elbows. **C.** Release.

Lateral Toss

Starting Position

The athlete stands with the feet a shoulder width apart and holding a medicine ball by the hips with the arms fully extended.

Movement Sequence

The athlete rotates the torso to the left while simultaneously slightly flexing the hips and knees (Fig. 15.12A). During the return, the hips and knees are extended and the ball is released toward the wall at a slight angle (Fig. 15.12B). As the ball rebounds off the wall, the athlete catches and perform the same action to the opposite side of the body (Fig. 15.12C).

Variations

Perform this drill with a partner. Maintain the rotation to the same side of the body.

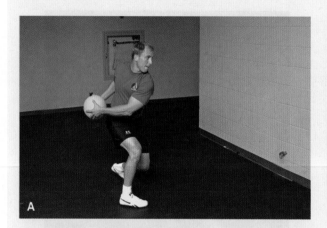

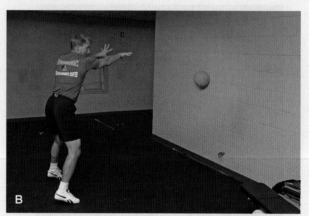

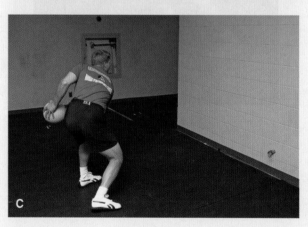

FIGURE 15.12 Lateral toss. **A.** Starting position with rotated torso. **B.** Release. **C.** Catch.

Two-Handed Put Throw

Starting Position

The athlete stands with the feet a shoulder width apart, holding a medicine ball in the center of the chest.

Movement Sequence

Begin by rotating the torso to the right (Fig. 15.13A) and flexing the hips and knees into a deep squat position (Fig. 15.13B). Once at the bottom, immediately extend the hips and knees while simultaneously rotating toward the starting position. The medicine ball will be thrown with the right hand (guide with the left). Fully extend the hips, knees, and right elbow, attempting to maximize the vertical height of the ball (Fig. 15.13C). Follow through completely by rotating to the left (Fig. 15.13D).

Variation

Perform this drill with a partner.

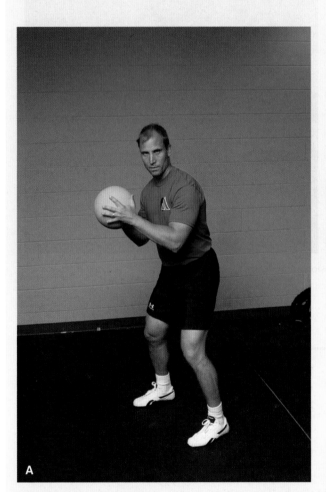
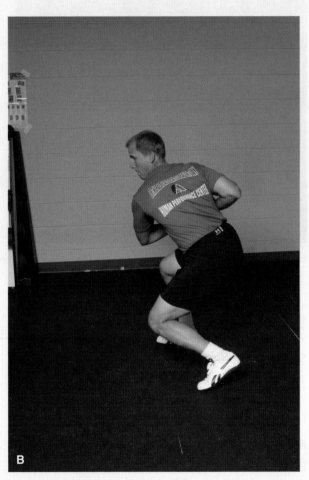

FIGURE 15.13 Two-handed put throw. **A.** Starting position with rotated torso. **B.** Deep squat position.

(continued)

Two-Handed Put Throw *(continued)*

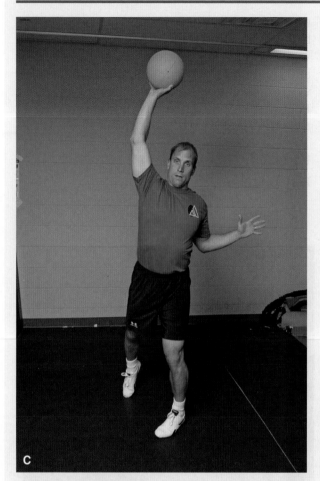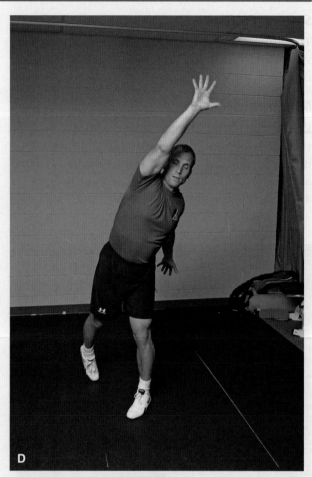

FIGURE 15.13 *(continued)* Two-handed put throw. **C.** Full extension and release. **D.** Follow-through.

Wood Chop Throw

Starting Position

The athlete stands with the feet a shoulder width apart, holding a medicine ball at the center of the chest (Fig. 15.14A).

Movement Sequence

Begin by rotating the torso to the right and flexing the hips and knees into a semisquat position (Fig. 15.14B). Move the ball in an arc from knee height to slightly above the head (Fig. 15.14C). Rotate the torso toward the start position, throwing the ball toward the ground (Fig. 15.14D).

Variation

Attempt to move and position yourself to catch the ball to initiate the next repetition.

Wood Chop Throw *(continued)*

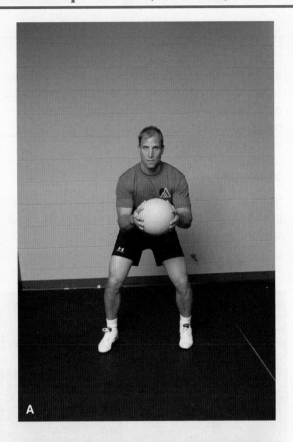

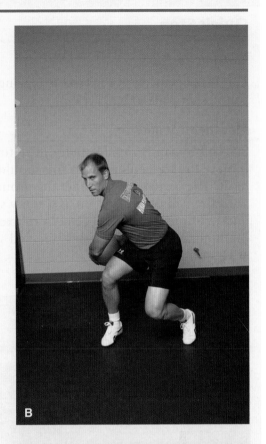

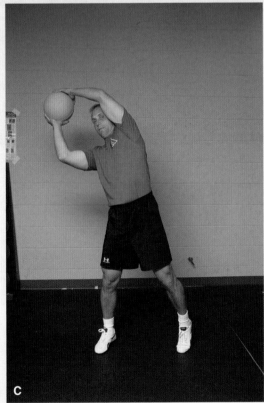

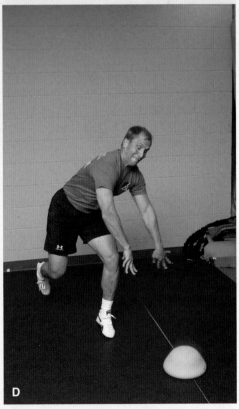

FIGURE 15.14 Wood chop throw. **A.** Starting position. **B.** Semisquat position. **C.** Arc movement. **D.** Release.

SPRINT MECHANIC DRILLS

Quick Step

Starting Position

This drill begins with the athlete jogging/running in place (Fig. 15.15A).

Movement Sequence

Swing the hands rapidly, being sure to initiate the movement from the shoulder joint. The feet should contact the ground with the ball of the foot during every support phase. Shoulders should remain relaxed. Maintain a visual focal point directed straight ahead (Fig. 15.15B).

The purpose of this drill is to enable the athlete to establish proper movement patterns (e.g., body alignment, support foot position, arm swing) without the mechanical or metabolic loads associated with high-speed horizontal movement.

Variation

Start at slower movement speeds and increase gradually from a jog into a run and finally a sprint.

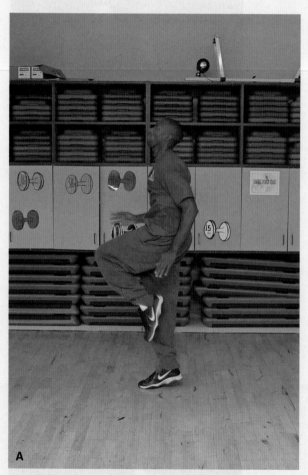

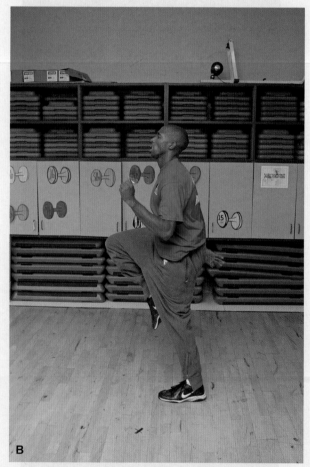

FIGURE 15.15 Quick step. **A.** Starting position. **B.** Step movement.

B-March

Starting Position

The athlete should begin this drill in a "marching" posture facing straight ahead (Fig. 15.16A).

Movement Sequence

Lift the knee (Fig. 15.16B) and pull the knee back to the ground. Although the knee is lifted and pulled back, it must be understood that the motion originates and is designed to accentuate the action about the hip. Keep the lower leg relaxed (do not kick; the lower leg will naturally have a whip-like motion when relaxed). Contact the ground with the ball of the foot and concentrate on "pulling" the body horizontally. Maintain visual focal point directed straight ahead. Keep shoulders relaxed. Proper arm swing should be maintained throughout.

The purpose of this drill is to create the appropriate muscle activation patterns during late swing through midsupport.

Variation

Start with a marching action and advance into skipping and finally skipping with a transition to a short sprint.

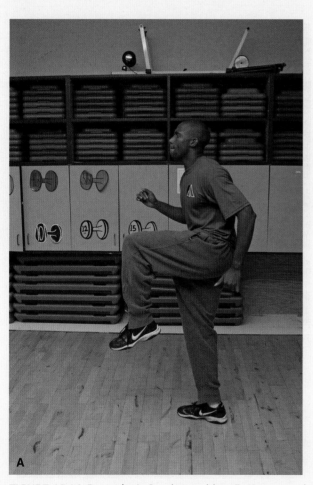
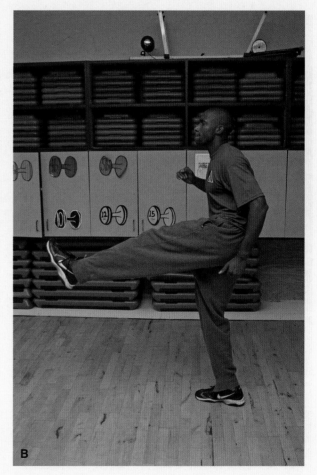

FIGURE 15.16 B-march. **A.** Starting position. **B.** Knee extension.

Stride Cycles

Starting Position

The athlete begins this drill by jogging or running forward (Fig. 15.17A).

Movement Sequence

Jog or run on the balls of the feet over a predetermined distance (e.g., 20 to 30 yd) (Fig. 15.17B). At a prescribed number of steps, perform a complete sprint cycle with one leg. Complete this repetition at a higher speed, contacting the ground on the ball of the foot and again "pulling" the body horizontally with hip extension (Fig. 15.17C). Allow the athlete

to transition into maximum effort linear sprinting by integrating single-leg full sprint cycles (swing and support phase) at prescribed intervals. All cycles should be performed near or at maximum speed.

Variation

Start with a high number of jogging/running steps (five to seven) between cycles, gradually reducing this (to one to three), and finally coupling into a double cycle (both the left and the right foot complete a cycle without jogging/running steps in between).

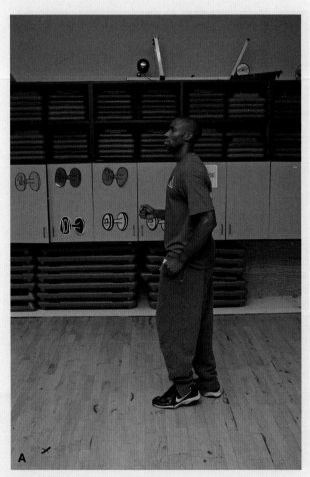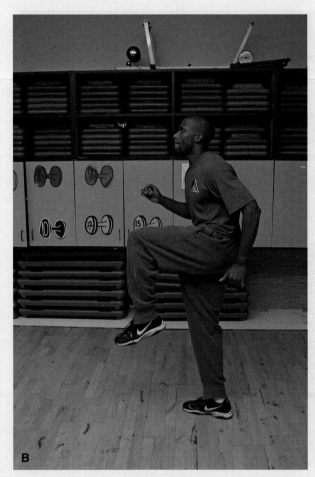

FIGURE 15.17 Stride cycle. **A.** Starting position. **B.** Jogging movement.

Stride Cycles *(continued)*

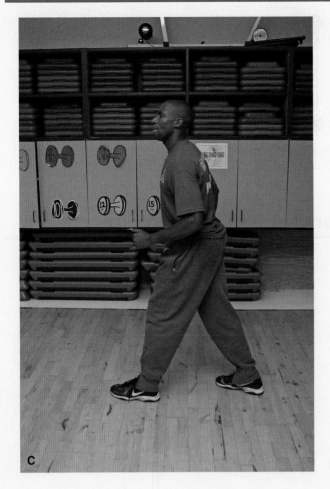

C.

FIGURE 15.17 *(continued)* Stride cycle. **C.** Hip extension.

Five-Point Agility Run

Starting Position

The athlete should start in an athletic "ready" position facing the direction of the first sprint.

Movement Sequence

Start at position X and run to position 1 as quickly as possible, returning to position X. Continue running to positions two to five, always returning to position X after each one (Fig. 15.18). The purpose of this drill is to improve agility by requiring quick stops, quick starts, rapid accelerations, and changes of direction.

Focus on an explosive start and accelerate to maximum speed as rapidly as possible, keeping the center of gravity low to stop quickly, and keeping the center of gravity on the back edge of the base of support.

Variation

This drill can be performed with various movements including sprinting, shuffling, and backpedaling. It can also be performed both clockwise and counterclockwise, and the distance of each sprint can be varied.

(continued)

Five-Point Agility Run *(continued)*

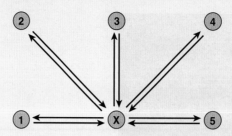

FIGURE 15.18 Five-point agility run.

T-Drill for Combining Lateral and Forward/Backward Movement

Starting Position

The athlete should start in an athletic "ready" position facing the direction of the first sprint.

Movement Sequence

Start at cone 1 and sprint to the left side of cone 2. Move around cone 2 and shuffle to the right to and around cone 3. Then shuffle to the left all the way back across to and around cone 4. Then shuffle to the right back to cone 2, then backpedal backward to cone 1 (Fig. 15.19). The purpose of the T-drill is to train the athlete to rapidly and effectively transition from forward/backward, forward/lateral, and backward/lateral movement patterns.

The focus of this drill is not only forward/backward/lateral movements but also the ability to transition from one to the other.

The center of gravity should be kept low, and on the back edge of the base of support when changing direction.

Variation

The footwork patterns and the distance between cones can be altered.

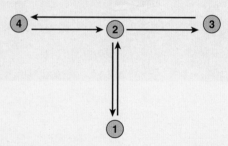

FIGURE 15.19 T-drill for combining lateral and forward/backward movement.

Five Dot Drill

Starting Position

The athlete should start in an athletic "ready" position facing forward.

Movement Sequence

There are various movement patterns for this drill. One common pattern is for the athlete to start with one foot on each of the two nearest dots, approximately 2 ft apart. She then jumps in a hop-scotch pattern to the two farthest dots, approximately 3 ft away. The athlete then

jumps backward in the same manner to the starting position (Fig. 15.20). This movement is repeated as many times as desired.

The athlete should maintain her center of gravity as close as possible to the center dot to facilitate rapid movement and maintaining balance. The athlete should maintain an athletic position during the drill with the center of gravity low. Encourage the athlete to move her feet as rapidly as possible. The purpose of the five-dot drill is to develop the

Five Dot Drill *(continued)*

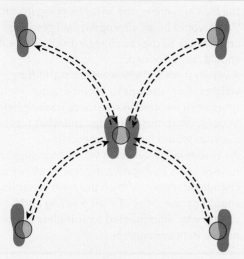

FIGURE 15.20 Five-dot drill.

ability to move the feet quickly while maintaining an athletic balanced position, using both single and double leg movements in forward/backward patterns.

Variation

Other movement patterns can be used for this drill, such as jumping with both feet together and jumping to each dot individually. The spacing of the dots can also be increased or decreased. Any variation or combination of movements can be used in one specific drill. The length of time the athlete performs the drill can be modified, or the number of single or double leg foot contacts can be used as an estimate of workload.

Hexagon Drill

Starting Position

The athlete should start in an athletic "ready" position facing forward in the middle of a hexagon.

Movement Sequence

Jump over one side of the hexagon and return back to the middle. Then jump over each of the six sides of the hexagon in order, always returning to the inside of the hexagon following each jump (Fig. 15.21). The purpose of the hexagon drill is to develop the ability to move the feet quickly while maintaining an athletic balanced position using both single and double leg movement patterns.

Variation

The pattern can be performed clockwise or counterclockwise. The size of the hexagon can also be varied.

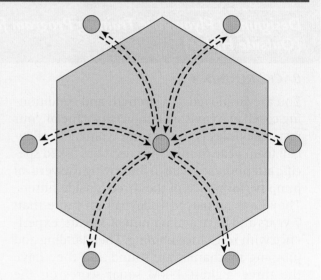

FIGURE 15.21 Hexagon drill.

SUMMARY

Sprinting, jumping, and changing directions are integral to almost all sports. Each of these basic motor skills utilizes the SSC, coupling eccentric and concentric muscle actions, to increase power output and ultimately enhance performance. Scientific evidence indicates that both mechanical and neural factors regulate SSC ability. In addition, fiber-type distribution, the use of the upper extremities, gender, age, agonist and antagonist strength, and fatigue can either attenuate or augment the SSC.

More importantly, program design and drill selection should weigh heavily on the experience of the athlete(s), with a focus on general motor development for younger athletes and greater sport specificity for advanced athletes. Training programs utilizing plyometric, sprint, and agility drills should address these factors as well as consider the intended outcomes in providing instructions to athletes on exercise performance.

MAXING OUT

1. A high school basketball coach asks the new strength and conditioning coach if she will watch his athletes perform their plyometric routine, which includes depth jumps. When they perform the depth jumps, she notices that many of them have poor landing mechanics (e.g., little flexion of the hips and knees, the knees buckling inward). What would be an appropriate suggestion she could make to the coach regarding how the drills should be performed?

2. A varsity track sprinter wants to start lifting weights in an attempt to become faster. He has never been involved in resistance training before. Initially, what muscle groups and what types of exercises would be most beneficial?

3. An elite-level soccer team wants your suggestions for new ways to improve the team's ability to change directions. Which program variables should be the focus of their training and how can they be manipulated to stimulate performance improvements?

CASE EXAMPLE

Designing a Plyometric Training Program for a Women's College Volleyball Player (Outside Hitter)

BACKGROUND

You are employed as a strength and conditioning coach at a Division I university. One of your responsibilities is to train the women's volleyball team year round. The coach has asked specific attention be given to improving the vertical jump performance of the three outside hitters. They have all played volleyball for more than 7 years and have a minimum of 3 years' experience with resistance training. Their landing and jumping mechanics are sound and they have the three highest 1-RM squat scores on the team. Using a needs analysis, identify the jumping characteristics of collegiate women's outside hitters and develop an 8-week plyometric cycle leading into the preseason.

RECOMMENDATIONS/CONSIDERATIONS

Begin with a needs analysis of jumping volume for the group of players. Watching several videos from the previous season should provide you with a very reasonable understanding of the types and volumes of jumps performed. You find the maximal number of spikes and blocks performed per game is approximately 34 and 27, respectively. If it is necessary to play four games to determine the outcome of a match, then an outside hitter could expect to perform nearly 250 jumps per match (136 spikes and 108 blocks). A movement analysis indicates that to perform a spike, the athlete must first generate horizontal velocity and transfer it to vertical motion. On the other hand, a block begins from a quasistatic squat position and has only vertical motion.

IMPLEMENTATION

Select exercises that are closely associated with the motor skills. For example, power skips performed for linear distance or maximal height would both provide a suitable stimulus for this group of athletes. Depth jumps could also be used sparingly to develop the ability to decelerate and change directions rapidly, as is found during the spike. Any type of vertical jumping drill would be appropriate to focus on blocking ability. More specifically, the block is started from a quasistatic position; therefore a drill such as box jumps would fit into the training program. The athletes should be instructed to perform all exercises with maximal takeoff velocity throughout the entire training cycle. An attempt is made to equate the actual volume observed during competition to what is prescribed during training. This should occur over several weeks and only be implemented during select training sessions. Progressive overload and a periodized schedule will allow for proper recovery between training stimulus.

RESULTS

Using appropriate progressions for volume and intensity and providing adequate rest should provide the necessary stimulus for improved performance and greater jumping ability. Regular assessment (approximately every 2 to 3 weeks) of performance using volleyball-specific vertical jump tests will provide the necessary feedback to monitor your program.

REFERENCES

1. Adams K, O'Shea J, O'Shea K, et al. The effect of six weeks of squat, plyometric, and squat-plyometric training on power production. J Appl Sports Sci Res 1992; 6:36–41.
2. Ashby BM, Heegaard JH. Role of arm motion in the standing long jump. J Biomech 2002;35:1631–1637.
3. Avela J, Komi PV. Interaction between muscle stiffness and stretch reflex sensitivity after long-term stretch-shortening cycle exercise. Muscle Nerve 1998;21:1224–1227.
4. Avela J, Komi PV. Reduced stretch reflex sensitivity and muscle stiffness after long-lasting stretch-shortening cycle exercise in humans. Eur J Appl Physiol Occup Physiol 1998;78:403–410.
5. Avela J, Kyrolainen H, Komi PV. Neuromuscular changes after long-lasting mechanically and electrically elicited fatigue. Eur J Appl Physiol Occup Physiol2001; 85:317–325.
6. Avela J, Kyrolainen H, Komi PV, et al. Reduced reflex sensitivity persists several days after long-lasting stretch-shortening cycle exercise. J Appl Physiol 1999;86: 1292–1300.
7. Belli A, Kyrolainen H, Komi PV. Moment and power of lower limb joints in running. Int J Sports Med 2002; 23:136–141.
8. Bencke J, Naesborg H, Simonsen EB, et al. Motor pattern of the knee joint muscles during side-step cutting in European team handball. Scand J Med Sci Sports 2000; 10:68–77.
9. Besier TF, Lloyd DG, Ackland TR. Muscle activation strategies at the knee during running and cutting maneuvers. Med Sci Sports Exerc 2003;35:119–127.
10. Besier TF, Lloyd DG, Ackland TR, et al. Anticipatory effects on knee joint loading during running and cutting maneuvers. Med Sci Sports Exerc 2001;33:1176–1181.
11. Besier TF, Lloyd DG, Cochrane JL, et al. External loading of the knee joint during running and cutting maneuvers. Med Sci Sports Exerc 2001;33:1168–1175.
12. Bobbert MF. Dependence of human squat jump performance on the series elastic compliance of the triceps surae: a simulation study. J Exp Biol 2001;204: 533–542.
13. Bobbert MF, Gerritsen KG, Litjens MC, et al. Why is countermovement jump height greater than squat jump height? Med Sci Sports Exerc 1996;28:1402–1412.
14. Bobbert MF, Van Soest AJ. Effects of muscle strengthening on vertical jump height: a simulation study. Med Sci Sports Exerc 1994;26:1012–1020.
15. Bobo M, Yarborough M. The effects of long-term aerobic dance on agility and flexibility. J Sports Med Phys Fit 1999;39:165–168.
16. Bosco C, Vittori C. Biomechanical characteristics of sprint running during maximal and supra-maximal speed. NSA 1986;1:39–45.
17. Brown ME, Mayhew JL, Boleach LW. Effect of plyometric training on vertical jump performance in high school basketball players. J Sports Med Phys Fit 1986;26:1–4.
18. Bushey SR. Relationship of modern dance performance to agility, balance, flexibility, power, and strength. Res Q Exerc Sport 1966;37:313–316.
19. Caraffa A, Cerulli G, Projetti M, et al. Prevention of anterior cruciate ligament injuries in soccer. A prospective controlled study of proprioceptive training. Knee Surg Sports Traumatol Arthrosc 1996;4:19–21.
20. Caserotti P, Aagaard P, Simonsen EB, et al. Contraction-specific differences in maximal muscle power during stretch-shortening cycle movements in elderly males and females. Eur J Appl Physiol 2001;84:206–212.
21. Clutch M, Wilton M. The effect of depth jumps and weight training on leg strength and vertical jump. Res Q Exerc Sport 1983;54:5–10.
22. Creer AR, Ricard MD, Conlee RK, et al. Neural, metabolic, and performance adaptations to four weeks of high intensity sprint-interval training in trained cyclists. Int J Sports Med 2004;25:92–98.
23. Corn RJ, Knudson D. Effect of elastic-cord towing on the kinematics of the acceleration phase of sprinting. J Strength Cond Res 2003;17:72–75.
24. Diallo O, Dore E, Duche P, et al. Effects of plyometric training followed by a reduced training programme on physical performance in prepubescent soccer players. J Sports Med Phys Fit 2001;41:342–348.
25. Dietz V, Schmidtbleicher D, Noth J. Neuronal mechanisms of human locomotion. J Neurophysiol 1979;42: 1212–1222.
26. Drabik J. Children & Sports Training: How Your Future Champions Should Exercise to be Healthy, Fit, and Happy. Island Pond, VT: Stadion, 1996.
27. Dupont G, Akakpo K, Berthoin S. The effect of in-season, high-intensity interval training in soccer players. J Strength Cond Res 2004;18:584–589.

28. Ellis L, Gastin P, Lawrence S, et al. protocols for the physiological assessment of team sports players. In: Gore CJ, ed. Physiological Tests for Elite Athletes. Champaign, IL: Human Kinetics, 2000.

29. Ettema GJ. Muscle efficiency: the controversial role of elasticity and mechanical energy conversion in stretch-shortening cycles. Eur J Appl Physiol 2001;85:457–465.

30. Fatouros IG, Jamurtas AZ, Leontsini D, et al. Evaluation of plyometric exercise training, weight training, and their combination on vertical jumping performance and leg strength. J Strength Cond Res 2000;14:470–476.

31. Finni T, Ikegawa S, Lepola V, et al. Comparison of force-velocity relationships of vastus lateralis muscle in isokinetic and in stretch-shortening cycle exercises. Acta Physiol Scand 2003;177:483–491.

32. Fox SI. Human Physiology. 8th ed. New York: McGraw-Hill, 2004.

33. Gallahue DL, John CO. Understanding Motor Development. 6th ed. New York: McGraw-Hill, 2006.

34. Gehri DJ, Ricard MD, Kleiner DM, et al. A comparison of plyometric training techniques for improving vertical jump ability and energy production. J Strength Cond Res 1998;12:85–89.

35. Griffin LY. The Henning Program. In Griffin LY, ed. Prevention of Noncontact ACL Injuries. Rosemont, IL: American Academy of Orthopaedic Surgeons, 2001.

36. Harman EA, Rosenstein MT, Frykman PN, et al. The effects of arms and countermovement on vertical jumping. Med Sci Sports Exerc 1990;22:825–833.

37. Harrison AJ, Gaffney S. Motor development and gender effects on stretch-shortening cycle performance. J Sci Med Sport 2001;4:406–415.

38. Haywood KM, Getchell N. Life Span Motor Development. 3rd ed. Champaign: Human Kinetics, 2001.

39. Hewett TE, Stroupe AL, Nance TA, et al. Plyometric training in female athletes. Decreased impact forces and increased hamstring torques. Am J Sports Med 1996; 24:765–773.

40. Hill AV. Mechanics of the contractile element of muscle. Nature 1950;166:415–419.

41. Horita T, Komi PV, Hamalainen I, et al. Exhausting stretch-shortening cycle (SSC) exercise causes greater impairment in SSC performance than in pure concentric performance. Eur J Appl Physiol 2003;88:527–534.

42. Jacobs R, van Ingen Schenau GJ. Intermuscular coordination in a sprint push-off. J Biomech 1992;25:953–965.

43. Jaric S. Changes in movement symmetry associated with strengthening and fatigue of agonist and antagonist muscles. J Motor Behav 2000;32:9–15.

44. Jaric S, Ropret R, Kukolj M, et al. Role of agonist and antagonist muscle strength in performance of rapid movements. Eur J Appl Physiol Occup Physiol 1995;71:464–468.

45. Johnson MD, Buckley JG. Muscle power patterns in the mid-acceleration phase of sprinting. J Sports Sci 2001; 19:263–272.

46. Kearney JT, Rundell KW, Wilber RL. Measurement of work and power in sport. In: Kirkendall DT, ed. Exercise and Sport Science. Philadelphia: Lippincott Williams & Wilkins, 2000.

47. Kivi DM, Maraj BK, Gervais P. A kinematic analysis of high-speed treadmill sprinting over a range of velocities. Med Sci Sports Exerc 2002;34:662–666.

48. Kurokawa S, Fukunaga T, Fukashiro S. Behavior of fascicles and tendinous structures of human gastrocnemius during vertical jumping. J Appl Physiol 2001;90: 1349–1358.

49. Kyrolainen H, Komi PV, Belli A. Changes in muscle activity patterns and kinetics with increasing running speed. J Strength Cond Res 1999;13:400–406.

50. Lees A, Rojas J, Ceperos M, et al. How the free limbs are used by elite high jumpers in generating vertical velocity. Ergonomics 2000;43:1622–1636.

51. Little T, Williams AG. Specificity of acceleration, maximum speed, and agility in professional soccer players. J Strength Cond Res 2005;19:76–78.

52. Lockie RG, Murphy AJ, Spinks CD. Effects of resisted sled towing on sprint kinematics in field-sport athletes. J Strength Cond Res 2003;17:760–767.

53. Luebbers PE, Potteiger JA, Hulver MW, et al. Effects of plyometric training and recovery on vertical jump performance and anaerobic power. J Strength Cond Res 2003;17:704–709.

54. MacDougall JD, Hicks AL, MacDonald JR, et al. Muscle performance and enzymatic adaptations to sprint interval training. J Appl Physiol 1998;84:2138–2142.

55. Mandelbaum BR, Silvers HJ, Watanabe DS, et al. Effectiveness of a neuromuscular and proprioceptive training program in preventing anterior cruciate ligament injuries in female athletes: 2-year follow-up. Am J Sports Med 2005;33:1003–1010.

56. Mann R, Sprague P. A kinetic analysis of the ground leg during sprint running. Res Q Exerc Sport 1980;51: 334–348.

57. Mann RA, Moran GT, Dougherty SE. Comparative electromyography of the lower extremity in jogging, running, and sprinting. Am J Sports Med 1986;14:501–510.

58. Mann RV. A kinetic analysis of sprinting. Med Sci Sports Exerc 1981;13:325–328.

59. Martin RJ, Dore E, Twisk J, et al. Longitudinal changes of maximal short-term peak power in girls and boys during growth. Med Sci Sports Exerc 2004;36:498–503.

60. Mayhew JL, Piper FC, Schwegler TM, et al. Contributions of speed, agility, and body composition to aerobic power measurement in college football players. J Appl Sports Sci Res 1989;3:101–106.

61. McBride JM, Triplett-McBride T, Davie A, et al. The effect of heavy- vs light-load jump squats on the development of strength, power, and speed. J Strength Cond Res 2002;16:75–82.

62. McNair PJ, Prapavessis H, Callender K. Decreasing landing forces: effect of instruction. Br J Sports Med 2000; 34:293–296.

63. Moritani T. Motor Unit and motorneurone excitability during explosive movements. In: Komi PV, ed. Strength and Power in Sport. Oxford, UK: Blackwell, 2003.

64. Neptune RR, Wright IC, van der Bogert AJ. Muscle coordination and function during cutting movements. Med Sci Sports Exerc 1999;31:294–302.

65. Nummela A, Mero A, Rusko H. Effects of sprint training on anaerobic performance characteristics determined by the MART. Int J Sports Med 1996;17(Suppl 2):S114–119.

66. Onate JA, Guskiewicz KM, Sullivan RJ. Augmented feedback reduces jump landing forces. J Orthop Sports Phys Ther 2001;31:511–517.

67. Paradisis GP, Cooke CB. Kinematic and postural characteristics of sprint running on sloping surfaces. J Sports Sci 2001;19:149–159.

68. Potteiger J, Lockwood R, Daub M, et al. Muscle power and fiber characteristics following 8 weeks of plyometric training. J Strength Cond Res 1999;13:275–279.

69. Prapavessis H, McNair PJ, Anderson K, et al. Decreasing landing forces in children: the effect of instructions. J Orthop Sports Phys Ther 2003;33:204–207.

70. Pratt CA. Evidence of positive force feedback among hindlimb extensors in the intact standing cat. J Neurophysiol 1995;73:2578–2583.

71. Radcliffe JC, Farentinos RC. High-Powered Plyometrics. Champaign, IL: Human Kinetics, 1999.

72. Rand MK, Ohtsuki T. EMG analysis of lower limb muscles in humans during quick change in running directions. Gait Posture 2000;12:169–183.

73. Silvers HJ, Mandelbaum BR. Preseason conditioning to prevent soccer injuries in young women. Clin J Sport Med 2001;11:206.

74. Sinning WE, Forsyth HL. Lower-limb actions while running at different velocities. Med Sci Sports 1970;2:28–34.

75. Strojnik V, Komi PV. Fatigue after submaximal intensive stretch-shortening cycle exercise. Med Sci Sports Exerc 2000;32:1314–1319.

76. Strojnik V, Komi PV. Neuromuscular fatigue after maximal stretch-shortening cycle exercise. J Appl Physiol 1998;84:344–350.

77. Swanson SC, Caldwell GE. An integrated biomechanical analysis of high speed incline and level treadmill running. Med Sci Sports Exerc 2000;32:1146–1155.

78. Takarada Y, Iwamoto H, Sugi H, et al. Stretch-induced enhancement of mechanical work production in frog single fibers and human muscle. J Appl Physiol 1997;83:1741–1748.

79. Trimble MH, Kukulka CG, Thomas RS. Reflex facilitation during the stretch-shortening cycle. J Electromyogr Kinesiol 2000;10:179–187.

80. van Ingen Schenau GJ, Bobbert MF, de Haan A. Does elastic energy enhance work and efficiency in the stretch-shortening cycle? J Appl Biomech 1997;13:389–415.

81. Van Praagh E. Development of anaerobic function during childhood and adolescence. Pediatr Exerc Sci 2000;12:150–173.

82. Verstegen M, Marcello B. Agility and coordination. In: Foran B, ed. High Performance Sports Conditioning. Champaign, IL: Human Kinetics, 2001.

83. Walshe AD, Wilson GJ, Ettema GJ. Stretch-shorten cycle compared with isometric preload: contributions to enhanced muscular performance. J Appl Physiol 1998;84:97–106.

84. Wiemann K, Tidow GN. Relative activity of hip and knee extensors in sprinting: implications for training. New Studies Athletics 1995;10(1):29–49.

85. Wilson GJ, Murphy AJ, Giorgi A. Weight and plyometric training: effects on eccentric and concentric force production. Can J Appl Physiol 1996;21:301–315.

86. Wilson GJ, Newton RU, Murphy AJ, et al. The optimal training load for the development of dynamic athletic performance. Med Sci Sports Exerc 1993;25:1279–1286.

87. Wroble RR, Moxley DP. The effect of winter sports participation on high school football players: strength, power, agility, and body composition. J Strength Cond Res 2001;15:132–135.

88. Young WB, McDowell MH, Scarlett BJ. Specificity of sprint and agility training methods. J Strength Cond Res 2001;15:315–319.

89. Young WB, Wilson GJ, Byrne C. A comparison of drop jump training methods: effects on leg extensor strength qualities and jumping performance. Int J Sports Med 1999;20:295–303.

90. Zafeiridis A, Saraslanidis P, Manou V, et al. The effects of resisted sled-pulling sprint training on acceleration and maximum speed performance. J Sports Med Phys Fit 2005;45:284–290.

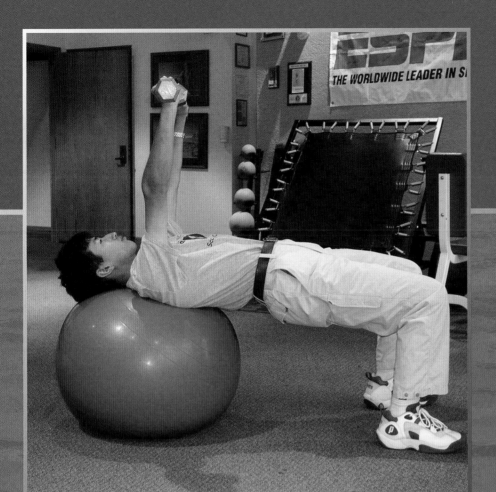

Special Topics

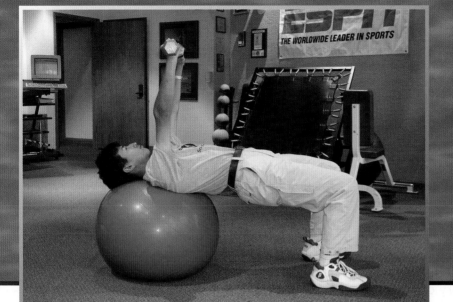

Foundations of Strength Training for Special Populations

MOH H. MALEK
ANN M. YORK
JOSEPH P. WEIR

Introduction

People are living longer, often with one or more chronic diseases. Athletes with disabilities are shattering stereotypes. Physicians are prescribing exercise for their patients to manage medical conditions such as cardiovascular disease and diabetes. Limited insurance coverage may lead a person with hemiplegia out of the physical therapy clinic and into the gym. These are just some of the reasons why exercise management for special populations has become so important.

Venues such as hospital-based wellness centers, fitness centers, and assisted living facilities have a wide mix of clients with special needs. A survey of health fitness instructors in southern California revealed that most of these instructors lacked the level of knowledge needed to safely train special populations (105). Therefore, the purpose of this chapter is to introduce the reader to a variety of special populations and the current findings related to exercise as a form of intervention. This chapter should be used as a reference by the health fitness instructor rather than a strict guideline. Table 16.1 lists Internet resources for the disorders discussed in this chapter, for further reference.

As in the case of any training regimen, the health fitness instructor needs to design an individualized program in close consultation with the client. For example, one client with a spinal cord injury may desire the strength and endurance to enter athletic competition; another may desire the strength and endurance to be able to get out of bed independently. In any case, it is imperative to work in close communication with the physician, physical therapist, or other primary care personnel to ensure the safety of the special population client. The health fitness instructor must understand the client's needs and precautions, where to get more information, and most importantly, be alert to problems and know when to take action or call for medical help. Although caution is essential, it is equally important not to deny those with spe-

cial needs the opportunity to reap the benefits of exercise.

Although this chapter touches on cardiovascular exercise and flexibility, the focus is on resistance training. **Resistance training** has become a critical component of exercise programs for athletes, in marked contrast to previous generations who were instructed to avoid resistance training for fear of becoming "muscle bound." More importantly, resistance training has become recognized as an important component for overall health and fitness in the general population (2). For some groups of individuals, however, participation in resistance training requires special scrutiny. In this chapter, resistance training for several populations with special needs is discussed, and unique aspects and possible contraindications for resistance training are considered. For those populations where resistance training is appropriate, the general principles of program design are the same as for the general population. That is, factors such as proper warm-up, periodization, and specificity need to be incorpo-

TABLE 16.1	INTERNET RESOURCES
DISEASE	**WEBSITE**
Sarcopenia	www.nia.nih.gov/
Osteoporosis	www.nof.org/
Arthritis	www.arthritis.org/ www.niams.nih.gov/
Cerebral palsy	www.ninds.nih.gov/health_and_medical/ disorders/cerebral_palsy.htm
Mental retardation/Down's syndrome	www.ndss.org/
Muscular dystrophy	www.mdausa.org/ www.ninds.nih.gov/health_and_medical/disorders/md.htm
Stroke	www.ninds.nih.gov/health_and_medical/disorders/stroke.htm
Fibromyalgia	http://fmaware.org/
Postpolio syndrome	www.ninds.nih.gov/health_and_medical/ disorders/post_polio_short.htm
Multiple sclerosis	www.nmss.org/
Spinal cord injury	www.asia-spinalinjury.org/ www.spinalcord.uab.edu/
AIDS/HIV	www.sis.nlm.nih.gov/HIV/HIVMain.html
Chronic obstructive pulmonary disease	www.nhlbi.nih.gov/health/public/lung/other/copd_fact.htm
Obesity	www.nhlbi.nih.gov/health/public/heart/obesity/lose_wt/ www.cdc.gov/nccdphp/dnpa/obesity/index.htm
Diabetes mellitus	diabetes.niddk.nih.gov/dm/pubs/statistics/index.htm
Cancer	www.nci.nih.gov/

rated into all programs. Although caution needs to be employed to avoid injury and overwork, it should be noted that the benefits of resistance training occur only through the application of progressive overload, and high intensity training (in terms of % of 1 RM) is often necessary for optimal benefits even in special populations.

GERIATRICS

In 2003, there were almost 36 million people aged 65 and over living in the United States, accounting for just over 12% of the total population, or about one in every eight people. This number will continue to grow over the next two decades as the baby boomers age. Persons reaching age 65 have an average life expectancy of an additional 18.2 years, yet many will be dealing with at least one chronic condition that will impact their quality of life. Among those 65 to 74 years old, almost 20% have difficulties with activities of daily living (ADLs), and over half of those 85 years of age and older have difficulties with ADLs. Unfortunately, only 26% of persons aged 65 to 74 and 16% of persons over age 75 report that they engage in regular leisure-time physical activity. Owing to the size of this demographic and their need for physical activity, health fitness professionals will increasingly interact with the geriatric population. The emphasis for many of these clients will be to maintain or improve their ability to perform ADLs.

Normal Aging and Sarcopenia

The typical aging process has deleterious effects on human skeletal muscle and is associated with loss of muscle mass, muscle strength and power, and eventually difficulty with ADLs. The progressive loss of muscle mass with advancing age is referred to as **sarcopenia** (50). Age-associated loss of lean body mass and function may not only impact an older person's quality of life but also lead to preventable injuries such as hip fractures. The rate of change in strength can be quite dramatic. Decreases in isokinetic strength occur at a rate of about 1.4% to 2.5% per year after age 65, depending on muscle group and contraction velocity (69). From ages 20 to 80, there is a loss of muscle fiber number of approximately 40%, which is also accompanied by a general reduction in muscle fiber size (97). Some studies have found that between the ages of 20 and 80 years, skeletal muscle mass decreases by 35% to 40% (49,51). The fiber atrophy tends to be greater in type II fibers (97). In addition, sarcopenia is accompanied by loss of motor units. Reinnervation of orphaned muscle fibers by surviving alpha motor neurons leads to whole muscles with fewer total motor units but with motor units that contain more fibers. Much of the decline in strength results from the loss of muscle mass, but muscle quality (strength per unit of muscle) may also decline (68). The overall effects of sarcopenia likely contribute to the decline in basal metabolic rate with age and a progressive increase in percent body fat. It appears that the relative (%) changes in muscle mass and upper body strength may be greater in males than females (79); however, the absolute effects of sarcopenia may be more severe in women. Indeed, approximately 50% of women above age 65 cannot lift 4.5 kg above their heads (83).

To counteract the effects of sarcopenia, researchers have focused on the effects of resistance training in the elderly (95,171,183). Fortunately, resistance exercise is a powerful stimulus to ameliorate the effects of sarcopenia in the elderly (50). A 1980 study was the first to show that resistance exercise could result in significant increases in muscle strength in the elderly (116). Since then, numerous studies have shown that resistance training results in significant improvements in muscle strength in older persons. In addition, resistance training can result in significant increases in muscle mass, even in individuals in their nineties (60). For example, one study examined the effects of a 3-month resistance training program in seventeen 76- to 92-year-old frail adults (184). The training program was performed on weight machines and consisted of eight different exercises (Fig. 16.1). Subjects lifted weights at 65% to 75% of their 1 RM and gradually progressed to 85% to 100% of their initial 1 RM. The investigators found a significant increase in muscle mass in their subjects after 3 months of resistance training, concluding that skeletal muscle proteins are able to adapt to increased contractile demand even in older adults (184). Another study examined the effects of maintaining muscle strength and size in the quadriceps muscle following 12 weeks of resistance training in 10 older males (70 ± 4 years) (166). The subjects performed isotonic leg extensions at 80% of their concentric 1-RM leg extension three times per week. At the end of 12 weeks, the subjects were divided into two groups, one performing strength training once a week and the other performing no

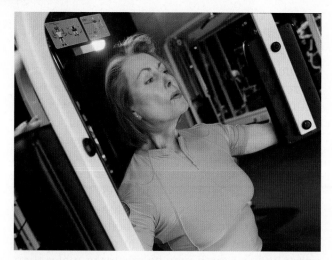

FIGURE 16.1 Weight training among the elderly has been shown to increase muscle mass and preserve strength.

exercise for 5 months. The investigators found an 11% decrease in 1-RM strength in the no exercise group but no decrease in the group that exercised once a week, concluding that training at 80% of 1 RM for 12 weeks [i.e., **progressive resistance training (PRT)**] will preserve both muscle mass and strength characteristics in older adults (166).

It is clear that resistance training can elicit significant improvements in muscle strength and muscle mass in the elderly. It is less clear whether resistance training improves function in older persons, but measures such as gait speed and the 6-minute walk test tend to show modest improvements with resistance training (96). Given the well-documented benefits of resistance training in older persons, resistance training exercise is now recognized as a critical component of fitness for adults of all ages (2,51). Indeed, it has been noted that increasing muscular strength and mass in the elderly improves not only functional status and independence but also quality of life (51). In addition, exercises should specifically target large muscle groups used in daily activities (51).

> *A progressive resistance training program for elderly individuals can reduce the effects of sarcopenia by increasing both muscle mass and functional capacity and improving quality of life.*

Osteoporosis

Osteoporosis is a systemic process of diminishing bone mass and deterioration of internal bone structure that results in an increased risk of fracture. It is known as a "silent disease," because the first sign of disease may be a fracture; therefore awareness of risk factors is important (Box 16.1). The diagnosis of osteoporosis is improving, however, with the advent of bone mineral density (BMD) testing. Approximately 44 million Americans, or 55% of the people 50 years of age and above, have osteoporosis, and almost 34 million more are estimated to be at increased risk. Women are at greater risk owing to hormonal changes that lead to the rapid depletion of bone mineral density with menopause.

More than 1.5 million fractures annually are attributed to osteoporosis, with wrist, hip, and vertebral fractures being the most common. Hip fractures often carry severe consequences; an average of 24% of hip fracture patients aged 50 and above die in the year following their fracture (122). The estimated national direct expenditure (hospitals and nursing homes) for osteoporosis-related fractures was $18 billion dollars in 2002, and the cost is rising; hence, this is clearly a public health concern (122).

Exercise has become a primary treatment recommendation for osteoporosis. To understand how exercise might affect osteoporosis, consider the process of bone remodeling. Bone is a dynamic tissue in which old, weakened tissue is resorbed and then replaced by new, stronger material. Peak bone mass is reached during young adult life; thereafter it gradually diminishes as more bone is resorbed than is created. **Osteopenia** is defined as low bone

16.1 RISK FACTORS FOR OSTEOPOROSIS

- Female
- Thin and/or small frame
- Advanced age
- Family history of osteoporosis
- Postmenopausal (including surgically induced)
- Amenorrhea (abnormal absence of menstrual periods)
- Anorexia nervosa
- Low lifetime calcium intake
- Vitamin D deficiency
- Medications (corticosteroids, chemotherapy, and others)
- Inactive lifestyle
- Cigarette smoking
- Excessive use of alcohol
- Low testosterone levels in men

mass, or BMD between 1.0 and 2.5 standard deviations below the mean of young normal adults. Osteoporosis is defined as BMD less than 2.5 standard deviations below the norm. Since bone responds to physical forces by building more tissue, it would be logical to assume that the stresses created during exercise could lead to increased bone density. Research supports this assertion in general, but there is still some variability in the findings.

In a meta-analysis that included 18 randomized controlled trials, aerobics, weight-bearing, and resistance exercises were all effective on the BMD of the spine. Studies of resistance-training programs varied in intensity, mode, and duration, however, leading to some variability in the findings (24). Nevertheless, the evidence is strong enough to suggest that resistance training and weight-bearing exercise are essential for the client with osteoporosis.

Although the ideal training program to improve BMD has yet to be defined, there are practical guidelines that can be incorporated into a structured fitness regime. Avoid spinal flexion during exercise and ADLs by maintaining a straight spine with erect posture. This will minimize increased loads on the vertebral bodies, which might cause compression fractures leading to kyphosis. Overhead compressive loads and twisting postures may also jeopardize the spine. Cardiovascular activity should emphasize safety and avoid ballistic movements. Flexibility exercises that improve posture and balance are indicated. Reduce the risk of falling by implementing facility safety strategies. Focus on functional exercises that improve leg and core strength as well as balance to prevent falls. Bone mass attained early in life and maintained with exercise, diet, and lifestyle choices is the best way to prevent osteoporosis, but improvements can be made with a comprehensive program, including resistance training (77).

Evidence suggests that resistance training and weight-bearing exercise are essential for the client with osteoporosis.

Arthritis

Musculoskeletal diseases account for approximately 240 billion U.S. dollars or 2.9% of the gross national product (44,185). In particular, arthritis is one of the most prevalent chronic conditions worldwide (44) and is projected to affect 60 million individuals by the year 2020 in the United States alone (44). The two most common types are rheumatoid arthritis and osteoarthritis.

Rheumatoid arthritis (RA) is a chronic, systemic, multijoint disease. It typically affects the joints of the hands, wrists, elbows, shoulders, knees, feet, and cervical spine in a symmetrical pattern. Marked inflammation of the joint synovium can lead to chronic pain, joint damage and deformity, and loss of function. In 20% of the cases, other organ systems such as the heart and lungs are involved (57). The onset of RA is primarily between the ages of 30 and 50, but the range extends from childhood to old age. RA affects 1% of the U.S. population or 2.1 million Americans, with 70% being women (14). Although the etiology of RA is unknown, it is classified as an autoimmune disorder (57). Because there is no known cure for RA, medical management of the disease focuses on controlling the inflammation with a combination of medications, including nonsteroidal anti-inflammatory drugs (NSAIDs), glucocorticoids or prednisone, disease-modifying antirheumatic drugs (DMARDs), biological response modifiers, and analgesics (14).

Traditionally, the exercise management of RA focused on preserving joint mobility and minimizing the stress placed on the joint. Therefore, range-of-motion exercises and/or non-weight-bearing workouts were the predominant modes of exercise prescribed by health care professionals. The use of dynamic exercise therapy, however, has started to become an alternative approach to treating RA patients (170). Although resistance training may seem counterintuitive as a training mode for RA patients, a study has shown that dynamic exercise therapy is effective in increasing muscle strength with no negative effects or increase in pain (170). Evidence regarding the beneficial effects of resistance training is increasing in the literature and this may, in the long term, be an alternative to traditional drug therapies, which result in substantial cost to the patient (44,185).

More recently, a multicenter clinical trial called Rheumatoid Arthritis Patients in Training (RAPIT) examined the long-term effects of a high-intensity exercise program (40). For this study, 309 RA patients were recruited and randomly assigned to either a usual-care group or the RAPIT group. The RAPIT group performed an 80-minute exercise regimen twice weekly. Each session included an aerobics cycling component (20 minutes), circuit training (20 minutes), and a sport activity/game (20 minutes), such as badminton. The circuit training regimen included exercises to enhance functional living (i.e., turning around in bed) along with resistance training with a light load and high repetitions. The investigators found that muscle strength increased significantly in the RAPIT group as compared to the usual-care group (25% versus 10%) over the 2-year period (40). The investigators also found that functional ability and physical capacity increased, and levels of psychological stress as measured by the Hospital Anxiety and Depression Scale (HADS)were reduced, thus significantly improving these aspects in the RAPIT group (40). Another study evaluated adherence and satisfaction in 146 RA patients who were enrolled in the RAPIT program and found that attendance after 2 years was 74%; at the end of the fifth year, 78% of the participating patients recommended the program to other RA patients (118).

In further support of exercise management of RA, yet another study examined the effects of a 2-year home-based strength-training program in 70 RA patients who were randomly assigned to either strength-training or a control group (75). Patients in the strength-training group performed two sets of 8 to 12 repetitions at 50% to 70% intensity for all muscle groups of the arms, legs, and trunk using rubber bands and dumbbells as resistance, whereas the control group performed range-of-motion and stretching exercises. Both groups performed their exercise regimens twice a week. The investigators found that strength training significantly increased knee extension strength (59%), grip strength (50%), trunk extension strength (19%), and trunk flexion strength (24%) as compared to the control group (75). Although the control group had an increase in the above-mentioned variables from baseline, this increase was substantially lower than that of the strength-training group. Also, the investigators found that strength levels remained as much as 50% above the baseline levels during a 5-year follow-up period (75). These findings were similar to those of another study that examined the effects of concurrent strength and endurance training in women with early and long-standing rheumatoid arthritis (73). As such, researchers have concluded that an individually tailored strength regimen should be part of standard care in working with clients with RA. Since RA is characterized by periods of exacerbation, joints that are inflamed should be rested

other than performing pain-free range of motion. Dumbbells or handles may be modified to assist those with a weakened grip.

Another common form of arthritis, especially in the older population, is **osteoarthritis**, also referred to as degenerative joint disease. Osteoarthritis affects more than 20 million individuals in the United States and is predicted to affect 70 million by 2030 (94,98,149). The disease is characterized by the degeneration of cartilage, which covers the ends of bones in a joint. Although the mechanism causing osteoarthritis is still under investigation, researchers have hypothesized that factors such as being overweight, joint injuries, and the aging process may contribute to its development (111). Although a number of treatment approaches such as pain relief techniques, surgery, and/or pharmaceutical interventions exist, recent research has found that exercise is one of the better treatments for osteoarthritis (141), and this may also be cost-effective.

Recently, a study examined the effectiveness and cost of providing a home-based exercise program versus home-based exercise supplemented with an 8-week class-based exercise program (111). Over 200 patients who had been diagnosed with knee osteoarthritis, as classified by the American College of Rheumatology, were given the home-based exercise program or supplemented with the 8-week class-based exercise program. Both programs involved exercise modalities including increasing strength of the lower limb as well as improving balance and mobility. All patients were assessed at 6 and 12 months following the exercise intervention. Patients in the supplemented group demonstrated greater improvements in strength, balance, and pain reduction during walking than those who received only the home-based exercise program. Additionally, the investigators suggested that the supplement program may be cost-effective for the management of patients with knee osteoarthritis (111).

Another study conducted a meta-analysis of 17 randomized clinical trials published in 2002 that examined the effects of various interventions for treating 2,562 osteoarthritis patients (65). With regard to self-reported physical function and pain rating, the results indicated that class-based programs had a greater effect for the two indices when compared to individual treatments or home-based programs. Regardless of the type of program prescribed, patients with chronic musculoskeletal disease should focus on the development of flexibility, coordination, muscular strength, balance and mobility, and overall aerobic fitness.

> *Although strength training for RA patients may seem counterintuitive, studies show increases in functional capacity that can be maintained for up to 5 years following training.*

PEDIATRICS

Many children are active in competitive sports, but there are a growing number who are sedentary and overweight. The prevalence of obesity among adolescents has more than doubled over the past 25 years. According to the American Obesity Association, approximately 30% of children and adolescents are overweight, and about 15% are obese (7). With this trend comes an increase in risk factors for conditions such as asthma, diabetes, and hypertension, which can follow a child into adulthood and possibly result in disease and disability.

Some children are born with a disability, such as cerebral palsy, Down's syndrome, or muscular dystrophy. Whereas these conditions are also found in adults, they are included in this section as they significantly affect physical functioning during childhood. Families and schools may turn to fitness centers as exercise outlets for these children as an adjunct to physical therapy or when insurance funds are depleted. Health fitness professionals can play a key role in getting the pediatric population started on a lifelong path of physical fitness (Fig. 16.2).

Healthy Children and Adolescents

The process of growth and development in **children** (prepuberty) and **adolescents** (postpuberty) results in increases in muscle size and strength (52–56). Much of the strength increase across age groups is simply due to increases in muscle size. The maturation of skeletal muscle and the nervous system, however, lead to increases in muscle strength in individuals of all ages that are larger than can be completely accounted for simply by increased muscle mass (52–56). That is, there is an "age effect" in this regard, which means that older children and adolescents will be stronger, pound for pound, than younger individuals (173).

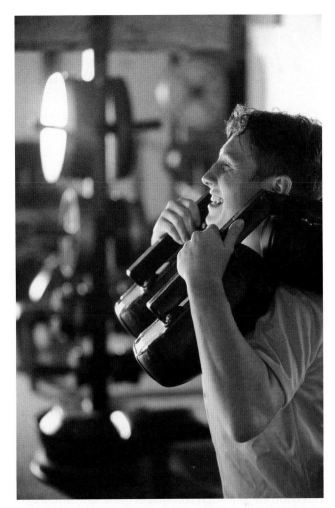

FIGURE 16.2 Encouraging adolescents to weight train will start them on a lifelong path of physical fitness.

Of interest have been the effects of resistance training in the context of growth and development. Specifically, resistance training can enhance strength development beyond what would be expected as a normal consequence of growth and development. Numerous studies have shown that resistance training in children and adolescents effectively increases muscle strength (54,56,132), and the benefits appear to transfer to other motor skills, such as those needed for the vertical jump (54). Prior to puberty, anabolic hormone concentrations are quite low, which limits the potential for resistance training to cause significant hypertrophy. Despite this, resistance training does increase muscle strength in this population. This suggests that the dominant effect occurs through neurological adaptations (21,54). After puberty, both males and females are capable of inducing substantive changes in both muscle size and strength with properly implemented resistance-training programs.

Q & A from the Field

A high school athlete wants to improve his strength by beginning a progressive resistance-training program. However, his parents have read in a popular fitness magazine that resistance training at a young age can be detrimental to the epiphyseal plate. Is it true that resistance training can stunt an adolescent's bone growth?

Although popular belief is that resistance training for adolescences can negatively affect bone growth, research does not support this position. Several studies have shown that a properly supervised progressive resistance training program does not negatively affect the epiphyseal plate. However, studies have shown that improper techniques and lifting excessive amounts of weight can result in damage to the epiphyseal plate. Therefore, the high school athlete would benefit from a training program consisting of lifting low to moderate amounts of weight that can be performed for 8 to 12 repetitions.

A primary concern with youth resistance training is safety; specifically, improper resistance training has the potential to cause damage to the **epiphyseal plates** (growth plates) at the ends of long bones (53). Fracture of these epiphyseal plates will lead to improper growth of the long bones. In addition, strains and sprains, especially of the low back, are risks associated with resistance training in youths (and adults). Several studies conducted examining resistance training in youths, however, have found that such training is quite safe and associated with a risk of injury comparable to that of resistance training in adults (21,53,54). The position statement of the National Strength and Conditioning Association (NSCA) regarding youth resistance training notes that "There are no justifiable safety reasons to preclude pre-pubescent [individuals] or adolescents from participating in a properly designed and supervised resistance training program" (54). The key to safe resistance training in youths is to ensure that there is proper supervision for training and that 1-RM or near 1-RM lifts are generally avoided (21). Instead, lighter weights that allow for relatively high repetitions are preferred for training, although some studies have shown that 1-RM testing is safe (53) and reliable (55). It may also be that resistance training can decrease injury risk. In adults, resistance training strengthens structures such as ligaments, tendons, and bones, which lessens the risk of injury. In addition, strength training can be used to correct strength imbalances. Similar outcomes are likely in youths, but limited data are available regarding reduction of injury risk with resistance training in youths.

A properly designed and supervised resistance training program should incorporate periodization principles to vary volume and intensity throughout the year. Each session should include a comprehensive warm-up period. Training programs should target all the major muscle groups and predominantly include compound multijoint exercises. Initial intensity and volume should be relatively light but progress toward 2 to 3 days per week with one to three sets per exercise at loads that allow 6 to 15 repetitions per set (54). A variety of different training modalities are appropriate, including free weights, body-weight resisted calisthenics, and machines. Progression should emphasize increases in repetitions relative to increases in resistance, and very light loads should be employed when new movements are being learned to ensure the learning of proper technique. Indeed, use of a broomstick in lieu of a weight bar may be appropriate in initially learning proper technique for complex free-weight exercises.

A properly supervised resistance-training program has been found to be beneficial in the pediatric population, with no harm to the epiphyseal plates.

Cerebral Palsy

Cerebral palsy (CP) is an umbrella term used to describe a group of nonprogressive infant-onset motor disorders typically caused by various sources of cerebral ischemia during the prenatal, perinatal, or postnatal period. Factors such as physical trauma during delivery and metabolic disturbances can lead to CP. Common motor problems include spasticity, hyperreflexia, difficulties with fine motor control, and gait dysfunction (e.g., crouch gait) (129). Cerebral palsy is the most common cause of childhood physical disability and occurs at a rate of between 2.0 and 2.5 cases per 1,000 live births (137).

Muscle weakness is often present in one (hemiplegia) or both limbs (diplegia) in individuals with CP. Quadriceps weakness has been shown to be correlated with poor gait performance in CP (36,37), suggesting that strength training may help improve gait function in CP. A variety of factors appear to contribute to this weakness. Two neural factors seem to be involved. First, individuals with CP have been shown to have higher levels of antagonist cocontraction (47), so that antagonist activation creates an opposing torque across the joint and diminishes the torque expressed at the joint by the agonist. Second, agonist activation appears to be diminished relative to age-matched controls (47) (i.e., individuals with CP are less able to recruit the motor units available in the motor unit pool). In addition, differences in muscle tissue characteristics likely influence strength. First, muscle size tends to be smaller in individuals with CP (47). In addition, higher levels of collagen are present in muscle from individuals with CP (26). Collectively, these observations indicate that less contractile protein can be brought to bear in creating force. Lower levels of specific tension (force per unit of muscle mass) are present in CP, which may reflect changes at both the muscle tissue and in neural activation (recruitment and cocontraction) (47).

Historically, resistance training has been discouraged for individuals with CP, often based on fears that it would exacerbate spasticity (velocity-dependent resistance to stretch). No evidence in the literature indicates that resistance training increases spasticity, however, and several studies have shown that resistance training results in increases in muscle strength in children with CP. One study showed that a 6-week strength training program (with three sessions per week) of the quadriceps using ankle weights for resistance (four sets of five repetitions at 65% of 1 RM) resulted in significant gains in strength (about 50% over pretraining values) in children (age range, 6 to 14 years) with CP who exhibited spas-

ticity and diplegia (37,38). Selected indices of gait function were also improved; however, the effects were much smaller than for the strength gains. Similar results were reported in children with CP exhibiting either hemiplegia or diplegia (36). Improvements in gait speed with resistance training were primarily influenced by increases in stride frequency with no change in stride length.

Cerebral palsy occurs in infancy, and the effects last throughout life. As noted previously, cerebral palsy is a disease characterized by symptoms such as spasticity, weakness, elevated antagonist cocontraction, and generally poor motor coordination. Most research regarding resistance training in cerebral palsy has examined its effects in children and adolescents. It is common for individuals with CP to stop training once they reach adulthood because of the amount of physiotherapy they went through during childhood (11). To date, there is little published research regarding the effects of resistance training in adults with CP. One study has shown that 10 weeks of twice-weekly training resulted in significant increases in muscle strength (11). More importantly, there were significant improvements in indices of range of motion, motor function, and the ability to ambulate. Further, there were no increases in spasticity. Although the adult data are limited to one study, it appears that resistance training is effective in improving both muscle strength and functional ability in adults with CP.

> *Resistance training in individuals with CP has been shown to increase muscle strength. These increases in strength do not exacerbate symptoms of CP such as spasticity. They may, however, help improve the performance of ADLs.*

Mental Retardation and Down's Syndrome

Several studies have shown that persons with mental retardation have less muscle strength and endurance than age and sex matched controls (12,29). One of the major causes of mental retardation is Down's syndrome. **Down's syndrome** is a genetic disorder that affects approximately 1 in 600 to 1,000 live births (72,78), and is characterized by cognitive delay, distinct facial features such as epicanthal folds of the eyelids and a relatively flat occiput and nasal bridge, and short limbs (72). Among its manifestations are poor muscle tone (hypotonia) and joint laxity (59, 72). The latter factors can lead to increased risk of musculoskeletal and orthopaedic problems (72). In addition, individuals with Down's syndrome tend to be less physically active than controls and are at increased risk of obesity, diabetes, and cardiovascular disease (59). Increasing physical activity and fitness in individuals with Down's syndrome is an important goal in its management, especially since the lower fitness associated with the disorder, coupled with the typical decline in fitness with aging, will likely leave individuals at particular risk for premature loss of the physical ability to perform jobs requiring light work (59).

Individuals with Down's syndrome have been shown to be significantly weaker than both age- and sex-matched controls as well as relative to age- and sex-matched individuals with mental retardation other than Down's syndrome (12,29). This weakness is correlated with low bone mineral density; therefore, the risk of osteoporosis is elevated in those with Down's syndrome (12). To date, only a few studies have examined the effects of resistance training in persons with mental retardation generally or with Down's syndrome specifically. A 9-week machine-based resistance-training program has shown large increases in muscle strength (greater than 42%) in adults with mental retardation (IQ range, 40 to 70) other than Down's syndrome (138). Comparable increases in isokinetic strength have followed 12 weeks of resistance training (hydraulic machine exercise) in individuals with mild (IQ range, 52 to 67) to moderate (IQ, 36 to 51) mental retardation (159). Another study combined strength training with cardiovascular endurance training in a program for adults (mean age, 39 years) with Down's syndrome (139). Relative to untrained controls, a 12-week program (three times a week, 10 to 20 repetitions per set) of machine-based exercises, including the leg press and bench press, resulted in 1-RM strength increases of approximately 40%. Although the data are still limited, these studies suggest that persons with mental retardation are capable of making substantive improvements in muscle strength with resistance training. Given the importance of strength in the vocational skills of persons with mental retardation, the potential for improvement in strength with training is an important observation.

 The benefit of resistance training for individuals with Down's syndrome is an increase in muscle tone and motor activity.

Muscular Dystrophy

Muscular dystrophy is an umbrella term that describes a family of genetic muscular diseases that involve dysfunction of the dystrophin glycoprotein complex in skeletal muscle. The muscular dystrophies lead to progressive muscle wasting, weakness, and disability. Of these, by far the most common form is **Duchenne muscular dystrophy** (DMD). DMD is the most common fatal childhood genetic disease (1 in 3,500 births) and is found only in boys. The gene for the muscle protein dystrophin is found on the X chromosome and is defective in DMD, resulting in a lack of dystrophin. Dystrophin is a filamentous cytoskeletal protein that serves to bind the contractile protein actin to the basement membrane via the dystrophin glycoprotein complex, located in the muscle cell membrane (sarcolemma). A lack of dystrophin therefore affects force transmission from the muscle cell to the connective tissue. Dystrophin is present in skeletal muscle, smooth muscle, cardiac muscle, and brain tissue. Because of the lack of dystrophin, forceful muscle contractions lead to excessive structural damage to the muscle, including the sarcolemma. A hallmark of DMD is high levels of creatine phosphokinase in the blood, which is evidence of sarcolemmal damage, since such damage allows muscle proteins to leak into the blood [this is also symptomatic of muscle damage associated with delayed-onset muscle soreness (DOMS) in healthy muscle]. In DMD, much of the muscle damage is likely mediated by calcium-activated proteases, which are activated by calcium influx following damage to the sarcolemma. Over time, repeated cycles of muscle degeneration and regeneration lead to a net degeneration of the muscle tissue (replaced by fat and connective tissue), weakness, loss of mobility, and eventually death. Death is usually due to secondary complications affecting the pulmonary and cardiac systems. Relatively few studies have examined the effects of resistance exercise in DMD (89), and the data are not suggestive of a significant benefit. Indeed, individuals with DMD are especially susceptible to damage from eccentric contractions, and resistance training incorporating eccentric contractions may accelerate the progression of DMD; it should therefore be avoided.

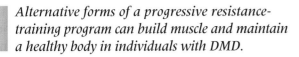

Alternative forms of a progressive resistance-training program can build muscle and maintain a healthy body in individuals with DMD.

NEUROMUSCULAR DISEASE

Neuromuscular diseases can be due to damage or dysfunction in the CNS, the peripheral nerves (**neuropathies**), or the muscle tissue itself (**myopathies**). In addition, complex multiple-system conditions can occur, such as stroke and fibromyalgia. Whereas specific diseases have primary effects on certain tissues, neurological effects will also lead to changes in the muscle tissue. Common symptoms of neuromuscular diseases include spasticity, which is a velocity-dependent resistance to stretch, rigidity, weakness, and sensory loss. These symptoms can further lead to inactivity and deconditioning, which can then exacerbate motor dysfunction. Historically, activities like resistance exercise have been discouraged for those with neuromuscular diseases owing to concerns about overwork and possible exacerbation of spasticity. It is now becoming clear, however, that in many cases the risk of overwork is much less than previously feared and that concerns regarding the exacerbation of spasticity are unfounded (34,64). Indeed exercise, in particular resistance exercise, can be a useful tool in the rehabilitation and subsequent management of many neuromuscular conditions, especially those where weakness is a primary contributor to loss of motor function.

Stroke

A **stroke** is the death of brain cells as a result of impaired blood flow to the brain. It is typically reported that approximately 500,000 people experience a stroke each year in the United States (19,109). More recent estimates increase this by 50% to approximately 750,000 (180). Strokes are the third leading cause of death (after heart disease and cancer) in the United States (19,93) and the leading cause of disability in adults (109). Stroke is the second leading cause of death, behind heart disease, worldwide (145). Approximately 31% of first-time strokes result in death within 1 year (42), with the greatest mortality risk occurring within the first 30 days following stroke (144); however

the overall death rate from stroke in the United States has been decreasing (25). The combined direct and indirect costs of stroke are estimated at $30 billion annually (108).

Strokes fall within two general categories. An ischemic stroke is conceptually similar to a myocardial infarction in that occlusion of a cerebral artery occurs as a consequence of plaque formation. In contrast, a hemorrhagic stroke results from the loss of structural integrity of a cerebral blood vessel and subsequent bleeding. Both types of stroke can lead to significant changes in muscle function, including weakness and spasticity. The motor symptoms are typically most severe on one side of the body (contralateral to the side of the lesion in the brain), so hemiplegia is common, although even the "good" side frequently shows motor deficits. It was previously thought that motor deficits that were not corrected within the first 6 months of rehabilitation following a stroke were permanent, and there was limited neural plasticity with which improvements in motor function could be effected. It is now clear, however, that the extent of neural plasticity is greater than previously thought and that significant improvements can occur well after the acute stage of stroke recovery.

Historically, resistance training had been discouraged for people following a stroke, often on the argument that resistance training might lead to increased spasticity. Several studies in individuals following the acute phase of stroke rehabilitation (> 6 months poststroke), however, have shown that spasticity, characterized by a velocity-dependent resistance to passive stretch, is not exacerbated by resistance training (18,150), and individuals who have had a stroke are capable of significant improvements in strength (18,48,150, 163). Further, several studies have shown that strength training has the potential to improve function. One such study reported that eccentric-only isokinetic knee extension training of the paretic quadriceps not only increased muscle strength but also decreased the asymmetry of body-weight distribution across the legs during sit-to-stand, while concentric-only isokinetic training improved indices of gait performance (48). Another study showed that 10 weeks (three times a week) of combined resistance training and endurance exercise (walking, stepping, cycling) resulted in significant improvements in gait speed, gait kinematics, and questionnaire-based estimates of physical activity and quality of life (162,163). In contrast,

6 months of resistance exercise using wrist and leg weights did not result in significant improvements in the 2-minute walk test or a disability index relative to a control group performing the same exercises with only body-weight resistance (115). No information regarding intensity (% of 1 RM) or progression of resistance was reported, so it is difficult to judge the efficacy of the intervention.

As with other populations, much of the improvement in strength can be attributed to adaptations in neural control. On electromyography, eccentric- and concentric-only training has shown an increase in agonist strength from 24% to 33% (48). The hypertrophic potential of paretic muscle due to stroke has not yet been examined. It seems likely, however, that significant adaptations at the muscle level occur, especially given that paretic muscle is significantly deconditioned and would be highly responsive to increased loading. Indeed, significant improvement in isokinetic strength has occurred following treadmill gait training in persons with stroke (153).

To date, most studies have employed relatively short training periods (10 weeks or less), and longer-term effects are unknown. Further, studies are limited by the lack of control groups (18,48, 150) or poorly defined resistance-training protocols (115). More research needs to be performed to further define the effects of resistance training on motor function poststroke and to improve our understanding of the different resistance-training protocols (e.g., optimal intensity range, appropriate frequency and volume of training, unilateral versus bilateral training) on outcomes. In the meantime, an individualized program focusing on functional activities appears to be a viable option. Particular attention should be paid to safety and the prevention of falls; exercise modification may be necessary for persons with hemiplegia.

Structured resistance training programs may improve a stroke patient's cardiovascular and respiratory efficiency, thus improving quality of life.

Fibromyalgia

Fibromyalgia is not a disease per se but rather is a chronic pain syndrome (fibromyalgia syndrome, or FMS) with a variety of symptoms (71). Chief among these is the widespread presence of tender points at sites throughout the body (71,182), typically in muscle tissue. It is estimated that the prevalence of FMS is 2% of the population, predominately in women (182). The prevalence increases with age (182). Individuals with FMS generate over twice the yearly health care costs than those without FMS (140). The diagnosis of FMS is difficult and requires pain to be present in at least 11 of 18 common sites throughout the body (71,182). In addition, other symptoms—such as fatigue (physical and mental), sleep disturbances, and problems with vision—are common. A variety of physiological manifestations are also present in FMS. These include endocrine indices such as elevated levels of substance P, diminished levels of serotonin, and low levels of thyroid hormone (182). In addition, symptoms involving the autonomic nervous system include elevated heart rate, low blood pressure, and altered control of blood flow during exercise (71). A deconditioning/pain cycle is frequently seen in FMS, as individuals with this condition often avoid physical activity owing to their muscular pain. This inactivity leads to deconditioning, which makes the muscles more susceptible to damage and further pain (84).

The pathophysiology of FMS is still poorly understood, but it appears to be linked with altered processing of afferent information in the central nervous system, often secondary to previous pain, as from trauma or a chronic illness, like cancer. The exposure to the initial pain is believed to cause "central sensitization" of dorsal horn neurons, triggering hyperalgesia (an exaggerated response to nociceptive input) and allodynia (interpretation of nonnociceptive input as painful) (20).

Exercise is frequently prescribed as an intervention for FMS (84). Aerobic exercise has been shown to alleviate pain in some individuals with FMS. Exercise, however, may also exacerbate muscle pain in FMS. Microtrauma to skeletal muscle, as occurs with eccentric exercise, may lead to increased sensory pain input to the central nervous system and increase pain sensation via nociceptive processing (i.e., central sensitization) (84).

Studies have been conducted examining the effects of resistance exercise in FMS. One study found that 21 weeks of traditional weight training (twice a week) in premenopausal women with FMS using exercises such as the squat and bench press resulted in strength increases comparable to those in age-matched subjects who did not have FMS (74). These adaptations were accompanied by significant improvements in vertical jump and rate of isometric force development. In addition, the FMS subjects showed significant decreases in neck pain, fatigue, and depression. Similar results came from a comparable training program in older women (about 60 years old) with FMS (169). In contrast, another study did not find significant differences between a strength-training group and a strengthening group (85); however, the strength training intervention was extremely mild (1- to 3-lb hand weights) relative to the protocols of the previous two studies (74,169). This suggests that benefits are acquired only when sufficient overload is applied. Although more research is needed to further delineate the optimal training protocol and define the long-term benefits and risks of resistance training in FMS, it appears that resistance training is a promising intervention.

▌ *A resistance-training program for FMS patients may help reduce pain and maintain muscle tone.*

Postpolio Syndrome

Poliomyelitis is a viral disease in which the polio virus attacks alpha motor neuron cell bodies in the spinal cord and brainstem. Individuals who contracted the virus might be asymptomatic, might develop mild flu-like symptoms with possible gastrointestinal distress, or might develop "paralytic" symptoms. Those with the paralytic form developed symptoms that varied depending on the degree of neuronal damage. Although death due to respiratory failure was not uncommon, most individuals achieved some level of recovery, ranging from various degrees of paralysis to apparent complete recovery. Many of the muscle fibers innervated by degenerated motor neurons were reinnervated by surviving motor neurons, resulting in a smaller total motor unit pool but with larger motor units (more muscle fibers per alpha motor neuron) due to reinnervation. With the advent of effective vaccines (e.g., Salk vaccine) in the 1950s and 1960s, new cases of poliomyelitis became extremely rare (154).

Individuals with **postpolio syndrome** (PPS) are those who have recovered function after the initial poliomyelitis only to develop symptoms of weakness and fatigue 30 or more years later (89). The development of PPS seems to be a consequence of the prolonged effects of reinnervation. Specifically, because polio survivors have fewer motor units and each surviving motor unit contains many more muscle fibers than motor units from control subjects, the consequences of the normal age-related loss of motor neurons are more severe in those with PPS. Further, over time surviving motor units appear to lose the ability to adequately service the large number of muscle fibers that each alpha motor neuron innervates; thus, neuronal "exhaustion" may contribute to the "new" weakness of PPS. Of primary concern regarding resistance training in PPS has been the possibility of exacerbating symptoms. Specifically, it has been suggested that fatiguing exercise may further contribute to motor neuron loss. In general, however, resistance training has been shown to improve muscle strength in postpolio syndrome (5,32,89,156). A significant portion of the strength increase appears to be due to an increase in the ability to maximally recruit the available motor units (32). Further, estimates of motor unit numbers have not been shown to be affected by resistance training (32), indicating that resistance training is unlikely to increase the rate of disease progression. Because the literature addressing resistance training in PPS is quite sparse, specific training guidelines are not yet available; it therefore seems prudent to err on the side of caution, so that the initial training intensity is low and progression occurs slowly.

▌ *Studies have found that exercise is safe and effective for individuals with PPS as long as individual tolerance (i.e., one starts to have fatigue or discomfort) is used to monitor exercise intensity.*

Multiple Sclerosis

Multiple sclerosis (MS) is a chronic inflammatory autoimmune disease of unknown etiology that affects the central nervous system. It causes a loss of myelin, the fatty sheath that insulates nerves, resulting in disruption of nerve conduction. Symptoms may include weakness, spasticity, tremor, fatigue, sensory disturbance, heat sensitivity, and impairment of balance, coordination, vision, speech, swallowing, cognition, and bowel and bladder function. Functional losses can range from mild to severe, often exhibit an exacerbation-remission pattern, and are ultimately progressive (90). MS affects approximately 400,000 people in the United States, with 200 new cases diagnosed each week and 2.5 million worldwide. Age of onset is typically 20 to 50 years, the majority of those affected being women. There is no known cure, but symptomatic treatment includes the use of disease-modifying drugs such as interferons, medication for exacerbations such corticosteroids, rehabilitation, and complementary and alternative medicine treatments including diet, yoga, and guided imagery (127).

A number of studies have been conducted to support anecdotal reports that exercise is beneficial for people with MS. Individual aerobic exercise programs using stationary cycling were shown to improve the fitness and quality of life of patients with MS (117,133). Group exercise sessions consisting of a 1-hour classes of warm-up, stretch, standing, and mat exercises over 10 weeks were also found to be beneficial (66). Results indicated short-term positive changes on standardized tests for balance, endurance, and fatigue in a group of 10 ambulatory MS patients. Resistance training in combination with aerobic exercise was studied in a randomized controlled trial of 95 individuals with MS (160). The 47 people in the exercise group completed five supervised 30-minute sessions of aerobic activity in a pool or on a bicycle ergometer at 65% to 70% of age-predicted maximal heart rate. Five supervised resistance-training sessions were alternated with the aerobic sessions consisting of circuit training by performing 10 to 15 repetitions at 50% to 60% of 1 RM of circuit training on 10 weight machines that targeted major muscle groups. These sessions were followed by 23 weeks of a home exercise program using elastic bands to work the same muscle groups targeted in the resistance-training sessions, along with mild aerobic exercise. The 48-member control group continued with their normal ADLs throughout the study. Results indicated that the motor fatigue of knee flexors and extensors of persons in the exercise group was reduced in mildly impaired women with MS as compared with the control group. The clinical message suggested by the authors was that exercise should be as specific as possible, and the outcome will be better in persons with mild to moderate disability.

In summary, studies indicate that people with MS can improve strength, fitness, and quality of life through aerobic and resistance training. Exercise programs should be tailored to the individual, taking into account the variability of the disease symptoms, such as balance, sensory loss, spasticity, cognition, and symptom exacerbation. In the case of an exacerbation, the focus should be on stretching and gentle active range of motion; resistance and aerobic exercise should be discontinued until the symptoms have remitted. A potential contraindication for exercise is overheating, as persons with MS may have an attenuated or absent sweating response that can result in a temporary exacerbation of symptoms and cause fatigue. The use of air conditioning, fans, and proper hydration and clothing will help to avoid this problem. For pool therapy, water temperatures of 80° to 84°F are recommended (178). Periods of activity may be alternated with periods of rest to avoid overheating and fatigue. Resistance exercises should target large muscle groups in closed-chain functional exercises.

 An aerobic and strength-training program may help improve fitness and quality of life in people with MS.

Spinal Cord Injury

Spinal cord injury (SCI) most often results from motor vehicle accidents (50.4%) and falls (23.8%), followed by violence (11.2%) and sports injuries (9%). According to The Spinal Cord Injury Information Network, there are approximately 247,000 people living with SCI in the United States today, with 11,000 new cases per year in a 3:1 ratio of males to females. The estimated lifetime cost for a 25-year-old who survives a SCI ranges from $600,000 to over $2.5 million for complex cases.

Categorization of SCI is complex and depends not only on the level of the injury but also on whether it is complete or incomplete. For a detailed explanation, consult the American Spinal Injury Association's *International Standards for Neurological Classification of Spinal Cord Injury,* updated in 2002. Briefly, C1 to T1 injuries result in tetraplegia (formerly called quadriplegia) and cause impairments in the arms, trunk, legs, and pelvic organs; T2 to T12 injuries result in paraplegia and causes impairment of the trunk, legs, and pelvic organs. These two groups are considered upper motor-neuron injuries and are typified by spastic paralysis and hyperreflexia below the injury. Injuries at T12 and below result in paraplegia with impairment of the trunk, legs, and pelvic organs and are considered lower-motor-neuron injuries, typified by flaccid paralysis and areflexia below the level of the injury.

In addition to these primary deficits, those with SCI are at high risk for secondary problems like cardiovascular disease, circulatory insufficiencies, osteoporosis, skin breakdown, musculoskeletal dysfunction, and pain (81). Research has indicated that some of these problems may be mitigated with a structured exercise program incorporating appropriate precautions; however, the effects of exercise conditioning are inversely proportional to the severity of the primary injury (81). For example, those with tetraplegia may require electrical stimulation or passive movements to use an upper body ergometer, resulting in a markedly reduced aerobic training effect (61).

Research on resistance training with SCI has focused on those with paraplegia. Shoulder girdle pain is a common complaint among those with paraplegia, apparently due to the stresses of wheelchair propulsion and transfers, and would indicate the need for strength training (81). Arm ergometry is a common method of endurance training, but used alone it was not sufficient to provide a functional strength gain because it failed to target the scapular muscles necessary for ADLs (39). Improvement in shoulder strength and pain was noted in a study that employed shoulder resistance exercises using elastic bands (35). Circuit resistance training, which incorporates periods of low-intensity high-repetition movements (such as a free-wheel arm ergometry) interspersed with a series of resistance-training exercises (such as free weights, weight machines, or elastic bands), has been shown to be the most effective method of improving strength and decreasing pain (81) (Fig. 16.3).

In general, the recommendations for resistance and aerobic training for those with SCI are not significantly different from those for the general population and should take into consideration specificity, overload, progression, and regularity (61). Several precautions, however, must be heeded due to the motor and sensory deficits that result from an SCI. One precaution in working with persons with a T6 or higher SCI is awareness of the potential life-threatening condition known as autonomic dysreflexia (Box 16.2). Symptoms include excessive rise in blood pressure, slowed heart rate, headache, blurred vision, and congestion. It can be set off by a noxious stimulus below the level of the injury, such as pressure to a limb or a full bladder. Immediate intervention consists of identifying and removing the noxious stimulus, monitoring blood pressure, and seeking medical help (61). Other precautions should consider risk of fracture due to osteoporosis, overuse pain due

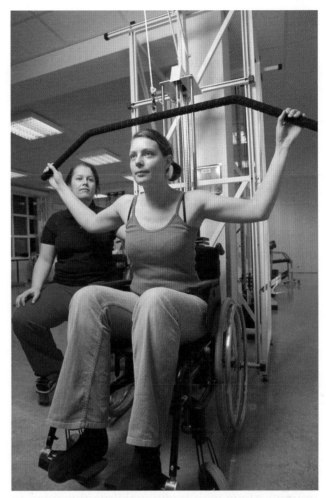

FIGURE 16.3 Resistance training exercises can be an effective way for those with spinal cord injuries to improve their strength and decrease their pain.

to muscle imbalance, hypotension, and difficulty maintaining thermal stability (81).

> *Knowledge of the type of injury and related precautions can minimize the risks and enhance the outcome of exercise programming for persons with SCI.*

16.2 SIGNS AND SYMPTOMS OF AUTONOMIC DYSREFLEXIA

■ Pounding headache
■ Blurred vision
■ Nasal congestion
■ Piloerection (goose bumps)
■ Profuse sweating above level of injury
■ Anxiety
■ Sudden increase in systolic blood pressure
■ Cardiac dysrhythmias

AIDS/HIV

Human immunodeficiency virus (HIV), which may lead to **acquired immunodeficiency syndrome (AIDS),** is a pandemic disease that currently has no cure (174). By the end of 2003, approximately 40 million individuals worldwide had been diagnosed with HIV/AIDS (31,63,168). Furthermore, reports estimate that 5 million new HIV infections occurred worldwide in 2003 alone (168). In the United States, approximately 40,000 new cases of HIV/AIDS occur each year, mostly among males (70%) (31,168). Notwithstanding the effects of HIV/AIDS on the immune system, the disease is also associated with weight loss (i.e., wasting) which is reported to be a strong predictor of mortality (151,175,176). Wasting is defined as a progressive and unintended loss of more than 10% of the individual's body weight (31). Symptoms of wasting include but are not limited to fever, poor appetite, and diarrhea (99–101). Most notably, wasting affects the musculoskeletal system, which results in weakness. As discussed in previous chapters, resistance training increases lean body weight, strengthens connective tissue, and increases skeletal muscle size. Therefore, researchers have examined the effects of resistance training, along with traditional drug therapies, to counteract the effects of wasting in this population (22,43,113,142,143,146).

One study examined the effects of a progressive resistance-training program on functional status in individuals with HIV both with and without muscle wasting (143). All subjects trained the major muscle groups of the upper and lower body three times per week for 8 weeks. The investigators found a 5.2% increase in lean body mass following the 8 weeks of training in the group that was experiencing muscle wasting. Additionally, this group increased their strength, as measured by 1 RM, by as much as 57% compared to baseline. The investigators concluded that progressive resistance training is beneficial in increasing the functional status of individuals with HIV experiencing muscle wasting (143). Similarly, another study found that testosterone treatment and resistance exercise increased gains in lean body weight and muscle mass in HIV-infected men with weight loss and low levels of testosterone (23). The investigators concluded, however, that the combination of testosterone treatment and resistance exercise

resulted in no additional gains when compared to either intervention alone (23).

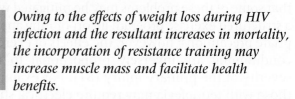 *Owing to the effects of weight loss during HIV infection and the resultant increases in mortality, the incorporation of resistance training may increase muscle mass and facilitate health benefits.*

CHRONIC OBSTRUCTIVE PULMONARY DISEASE

Chronic obstructive pulmonary disease (COPD) is a progressive respiratory illness that is not completely reversible (16). The primary pathology of COPD is expiratory airflow limitation (17). Approximately 12.1 million adults 25 years of age or older were diagnosed with COPD in 2001 (119). Furthermore, a recent economic analysis revealed that the annual societal cost for treating a single COPD patient in the United States and Europe was $5,646 (76, 136). It should be noted that COPD encompasses a number of pulmonary conditions such as asthma, emphysema, and chronic bronchitis. Although the condition is mostly associated with chronic cigarette use, other factors such as infection, environmental pollution, and heredity can also bring about COPD (167). Biopsies from the quadriceps muscle of COPD patients have revealed a loss of type I muscle fibers as well as a reduction in oxidative enzymes (82,107). This finding and the increased work of breathing often experienced by COPD patients may partly explain the associated fatigue from performing ADLs. The symptoms associated with COPD also include dyspnea on mild exertion and a reduced quality of life. Depending on the severity of this condition, traditional treatments have included pharmacological intervention, oxygen therapy, lung transplantation, or lung volume reduction surgery (16,17). More recently, pulmonary rehabilitation clinics are incorporating exercise training as a standard part of treating COPD patients.

Interestingly, exercise has been found to have only a moderate effect on pulmonary function (92). Whereas most studies have focused on the effects of endurance training involving upper and lower extremities (103,106), a few studies have examined the effects of resistance training (130,157) as a modality for increasing functional ability and quality of life. Because COPD patients have weakened peripheral and respiratory muscles, resistance training can be used as a countermeasure to stimulate and strengthen the affected musculature (102). Although the benefits of this type of exercise have been well documented with other clinical populations (58,95), there is still debate as to the effectiveness of strength training for COPD patients.

One study examined the effects of strength and endurance training in 47 patients with moderate to severe COPD ($FEV_1 \leq 41\% \pm 11\%$ of predicted) over a 12-week period (128). Patients were randomly assigned to endurance training only, strength training only, or combined endurance and strength training. The strength training protocol consisted of five exercises: chest pull, butterfly, neck press, leg flexion, and leg extension. Patients performed four sets of six to eight repetitions for each exercise at an intensity ranging from 70% to 85% of their 1 RM. Adjustments to the workload were made every 2 weeks as the patient's strength increased. The investigators found that patients in the strength training group significantly improved their distance walking (561 m) compared with the other two training modalities (501 and 493 m, respectively) (128). Additionally, the investigators found that patients rated their fatigue, dyspnea, and functional impairment scores (as measured by questionnaires) lowest in the strength training group after 12 weeks.

Another study evaluated the effectiveness of 12-weeks of full-body progressive resistance training in nine COPD patients ($FEV_1 \leq 41.9\% \pm 16\%$ of predicted) who were undergoing aerobic training as part of their pulmonary rehabilitation (130). Patients performed three sets of 8 to 12 repetitions at 32% to 64% of their 1 RM on 12 resistance-training machines. Exercises included multijoint (i.e., chest press) as well as single-joint (i.e., biceps curl) movements. Patients had an increase 5 and 29.2% in lean body mass and total distance completed during the 6-minute walk test, respectively. More importantly, COPD patients who received resistance training improved significantly more than the control group on three of the five physical function assessments (e.g., total arm raises in 1 minute, total standing up and sitting down in 1 minute, and timed stair climbing). Based on their results, the investigators recommended that whole-body resistance training be incorporated with the aerobic training regimen for pulmonary rehabilitation of COPD patients (130).

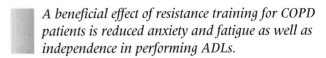

> *A beneficial effect of resistance training for COPD patients is reduced anxiety and fatigue as well as independence in performing ADLs.*

CARDIOVASCULAR DISEASE

Cardiovascular disease, which includes coronary heart disease and stroke, remains the leading cause of death among Americans and is estimated to have an economic cost of over $350 billion (33). The major risk factors for cardiovascular disease included hypertension, elevated serum total cholesterol, cigarette smoking, and diabetes mellitus (8). Data indicate that approximately 40% of deaths in the United States during 1999 were caused by cardiovascular disease (10,121) To reduce the mortality and morbidity associated with cardiovascular disease, researchers have examined the effects of exercise (2,88). A recent meta-analysis examined the dose-response relationship of physical activity on cardiovascular risk factors (124). The investigators systematically reviewed studies published from 1966 to 2003 in which the effect of exercise on cardiovascular risk factors was evaluated. They found that exercise is associated with reduced cardiovascular risk factors in a dose-response manner (124). That is, higher levels of physical activity were associated with a lower risk of developing cardiovascular disease. Furthermore, the investigators found that even 1 hour of walking per week tended to reduce cardiovascular risk factors (124).

The effects of resistance exercise may also reduce cardiovascular risk factors (134). One study found that resting systolic and diastolic blood pressure decreased by 2% to 4% following dynamic resistance training exercise in adults (86). Similar results were found for reductions in resting blood pressure in children and adolescents (87). In addition, resistance training improves insulin sensitivity and glucose tolerance, and improved muscle strength likely decreases the physiological stress of ADLs (70,112,134).

In addition to reducing cardiovascular disease risk factors, resistance training is increasingly incorporated into comprehensive cardiac rehabilitation programs in those with coronary artery disease. For example, one study examined the effects of resistance training on functional capacity in older women with coronary heart disease (CHD) (4). Forty-two CHD subjects were divided into two groups, which either performed two sets of eight exercises for the major muscle groups or met three times a week for 40 minutes with a cardiac rehabilitation specialist. The investigators found that the women in the weight-training group improved their functional capacity and therefore were able to perform ADLs without adverse effects (4). The principles of resistance training do not differ in those with coronary artery disease versus those without, but particular attention must be paid to minimize risk of cardiovascular events during training. Contraindications to resistance training include unstable angina, uncontrolled hypertension (systolic blood pressure equal to or greater than 160 mm Hg, diastolic equal to or greater than 100 mm Hg), uncontrolled dysrhythmias, severe valvular disease, hypertrophic cardiomyopathy, left ventricular outflow tract obstruction, and untreated congestive heart failure (9,134). Patients need physician approval prior to training, initial intensity should be low, and progression should be relatively slow. Following surgery, a recovery period of up to 3 months may be required before starting resistance training (134).

For those with congestive heart failure (CHF), resistance training may also be a benefit. Individuals with CHF have significant fatigue and shortness of breath with physical activity; much of these effects appear to be due to changes in skeletal muscle tissue, including type I muscle fiber atrophy. One study found that 10 weeks of resistance training improved muscle strength (43%), muscle endurance (299%), and performance on the 6-minute walk test (13%) in 16 women with CHF (135). Another study found that combined endurance plus resistance training improved peak Vo_2 and left ventricular function more than training with only endurance exercise (41). A third study examined the effects of 8 weeks of aerobic and resistance training on peripheral skeletal muscle vessel function in the forearm in 12 males with CHF (104). The training sessions consisted of resistance exercise for the upper and lower limbs, whereas cycling on a stationary bicycle comprised the aerobic component of the training intervention. The investigators found that forearm vascular function improved in the trained limb when compared with the untrained limb (104). These find-

ings demonstrate that a combination of aerobic and resistance-training exercises are beneficial for improving vascular function in patients with CHF.

A combination of aerobic exercise and circuit resistance training improves skeletal muscle function, vasculature to skeletal muscle, as well as functional capacity in patients with cardiovascular disease.

OBESITY

Overweight and obesity are health issues that have reached epidemic proportions within the United States (28). Overweight is defined as having a body mass index (BMI) of 25–29.9; obesity is defined as a BMI greater than 30 (120). A recent study of national costs attributed 5.5% to 9.1% of total U.S. medical expenditures to overweight and obesity treatment, which is considerably higher than the 2% to 3.5% reported for other countries (62,164). On the state level, obesity-attributed Medicare estimates ranged from $15 million (Wyoming) to $1.7 billion (California) (62). Obesity in the United States is associated with many diseases, such as cancer, type II diabetes, hypertension, hyperinsulinemia, and coronary heart disease (28,123,158). Although body size, shape, and composition are influenced by genetic factors (147,148,177), studies have found success with a regimen of caloric restriction (161). The use of resistance training in conjunction with caloric restriction may further aid in the battle against obesity (Fig. 16.4).

One study investigated the effects of exercise training on resting metabolic rate in moderately obese women (27). Subjects were divided into one group that underwent resistance training and another that received resistance training as well as a walking regimen. The resistance-training program was developed to promote increases in strength and fat-free mass. The investigators found that those in the group doing only resistance training significantly increased their resting metabolic rate following the training intervention (27). Thus, it was concluded that resistance training has the potential to increase resting metabolic rate through an increase in fat-free mass. A separate systematic analysis of studies examining the effects of exer-

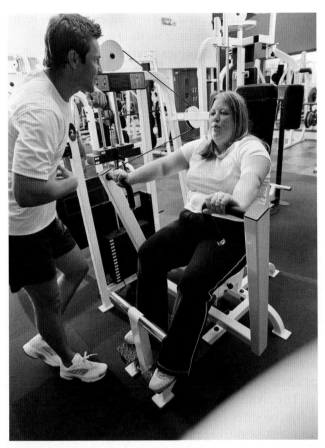

FIGURE 16.4 Resistance training and caloric restriction work together to battle obesity.

cise regimens in pediatric obesity found that exercise, whether aerobic and/or resistance training, accounted for as much as 86% of the variance in changes in body fat percentage at 1 year (110). The benefits of exercise programs are not limited to body composition. Another study examined the effects of an 8-week circuit-training regimen on conduit vessel function in 19 obese adolescents (172). In addition to the reduction in percent body fat, the investigators found that vascular flow, which was impaired prior to the intervention, normalized after 8 weeks of circuit training (172). Although we have focused on the benefits of resistance training, it should be noted that the combination of aerobic and resistance training exercise (131) as well as caloric restriction constitutes the best approach to reducing body fat in a safe and effective manner (181).

A combination of resistance training, aerobic exercise, and caloric restriction is the optimal method of reducing body fat in a safe and effective manner in obese individuals.

DIABETES MELLITUS

There are two general categories of diabetes mellitus. **Type I diabetes** is a disease characterized by pancreatic damage, resulting in diminished insulin secretion from the pancreas. It is typically due to an autoimmune condition in which the immune system attacks the pancreas, but it may also stem from pancreatic damage due to other diseases, such as pancreatic cancer. Individuals with type I diabetes, often referred to as juvenile-onset diabetes, require insulin injections to control blood glucose levels. In contrast, **Type II diabetes** is a condition characterized by insulin resistance. That is, a given glucose challenge requires a greater insulin response. Obesity is a prime cause of type II diabetes, and the increasing prevalence of obesity is leading to higher incidence of type II diabetes. Notably, increasing rates of childhood obesity are leading to ever more cases of type II diabetes in childhood. In advanced cases, type II diabetes leads to diminished pancreatic function and, eventually, often to the need for exogenous insulin.

It is well established that aerobic exercise can both decrease the risk of developing type II diabetes and aid in glycemic control. In addition to the effects of aerobic exercise on body composition and weight, which decrease insulin resistance, the effects of aerobic exercise on muscle metabolism also have beneficial effects. Specifically, increases in GLUT4 glucose transporter levels at the muscle cell membrane in response to exercise, and the effects of aerobic exercise on cellular glucose metabolism, contribute to the prevention and treatment of type II diabetes.

It is less well appreciated that resistance training can also have significant benefits in the prevention and treatment of type II diabetes (179). Studies have shown that resistance exercise, like aerobic exercise, improves insulin sensitivity and glucose tolerance (80) and decreases levels of glycosylated hemoglobin (30,45), resulting in improve glycemic control. Resistance exercise is recommended for those with type II diabetes by both the American Diabetes Association (15) and the American College of Sports Medicine (6). The specific characteristics of resistance training protocols that optimize the benefits on glucose tolerance, insulin sensitivity, and glycemic control are still unknown; however, it has been suggested that high-intensity resistance training may be more effective than low-intensity, high-volume training (30,179). Nonetheless, significant effects can be had with lower intensity (40% to 50% of 1 RM) training (80), at least in the short term.

The control of overall blood glucose in diabetic patients can be improved with a regular exercise regimen.

CANCER

In the year 2000, **cancer** was the second leading cause of death in the United States, behind heart disease (114). In 2003, it was estimated that 1,334,100 new cases and 556,500 deaths were associated with cancer (155). Despite these figures, the 5-year relative survival rate for all cancers combined is 62% (155). Generally, the treatment of cancer involves a certain level of radiation, chemotherapy, surgery, or a combination of the above. Because many of these treatments are intensive and affect the individual's physiologic function, fatigue, muscle wasting, and energy loss often result (3,126). Studies have found that various forms of physical activity, such as aerobic exercise and resistance training, are beneficial in minimizing the effects of cancer treatment (3,67).

One study examined the effects of a 10-week outpatient wellness program on variables of fitness in 20 cancer patients with a mean age of 50 years (46). In addition to performing aerobic exercises, the patients were supervised through a progressive resistance-training exercise using strength machines. They found that, after 10 weeks of training, muscular strength increased by 45% to 98%, depending on the muscle being exercised. Additionally, patients rated their functional capacity to perform ADLs (e.g., household tasks, preparing food, etc.) as significantly greater following the 10-week training program. Similar results came from a study of 23 cancer patients between the ages of 18 and 65 years (3). Patients engaged in 9 hours per week of supervised exercise, which included a combination of aerobic and resistance training. The investigators found significant increases in cardiorespiratory endurance and muscular strength (3). For a more extensive review of the effects of physical activity on cancer, we recommend two recent articles (165,125).

Resistance training and aerobic exercise can help counteract the muscle wasting and fatigue associated with cancer treatment.

PREGNANCY

Concerns about exercise during **pregnancy** focus on the potential problems of increased body temperature, impaired uterine blood flow and nutrient supply, and the risk of preterm labor. Studies have shown that for the mother, the benefits outweigh the risks. Moderate, regular exercise during pregnancy has many benefits for the mother, including decreased weight gain, more rapid weight loss after pregnancy, improved sense of well-being, and decreased risk of musculoskeletal pain and gestational diabetes. There are some mild risks for the fetus, but fortunately the adverse effects of a proper exercise program will be minimal if it is prudently administered (1,91,152).

The American College of Obstetricians and Gynecologists (ACOG) has established guidelines for exercise during pregnancy. A pregnant woman should always seek guidance from her physician prior to proceeding with an exercise program. If a woman has been exercising prior to pregnancy, she should be able to continue with her program with minor modifications. If a woman has not exercised previously, she may cautiously begin a gentle exercise program during pregnancy and must be alert to overexertion and complications.

Cardiovascular exercise should consist of 30 minutes or more of moderate exercise on most days. Exercise intensity should be judged by ratings of perceived exertion (RPE) in the light to somewhat hard range (RPE 11–13) rather than effect on heart rate and should allow the participant to pass the "talk test" during exercise. Women may find low-impact activities and water exercise more comfortable due to the increased weight and postural changes that occur with advancing pregnancy. Another musculoskeletal change that occurs during pregnancy is increased ligamentous laxity due to increased levels of the hormones estrogen and relaxin. Although research on resistance training is sparse, it appears safe. It is prudent, however, to minimize the possibility of strains and sprains by using proper form and a variety of exercises to avoid overuse injuries. Dynamic lifting with lighter weights and multiple repetitions is recommended, while avoiding repetitive isometric or heavy lifting, which may result in a Valsalva maneuver (13). Supine exercises should be avoided after the first trimester, because this position causes mild obstruction of venous return, which can affect cardiac output. Motionless standing can lead to venous pooling, so this position too should be minimized. Appropriate hydration, avoidance of overheating, and adequate nutrition should be observed.

The ACOG guidelines suggest avoidance of activities the have the potential for impact or falling, such as ice hockey, horseback riding, vigorous racquet sports, kickboxing, and soccer. Exertion at high altitudes or scuba diving are also cautioned against. Exercise of any sort should be terminated immediately if any of the following occurs: vaginal bleeding, dizziness, shortness of breath, headache, chest pain, calf pain or swelling (possible thrombophlebitis), preterm labor, leakage of amniotic fluid, or muscle weakness (Box 16.3). A pregnant woman with diabetes, morbid obesity, hypertension, or other high-risk conditions should not exercise until she has been carefully evaluated by her physician, and then only with an individualized program.

> *With her physician's approval, a healthy pregnant woman without obstetric or medical risks may safely engage in a moderate regular exercise program.*

SUMMARY

Resistance exercise in concert with cardiovascular and flexibility exercise is an important component of exercise programs in the general population. It is increasingly apparent that resistance exercise provides significant benefits to children, adolescents, and the well elderly. Furthermore, resistance exercise appears to provide significant benefits to individuals with a variety of conditions such as COPD, AIDS, diabetes, and neuromuscular diseases. With few exceptions (Duchenne muscular dystrophy), the benefits of resistance exercise far outweigh the potential risks, especially when properly designed and supervised. Nonetheless, caution should be applied in introducing progression into a program. Using a team approach with appropriate health care providers can enhance the safety and effectiveness of a program. Future research needs to further delineate the program design variables (intensity, frequency, volume, etc.) that maximize benefits (including functional outcomes) while minimizing deleterious effects for different diseases and syndromes. In addition, longer-term studies need to be performed to assess the benefits and risks of prolonged resistance exercise for these special populations.

MAXING OUT

1. A 32-year-old woman wants assistance in designing an exercise program. She is 100 lb overweight, smokes one pack of cigarettes per day, and complains of knee pain when climbing stairs. What parameters should her program have? Are there any special considerations?

2. An 82-year-old man had a stroke 5 years earlier and has some residual right-sided weakness with mild spasticity, although he is able to walk independently and lives alone. His daughter has brought him to the gym and wants him to start an exercise program. His goal is to stay as independent as possible. Is it safe to start him on resistance training program? What types of exercise would be most appropriate for him?

3. A 52-year-old female with a history of type II diabetes wants to start exercising. What types of physical problems might this woman have? Are there any precautions that should be considered? Design an appropriate fitness program for this woman.

4. A 44-year-old male volunteer coach for the high school football team wants to start working out with his son, who is on the team. He had a heart attack 6 months earlier and has completed cardiac rehabilitation phases 1, 2, and 3. Now he wants to stay fit and asks for some advice. What are some guidelines and precautions for an exercise program?

16.3 WARNING SIGNS TO STOP EXERCISING DURING PREGNANCY

■ Excessive fatigue
■ Pain (particularly in the back or pubic area)
■ Dizziness
■ Shortness of breath
■ Heart palpitations
■ Decreased fetal movement
■ Persistent contractions
■ Rupture of membranes
■ Vaginal bleeding

CASE EXAMPLE
Improving the Quality of Life in Older Adults

BACKGROUND

Mr. Smith, a 76-year-old avid golfer, complains that he is having increasing difficulty with bending, walking on hills and uneven ground, and getting in and out of the golf cart. He has a history of bilateral knee osteoarthritis controlled with NSAIDs and hypertension controlled with medication. He admits that he has not adhered to exercise programs in the past but is now motivated because he wants to continue golfing.

RECOMMENDATIONS/CONSIDERATIONS

After having Mr. Smith complete a health screen questionnaire and getting clearance from his physician, exercise testing is performed, as outlined in Chapter 8. The components of the fitness program should focus on strength and flexibility of the lower extremities, targeting major muscle groups used in ADLs including golf, aerobic conditioning, and balance and coordination activities. Review the preceding sections on sarcopenia, osteoarthritis, and cardiovascular disease for more information.

IMPLEMENTATION

For resistance training, a 5- to 10-minute warm-up should be followed by strength training for major muscle groups, focusing on the lower extremities but including the upper extremities and trunk, as all are important for golf and other ADLs. Begin with 65% to 75% of 1 RM, and progress to 85% to 100% of 1 RM as tolerated two to three sessions per week, with 8 to 12 repetitions. Knee pain should be monitored and activities modified if increased pain and inflammation is reported. For example, open-chain knee extensions could be replaced with closed-chain leg presses, load could be reduced, or arc of motion modified to a pain-free range. The session would end with stretching of the major muscle groups.

For aerobic conditioning, a combination of activities could be used including treadmill walking, stationary bicycling, and water activities. Treadmill walking is functional and inclines can be gradually introduced to simulate hill walking. Stationary bicycling has the advantage of providing knee range of motion, which can be increased by lowering the seat height. Water aerobics can provide cardiovascular conditioning while minimizing joint stresses. Mr. Smith should be taught perceived level of exertion, age-related target heart rate, and how to monitor his blood pressure. He could be encouraged to join an exercise group to enhance adherence. Supervised but simple balance and coordination activities such as grapevine walking, single leg balance, and walking on an exercise mat to simulate uneven ground can become independent once safety is established. Mr. Smith should be educated on the importance of an ongoing program, warning signs for cardiovascular disease, and osteoarthritis precautions.

RESULTS

Mr. Smith will develop both muscular strength and endurance. As a result, he will have improved balance and mobility, which will enhance his golf swing. Furthermore, Mr. Smith may have less difficulty walking on hills and uneven ground and getting in and out of the golf cart.

REFERENCES

1. ACOG. ACOG Committee opinion. Number 267, January 2002: exercise during pregnancy and the postpartum period. Obstet Gynecol 2002;99:171–173.
2. ACSM. American College of Sports Medicine Position Stand. The recommended quantity and quality of exercise for developing and maintaining cardiorespiratory and muscular fitness, and flexibility in healthy adults. Med Sci Sports Exerc 1998;30:975–991.
3. Adamsen L, Midtgaard J, Rorth M, et al. Feasibility, physical capacity, and health benefits of a multidimensional exercise program for cancer patients undergoing chemotherapy. Support Care Cancer 2003;11: 707–716.
4. Ades PA, Savage PD, Cress ME, et al. Resistance training on physical performance in disabled older female cardiac patients. Med Sci Sports Exerc 2003;35:1265–1270.
5. Agre JC, Rodriquez AA, Franke TM. Strength, endurance, and work capacity after muscle strengthening

exercise in postpolio subjects. Arch Phys Med Rehabil 1992;78:681–686.

6. Albright A, Franz M, Hornsby G, et al. American College of Sports Medicine position stand: exercise and type 2 diabetes. Med Sci Sports Exerc 2000;32:1345–1360.

7. American Obesity Association. Available at www. obesity.org. Accessed December 08, 2005.

8. American College of Sports Medicine. Franklin BA, Whaley MH, Howley ET, Balady GJ. ACSM's Guidelines for Exercise Testing and Prescription Philadelphia: Lippincott Williams & Wilkins, 2000:33–130.

9. American College of Sports Medicine. Whaley MH, Brubaker PH, Otto RM, Armstrong LE. ACSM's Guidelines for Exercise Testing and Prescription. 7th ed. 30th Anniversary ed. Philadelphia: Lippincott Williams & Wilkins, 2006:xxi, 366.

10. Anderson RN. Deaths: leading causes for 1999. Natl Vital Stat Rep 2001;49:1–87.

11. Andersson C, Grooten W, Hellsten M, et al. Adults with cerebral palsy: walking ability after progressive strength training. Dev Med Child Neurol 2003;45:220–228.

12. Angelopoulou N, Matziari C, Tsimaris V, et al. Bone mineral density and muscle strength in young men with mental retardation (with and without Down syndrome). Calcif Tiss Int 2000;66:176–180.

13. Artal R, O'Toole M. Guidelines of the American College of Obstetricians and Gynecologists for exercise during pregnancy and the postpartum period. Br J Sports Med 2003;37:6–12; discussion 12.

14. Arthritis Foundation. Disease Center: Rheumatoid Arthritis. Available at: www.arthritis.org/conditions/diseasecenter/RA/default.asp. Accessed December 19, 2004.

15. Association, American Diabetes. Diabetes mellitus and exercise. Diabetes Care 2002;25(Suppl):S64–S68.

16. ATS. Pulmonary rehabilitation 1999. American Thoracic Society. Am J Respir Crit Care Med 1999;159:1666–1682.

17. ATS/ERS. Skeletal muscle dysfunction in chronic obstructive pulmonary disease. A statement of the American Thoracic Society and European Respiratory Society. Am J Respir Crit Care Med 1999;159:S1–40.

18. Badics E, Wittman A, Rupp M, et al. Systematic muscle building exercises in the rehabilitation of stroke patients. Neurorehabilitation 2002;17:211–214.

19. Becker, RC. Editorial. Thromboneurology and the search for stroke therapies. Stroke. 1997;28:1657–1659.

20. Bennett RM. Emerging concepts in the neurobiology of chronic pain: evidence of abnormal processing in fibromyalgia. Mayo Clin Proc 1999;74:385–398.

21. Bernhardt DT, Gomez J, Johnson MD, et al. Strength training by children and adolescents. Pediatrics 2001;107:1470–1472.

22. Bhasin S, Storer TW. Exercise regimens for men with HIV. JAMA 2000;284:175–176.

23. Bhasin S, Storer TW, Javanbakht M, et al. Testosterone replacement and resistance exercise in HIV-infected men with weight loss and low testosterone levels. JAMA 2000;283:763–770.

24. Bonaiuti D, Shea B, Iovine R, et al. Exercise for preventing and treating osteoporosis in postmenopausal women. Cochrane Database Syst Rev 2002;CD000333.

25. Bonita R. Epidemiology of stroke. Lancet 1992;339:342–347.

26. Booth CM, Cortina-Borja MJ, Theologis TN. Collagen accumulation in muscles of children with cerebral palsy and correlation with severity of spasticity. Dev Med Child Neurol 2001;43:314–320.

27. Byrne HK, Wilmore JH. The effects of a 20-week exercise training program on resting metabolic rate in previously sedentary, moderately obese women. Int J Sport Nutr Exerc Metab 2001;11:15–31.

28. Calle EE, Rodriguez C, Walker-Thurmond K, Thun MJ. Overweight, obesity, and mortality from cancer in a prospectively studied cohort of U.S. adults. N Engl J Med 2003;348:1625–1638.

29. Carmeli E, Ayalon M, Barchad S, et al. Isokinetic leg strength of institutionalized older adults with mental retardation with and without Down's syndrome. J Strength Cond Res 2002;16:316–320.

30. Castaneda C, Layne JE, Munoz-Orians L, et al. An randomized controlled trial of resistance exercise training to improve glycemic control in older adults with type 2 diabetes. Diabetes Care 2002;25:2335–2341.

31. CDC. HIV and AIDS–United States 1981–2001. MMWR 2001;50:430–434.

32. Chan KM, Amirjani N, Sumrain M, et al. Randomized controlled trial of strength training in post-polio. Muscle Nerve 2003;27:332–338.

33. Chobanian AV, Bakris GL, Black HR, et al. Seventh report of the Joint National Committee on Prevention, Detection, Evaluation, and Treatment of High Blood Pressure. Hypertension 2003;42:1206–1252.

34. Curtis CL, Weir JP. Overview of exercise responses in healthy and impaired states. Neurol Rep 1996;20:13–19.

35. Curtis KA, Tyner TM, Zachery L. Effect of a standard exercise protocol on shoulder pain in long-term wheelchair users. Spinal Cord 1999;37:421–429.

36. Damiano DL, Abel MF. Functional outcomes of strength training in spastic cerebral palsy. Arch Phys Med Rehabil 1998;79:119–125.

37. Damiano DL, Vaughan CL, Abel MF. Muscle response to heavy resistance exercise in children with spastic cerebral palsy. Dev Med Child Neurol 1995;37:731–739.

38. Damiano DL, Kelly LE, Vaughn CL. Effects of quadriceps femoris muscle strengthening on crouch gait in children with spastic diplegia. Phys Ther 1995;75:658–671.

39. Davis GM, Shepard RJ. Strength training for wheelchair users. Br J Sports Med 1990;24:25–30.

40. de Jong Z, Munneke M, Zwinderman AH, et al. Is a long-term high-intensity exercise program effective and safe in patients with rheumatoid arthritis? Results of a randomized controlled trial. Arthritis Rheum 2003;48:2415–2424.

41. Delagardelle C, Feiereisen P, Autier P, et al. Strength/endurance training versus endurance training in congestive heart failure. Med Sci Sports Exerc 2002;34:1868–1872.

42. Dennis MS, Burn JP, Sandercock PA, et al. Long-term survival after first-ever stroke: the Oxfordshire Community Stroke Project. Stroke 1993;24:796–800.

43. Dudgeon WD, Phillips KD, Bopp CM, Hand GA. Physiological and psychological effects of exercise interventions in HIV disease. AIDS Patient Care STDS 2004;18:81–98.

44. Dunlop DD, Manheim LM, Yelin EH, et al. The costs of arthritis. Arthritis Rheum 2003;49:101–113.

45. Dunstan DW, Daly RM, Owen N, et al. High-intensity resistance training improves glycemic control in older patients with type 2 diabetes. Diabetes Care 2002;25: 1729–1736.

46. Durak EP, Lilliy PC. The application of an exercise and wellness program for cancer patients: a preliminary outcomes report. J Strength Cond Res 1998;12:3–6.

47. Elder GCB, Kirk J, Stewart G, et al. Contributing factors to muscle weakness in children with cerebral palsy. Dev Med Child Neurol 2003;45:542–550.

48. Engardt M, Knutsson E, Jonsson M, Sternhag M. Dynamic muscle strength training in stroke patients: effects on knee extension torque, electromyographic activity, and motor function. Arch Phys Med Rehabil 1995;76:419–425.

49. Evans WJ. Effects of exercise on body composition and functional capacity of the elderly. J Gerontol 1995;50A: 147–150.

50. Evans WJ. Effects of exercise on senescent muscle. Clin Orthop Rel Res 2002;403S:S211–S220.

51. Evans WJ. Exercise training guidelines for the elderly. Med Sci Sports Exerc 1999;31:12–17.

52. Faigenbaum AD, Milliken LA, LaRosa R, et al. Comparison of 1 and 2 days per week of strength training in children. Res Q Exerc Sport 2002;73:416–424.

53. Faigenbaum AD, Milliken LA, Westcott WL. Maximal strength testing in healthy children. J Strength Cond Res 2003;17:162–166.

54. Faigenbaum AD, Kraemer WJ, Cahill B, et al. Youth resistance training: position statement paper and literature review. Strength Cond J 1996;18:62–75.

55. Faigenbaum AD, Westcott WL, Long C, et al. Relationship between repetitions and selected percentages of the one-repetition maximum in healthy children. Pediatr Phys Ther 1998;10:110–113.

56. Falk B, Tenenbaum G. The effectiveness of resistance training in children. Sports Med 1996;22:176–186.

57. Fassbender HG. The Pathology and Pathobiology of Rheumatic Disease. 2nd ed. New York: Springer, 2002.

58. Fenicchia LM, Kanaley JA, Azevedo JL Jr, et al. Influence of resistance exercise training on glucose control in women with type 2 diabetes. Metabolism 2004;53: 284–289.

59. Fernhall B. Physical fitness and exercise training of individuals with mental retardation. Med Sci Sports Exerc 1993;25:442–450.

60. Fiatarone MA, Marks EC, Ryan ND, et al. High-intensity strength training in nonagenarians: effects on skeletal muscle. JAMA 1990;263:3029–3034.

61. Figoni SF. Spinal cord disabilities: paraplegia and tetraplegia. In: Durstine JL, Moore GE, eds. ACSM's Exercise Management for Persons with Chronic Diseases and Disabilities. Champaign, IL: Human Kinetics, 2003: 247–253.

62. Finklestein EA, Fiebelkorn IC, Wang G. National medical spending attributable to overweight and obesity: how much, and who's paying? Health Affairs 2003; W3:219–226.

63. Fleming PL, Byers RH, Sweeney PA, Daniels D, Karon JM, Janssen RS. HIV prevalence in the United States, 2000. In: 9th Conference on Retroviruses and Opportunistic Infections. Seattle, WA: 2002.

64. Forrest G, Qian X. Exercise in neuromuscular disease. Neurorehabilitation 1999;13:135–139.

65. Fransen MS, McConnell S, Bell M. Exercise for osteoarthritis of the hip or knee. Cochrane Database Syst Rev 2003;CD004286.

66. Freeman J, Allison R. Group exercise classes in people with multiple sclerosis: a pilot study. Physiother Res Int 2004;9:104–107.

67. Friedenreich CM, Courneya CS. Exercise as rehabilitation for cancer patients. Clin J Sport Med 1996;6:237–244.

68. Frontera WR, Suh D, Krivickas LS, et al. Skeletal muscle fiber quality in older men and women. Am J Physiol 2000;279:C611–C618.

69. Frontera WR, Hughes VA, Fielding RA, et al. Aging of skeletal muscle: a 12-year longitudinal study. J Appl Physiol 2000;88:1321–1326.

70. Goldberg LD, Elliot DL, Keuhl KS. Cardiovascular changes at rest and during mixed static and dynamic exercises after weight training. J Appl Sport Sci Res 1998;2:42–45.

71. Goodman CC. The immune system. In: Goodman CC, Boissonault WG, Fuller KS, eds. Pathology. Implications for the Physical Therapist. 2nd ed. Philadelphia: Saunders, 2003:153–193.

72. Goodman CC, Glanzman A. Genetic and developmental disorders. In: Goodman CC, Boissonault WG, Fuller KS, eds. Pathology. Implications for the Physical Therapist. 2nd ed. Philadelphia: Saunders, 2003:829–870.

73. Hakkinen A, Hannonen P, Nyman K, et al. Effects of concurrent strength and endurance training in women with early or longstanding rheumatoid arthritis: comparison with healthy subjects. Arthritis Rheum 2003; 49:789–797.

74. Hakkinen A, Hakkinen K, Hannonen P, Alen M. Strength training induced adaptations in neuromuscular function in premenopausal women with fibromyalgia: comparison with healthy women. Ann Rheum Dis 2001; 60:21–26.

75. Häkkinen A, Sokka T, Hannonen P. A home-based two-year strength training period in early rheumatoid arthritis led to good long-term compliance: a five-year follow-up. Arthritis Rheum 2004;51:56–62.

76. Halpern MT, Stanford RH, Borker R. The burden of COPD in the U.S.A.: results from the Confronting COPD survey. Respir Med 2003;97(Suppl C):S81–S89.

77. Helleckson KL. NIH releases statement on osteoporosis prevention, diagnosis, and therapy. Am Fam Phys 2002; 66:161–162.

78. Hook EB. Epidemiology of Down syndrome. In: Pueschel SM, Rynders JE, eds. Down Syndrome: Advances in Biomedicine and the Behavioral Sciences. Cambridge, UK: Ware Press, 1982:11–88.

79. Hughes VA, Frontera WR, Wood M, et al. Longitudinal muscle strength changes in older adults: influence of muscle mass, physical activity, and health. J Gerontol Biol Sci 2001;56A:B209–B217.

80. Ishii T, Yamakita T, Sato T, et al. Resistance training improves insulin sensitivity in NIDDM subjects without

altering maximal oxygen uptake. Diabetes Care 1998: 21:1353–1355.

81. Jacob PL, Nash MS. Exercise recommendations for individuals with spinal cord injury. Sports Med 2004;34: 727–751.

82. Jakobsson P, Jorfeldt L, Brundin A. Skeletal muscle metabolites and fibre types in patients with advanced chronic obstructive pulmonary disease (COPD), with and without chronic respiratory failure. Eur Respir J 1990: 3:192–196.

83. Jette AM, Branch LG. The Framingham Disability Study: II. Physical disability among the aging. Am J Public Health 1981;71:1211–1216.

84. Jones KD, Clark SR. Individualizing the exercise prescription for persons with fibromyalgia. Rheum Dis Clin North Am 2002;28:419–436.

85. Jones KD, Burckhardt CS, Clark SR, et al. A randomized controlled trial of muscle strengthening versus flexibility training in fibromyalgia. J Rheumatol 2002;29: 1041–1048.

86. Kelley GA, Kelley KS. Progressive resistance exercise and resting blood pressure: a meta-analysis of randomized controlled trials. Hypertension 2000;35:838–843.

87. Kelley GA, Kelley KS, Tran ZV. The effects of exercise on resting blood pressure in children and adolescents: a meta-analysis of randomized controlled trials. Prev Cardiol 2003;6:8–16.

88. Kelley GA, Kelley KS, Tran ZV. Walking and resting blood pressure in adults: a meta-analysis. Prev Med 2001;33:120–127.

89. Kilmer DD. Response to resistive strengthening exercise training in humans with neuromuscular disease. Am J Phys Med 2002;81(Suppl):S121–S126.

90. Klingbeil H, Baer HR, Wilson PE. Aging with a disability. Arch Phys Med Rehabil 2004;85:S68–S73.

91. Kramer MS. Aerobic exercise for women during pregnancy. Cochrane Database Syst Rev 2002;CD000180.

92. Lacasse Y, Wong E, Guyatt GH, et al. Meta-analysis of respiratory rehabilitation in chronic obstructive pulmonary disease. Lancet 1996;348:1115–1119.

93. Lackland D. Bacjam D:. Carter TD. et al. The geographic variation in stroke incidence in two areas of the southeastern stroke belt. Stroke 1998;29:2061–2068.

94. Lanes SF. Lanza LL, Radensky PW, et al. Resource utilization and cost of care for rheumatoid arthritis and osteoarthritis in a managed care setting: the importance of drug and surgery costs. Arthritis Rheum 1997;40: 1475–1481.

95. Latham NK, Bennett DA, Stretton CM, Anderson CS. Systematic review of progressive resistance strength training in older adults. J Gerontol A Biol Sci Med Sci 2004;59:48–61.

96. Latham NK, Bennett DA, Stretton CM, Anderson CS. Systematic review of progressive resistance strength training in older adults. J Gerontol Med Sci 2004; 59A:48–61.

97. Lexell J, Taylor CC, Sjostrom M. What is the cause of the ageing atrophy? Total number, size and proportion of different fiber types studied in whole vastus lateralis muscle from 15- to 83-year-old men. J Neurol Sci 1988; 84:275–294.

98. Liang MH, Cullen KE, Larson MG, et al. Cost-effectiveness of total joint arthroplasty in osteoarthritis. Arthritis Rheum 1986;29:937–943.

99. MaCallan DC. Metabolic abnormalities and the "wasting syndrome" in HIV infection. Nutrition 1996;12: 641–642.

100. Macallan DC. Wasting in HIV infection and AIDS. J Nutr 1999;129:238S–242S.

101. Macallan DC, Griffin GE. Metabolic disturbances in AIDS. N Engl J Med 1992;327:1530–1531.

102. Mador MJ. Muscle mass, not body weight, predicts outcome in patients with chronic obstructive pulmonary disease. Am J Respir Crit Care Med 2002;166:787–789.

103. Mador MJ, Kufel TJ, Pineda LA, et al. Effect of pulmonary rehabilitation on quadriceps fatigability during exercise. Am J Respir Crit Care Med 2001;163:930–935.

104. Maiorana A. O'Driscoll G, Dembo L, et al. Effect of aerobic and resistance exercise training on vascular function in heart failure. Am J Physiol Heart Circ Physiol 2000;279:H1999–2005.

105. Malek MH, Nalbone DP, Berger DE, Coburn JW. Importance of health science education for personal fitness trainers. J Strength Cond Res 2002;16:19–24.

106. Maltais F, LeBlanc P, Simard C, et al. Skeletal muscle adaptation to endurance training in patients with chronic obstructive pulmonary disease. Am J Respir Crit Care Med 1996;154:442–447.

107. Maltais F, Simard AA, Simard C, et al. Oxidative capacity of the skeletal muscle and lactic acid kinetics during exercise in normal subjects and in patients with COPD. Am J Respir Crit Care Med 1996;153:288–293.

108. Matchar DB, Duncan PW. The cost of stroke. Stroke Clinical Updates 1994;5:9–12.

109. Mayo NE. Stroke. 1. Epidemiology and recovery. Phys Med Rehabil 1993;7:1–25.

110. Maziekas MT, LeMura LM, Stoddard NM, et al. Follow up exercise studies in paediatric obesity: implications for long term effectiveness. Br J Sports Med 2003;37: 425–429.

111. McCarthy CJ, Mills PM, Pullen R, et al. Supplementation of a home-based exercise programme with a class-based programme for people with osteoarthritis of the knees: a randomised controlled trial and health economic analysis. Health Technol Assess 2004;8:1–76.

112. McCartney N, McKelvie RS, Martin J, et al. Weight training induced attenuation of the circulatory response of older males to weight lifting. J Appl Physiol 1993;74: 1056–1060.

113. McDermott AY, Shevitz A, Knox T, et al. Effect of highly active antiretroviral therapy on fat, lean, and bone mass in HIV-seropositive men and women. Am J Clin Nutr 2001;74:679–686.

114. Mokdad AH, Marks JS, Stroup DF, Gerberding JL. Actual causes of death in the United States, 2000. JAMA 2004;291:1238–1245.

115. Moreland JD, Goldsmith CH, Huijbregts MP, et al. Progressive resistance strengthening exercises after stroke: a single-blind randomized controlled trial. Arch Phys Med Rehabil 2003;84:1433–1440.

116. Moritani T, deVries HA. Potential for gross muscle hypertrophy in older men. Am J Phys Med 1980;35:672–682.

117. Mostert S, Kesselring J. Effects of a short-term exercise training program on aerobic fitness, fatigue, health perception and activity level of subjects with multiple sclerosis. Mult Scler 2002;8:161–168.

118. Munneke M, de Jong Z, Zwinderman AH, et al. Adherence and satisfaction of rheumatoid arthritis patients with a long-term intensive dynamic exercise program (RAPIT program). Arthritis Rheum 2003;49:665–672.

119. NHLBI. Chronic Obstructive Pulmonary Disease (COPD) Data Fact Sheet. U.S. NIH Publication No. 03-5229. Bethesda, MD: National Heart, Lung, and Blood Institute, 2003:1–6.

120. NIH. Clinical Guidelines on the Identification, Evaluation, and Treatment of Overweight and Obesity in Adults. Bethesda, MD: National Institutes of Health, National Heart, Lung, and Blood Institute, 1998.

121. NIH. NIH develops consensus statement on the role of physical activity for cardiovascular health. Am Fam Physician 1996;54:763–764, 767.

122. NIH. Osteoporosis Prevention, Diagnosis, and Therapy. NIH Consensus Statement. 2000;17:1–45.

123. NIH. The Surgeon General's Call to Action to Prevent and Decrease Overweight and Obesity 2001. Rockville, MD: U.S. Department of Health and Human Services, 2001:1–39.

124. Oguma Y, Shinoda-Tagawa T. Physical activity decreases cardiovascular disease risk in women: review and meta-analysis. Am J Prev Med 2004;26:407–418.

125. Oldervoll LM, Kaasa S, Hjermstad MJ, et al. Physical exercise results in the improved subjective well-being of a few or is effective rehabilitation for all cancer patients? Eur J Cancer 2004;40:951–962.

126. Oldervoll LM, Kaasa S, Knobel H, Loge JH. Exercise reduces fatigue in chronic fatigued Hodgkins disease survivors—results from a pilot study. Eur J Cancer 2003;39:57–63.

127. Olek ML. Multiple Sclerosis: Etiology, Diagnosis, and New Treatment Strategies. Totowa, NJ: Humana Press, 2005:xv, 245.

128. Ortega F, Toral J, Cejudo P, et al. Comparison of effects of strength and endurance training in patients with chronic obstructive pulmonary disease. Am J Respir Crit Care Med 2002;166:669–674.

129. Padget K. Alterations of neurologic function in children. In: McCance KL, Huether SE, eds. Pathophysiology. The Biological Basis for Disease in Adults and Children. St. Louis: Mosby, 1998:566–596.

130. Panton LB, Golden J, Broeder CE, et al. The effects of resistance training on functional outcomes in patients with chronic obstructive pulmonary disease. Eur J Appl Physiol 2004;91:443–449.

131. Park SK, Park JH, Kwon YC, et al. The effect of combined aerobic and resistance exercise training on abdominal fat in obese middle-aged women. J Physiol Anthropol Appl Human Sci 2003;22:129–135.

132. Payne VG, Morrow JR Jr, Johnson L, et al. Resistance training in children and youth: a meta-analysis. Res Q Exerc Sport 1997;68:80–88.

133. Petajan JH, Gappmaier E, White AT, et al. Impact of aerobic training on fitness and quality of life in multiple sclerosis. Ann Neurol 1996;39:432–441.

134. Pollock ML, Franklin BA, Balady GJ, et al. AHA Science Advisory. Resistance exercise in individuals with and without cardiovascular disease: benefits, rationale, safety, and prescription: An advisory from the Committee on Exercise, Rehabilitation, and Prevention, Council on Clinical Cardiology, American Heart Association; Position paper endorsed by the American College of Sports Medicine. Circulation 2000;101:828–833.

135. Pu CT, Johnson MT, Forman DE, et al. Randomized trial of progressive resistance training to counteract the myopathy of chronic heart failure. J Appl Physiol 2001;90:2341–2350.

136. Ramsey SD, Sullivan SD. The burden of illness and economic evaluation for COPD. Eur Respir J Suppl 2003;41:29s–35s.

137. Reddihough DS, Collins KJ. The epidemiology and causes of cerebral palsy. Aust J Physiother 2003;49:7–12.

138. Rimmer JH, Kelly LE. Effects of a resistance training program on adults with mental retardation. Adapt Phys Ed Q 1991;8:146–153.

139. Rimmer JH, Heller T, Wang E, Valerio I. Improvements in physical fitness in adults with Down syndrome. Am J Ment Retard 2004;109:165–174.

140. Robinson RL, Birnbaum HG, Morley MA, et al. Economic cost and epidemiological characteristics of patients with fibromyalgia claims. J Rheumatol 2003;30:1318–1325.

141. Roddy E, Zhang W, Doherty M, et al. Evidence-based recommendations for the role of exercise in the management of osteoarthritis of the hip or knee—the MOVE consensus. Rheumatology (Oxford) 2004.

142. Roubenoff R. Abad LW, Lundren N. Effect of acquired immune deficiency syndrome wasting on the protein metabolic response to acute exercise. Metabolism 2001;50:288–292.

143. Roubenoff R, Wilson IB. Effect of resistance training on self-reported physical functioning in HIV infection. Med Sci Sports Exerc 2001;33:1811–1817.

144. Sacco RL. Risk factors, outcomes, and stroke subtypes for ischemic stroke. Neurology 1997;49(Suppl 4):S39–S44.

145. Sacco RL, Wolf PA, Gorelick PB. Risk factors and their management for stroke prevention: outlook for 1999 and beyond. Neurology 1999;53(7 Suppl 4):S15–S24.

146. Sattler FR, Jaque SV, Schroeder C, et al. Effects of pharmacological doses of nandrolone decanoate and progressive resistance training in immunodeficient patients infected with human immunodeficiency virus. J Clin Endocrinol Metab 1999;84:1268–1276.

147. Schousboe K. Visscher PM, Erbas B, et al. Twin study of genetic and environmental influences on adult body size, shape, and composition. Int J Obes Rel Metab Disord 2004;28:39–48.

148. Schousboe K, Willemsen G, Kyvik KO, et al. Sex differences in heritability of BMI: a comparative study of results from twin studies in eight countries. Twin Res 2003;6:409–421.

149. Sevick MA, Bradham DD, Muender M, et al. Cost-effectiveness of aerobic and resistance exercise in seniors with knee osteoarthritis. Med Sci Sports Exerc 2000;32:1534–1540.

150. Sharp SA, Brouwer BJ. Isokinetic strength training of the hemiparetic knee: effects on function and spasticity. Arch Phys Med Rehabil 1997;78:1231–1236.

151. Sherlekar S, Udipi SA. Role of nutrition in the management of HIV infection/AIDS. J Indian Med Assoc 2002; 100:385–390.

152. SMA. SMA statement the benefits and risks of exercise during pregnancy. Sport Medicine Australia. J Sci Med Sport 2002;5:11–19.

153. Smith GV, Silver KHC, Goldberg AP, Macko RF. "Task-oriented" exercise improves hamstring strength and spastic reflexes in chronic stroke patients. Stroke 1999; 30:2112–2118.

154. Smith MB. The peripheral nervous system. In: Goodman CC, Boissonnault WG, Fuller KS, eds. Pathology. Implications for the Physical Therapist. Philadelphia: Saunders, 2003:1161–1162.

155. Society, American Cancer. Cancer Facts and Figures 2003. Atlanta: American Cancer Society, 2003:1–48.

156. Spector SA. Gordon PL, Feuerstein IM, et al. Strength gains without muscle injury after strength training in patients with postpolio muscular atrophy. Muscle Nerve 1996;19:1282–1290.

157. Storer TW. Exercise in chronic pulmonary disease: resistance exercise prescription. Med Sci Sports Exerc 2001; 33:S680–S692.

158. Stunkard AJ. Wadden TA. Obesity: Theory and therapy. New York: Raven Press, 1993.

159. Suomi R, Surburg PR, Lecius P. Effects of hydraulic resistance strength training on isokinetic measures of leg strength in men with mental retardation. Adapt Phys Ed Q 1995;12:377–387.

160. Surakka J, Romberg A, Ruutiainen J, et al. Effects of aerobic and strength exercise on motor fatigue in men and women with multiple sclerosis: a randomized controlled trial. Clin Rehabil 2004;18:737–746.

161. Taylor E, Missik E, Hurley R, et al. Obesity treatment: broadening our perspective. Am J Health Behav 2004; 28:242–249.

162. Teixeira-Salmela LF, Nadeau S, McBride I, Olney SJ. Olney. Effects of muscle strengthening and physical conditioning training on temporal, kinematic and kinetic variables during gait in chronic stroke survivors. J Rehabil Med 2001;33:53–60.

163. Teixeira-Salmela LF, Olney SJ, Nadeau S, Brouwer B. Muscle strengthening and physical conditioning to reduce impairment and disability in chronic stroke survivors. Arch Phys Med Rehabil 1999;80:1211–1218.

164. Thompson D, Wolf AM. The medical-care cost burden of obesity. Obes Rev 2001;2:189–197.

165. Thune I, Furberg AS. Physical activity and cancer risk: dose-response and cancer, all sites and site-specific. Med Sci Sports Exerc 2001;33:S530–550; discussion S609-S510.

166. Trappe S, Williamson D, Godard M. Maintenance of whole muscle strength and size following resistance training in older men. J Gerontol A Biol Sci Med Sci 2002;57:B138–B143.

167. Trupin L, Earnest G, San Pedro M, et al. The occupational burden of chronic obstructive pulmonary disease. Eur Respir J 2003;22:462–469.

168. UNAIDS. AIDS Epidemic Update. Geneva: UNAIDS Information Centre, 2003:1–39.

169. Valkeinen H, Alen M, Hannonen A, et al. Changes in knee extension and flexion force, EMG and functional capacity during strength training in older females with fibromyalgia and healthy controls. Rheumatology 2004; 43:225–228.

170. Van den Ende CH, Vliet Vlieland TP, Munneke M, Hazes M. Dynamic exercise therapy in rheumatoid arthritis: a systematic review. Br J Rheumatol. 1998;37:677–687.

171. Villareal DT, Steger-May K, Schechtman K, et al. Effects of exercise training on bone mineral density in frail older women and men: a randomised controlled trial. Age Ageing 2004;33:309–312.

172. Watts K, Beye P, Siafarikas A, et al. Exercise training normalizes vascular dysfunction and improves central adiposity in obese adolescents. J Am Coll Cardiol 2004; 43:1823–1827.

173. Weir JP, Housh TJ, Johnson GO, et al. Allometric scaling of isokinetic peak torque: the Nebraska Wrestling Study. Eur J Appl Physiol 1999;80:240–248.

174. Wheeler DA. The human immunodeficiency virus. Cutis 1995;55:81–83.

175. Wheeler DA. Weight loss and disease progression in HIV infection. AIDS Read 1999;9:347–353.

176. Wheeler DA, Gibert CL, Launer CA, et al. Weight loss as a predictor of survival and disease progression in HIV infection. Terry Beirn Community Programs for Clinical Research on AIDS. J Acquir Immune Defic Syndr Hum Retrovirol 1998;18:80–85.

177. Whitaker RC, Wright JA, Pepe MS, et al. Predicting obesity in young adulthood from childhood and parental obesity. N Engl J Med 1997;337:869–873.

178. White LJ, Dressendorfer RH. Exercise and multiple sclerosis. Sports Med 2004;34:1077–1100.

179. Willey KA, Fiatarone Singh MA. Battling insulin resistance in elderly obese people with type 2 diabetes. Bring on the heavy weights. Diabetes Care 2003;26: 1580–1588.

180. Williams W, Jiang JG, Matcher DB, Samsa GP. Incidence and occurrence of total (first-ever and recurrent) stroke. Stroke 1999;30:2523–2528.

181. Wing RR. Physical activity in the treatment of the adulthood overweight and obesity: current evidence and research issues. Med Sci Sports Exerc 1999;31:S547–S552.

182. Wolfe F, Ross K, Anderson J, et al. The prevalence and general characteristics of fibromyalgia in the general population. Arthritis Rheum 1995;38:19–28.

183. Yarasheski KE. Exercise, aging, and muscle protein metabolism. J Gerontol A Biol Sci Med Sci 2003;58: M918–M922.

184. Yarasheski KE, Pak-Loduca J, Hasten DL, et al. Resistance exercise training increases mixed muscle protein synthesis rate in frail women and men ≥76 yr old. Am J Physiol 1999;277:E118–E125.

185. Yelin, E. Cost of musculoskeletal diseases: impact of work disability and functional decline. J Rheumatol Suppl2003;68:8–11.

CHAPTER

17

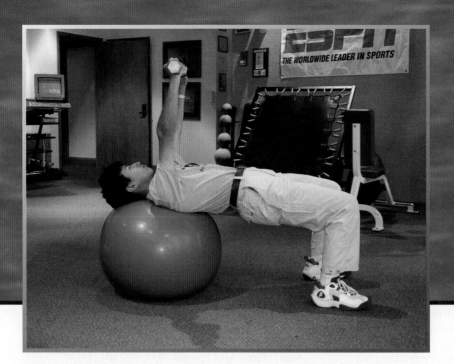

Principles of Injury Prevention and Rehabilitation

TODD S. ELLENBECKER
JAKE BLEACHER
ANNA THATCHER

Introduction

This chapter offers an overview of the role of strength and conditioning in the prevention of injuries and bridging the gap between rehabilitation and return to participation. Included in this chapter is an overview of the sports medicine professionals responsible for providing care for the athlete as well as the stages of recovery and healing from a musculoskeletal injury. Basic definitions of musculoskeletal injuries and more detailed descriptions of the anatomy and biomechanics of the shoulder, knee, and spine are included, along with common injury patterns and exercise implications applicable for strength and conditioning professionals working with athletes with a history of musculoskeletal injury, especially those hoping to prevent them.

Q & A from the Field

Should athletes perform open or closed kinetic chain lower extremity exercises during their strength programs?

There are advantages and disadvantages to both open and closed kinetic chain exercises. Since daily and sport activities occur in both the open and closed kinetic chains, both types of exercises should be included in a strengthening program. As described in the text, precautions may need to be taken at certain ranges of motion if there is a history of knee injury.

Although this chapter provides significant detail on rehabilitation as well as injury prevention for the strength and conditioning professional, such rehabilitation should be performed under the supervision of a physician and physical therapist. This chapter also includes information regarding the specific roles of each health care provider in a sports medicine team as well as an overview of all phases of the injury prevention and rehabilitation process to facilitate the understanding of each individual's role in the team approach to both preventing injury and returning an injured athlete to participation.

Some of the most basic principles of injury prevention have the most profound influence for strength and conditioning professionals as well as other clinicians in sports medicine. These include adequate preactivity development of muscular strength, endurance and balance, proper flexibility, and—often most importantly—proper sport biomechanics or technique (45).

Many injuries in athletes occur from overtraining and overuse (34). Improper levels of muscular strength and endurance are often cited as critical factors in the development of injuries such as rotator cuff tendonitis (17), humeral epicondylitis (40), and patellofemoral pain and shin splints (22).

Additionally, sports medicine research profiling various populations of athletes has also identified characteristic patterns of muscular development that create muscular imbalances and can lead to injury (9). A **muscular imbalance** occurs with adaptive changes to the length and strength of a muscle on one side of a joint, resulting in the asymmetrical forces across the joint. The result is diminished participation of one muscle, leading to disuse atrophy or excessive motion in the direction of the dominant muscle.

One example of a muscular imbalance identified with isokinetic testing of the glenohumeral joint of overhead athletes was reported by a study whereby significant increases in the strength of the internal rotators was measured on the dominant arm of professional baseball pitchers without concomitant increases in the strength of the external rotator musculature, thus creating a muscular imbalance (41). Studies in elite-level tennis players (18,20) have identified similar imbalances between the internal and external rotators.

Careful evaluation and application of stretching programs are other important factors in injury prevention. Although studies directly linking flexibility training and injury prevention are not clear cut, the general consensus among sports medicine professionals is that significant muscular inflexibility can inhibit optimal performance and lead to joint and muscle tendon injury in the repetitive environment where athletic individuals train and compete (45). Despite recent changes in the application of static and dynamic stretching programs, sport scientists still believe specific types of flexibility training to be important in both performance enhancement and injury prevention.

Finally, the use of proper sport technique and biomechanics is a critical factor in the prevention of injury. The link between improper use of the kinetic chain in throwing and racquet sports and arm injury has been outlined (27). The **kinetic chain** is made up of a series of rigid segments connected by movable joints. The entire body or any of its parts containing one or more joints could be considered a kinetic chain.

The use of sport technique that optimizes power generation from the lower extremity and trunk and allows for the transfer of force from the ground reaction forces up through the lower extremities

Q & A from the Field

A female high school athlete has developed knee pain in performing squats and lunges. What are some possible errors in technique she may demonstrate?

If hip weakness or decreased control is present, the hip on the non–weight-bearing side may lower during the exercise. Her femur(s) may rotate internally and her knee(s) might move medially into a valgus position. The athlete may have excessive foot pronation during movement.

and trunk to the upper extremity is recommended. Although in many cases the strength and conditioning professional cannot directly evaluate this facet of the injury prevention program, referral of athletes to qualified individuals such as high-level sport-specific coaches and sport biomechanists is highly recommended.

PREPARTICIPATION PHYSICALS

It is beyond the scope of this chapter to completely outline all facets of the preparticipation physical; however, the basic premise of the physical as well as its key components should be discussed. Several complete references on preparticipation physicals can serve as excellent resources in designing or developing such an examination (1,27). In general, the **preparticipation physical** is an integral part of the injury prevention process. The actual physical is designed to evaluate the athlete's body using a specific series of evaluation methods or tests that screen or identify key factors that could lead to an injury if the athlete were to participate in his or her sport without rehabilitation or other preparative measures.

Whereas some of the basic tests are included in nearly all physicals (measurement of height, weight, heart rate, blood pressure, etc.) most physicals are made specific to the sport or activity in which a given athlete or group of athletes is participating. One example would be the careful evaluation of rotator cuff strength and shoulder flexibility in baseball and tennis players as well as swimmers. This area would not be emphasized as heavily for soccer players or other primarily lower-body ath-

letes. Careful development of the actual components of the preparticipation physical with the entire sports medicine team is necessary, since many specialists and types of clinicians are needed to ensure that the most thorough evaluation is made. Additionally, the important roles follow-up, tracking, and ultimately retesting play cannot be overlooked.

> *Preparticipation physicals are an important part of the comprehensive care of the athlete. Using a structured evaluation process, key structural deficits and strength and flexibility deficiencies can be identified that can decrease the risk of injury or reinjury.*

ROLES OF HEALTH CARE PROFESSIONALS INVOLVED IN INJURY PREVENTION AND REHABILITATION

Numerous health care professions are involved in various aspects of sports injury management. Depending on the sports program (e.g., high school, college, professional team, community recreation), professionals in medicine, chiropractors, psychology, biomechanics, exercise physiology, nutrition, physical therapy, athletic training, and strength and conditioning may be involved in different stages of injury management. The diversity of health professionals involved in injury management allows the athlete to recover not only physically but also emotionally and socially.

The areas of injury prevention, recognition, and rehabilitation are common interests to professions including physicians, physical therapists, athletic trainers, and strength and conditioning professionals. These four professions commonly have extensive involvement throughout the rehabilitation process and are further discussed below.

- *Physicians.* The physician is responsible for the health care of an injured athlete, including diagnosing and treating injuries. When an injury occurs, the physician makes the ultimate decision on when it is safe to return to sport activities. The physician guides other members of the team throughout the rehabilitation process.
- *Physical Therapists.* According to the American Physical Therapy Association, the scope of practice for a physical therapist includes providing services to patients who have impairments, functional limitations, disabilities, or changes in physical function and health status resulting from injury, disease, or other causes; interaction and practicing in collaboration with a variety of professionals; addressing risk factors and behavior that may impede optimal functioning; providing prevention and promoting health, wellness, and fitness; consulting, educating, engaging in critical inquiry, and administration; and directing and supervising support personnel (2).
- *Athletic Trainers.* Performance domains of the certified athletic trainer as defined by the Board of Certification include prevention; clinical evaluation and diagnosis; immediate care; treatment, rehabilitation, and reconditioning; organization and administration; and professional responsibility (37). School districts, colleges and universities, sports medicine clinics, professional teams, and industrial settings may employ athletic trainers. The athletic trainer is often present at sport practices and games and is therefore likely to be the first person to evaluate an injury and provide acute treatment. His or her daily presence at sport practices also allows the athletic trainer extensive involvement throughout the entire rehabilitation process.
- *Strength and Conditioning Professional.* Strength and conditioning professionals have the knowledge of appropriate exercise techniques to work in conjunction with other members of the health care team to develop and supervise reconditioning programs. It is important strength and conditioning profes-

sionals be informed of injuries and any precautions to exercise, as they may be the only ones involved with the athlete once return to sport has occurred. Strength and conditioning professionals play an important role in the transition from a controlled, supervised rehabilitation program to a lifelong, independent exercise program as well as the return to participation for an athlete. The strength and conditioning professional can play a key role in prescribing exercises for injury prevention in the uninjured athlete.

> *The strength and conditioning professional plays a key role in injury prevention by prescribing sport-specific exercises that may decrease the risk of injuries common in a specific sport. The strength and conditioning professional, by working closely with the sports medicine team, also plays an important role in the transition from a rehabilitation program to full participation in the sport.*

Since sports injury management involves a multidisciplinary team, it is essential to have good communication to allow a safe return to athletic activity as soon as possible. Within each individual sports medicine team, there should be agreement on the specific roles for each member. The roles of sports medicine professionals are increasingly overlapping as practitioners extend from the "traditional" work settings, complete continuing education, and attain specialist certifications. Each professional brings his or her unique expertise to the sports medicine team that will enhance injury prevention, recognition, and rehabilitation. Despite research evidence, sports medicine (including injury management and return to play criteria) is not an exact science. The sports medicine team must discuss varying philosophies and theories to provide consistent, up-to-date care. Communication must also occur with the athlete, coach, team, and family members when appropriate. To allow optimal injury recovery, responsibilities of all professionals involved in injury management include communication, continuing education, promoting athlete safety, and understanding the mental and physical demands of sport.

> *To work in the field of sports medicine requires teamwork, and optimal knowledge and understanding of the roles of all of the members of the sports medicine team is required to best serve the athlete.*

INJURY CLASSIFICATION

Injuries occur on a regular basis in sporting activities. To treat such injuries successfully in a rehabilitation setting, the health professional must understand the mechanism and type of injury involved. In classifying an injury, we use various definitions to outline its extent and severity in order to adopt the appropriate methods of treatment at the appropriate stages of healing.

Overuse injuries are often a result of microtrauma, where the involved tissue becomes inflamed and painful over an indeterminate time secondary to forces exceeding the strength and healing rate of the tendon or involved structure. A **microtrauma** injury is an injury to a tissue or structure from the application of repetitive stress without adequate rest and recovery time. **Tendonitis** refers to inflammation of the tendon and associated sheath, whereas **tendonosis** involves degeneration of the tendon caused by chronic inflammation (30).

Acute injuries that occur on a given occasion, with an identifiable source, are termed **macrotrauma**. There are varying degrees of macrotraumatic events, and they can be categorized as intrinsic or extrinsic. Intrinsic injuries result from forces (mechanical, environmental, or situational) that supersede the ability of the athlete to respond and avoid injury (45). A shot-putter who ruptures his pectoralis tendon while attempting to best his opponent's distance has suffered an intrinsic injury. Extrinsic injuries occur when an identifiable source beyond the athlete's control is the primary cause of trauma. A running back tackled directly at his knee by an opponent's helmet, causing rupture of the knee ligaments, has suffered an extrinsic injury.

There is a continuum in classifying the severity of soft tissue injury. A **strain** occurs when the involved soft tissue(s) is subject to forces invoking a graded local inflammatory response without disrupting the structural integrity of the tissue. A baseball pitcher who throws 100 pitches at high velocities in a single game experiences local soreness in the shoulder girdle secondary to strain on the contractile tissue around the shoulder. Such a strain usually takes several days to a week to heal if further immediate stressors are avoided.

A **sprain** occurs when contractile or noncontractile soft tissue is subject to forces exceeding the inherent strength of the tissue, causing pain, local or diffuse inflammation, and varying degrees of functional and structural tissue loss. Different classification systems for sprains exist. They are typically classified with a numerical scale (30,43,45), the lower numbers indicating the least amount of tissue damage and the higher numbers usually pointing to a complete rupture or functional loss of the structure. For example, a grade I ankle sprain, according to Hershman and Nicholas, involves microscopic tearing of the ligament without loss of function and may take weeks to heal, whereas a grade III ankle sprain involves complete tearing of the ligament with complete loss of function and will probably require surgical intervention (43). Treatment of the athlete then varies based on the severity of the injury.

Contusions can occur to muscle, bone, and cartilage and are typically the result of a collision with an outside force such as an opponent, the ground, or a foreign object. Contusions to muscle tissue can also be classified by severity based on the amount of hemorrhage, pain, range-of-motion (ROM) limitations, and the extent of tissue involvement. The grading system is similar to that for ligamentous injuries, with grade I injuries involving mild pain and limitations and grade III injuries being the most severe, with herniation of the muscle through the fascial tissue, along with possible bruising of the underlying bone. Severe contusions may require surgery or evacuation of the hematoma. Care must be taken with moderate to severe muscle contusions to avoid further complications, such as functional loss of the muscle or myositis ossificans, which is a condition involving calcification within the muscle tissue as a result of additional inflammation or trauma. **Articular cartilage** is a thin layer of specialized tissue covering the surfaces of synovial joints such as the knee or hip. The cartilage promotes normal movement between joint surfaces and reduces potentially harmful forces such as shear or compression between them. Articular cartilage receives nutrition through components within the synovial fluid that bathe the joint during normal movement. Injuries to articular cartilage pose a challenge owing to the lack of a direct blood supply and limited ability to self-repair. When injuries to articular cartilage or synovial joints do occur, the goals should be to promote healing by decreasing joint effusion, maintaining ROM and movement between joint surfaces, and preventing overload to the joint surfaces.

Understanding the classification of many athletic injuries helps sports medicine professionals in the design of rehabilitation and prevention programs.

PHASES OF TISSUE HEALING: CLINICAL TREATMENT AND EXERCISE CONSIDERATIONS

Following an acute musculoskeletal injury, there are three phases of tissue healing: inflammation, proliferation/repair, and maturation/remodeling. Health professionals need to identify the healing phase to determine appropriate treatment and exercise. Although each phase is defined by certain characteristics, healing occurs along a continuum, and phases overlap. Phase durations are given only as guidelines and vary based on factors including type of tissue and injury severity. Clinical judgment must be used to determine appropriate treatment as healing progresses. Signs and symptoms should be continually monitored throughout the healing phases and treatment adjusted as necessary. The physiology, signs and symptoms, treatment, and exercise considerations for each phase are described below.

Inflammatory Phase

Inflammation is the body's response to injury to protect against and remove foreign materials (bacteria, damaged cells, dead tissue), and begin the process of tissue healing and regeneration. The **inflammatory phase** begins immediately after injury and can last up to approximately 6 days (21). The purposes of inflammation are to protect the body against foreign material, destroy and remove foreign materials (i.e., bacteria, damaged cells, dead tissue), localize the injury, and ultimately promote tissue healing and regeneration (21,28). Although the inflammatory response is a necessary phase of the healing process, it can become problematic if it occurs to excess. For example, the same inflammatory response occurs whether there is foreign material present (e.g., infection) or if no foreign material is present (e.g., an ankle sprain). Another example involves the inflammatory response of scar tissue formation. This response is useful when

damage such as a muscle tear occurs, but it can be detrimental to the tissue and decrease function in chronic inflammatory conditions. Prompt recognition and treatment of an injury will help control the inflammatory response, optimize the healing environment, and allow an earlier return to activity.

Following tissue damage and cell death from an injury, chemicals are released that cause several vascular and cellular changes. Immediately following trauma, the first cells to arrive at the injured site are platelets. Platelets release serotonin, which produce immediate vasoconstriction at the injured site. Following a brief period of vasoconstriction, histamine is released from mast cells (connective tissue cells). Histamine increases vascular permeability and causes vasodilation, resulting in increased swelling. Bradykinin is another chemical released by injured tissue that increases permeability. Increased vascular permeability increases swelling by allowing fluids and proteins out of the capillaries and into the tissues. An osmotic pressure imbalance is created as blood and plasma proteins enter the interstitial space. Swelling results as more fluid moves into the area to return pressure to normal. Prostaglandins and leukotrienes are two other chemicals causing increased permeability and vasodilation, resulting in swelling and pain. Prostaglandins are produced in nearly all tissues and released in response to damaged cells. Many pain and anti-inflammatory medications work by affecting prostaglandin synthesis.

The cellular response consists in the arrival of increased numbers of leukocytes (white blood cells) in the injured area due to increased permeability. Neutrophils and macrophages are two kinds of leukocytes found at the injury site. They are responsible for phagocytosis and the removal of debris. Neutrophils destroy bacteria when the latter are present (28).

To control the amount of fluid in the tissue area and localize injury, blood coagulation must occur. This process begins with damaged cells releasing thromboplastin, which causes prothrombin to be converted into thrombin. Next, fibrinogen is converted into a fibrin clot, which shuts off blood supply to the injured area. This prevents the spread of infection by blocking off the area, keeps foreign agents at the site with the greatest white blood cell activity, forms a clot to stop bleeding, and provides the framework for tissue repair (36).

Signs and symptoms used to identify the physiological changes of the inflammatory phase are remembered by using the acronym **SHARP**, which stands for **s**welling, **h**eat, **a**ltered function, **r**edness, and **p**ain. Swelling is assessed visually, through palpation, and with anthropometric measurements (measurements taken circumferentially around an extremity). The intensity of the inflammatory response and swelling are usually proportional to the amount of tissue damage; however, the amount of swelling is not always an accurate predictor of injury severity. Skin that is warm to the touch is another sign of the inflammatory process. Altered function is a consequence of damaged tissue, swelling, heat, and pain. Redness is assessed visually with bilateral comparison. Pain is a subjective measure. A quantitative pain-rating scale (e.g., a visual analogue scale rating pain on a scale from 0 to 10) can be used to monitor pain levels throughout the rehabilitation process.

Goals of clinical treatment and exercise during the inflammatory phase include the following:

- Prevent further injury
- Decrease swelling and pain
- Establish baseline measurements of signs and symptoms (pain level, swelling, ROM, strength, functional ability)
- Maintain overall fitness level

Many of these goals are accomplished by following the **PRICE** method, comprising **p**rotection, **r**est, **i**ce, **c**ompression, and **e**levation.

- *Protection.* Based on injury location and severity, protection of the injured area can be accomplished through the use of a splint, sling, brace, or assistive device (e.g., crutches). Splinting helps to decrease muscle guarding and breaking the pain-spasm-pain cycle.
- *Rest.* Rest is often applied as "relative rest" or "restricted function." Based on injury severity, clinical judgment is used to determine the balance between protection and safe, early mobilization. Although injured tissue needs to be protected and immobilized, prolonged rest can lead to tissue contractures and loss of ROM. Even if the injured area needs to be immobilized, appropriate exercise can be performed with uninjured areas to minimize losses in overall fitness level (see "Exercise Considerations," below).
- *Ice/Cryotherapy.* The primary goal of cryotherapy is to decrease tissue temperature (28). This subsequently results in other

physiological changes to promote healing. Decreased metabolism is one of the main benefits of cryotherapy used for acute injuries. Decreased metabolism minimizes secondary hypoxic injury by decreasing the oxygen need of the cell. Secondary hypoxic injury is tissue death that occurs after the initial injury due to lack of oxygen supply. Tissues near the injured site die because the inflammatory process decreases blood flow. With decreased blood flow, cells that survived the initial injury die because they cannot get enough oxygen or get rid of waste products. Other benefits of cryotherapy are decreased vascular permeability and vasoconstriction. Cryotherapy should be applied as soon as possible after evaluation of an acute injury. It is important, however, to do an adequate evaluation before muscle spasm, pain, and stiffness increase. Prompt application of cryotherapy cannot reverse the initial trauma, but decreasing secondary hypoxic injury will decrease the overall amount of injured tissue. Cryotherapy should be applied with a cooling-to-rewarming ratio of 1:2; initially ice may be applied approximately 30 minutes every 1 ½ to 2 hours (28).
- *Compression.* Compression can be applied via an intermittent compression pump or elastic bandage. Compression controls edema formation and decreases swelling by promoting reabsorption of fluid.
- *Elevation.* Elevation decreases capillary hydrostatic pressure, which forces fluid out of the capillary in an uninjured state.

The strength and conditioning professional should be aware of the PRICE method of treating injuries. Some of these treatment methods may also be utilized during the postinjury transition from rehabilitation to full participation in the sport.

In addition to the treatments already discussed, health care professionals may use a variety of other modalities to promote healing and control the inflammatory process. A common form of electrical stimulation used for control of acute pain is sensory level stimulation. Transcutaneous electrical nerve stimulation (TENS) units are devices that provide sensory-level stimulation. One disadvantage of this modality is that symptom relief occurs only while the TENS device is being used (42) (Fig. 17.1).

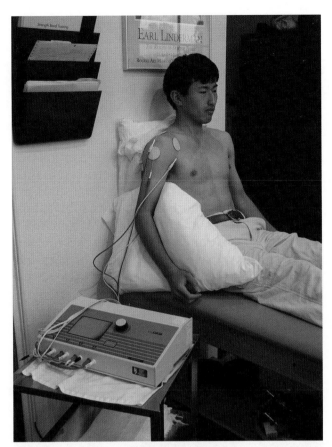

FIGURE 17.1 Electrical stimulation. TENS is used to control acute pain in patients with rotator cuff tendonitis.

Ultrasound is another modality that may be used to promote healing. During the inflammatory phase, pulsed ultrasound should be used for its nonthermal effects, including altered membrane permeability, to promote tissue healing (21). The use of continuous ultrasound produces heat in the tissues and is contraindicated during the inflammatory phase. Various applications of electrical stimulation and ultrasound may be used to facilitate delivery of a topical drug into the tissues, known as iontophoresis and phonophoresis, respectively. Use of any of the above modalities is decided on by an appropriately trained health care professional.

Based on injury severity, gentle range-of-motion (ROM) exercises may be indicated near the end of the inflammatory phase. Performing such exercises early will decrease the negative effects of immobilization. Each type of tissue responds differently to immobilization and remobilization. Negative effects of immobilization on muscle include decreased muscle fiber size, decrease in size and number of mitochondria, decrease in muscle tension pro-

duced, increase in lactate concentration with exercise, and a decrease in total muscle weight. Early controlled passive or active motion may be used postoperatively to retard muscle atrophy and tissue contracture. It also allows for diffusion of synovial fluid to nourish articular cartilage, meniscus, and ligaments. In postoperative cases, the physician's protocol must be followed in progressive ROM and strengthening exercises.

Although strengthening of the injured tissue is generally not indicated during this phase, maintenance of overall fitness, including strength, flexibility, and endurance, is important for both the physical and psychological return to sport (45). An athlete with a lower extremity injury may use an upper-body ergometer to minimize loss of cardiovascular endurance. Aquatic physical therapy may be an alternative if lower extremity weight-bearing restrictions are present. Strength exercises of noninvolved areas may be performed if they do not risk reinjury. A balance between strengthening for overall fitness and rest must be maintained to allow the body to heal and prevent fatigue.

Repair Phase

The **repair phase** begins once inflammatory debris has been removed, approximately 3 to 20 days after injury (21). According to some sources, the repair phase may last up to 6 weeks. Events during the repair phase include scar formation, tissue regeneration, and tissue repair, which increase strength at the injured site.

A lack of oxygen at the injured site stimulates neovascularization, or the formation of new capillaries. The formation of new capillaries increases blood flow, oxygen, and nutrients at the injured site. Collagen synthesis occurs as fibroblastic cells begin producing collagen fibers. During this phase, the collagen is laid down randomly and is weak in structure.

The formation of scar tissue after injury is a normal response; however, excessive collagen deposition and scar formation can hinder the healing process. As scar tissue matures, it becomes inelastic and firm as well as lacking in blood flow. This type of tissue forms adhesions, which decrease ROM and function. Therefore, it is important to promote proper healing and decrease the amount of scar tissue formation.

During the repair phase, the signs and symptoms of the inflammatory response subside. The amount of swelling remains constant or begins to subside. Skin temperature and color approach those of the contralateral side. Although pain decreases overall, palpable tenderness or pain with specific movements may still be present. Skin color is similar to that of the contralateral extremity; however, ecchymosis may be present. Function slowly improves throughout the repair phase.

Goals of treatment during the repair phase include the following:

- A continued decrease in inflammation
- Maintenance of ROM by minimizing contracture and adhesion formation
- Improvements in strength and function

Modalities should be used as needed to increase exercise tolerance and continue to promote healing. In addition to controlling pain, modalities are used to increase circulation prior to exercise and decrease circulation (and swelling) afterward. Thermotherapy, which was contraindicated in the inflammatory phase, is safe to use once active swelling has subsided. Monitoring of the signs and symptoms of the inflammatory response will help determine when swelling is no longer active and begins to decrease. Thermotherapy promotes healing by increasing circulation, decreasing pain, and increasing collagen extensibility. Common forms of thermotherapy include moist hot packs, warm whirlpools, and continuous ultrasound. After exercise, many of the same treatment interventions used during the inflammatory phase should be continued. Cryotherapy, electrical stimulation, compression, and elevation will control any pain and swelling that may result from exercise.

In addition to the modalities already mentioned, manual therapy techniques including passive ROM and joint mobilization may be used to further decrease pain and increase ROM. Joint mobilization will help restore normal joint motion when ROM is limited due to joint capsule tightness.

Active-assisted and active ROM exercises should be initiated if not already included in treatment at the end of the inflammation phase. ROM is performed under controlled, supervised conditions, as the collagen is still weak during this phase. As soon as pain and swelling are controlled, strengthening exercises for the injured area can be initiated. Proper exercise progression will aid healing by increasing circulation, increasing oxygen and optimizing collagen realignment. ROM and strengthening exercises promote optimal healing of soft tissue and collagen by causing realignment along

lines of stress in a similar manner as bone responds to stress according to Wolff's law.

Exercise should place progressively increasing amounts of stress on the healing tissues. One study described an exercise progression continuum to be used during rehabilitation (12). Although all stages are listed here, the later stages are not appropriate until the repair phase due to increased stress placed on the tissue. The exercise progression is as follows: submaximal multiple-angle isometrics, maximal multiple-angle isometrics, submaximal short-arc exercises, maximal short-arc exercises, submaximal full ROM exercises, maximal full ROM exercises.

Multiple-angle and short-arc exercises are performed to allow exercise throughout the pain-free ROM. In addition to strengthening muscles at the ROM where the exercise is performed, strengthening also occurs up to 10 degrees (isometric) or 15 degrees (isokinetic) on either side of the ROM at which the exercise is performed (12). Therefore, performing exercises in a safe, pain-free ROM will increase strength into the affected areas (Fig. 17.2). The pelvis is locked by the gluteal

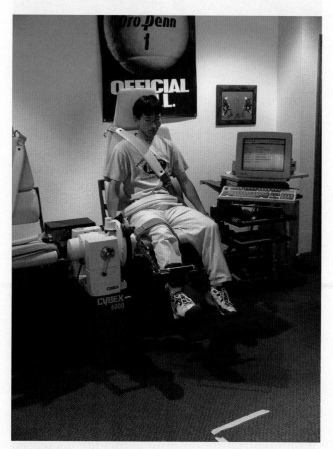

FIGURE 17.2 Cybex isokinetic knee extension exercise. Using a short arc of range of motion between 90 and 60 degrees provides a pain-free way to increase strength.

muscles in the first 60 degrees of movement. As the lumbar spine is gradually flexed, there is an increasing amount of activity of the erector spinae and superficial muscles of the back. In the next 25 degrees of motion (the second phase), relaxation of the pelvis occurs with respect to the femurs. In the fully flexed position, the weight of the trunk is borne by the ligaments and passive extension of the muscles as all the muscles are relaxed. Extension from full flexion to the neutral position is achieved in the reverse order: pelvic extension is followed by extension of the lumbar spine.

In addition to strengthening, proprioceptive exercises should be included. The term **proprioception** describes the sensation of joint movement (kinesthesia) and joint position (joint position sense) (31). Proprioception is decreased after trauma to tissues containing mechanoreceptors, such as muscles, ligaments, and joints. A joint with decreased proprioceptive feedback and joint position sense is at greater risk for reinjury. By incorporating proprioceptive exercises into a rehabilitation program, the neuromuscular control and dynamic joint stabilization needed for athletic activities are improved (31). Examples of basic proprioceptive exercises include single-leg balance and balance-board activities. The single-leg balance is illustrated in Figure 17.3.

Tissue response to exercise should be constantly monitored. Increased pain and swelling implies that too much stress has been placed on the tissue. When signs and symptoms of inflammation recur or increase, exercise should be decreased and treatment discussed during the inflammatory phase as indicated.

Remodeling Phase

The last stage in the healing process is the **remodeling phase**. Even though a person may have returned to his or her prior level of function, the remodeling phase can continue more than a year after the initial injury (36). Near the end of the repair phase, the tensile strength of the collagen increases and the number of fibroblasts diminishes, signaling the start of the maturation phase. According to Davis's law, realignment and remodeling of the collagen fibers results from tensile forces. As stress to the collagen is increased, the fibers realign in a position of maximum efficiency, parallel to the lines of tension. Collagen becomes more organized and its strength increases.

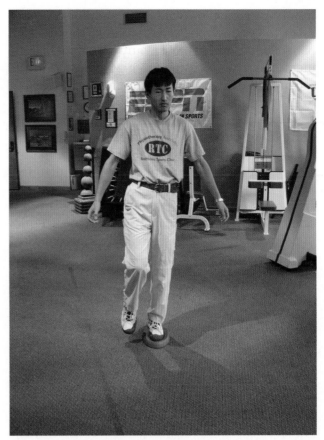

FIGURE 17.3 Single-leg balance. This unilateral lower extremity proprioception exercise using a Thera-band stability trainer improves neuromuscular control and dynamic joint stabilization.

Signs and symptoms present since the inflammatory phase will continue to decrease and will eventually disappear by the end of the remodeling phase. There will be minimal to no swelling, pain with motion, or pain with palpation. Function continues to approach preinjury levels. Initial measurements including swelling, ROM, and strength should be reevaluated.

The primary goal of treatment during the remodeling phase is to regain the prior level of function of the injured tissue. Modalities will be continued as in the repair phase as needed to maintain optimal healing environments and assist in regaining full ROM. Modality use is decreased, however, as exercise tolerance increases. Manual therapy and joint mobilizations should be continued until full ROM is achieved. Collagen will continue to realign along the lines of stress applied by ROM and strengthening activities.

Regaining full strength is an emphasis during the remodeling phase. It is during this phase that the role of the rehabilitation specialist is critical for restoring function through the application of appropriate forces through exercise, manual therapy, and patient education to prevent any long-term impairment. Exercises are progressed as discussed in the repair phase. Signs and symptoms are monitored to prevent placing too much stress on the tissue and risking reinjury. Proprioceptive exercise should also be progressed. As strength and proprioception are increased, functional activities simulating work or sport requirements should be included. Speed of movement, type of muscle contraction, and length of activity are important factors to consider in developing functional activities. Functional and sport-specific exercises are incorporated into the return-to-activity phase, discussed in the next section.

Phases of healing must be kept in mind as health professionals continue to push earlier return to sport. Clinical judgment will determine appropriate exercise and treatment progression through the healing phases to allow optimal return to sport. Since return to competitive sport activities often occurs before the healing phases are complete, continued strengthening and bracing should be incorporated as necessary to prevent further injury. A strength and conditioning professional is able to assist the transition from the controlled, supervised environment of a rehabilitation clinic to a lifelong independent exercise program for injury prevention.

RETURN-TO-ACTIVITY PHASE: THE ROLE OF THE INTERVAL PROGRAM

Of all the stages in the rehabilitation process, the return to sport or full activity is easily the most anticipated for all persons on the sports medicine team and clearly the most anticipated both physically and mentally by the patient. Despite the popularity of this stage of the recovery process, this phase is probably the least well defined and filled with guidelines and ambiguous rules that often are not predicated on research, functional outcomes, or evidence-based practice themes. Many methods can be used to define or determine whether the athlete is ready for a return to full activity. Most clinicians and sports scientists recommend the inclusion of as much objectively based testing as

possible. Use of clinical testing comes in two primary categories: subjective and objective. Subjective tests are designed to be completed by the patients themselves and typically involve questions geared at obtaining the patient's perceived level of function. Objective testing is performed in several areas to determine the appropriateness of a return to sport.

Determination of a return of ROM of the injured joint or joints is carefully performed with a goniometer, or additional flexibility testing can be done using standardized tests like the sit-and-reach maneuver, which measures low back and hamstring flexibility. Typically a return of ROM equal to that of the contralateral or uninjured extremity is striven for. Exceptions to matching ROM or strength to the opposite side include injury to the opposite side or the presence of exceptional ROM or strength on one side from playing a unilateral sport such as tennis or baseball. In most patients, however, using a goal of achieving at least the ROM or strength levels of the uninjured side is appropriate.

A determination of strength must also be made before the patient can be returned to sport or aggressive activities without injury. Typical strength comparisons use the opposite side as a baseline and employ either manual muscle testing techniques or more sophisticated equipment like isokinetic or hand-held dynamometers. These pieces of equipment further objectify strength levels and are capable of reliably testing strength at multiple velocities that more appropriately match the speeds of human movement in activities of daily living (ADLs) or some sport activities. Initiation of return-to-sport programs involving running and throwing is not recommended when deficits in muscular strength are 20% or more (12). Therefore, although these isolated types of muscle performance tests cannot simulate all functional demands, they provide the clinician with a valid and reliable measure or indicator of muscular performance around an injured joint.

In addition to the objective tests for strength and ROM, testing specifically designed to assess the function of the limb or individual as a whole are recommended. These are typically called functional tests. **Functional tests** are tests administered to assess whether an individual can safely return to sport and function without limitations. Examples of functional tests are hop-and-jump tests like the one-leg hop test and vertical jump test. The one-leg hop test is particularly popular. In the patient with an injured knee, this test can be performed simply in a clinic using a tape measure and piece of tape to delineate starting position. The patient takes off and lands on the same limb, and a comparison of one limb to the other is then performed. Failure to reach the distance generated on the contralateral side often indicates an inability to generate power in the lower extremity as well as hesitancy in landing and lack of the eccentric control necessary to absorb the load following the jump. In addition to the actual distance, quantitative assessment of these patients often provides valuable insight as to their readiness to absorb the impact load on landing and ability to land on one leg. Often patients will land on both legs in an effort to shield the injured extremity from the stress and eccentric overload inherent in landing. Information gleaned during functional testing is imperative for the clinical decision-making process that must be undertaken in considering a patient for a full return to activity.

> *The return-to-activity phase is an extremely critical part of the rehabilitation process that should be based on function rather than time or symptoms. The strength and conditioning professional should have a defined role in this phase of the recovery process.*

THE INTERVAL SPORT-RETURN PROGRAM

An **interval sport-return program** is a rehabilitative program designed to progress an athlete to return to sporting activity. It is a program of graded intensity and volume with emphasis placed on the athlete demonstrating adequate strength, endurance, and biomechanics to successfully advance through the program. Several key components are inherent in an interval sport-return program. These are warm-up, alternate-day performance scheduling, integration with conditioning, progressive stages of intensity, proper biomechanics and evaluation of mechanics, and cool-down or aftercare. Each of these is an important component of currently used interval sport-return programs and can easily be adapted into nearly any sport or activity.

Warm-Up

Despite the understandable anticipation that a patient has on returning to a sport following the hiatus required by injury or during rehabilitation, a proper warm-up must precede actual performance in the interval program. Despite recent evidence that the acute effects of stretching may diminish jump and power performance for a period of up to 20 minutes (2,29), the potential injury prevention or reinjury benefits of stretching and warm-up make this an important initial stage in the interval program. Typically, the warm-up consists of a light cardiovascular workout to elevate local tissue temperature and increase blood flow to the peripheral aspects of the limbs. This warm-up is then followed by static stretches with isolated positioning of the muscles' origins and insertions, such that controlled and static elongation occurs. Hold times of 15 to 30 seconds are generally used to produce plastic deformation of the tissue and enhance the flexibility and ROM of the hamstrings and other muscles.

Alternate-Day Performance Scheduling

Interval sport performance programs typically have an alternate-day performance schedule. This is designed to allow the musculature and static restraint mechanisms surrounding the injured joint or joints a period of recovery before sport activity is again administered. Additionally, the day off following performance allows the patient and clinician time to determine the tolerance of the body to the previous day's level of performance. Close monitoring of all subjective symptoms and objective signs is an important part of determining when the next stage or intensity of activity is initiated. Therefore, alternate-day performance of the interval program is recommended.

Integration with Conditioning

This is perhaps one of the most difficult aspects of returning patients to their sport. The importance of continuing with strength and ROM exercises during the interval program is widely recognized. Restoration of final muscular balance and obtaining the last few degrees of flexibility and motion around a formerly restricted joint are all aspects that require continued rehabilitative exercise and conditioning during this phase. Although there is limited work published in this area, several clinical suggestions or guidelines are typically followed. Performance of sport-specific activity is recommended before or prior to any strength or power training. This is to ensure that the body's musculature, which provides the dynamic stability for the joints, is properly functioning and not fatigued during the functional performance. Additionally, exercises to segments even far away from the injured segment may complicate functional performance.

Progressive Stages of Intensity

For a program to truly be interval in nature, it must contain progressive stages of gradually increasing intensity. These progressive stages allow patients and clinicians to responsibly progress the stresses applied to the postoperative or postinjury tissue. One example is an interval throwing program. The interval throwing program contains gradually progressive stages or steps of both increasing distance and volume (number of throws). Careful monitoring of patients through this program finds them increasing distance from as little as 30 to 45 ft initially to as much 120 to 150 ft based on the type of position played. Within each distance is a progression in the number of throws as well. This allows for independent increases in the intensity of the throwing (longer distance) as well as an increase in the number of repetitions, which challenges the patient's ability to withstand repeated stresses and builds endurance. For a complete description of an interval throwing program used in shoulder rehabilitation, see Andrews and Wilk (47). Interval tennis programs follow similar guidelines and are reviewed in Ellenbecker (17).

Proper Biomechanics and Evaluation of Mechanics

Another critical part of the interval return process is the emphasis on proper biomechanics. Many times returning from an injury or surgery leaves the athlete with deficits in muscle balance, ROM, and proprioception or kinesthetic awareness in the limb or affected joint and hence sets the athlete up for compensatory movement patterns. Often these movement patterns can lead to injury in the segment being rehabilitated or in adjoining segments. A perfect example of this is when someone is returning to tennis play after a knee arthroscopy and he or she develops tennis elbow because of problems with lower body movement and an increase in the contribution and loading on the arm. Another example would be the athlete returning to throw after a shoulder injury who, due to a loss in external rotation ROM, "shortarms" the ball, resulting in greater loading on the inside (medial aspect) of the elbow joint (33).

Therefore, careful monitoring of the athlete's mechanics are indicated during the return-to-activity phase. This can be accomplished by having the health care clinician observe the interval process as well as having the interval process performed in the presence of a coach or even sports biomechanist.

Cool-Down or Aftercare

Equally important as the warm-up, the cool-down or aftercare following the interval return program is an essential part of this process. In the earlier phases of the interval program, where a physical therapist or athletic trainer is often supervising the program being executed in the clinical setting, the remainder of a rehabilitation program is typically completed on the same day as the interval sport-return program. So, following the throwing or running or whatever the sport activity is, rehabilitation exercises geared at restoring optimal muscle balance and fatigue resistance and joint ROM as well proprioception and balance are commenced. This allows the athlete to continue perfecting the injured areas during the interval return process and ensures that a day of nearly complete recovery can be followed on the day after the interval program and rehabilitative exercise session. Aftercare in this situation is guided by the rehabilitation professional.

In the later stages of the interval program, athletes are typically performing these activities independently off site. Therefore, strict instruction regarding the amount, intensity, and duration of maintenance exercise must be shared with the athlete as well as the specific instructions for postsession stretching and icing. The use of ice to create vasoconstriction in the affected area is widely accepted in both clinical medicine and sports medicine. The amount of time that ice is used after an injury or following a return to full activity varies and has not been formally studied. Current recommendations are typically for application of ice following postworkout stretching. Following an organized and consistent program of aftercare will ensure that the execution of the off-site interval program mirrors the program initially designed in the clinical setting and is thought to minimize the risk of reinjury and facilitate the return to activity.

OVERVIEW OF JOINT BIOMECHANICS AND EXERCISE APPLICATIONS

Proper joint biomechanics during exercise performance are important to both the safety and efficacy of the exercises. With injured athletes, proper mechanics become even more important. These descriptions are meant to heighten the understanding of strength and conditioning professionals and allow for safe and optimal application of resistive exercise. Specific reference to common athletic injuries is included to understand the modifications to traditional exercise based on joint biomechanics.

The strength and conditioning professional should have a basic understanding of the biomechanical concepts of the knee, shoulder, and spine and be able to provide specific exercise applications based on these inherent joint biomechanical characteristics.

Overview of Knee Biomechanics and Exercise Applications

The knee joint is commonly injured during athletic activities. Knowledge of knee anatomy and biomechanics should be considered when designing exercise programs to prevent and rehabilitate lower extremity injuries. The knee joint is classified as a synovial joint and consists of the tibiofemoral and patellofemoral articulations. Motion at the tibiofemoral joint occurs in flexion, extension, and internal and external rotation. The screw home mechanism occurs at terminal knee extension and involves the tibia externally rotating on a fixed femur in open kinetic chain activity.

Four main ligaments provide stability to the knee joint: anterior cruciate ligament, posterior cruciate ligament, medial collateral ligament, and the lateral collateral ligament. Another commonly injured structure in the knee is the meniscus. The knee has a lateral and medial meniscus, with the medial meniscus having a higher incidence of injury. The meniscus functions are to absorb shock by dissipating forces over a larger surface area, aid in joint lubrication, and increase joint congruency and stability (7).

In general, rehabilitation for knee injuries will include strengthening exercises for the quadriceps and hamstring muscles, total leg strengthening, and proprioceptive exercises. Restoring the balance between knee flexion and extension strength is an important rehabilitation goal. A 2:3 ratio of knee flexion to extension strength is desirable (13). Total leg strengthening is indicated, as proximal muscle weakness is often found with distal lower extremity injuries. Proprioceptive exercises are often indicated after a lower extremity injury because trauma to tissues containing mechanoreceptors will decrease proprioception. These rehabilitation principles are further discussed below in relation to two common knee injuries, patellofemoral pain syndrome and anterior cruciate ligament (ACL) injury.

PATELLOFEMORAL PAIN SYNDROME AND RESISTANCE EXERCISES

The patella is a sesamoid bone that functions to optimize the extensor mechanism by increasing the force capability of quadriceps muscles (7). Different areas of the patella contact the femur as the knee joint moves through full ROM. The injured area of the patellar surface will determine the symptomatic ranges of motion. Symptoms occur because of a compressive force on the patellofemoral joint as the quadriceps muscle contracts to extend the knee. The quadriceps muscle pulls the patella superiorly and the resistance from the patellar tendon pulls the patella inferiorly. The resultant force is compression of the patella against the femur. Dynamic and static restraints, such as the quadriceps muscles and retinaculum, will affect patellar tracking.

Patellofemoral pain syndrome is the name often given to the symptom of anterior knee pain. There are several possible causes of such pain. Specific diagnoses that may be included under this general term include chondromalacia patella, patellar tendonitis, patellofemoral malalignment, plica syndrome, and Osgood Schlatter's disease (14).

Success in treating this syndrome is dependent on determining the cause of the pain, which can often be multifactorial. Only after identifying the cause(s) of patellofemoral pain can appropriate treatment be determined. A classification system of patellofemoral disorders has been developed to serve as a foundation for clinical interventions (50). Categories within this classification system include patellar compression syndromes, patellar instability, biomechanical dysfunction, direct patellar trauma, soft tissue lesions, overuse syndromes, osteochondritis, and neurologic disorders. Pathological findings that may need to be addressed when treating patellofemoral pain syndrome include: patellar alignment, patellar hypo- or hypermobility, vastus medialis oblique weakness, muscle strength/flexibility imbalances. The **vastus medialis oblique** (VMO) is the most medial of the quadriceps muscles and is often implicated in many patterns of patellofemoral pain syndromes.

Rehabilitation for patellofemoral pain syndrome commonly includes the following: quadriceps strengthening, addressing muscle strength and flexibility imbalances throughout the entire lower extremity, orthotic devices, stretching the lateral retinaculum, aerobic conditioning, taping, and bracing (22). Patellofemoral pain often occurs as a secondary injury. Therefore, it is necessary to consider the patellofemoral joint during all knee joint rehabilitation programs to prevent causing additional injuries.

Exercises for patellofemoral pain syndrome should be related to the specific pathological findings of the evaluation. The following are general exercise suggestions that apply to developing strength programs to treat and prevent patellofemoral pain syndrome.

- *Perform exercises only through pain-free ROMs.* Relatively safe ROMS in which to perform patellofemoral rehabilitation have been recommended. Due to the different effects of gravity in the open- and closed-kinetic-chain positions, it has been recommended to perform open-kinetic-chain exercises between the angles of 90 and 50 degrees and 10 to 0 degrees of knee flexion. Activities in the closed kinetic chain should be performed between 50 and 0 degrees. There can be an increase in patellofemoral joint reaction forces as flexion angle increased during a squat exercise (47). These researchers also recommend avoiding knee flexion angles greater than approximately 60 degrees in attempts to reduce patellofemoral compression during closed-kinetic-chain activities such as the squat exercise. Multiple-angle isometrics and short-arc exercises can be used for strengthening in pain-free ranges of motion.

- *Emphasize quadriceps/VMO strengthening.* After an injury, pain and swelling lead to selective reflex inhibition of the quadriceps, specifically the VMO muscle. Despite numerous research studies, there is little consensus on the most effective exercises to maximize VMO muscle recruitment. Suggested exercises for VMO strengthening include biofeedback to monitor VMO contraction used in conjunction with open and closed kinetic chain exercises, short-arc quadriceps exercises, and hip adduction performed in conjunction with a squat exercise (14).

- *Incorporate exercises for core and total leg strengthening.* Exercises for proximal lower extremity muscles should be included as indicated by the evaluation. Strengthening of the hip flexor muscles and hamstring muscles is often indicated (14). It has also been shown that the hip external rotators (22,25) and hip abductors (25) may require strengthening, especially in females. Strengthening the hip muscles will increase proximal stability and minimize femoral internal rotation and valgus knee motion, which alters stress on the patellofemoral joint. Examples of exercises for total leg strengthening that often do not increase symptoms include stationary bicycling with a high seat, supine straight leg raises, lateral step-ups, and retro step-ups.

ANTERIOR CRUCIATE LIGAMENT INJURY AND RESISTANCE EXERCISES

One of the most common injuries to the knee during athletic injuries is a torn anterior cruciate ligament (ACL). The ACL is the primary restraint to anterior translation of the tibia on the femur in the open kinetic chain. In the closed kinetic chain, the ACL functions to prevent posterior displacement of the femur on the tibia. Depending on the direction and amount of force, injury to the medial collateral, lateral collateral, and posterior cruciate ligaments or menisci may also occur with a torn ACL. Depending on the severity of injury and activity level of an individual, operative or nonoperative treatment may be chosen. For active individuals with a torn ACL, surgical reconstruction is usually the treatment of choice.

After reconstructive surgery, the emphasis of rehabilitation progresses from ROM to strength and proprioception. Regaining full knee extension is important for normal knee biomechanics during gait and to prevent secondary complications. Once strengthening exercises are initiated, it is important to consider strain on the ACL during lower extremity strength exercises. The greatest amount of strain is placed on the ACL between 0 and 30 degrees of knee flexion. Guidelines for strengthening exercises are discussed below.

Goals of ACL reconstruction and rehabilitation include restoration of knee stability, preservation of knee cartilage, expedient return to daily activities including sport participation, and early recognition of complications (15). Exercise progression will be based on the orthopedic surgeon's protocol. Factors that may influence healing rate and exercise progression are preoperative condition of the knee, type of graft used, and concomitant injuries. General exercise guidelines after ACL reconstruction are as follows:

■ *Regain knee flexion and extension strength.* The hamstring muscles are the dynamic restraint to anterior translation of the tibia on the femur. Increasing the strength and control of the hamstring muscles will increase dynamic stability of the knee joint and decrease ACL strain. The quadriceps must also be strengthened as atrophy occurs due to pain and swelling. Regaining strength of the quadriceps muscles is needed for control of the knee joint. As mentioned above, the ratio of knee flexion to extension strengthening should be at least 2:3 (13).

■ *Incorporate proprioceptive exercises.* Lower extremity proprioceptive exercises are indicated, since decreased proprioception occurs after ACL injury. Mechanoreceptors, which provide input from the knee to the central nervous system, are injured after a torn ACL. This causes decreased input from the knee joint to the central nervous system (5). The resulting decreased neuromuscular control and proprioception increase reinjury risk. Numerous exercises can improve proprioception, including single-leg balance activities on surfaces such as foam and balance boards.

■ *Include unilateral exercises.* One study found subjects who had undergone ACL reconstruction significantly unloaded the involved extremity in performing a parallel squat exercise 6 to 7 months postoperatively (39). Not until 12 to 15 months postoperatively did bilateral weight bearing normalize. Therefore, unilateral strength exercises should be performed to achieve maximal strength gains in the involved extremity.

■ *Strengthen muscles in both the closed and open kinetic chain.* Strengthening exercises should simulate functional activities. Both regular daily activities such as gait and sport activities require muscles to function in the closed kinetic chain and open kinetic chains. **Closed-kinetic-chain** (CKC) exercises involve cocontraction of the muscles surrounding a joint and are characterized by a linear stress pattern and fixture of the distal segment of the extremity to the ground of supportive surface (19). CKC exercises utilize multiple joints and joint axes. One prime example of a CKC exercise is the squat or lunge. CKC exercise in lower extremities involves cocontraction of the quadriceps and hamstring muscles. Anterior translation of the tibia on the femur is minimized by hamstring contraction, decreasing strain on the ACL. **Open-kinetic-chain** (OKC) exercise is characterized by a rotator stress pattern and isolated joint and muscle function. The distal aspect is technically allowed to swing freely in space. One example of an OKC exercise is the knee-extension exercise. Open kinetic chain exercises are needed provide isolated quadriceps strengthening. Due to increased strain on the ACL from approximately 0 to 30 degrees of knee extension in the open kinetic chain, exercises must be performed with appropriate modifications (limit last 30 degrees of knee extension) (Fig. 17.4).

Nonoperative treatment is usually only chosen by less active individuals. The laxity from a torn ACL increases the risk of future meniscal and articular cartilage damage. Cartilage damage will continue to increase knee pain and limit function over time. Like the postoperative rehabilitation goals, nonoperative goals include regaining hamstring and quadriceps muscle strength and lower

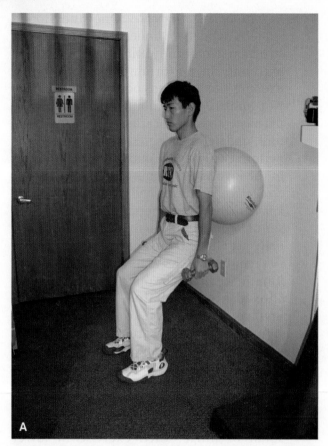
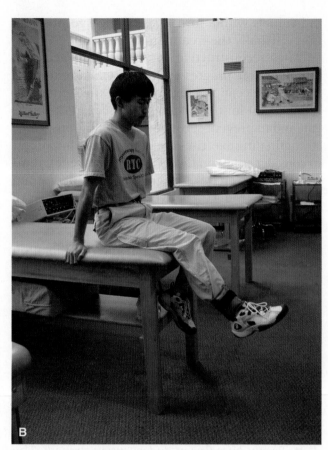

A

B

FIGURE 17.4 Closed and open kinetic chain exercises. **A.** A closed kinetic chain exercise using a stability ball. **B.** An open knee extension exercise.

extremity proprioception. The same exercise principles discussed above for postoperative strengthening can be applied.

Overview of Shoulder Biomechanics and Exercise Applications

The shoulder or glenohumeral joint is the most mobile joint in the human body. The shoulder complex is composed of several joints; however the discussion here focuses primarily on the glenohumeral and scapulothoracic joints. One early researcher identified the delicate balance during upper extremity elevation between the glenohumeral and scapulothoracic joints (10). He termed this the **scapulohumeral rhythm**: for every 2 degrees of glenohumeral joint motion, 1 degree of scapulothoracic motion occurs. This relationship points out the important role that the scapulothoracic joint plays in shoulder function and how

important proper strength and endurance of the muscles that stabilize the scapula are for normal function. The muscles that stabilize the scapula include the serratus anterior, trapezius, rhomboids, and levator scapulae. The important upward rotation of the scapula that the serratus anterior and trapezius perform is required to optimize the length-tension relationship of the rotator cuff muscle tendon units as well as to move the acromion from the path of the elevating humerus (27).

The stability of the glenohumeral joint's ball-and-socket articulation is provided by both static and dynamic elements. The static elements include the glenoid labrum and articular capsule as well as negative intra-articular pressure (49). The dynamic stabilizers of the glenohumeral joint include the four rotator cuff muscle tendon units and the biceps long head.

One of the most important biomechanical principles in shoulder function is the deltoid rotator cuff force couple. A **force couple** is the combination of muscle force(s) acting across a joint and causing rotational movement around an axis. This phenomenon explains how the rotator cuff and deltoid muscles work together to provide arm movements (24). The deltoid provides force primarily in a superior direction in contracting unopposed during arm elevation. The rotator cuff must provide both compressive force as well as an inferiorly directed force to prevent impingement of the rotator cuff tendons against the overlying acromion. Failure of the rotator cuff to maintain humeral congruency leads to glenohumeral joint instability, rotator cuff tendon pathology, and labral injury (49). Imbalances in the deltoid–rotator cuff force couple primarily occur during inappropriate training and development of the deltoid without strengthening of the rotator cuff and exacerbate the superior migration of the humeral head provided by the deltoid and lead to impingement. The exercises listed below can be applied to ensure that a balanced training program for the shoulder and upper extremity is followed and is particularly important for athletes who make overhead movements with their arms, such as baseball players, tennis players, and swimmers.

COMMON INJURIES OF THE SHOULDER
The early 1970s saw the introduction of the concept of **shoulder impingement**, which refers to the mechanical impingement or compression of the rotator cuff tendons between the humeral head and the acromion (38). The subacromial space is only reported at 6 to 14 mm in normal subjects (11). With muscular imbalance and/or fatigue, capsular ROM restriction, and repeated overuse in overhead positions, rotator cuff impingement occurs, producing a progression of disability. This progression starts with edema and hemorrhage initially and, with continued overuse, can lead to partial- and full-thickness tears from the mechanical stresses of compression and impingement (38). Impingement typically responds to nonoperative rehabilitation, which consists of modalities to decrease inflammation and pain as well as proper exercises, which activate and strengthen the rotator cuff muscles using positions that do not place the rotator cuff in a compressed or impinged position, thus allowing for healing.

Most recently, medical professionals and scientists have understood the important role that instability of the glenohumeral joint plays in rotator cuff disease. Impingement of the rotator cuff against the acromion may occur secondary to glenohumeral joint instability from attenuation of the static stabilizers, such as capsular laxity, labral pathology, and abnormal work or sport biomechanics (8,26). Excessive translation or subluxation of the humeral head relative to the glenoid can occur in athletes and individuals with capsular laxity, often developed from repetitive overuse in the overhead movement patterns used in throwing or serving (26). Additionally, shoulder instability can occur from a traumatic event such as a fall on an outstretched arm or the combined movement of abduction and external rotation in contact sports. This can result in a full dislocation of the humeral head from the glenoid. Careful application of rotator cuff and scapular exercises are again indicated in these patients to improve dynamic stabilization.

APPLICATION OF RESISTIVE EXERCISE FOR THE GLENOHUMERAL JOINT
The anatomical and biomechanical concepts outlined earlier in this chapter provide framework for the clinician to choose exercise positions and movement patterns to increase both strength and muscular endurance in patients and individuals with shoulder injury or weakness. In addition to the concepts such as the scapular plane position, avoidance of impingement positions, and the important role force couples play in producing controlled glenohumeral joint motion are electromyographic (EMG) studies that specifically measure individual muscular activity patterns with traditionally utilized exercise patterns.

Blackburn et al. (6) used electromyography to measure muscular activity in the posterior rotator cuff during traditional shoulder exercise using isotonic weights. The authors identified a position that has been referred to as the "Blackburn position," which consists of prone horizontal abduction with 100 degrees of abduction and an externally rotated humeral position. This position was reported to involve high levels of muscular activity in the supraspinatus muscle, infraspinatus, teres minor, and scapular stabilizers (4,6,46). This prone position has become a classic exercise in many rehabilitation programs for both glenohumeral joint impingement and instability (6). Modification of this exercise using only 90 degrees of abduction to decrease potential subacromial contact and compression has been recommended (16,17).

In addition to the study of Blackburn et al. (6), another study has provided the most comprehensive analysis of shoulder muscle activity during traditional exercises used during rehabilitation programs (46). Examples of exercises used during rotator cuff rehabilitation are pictured in Figure 17.5. These exercises utilize positions outlined in this chapter and have confirmed high levels of muscle activation of the rotator cuff while placing the shoulder in a comfortable "nonimpingement position." Exercises to improve strength and muscular endurance are also recommended for the scapular stabilizers. Another group of researchers has outlined the muscular activation patterns of the scapular muscles during rehabilitation exercises (35). Application of seated rows and push-up with a "plus," which involves accentuating scapular protractions, are considered "core scapular" exercises based on this research.

Exercises with 90 degrees of abduction are indicated to provide sport-specific conditioning of the rotator cuff (17). Figure 17.6 shows how external rotation can be performed with the shoulder elevated 90 degrees in the scapular plane. The **scapular plane position** is the plane 30 degrees anterior to the frontal plane of the body and is a position characterized by high levels of bony congruity between the humeral head and glenoid as well as neutral tension in the glenohumeral capsule (44). The use of the scapular plane position is highly recommended during rehabilitation.

Finally, modification of traditional exercises performed by many athletes and active individuals in the gym is followed and recommended. Limiting shoulder forward and lateral raises to only 90 degrees is highly recommended along with performing lat pull-downs in front of the head rather than behind (23). Limiting the ROM during bench presses and "pec deck" exercise to positions in front of the scapular plane to decrease stress on the front of the shoulder is also widely recommended (23).

Overview of Spine Biomechanics and Exercise Applications

The spine consists of 33 segments divided into five regions (cervical, thoracic, lumbar, sacral, and coccygeal), with the first 24, or presacral, vertebrae having the most clinical relevance. The S-shaped curve of the spine allows increased shock absorption and overall flexibility, and is due to the cervical and lumbar lordosis combined with the thoracic

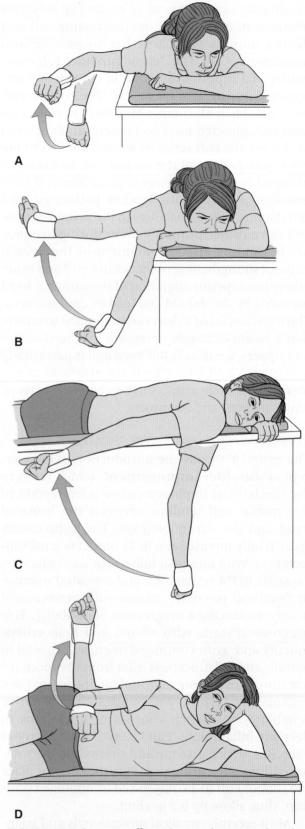

FIGURE 17.5 Rotator cuff exercises used to strengthen the rotator cuff and scapular stabilizers based on EMG research. **A.** 90/90 external rotation. **B.** Prone horizontal abduction. **C.** Shoulder extension. **D.** Side-lying external rotation.

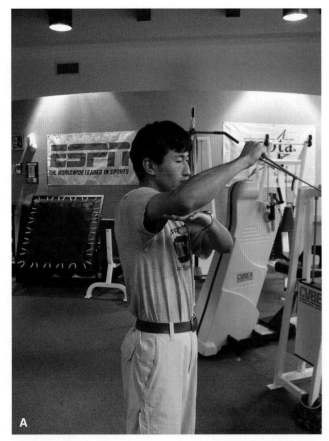
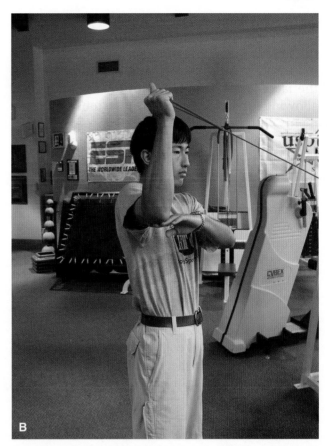

FIGURE 17.6 External rotation exercise with Thera-band using 90 degrees of elevation in the scapular plane.
A. Starting position. **B.** Ending position.

and sacral kyphosis. The spine has several key functions from an anatomical and biomechanical standpoint. It serves to house and protect the spinal cord and vital organs. It functions to dissipate weight-bearing forces of the head and trunk to the pelvis, and allows controlled movement of the spine against gravity. The spine can be divided into individual blocks or units called spinal segments. The **spinal segment** is considered the functional unit (Fig. 17.7) within the spinal column and consists of the disc–vertebral body interface, the facets or zygapophyseal joints, and the ligaments, muscles, and vessels that compose the segment. Together the individual functional units or spinal segments function as a whole to allow for coordinated movement.

The size and mass of the spinal segment increases from the cervical to the lumbar spine to allow for increased weight bearing on the lower segments. In addition, regional differences in the structure of the spine exist to accommodate the functional demands and movement patterns unique to a particular area of the spine. In the cervical spine, for example, the orientation and shape

of the joint surfaces allows for greater freedom of movement and positioning of the head in space. In contrast, the thoracic spine has significantly less total ROM, due to the articulation of the ribs and the shape of the spinal motion segment; this is

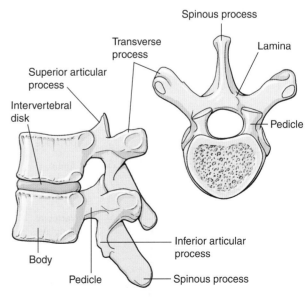

FIGURE 17.7 Anatomy of the vertebrae.

because of its primary role in protecting the vital organs and increasing respiratory efficiency. In the lumbar spine, the discs are larger to allow for increased weight bearing, and the orientation of the facet joints is primarily in the sagittal plane, allowing for greater flexion and extension movements with minimal rotation.

In a normal upright standing posture, 84% of the weight-bearing forces are transmitted through the vertebral body and disc–vertebral body interface, with the remaining 16% borne by the articular facet joints. The intervertebral disc interface consists of the cartilaginous vertebral endplates on the superior and inferior surfaces of the vertebral body and the interposed discs. The disc consists of the nucleus pulposus at the center, composed of a mucoid material with a water-binding capacity, giving it a gelatinous composition. The nucleus is surrounded by the annulus fibrosus comprising concentric layers of collagen and fibrocartilage designed to resist tensile, torsion, and compressive loads on the disc (Fig. 17.8). The oblique orientation of the annular fibers reinforces the strength of the disc, allowing resistance to the directional forces and movements exerted by the nucleus. Based on the design of the disc, it is thought to have the characteristics of a hydraulic system, where the self-contained nucleus cannot be compressed and therefore exerts pressure outward toward the vertebral endplates and annular rings. Owing to the relative avascularity of the disc, most disc nutrition occurs through diffusion via the vertebral endplate during cycles of loading and unloading, allowing for adequate exchange of nutrients and waste products. With age, the composition of the nucleus becomes less distinct from that of the annular fibers because of changes in the chemical composition in the nucleus.

Movement in the spine occurs three-dimensionally, with the individual segments having six degrees of freedom or motion components. On a basic level, movement at the spinal segments involves varying degrees of translation and rotation that occur when movement is produced in cardinal movements, such as flexion, extension, side bending, and rotation. The accompanying movements between the vertebrae as primary movements are produced are termed **coupling patterns**. The coupling patterns are the result of the geometry of the individual vertebrae, connecting ligaments, and discs. For example, when the spine is flexed, there is accompanying superior and inferior translation or gliding of the individual segments, which accounts for the coupling movements. Another example of coupling occurs when the cervical spine is bent to the side or laterally flexed; then the vertebral segments will rotate in the same direction as the side-bending motion (48). Coupling patterns need to occur for normal spinal movement, and the degrees and types of patterns vary based on the region of the spine and spinal posture when the movement is produced (48).

REAL-WORLD APPLICATION
Spine

The sit-and-reach test and the straight-leg-raise (SLR) test measure the ROM of the hamstrings and lumbar paraspinals. To perform the SLR test, the client is asked to lie supine with both legs straight out. You grasp the leg below the ankle with the knee extended and slowly raise the leg back toward the client. When movement of the pelvis is detected, indicating the end of the ROM, the test is complete. The normal range of motion is considered 80 degrees.

The sit-and-reach test is performed by having the person assume a long sitting position with the legs straight out in front. He or she is then asked to bend forward and reach for the toes. If the pelvis flexes toward the thigh at an 80-degree angle between the sacrum and table, a normal movement has occurred. Note that this is the same angle as that between the leg and the table in the SLR test. When hamstring length is restricted, the pelvis will be in a posterior orientation, with movement occurring through the lumbar spine.

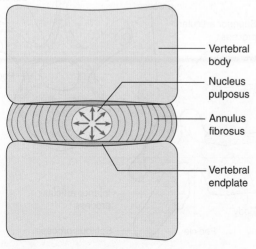

FIGURE 17.8 Structure of the intervertebral disc.

Clinical manifestations of coupling patterns become relevant when dysfunction occurs either due to degeneration or mechanical locking of the joint. This frequently happens when one attempts to perform a combined movement, such as retrieving an object by bending forward and rotating, causing mechanical locking of the facet joint. This biomechanical alteration causes pain and restriction with movement.

MUSCLES OF THE SPINE

Humans rely heavily on the muscles of the spinal column for movement, postural control, and stability of the individual segments as we perform activities from a very basic level to highly advanced movements, as in sports. The role of the various vertebral muscles is based on their size, attachments, and location. The complex interaction of muscle activity to concurrently produce movement while affording stability is the foundation of efficient spinal motion.

The anterior muscles in the abdominal wall consist of the rectus abdominis, external and internal obliques, and transverse abdominis. Collectively, the primary movements produced by these muscles are flexion and rotation of the trunk, with minimal muscle activity during normal erect standing. These muscles also act to regulate pelvic position by counterbalancing the pull of the back extensors.

The transverse abdominis plays a key role in achieving spinal stabilization by forming a rigid cylinder, increasing intra-abdominal pressure when contracted. The horizontal orientation of the fibers, and the attachment into the thoracolumbar fascia provides this stabilizing role. In both heavy resistance lifting and in an athlete lifting himself off the floor on his fingertips and toes, extreme abdominal and paraspinal muscle forces are needed to stabilize the spine (Figure 17.9).

The erector spinae muscles are posteriorly situated to the spine, run the entire length of the spine, and consist of the superficial and deep divisions. Together, the erector spinae muscles act to extend the spine while lifting and consequently are intermittently active to counteract the gravitational flexion line of pull on the body.

The stabilizing role of the deep erector spinae is evident in considering the line of pull of the deep erector spinae and the opposing iliopsoas. The contralateral anteroposterior line of pull in these muscles acts as a guy-wire check system for stability of the lumbar spine in the sagittal plane. The multifidus is an important segmental stabilizer in the lumbar spine. It is present throughout the entire spine but is thickest in the lumbar region. With the segmental attachment, along with their orientation of pull, the multifidus muscles are thought to act as important stabilizers in the lumbar spine

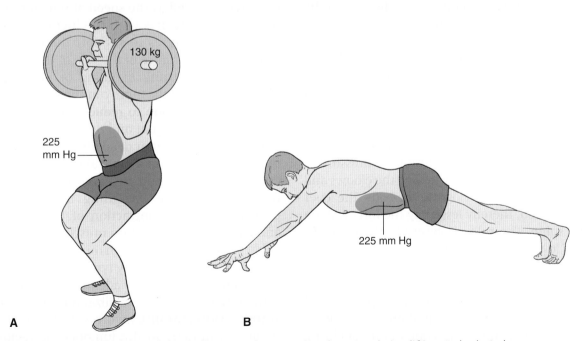

FIGURE 17.9 Role of intra-abdominal pressure in protecting the spine during lifting. In both **A.** heavy-resistance lifting and **B.** lifting of body weight, extreme intra-abdominal pressures are necessary to stabilize the spine.

during lifting and rotational movements of the trunk (32).

FUNCTIONAL TRAINING AND REHABILITATION OF THE BACK

Injuries in the spine occur frequently, with an estimated 80% of the general population experiencing low back pain at some point in their lives (43). The etiology of back pain is not clearly understood; often, it is difficult to identify the source or cause of such pain. In many cases, however, mechanical back pain is a result of faulty body mechanics, postural habits, and repetitive stresses that can be avoided.

The **neutral spine** is a posture that reduces the stress to the static structures of the spine and minimizes muscular effort by optimally aligning the segments in their most natural resting position. The neutral spine is achieved through finding the neutral position of the pelvis. This is done by flexing and extending the pelvis to end ranges, appreciating the sense of the extremes, and finding the middle range, where there is the least amount of strain to the spine. Maintenance of this neutral spine position provides the optimal position of the spinal curves for muscle length and joint position sense as well as distributing the forces along the spinal segment(s) equally.

When lifting weights or performing functional lifting, several concepts should be followed to avoid risk of injury. Minimizing the distance of the object to be lifted by keeping it close to the body reduces the joint reaction forces and intradiscal pressure within the spine. By holding a weighted object away from the body, the lever arm is dramatically increased, requiring higher muscle forces to maintain equilibrium while significantly increasing intradiscal pressure (Fig. 17.10). For example, in performing front raises with dumbbells with the elbows extended, the intradiscal pressure is exceedingly high. By simply flexing the elbows and keeping the dumbbells closer to the body, the lever arm is reduced, thereby lessening the forces acting on the spine. The role of obesity in the development of lower back problems is also related to having a larger lever arm acting on the low back when the abdomen protrudes anteriorly.

Studies have demonstrated the importance of generating large intra-abdominal pressures within the spine through the contraction of the stabilizing muscles of the paraspinals and abdominals in lifting heavy weights and in performing pushing

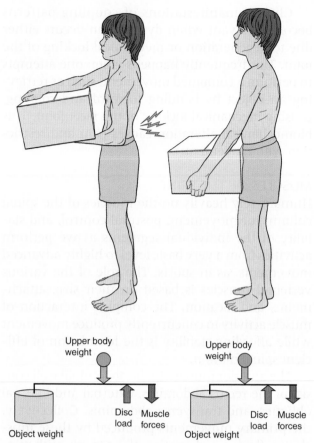

FIGURE 17.10 Proper lifting mechanics. Minimizing the distance of the object being lifted to the body reduces joint reaction forces and intradiscal pressure within the spine.

movements against heavy resistance. The amount of weight, as well as the speed at which the lift is performed, correlates with the increase in intra-abdominal pressures to support the spine, reinforcing the importance of the role of the stabilizing muscles of the trunk in lifting or pushing (see Fig. 17.9) Some of the more common lifts requiring adequate stabilization to reduce the risk of injury are the weighted squat and dead lift. In performing a weighted squat or dead lift, it is important to maintain the spine in a neutral position, avoiding excess lumbar flexion or extension throughout the movement by increasing intra-abdominal pressure through contraction of the abdominal and paraspinal stabilization muscles. This concept of back stabilization through muscular contraction should be utilized with any type of resistance training where the spine lacks adequate stabilization; it is the forefront of core-stabilization training. **Core stabilization training** involves strengthening the stabilizing muscles in the lumbopelvic region for adequate force generation and energy dissipation to the distal segments of the kinetic chain.

Core stabilization is an important concept for the strength and conditioning professional in terms of both performance and injury prevention. A number of appropriate methods can be utilized to train the core.

Core stabilization training has reached new levels of popularity within athletic and exercise training circles because it has been shown that this type of training not only reduces the risk of injury through focusing on the important role of the stabilization muscles but also enhances muscular control and efficiency. Traditional lifting methods have been supplemented with exercises utilizing core training to improve performance. Supplemental core exercises should be included with traditional lifting exercises during daily workouts to engage these very important trunk muscles. Some of the more common exercises include the following:

1. Pushups with feet or hands on a ball (Fig. 17.11A)
2. Bench press with back on ball, unsupported at the hips (Fig. 17.11B)
3. Reverse sit-up with feet on ball
4. Trunk rotation in standing or sitting on a ball
5. Opposite arm and leg in quadruped
6. Prone isometric abdominals
7. Bridging with feet on a ball (Fig 17.11C,D)
8. Lunges with trunk rotation
9. Thera-band sidestepping
10. Side-lying plange with unilateral row (Fig. 17.11E,F)

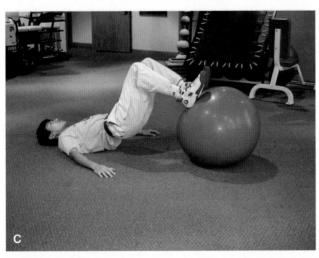

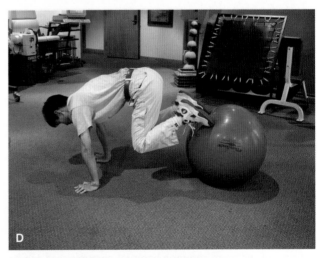

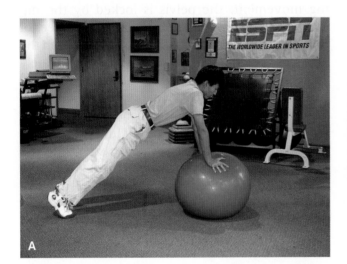

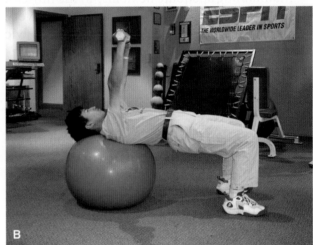

FIGURE 17.11 Core stabilization exercises. **A.** Push-up over a stability ball. **B.** Bench press exercise on a stability ball. **C.** Bridging with feet on a stability ball. **D.** Knee-to-chest exercise with feet on a stability ball.

(continued)

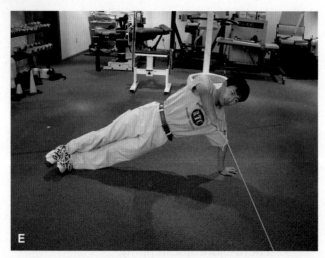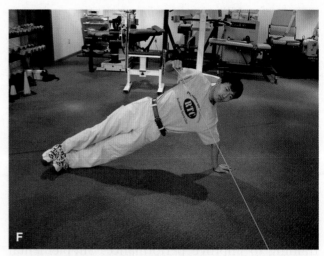

FIGURE 17.11 (*continued*) Core stabilization exercises. **E.** Starting position of plange with unilateral row using elastic resistance. **F.** Ending position of the row.

Maintaining adequate flexibility in the muscles of the low back and lower extremities is also very important because of their influence on pelvic alignment and control. Tight hamstrings, paraspinals, or hip flexors can adversely position the pelvis in too much flexion or extension, predisposing the individual to injury or degenerative changes over longer periods. An example of this need for adequate flexibility can be demonstrated in what is termed **lumbar-pelvic rhythm**, which is a sequential sharing of motion between the paraspinals and hip extensors in the act of bending forward to touch the toes. During the initial bend-

ing movement, the pelvis is locked by the hip extensors for approximately the first 60 degrees of motion, with movement primarily coming from the lumbar segments. This is followed by approximately 25 degrees of hip motion when the paraspinal muscles become more active, to allow for the additional motion to achieve full forward bending. The reverse sequence occurs with return from full flexion, with lumbar extension followed by pelvic extension. The implications are that with inadequate ROM or muscle activation in either area, injury may result from motion compensations due to an abnormal lumbar-pelvic rhythm (Figure 17.12).

REAL-WORLD APPLICATION
Posture

Back pain is among the most common forms of musculoskeletal pain and disability. Many cases of back pain can be linked to muscular imbalances; more often, they are highly correctable with appropriate education and exercise. Often, patients will have vague complaints of back pain throughout the day without any remarkable history to explain their symptoms. They will demonstrate restricted muscle flexibility and poor postural habits.

Simply observing a person in his or her natural sitting and standing postures frequently reveals poor spinal alignment which, cumulatively, can lead to the general back pain they frequently complain of during static prolonged postures. Some of the more common habitual postures that can be

observed are sacral or "slumped" sitting and a forward posture of the head and shoulders.

The influence of muscle flexibility on back pain is considerable. In the lumbar spine, restricted length of the hamstrings and hip flexors can have a tremendous impact on back pain because of the attachment of these muscles to the pelvis and lumbar spine. Inadequate hamstring length will cause more motion and stress to be placed on the lumbar discs with the pelvis in a more posterior or kyphotic posture. With tight hip flexors, the lumbar spine is in a more arched or lordotic posture, causing stretch weakness to the abdominals as well as compressing the facets of the spine.

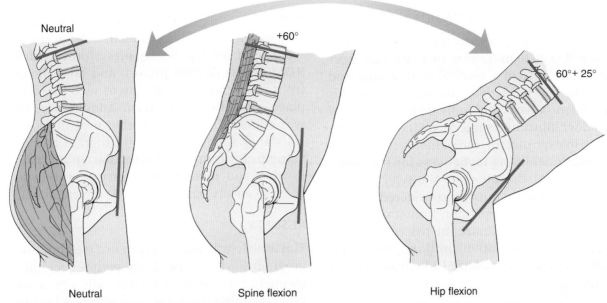

FIGURE 17.12 Muscle activity in forward bending. Bending forward is a two-part movement involving both the spine and the pelvis. Part one involves the first 60 degrees of movement, and part two involves an additional 25 degrees of forward trunk flexion.

SUMMARY

Injury prevention and rehabilitation involve a coordinated effort from various health care professionals. Strength and conditioning professionals must be aware of the stress placed on body tissues during strengthening exercises to minimize injury risk. When pain or injury does occur, activity needs to be modified and referral to an appropriate health care professional should be made as needed. Communication between sports medicine professionals is vital in transitioning an athlete from a supervised rehabilitation program to a return to sport interval program, and ultimately an independent conditioning program. Conduct-ing preparticipation physicals, identifying muscular strength and endurance deficits, awareness of joint and body mechanics during strengthening exercises, and appropriate activity progression after injury are all ways to minimize injury risk and maximize sport performance.

MAXING OUT

1. A basketball player at a rural high school sustains an ankle sprain. There is no health care professional present at the time of the injury. What actions should be taken?
2. What muscles should be addressed by exercises in a core stabilization program?

CASE EXAMPLE
Upper Extremity

BACKGROUND

A 45-year-old recreational athlete has a goal of returning to a weightlifting program for general fitness. He states that 5 years ago he had shoulder surgery, due to a long history of shoul-der tendonitis that began when he was in college playing baseball. He has no idea what type of lifting he should do for his upper body but feels very weak and wants to increase his strength and general fitness levels.

(continued)

RECOMMENDATIONS/CONSIDERATIONS

Since this athlete describes previous injuries, you will need to make sure that he is no longer under the care of a medical professional and that he has no activity restriction from his physician. Given this individual's history of shoulder injury and surgery, great care must be taken in exposing this individual to the stresses of traditional lifting maneuvers for the upper extremity. Modifications to the typical lifting recommendations must be considered. A low-resistance, higher-repetition format should be used initially to minimize the risk of injury, in addition to modifications in lifting ROM and movement patterns utilized (discussed in this chapter).

IMPLEMENTATION

This individual was placed on a twice-weekly program initially with a 15-RM load (a load that can be lifted 15 times but not 16) and a multiple-set training paradigm. Modifications were used for the bench press (only partial ROM on the descent phase), and lat pull (in front only); tricep press-downs were used in place of pull-overs or dips. Additionally, he was educated on the importance of the low-resistance higher-repetition program and its value in fostering local muscular endurance. Rowing and rotator cuff exercises were also given to ensure balanced muscle development.

RESULTS

This athlete was able to return to a weightlifting program for the upper body without reinjury owing to the use of an anatomically safe resistance-training program. This allowed him to gain the important benefits of resistance training without the typical stresses and overloads inherent in many traditional lifting patterns.

REFERENCES

1. American College of Sports Medicine. Current Comment, Preparticipation Physical Examinations. Indianapolis, IN: ACSM, 1999.
2. American Physical Therapy Association. Guide to Physical Therapist Practice. 2nd ed. Alexandria VA: American Physical Therapy Association, 2001.
3. Avela J, Kyrolainen H, Komi PV. Altered reflex sensitivity after repeated and prolonged passive muscle stretching. J Appl Physiol 1999;86:1283–1291.
4. Ballantyne BT, O'Hare SJ, Paschall JL, et al. Electromyographic activity of selected shoulder muscles in commonly used therapeutic exercises. Phys Ther 1993;73;668.
5. Beynnon BD, Ryder SH, Konradsen L, et al. Effect of anterior cruciate ligament trauma and bracing on knee proprioception. Am J Sports Med 1999;27:2:150–155.
6. Blackburn TA, McLeod WD, White B, et al. EMG analysis of posterior rotator cuff exercises. Athl Train 1990; 25:40.
7. Brindle T, Nyland J, Johnson DL. The meniscus: review of basic principles with application to surgery and rehabilitation. J Athl Train 2001;36(2):160–169.
8. Burkhart SS, Morgan CD, Kibler WB. The disabled throwing shoulder: spectrum of pathology: Part I. Pathoanatomy and biomechanics. Arthroscopy 2003; 19(4):404–420.
9. Chandler TJ, Kibler WB, Stracener EC, et al. Shoulder strength, power, and endurance in college tennis players. Am J Sports Med 1992;20:455–458.
10. Codman EA. The Shoulder, Boston: privately printed, 1934.
11. Cotton RE, Rideout DF. Tears of the humeral rotator cuff: a radiological and pathological necropsy survey. J Bone Joint Surg 1964;46B:314.
12. Davies GJ. A Compendium of Isokinetics in Clinical Usage and Rehabilitation Techniques. 4th ed. Onalaska, WI: S and S Publishers, 1992.
13. Davies GJ, Heidersceit BC, Clark M. Open kinetic chain assessment and rehabilitation. Athl Train Sports Health Care Perspect 1995;1(4):347–370.
14. Davies GJ, Manske RC, Slamma K, et al. Selective activation of the vastus medialis oblique: what does the literature really tell us? Physiother Canada 2001;100–115.
15. DeCarlo M, Klootwyk T, Oneacre K. Anterior cruciate ligament. In: Ellenbecker TS, ed. Knee Ligament Rehabilitation. Philadelphia: Churchill Livingstone, 2000.
16. Ellenbecker TS. Clinical Examination of the Shoulder. Philadelphia: Saunders, 2004.
17. Ellenbecker TS. Rehabilitation of shoulder and elbow injuries in tennis players. Clin Sports Med 1995;14(1):87–109.
18. Ellenbecker TS. Shoulder internal and external rotation strength and range of motion in highly skilled tennis players. Isokinet Exerc Sci 1992;2:1–8.
19. Ellenbecker TS, Davies GJ. The application of isokinetics in testing and rehabilitation of the shoulder complex. J Athl Train 2000;35(3):338–350.
20. Ellenbecker TS, Roetert EP. Age specific isokinetic glenohumeral internal and external rotation strength in elite junior tennis players. J Sci Med Sport 2003;6(1):63–70.
21. Fulcher SM, Kiefhaber TR, Stern PJ. Upper-extremity tendinitis and overuse syndromes in the athlete. Clin Sports Med 1998;17:3:433–448.

22. Fulkerson JP. Diagnosis and treatment of patients with patellofemoral pain. Am J Sports Med 2002;30(3): 447–456.

23. Gross ML, Brenner SL, Esformes I, Sonzogni JJ. Anterior shoulder instability in weight lifters. Am J Sports Med 1993;21(4):599–603.

24. Inman VT, Saunders JB, Abbott LC. Observations on the function of the shoulder joint. J Bone Joint Surg 1944; 26(1):1–30.

25. Ireland ML, Willson JD, Ballantyne BT, Davis IM. Hip strength in females with and without patellofemoral pain. J Orthop Sports Phys Ther 2002;33(11):671–676.

26. Jobe FW, Kivitne RS. Shoulder pain in the overhand or throwing athlete. Orthop Rev 1989;18:963–975.

27. Kibler WB. The role of the scapula in athletic shoulder function. Am J Sports Med 1998;26(2):325–337.

28. Knight KL. Cryotherapy in Sports Injury Management. Champaign IL: Human Kinetics, 1995.

29. Kokkonen J, Nelson A, Cornwell A. Acute muscle stretching inhibits maximal strength performance. Res Q Exerc Sport 1998;69(4):411–415.

30. Kraushaar BS, Nirschl RP. Tendonosis of the elbow (tennis elbow): Clinical features and findings of histological, immunohistochemical, and electron microscopy studies. J Bone Joint Surg 1999;81-A(2):259–278.

31. Lephart SM, Pincivero DM, Giraldo JL, et al. The role of proprioception in the management and rehabilitation of athletic injuries. Am J Sports Med 1997;25:130–137.

32. Macdonald DA, Lorimer Moseley G, Hodges PW. The lumbar multifidus: does the evidence support clinical beliefs? Man Ther 2006;11:254–263. PMID: 16716640 [PubMed—as supplied by publisher].

33. Marshall RN, Elliott BC. Long-axis rotation: the missing link in proximal to distal sequencing. J Sports Sci 2000; 18:247–254.

34. Marx RG, Sperling JW, Cordasco FA., Overuse injuries of the upper extremity in tennis players. Clin Sports Med 2001;20(3):439–451.

35. Moseley JB, Jobe FW, Pink M. EMG analysis of the scapular muscles during a shoulder rehabilitation program. Am J Sports Med 1992;20:128–134.

36. Mosesson MW. Fibrinogen and fibrin structure and functions. J Thromb Haemost 2005:8:1894–1904.

37. National Athletic Trainers' Association. Athletic Training Educational Competencies. 3rd ed. Dallas: National Athletic Trainers' Association, 1999.

38. Neer CS. Anterior acromioplasty for the chronic impingement syndrome in the shoulder. J Bone Joint Surgery (Am) 1972;54A:41–50.

39. Neitzel JA, Kernozek TW, Davies GJ. Loading response following anterior cruciate ligament reconstruction during the parallel squat exercise. Clin Biomech 2002;7(7): 551–554.

40. Nirschl RP, Sobel J. Conservative treatment of tennis elbow. Phys Sports Med 1981;9:43–54.

41. Noffal GJ. Isokinetic eccentric-to-concentric strength ratios of the shoulder rotator muscles in throwers and nonthrowers. Am J Sports Med 2003;31(4):537–541.

42. Nyland J, Nolan MF. Therapeutic modality: rehabilitation of the injured athlete. Clin Sports Med 2004;23(2): 299–313, vii.

43. Richardson JK, Iglarsh, A. Clinical Orthopaedic Physical Therapy. Philadelphia: Saunders, 1994.

44. Saha AK: Mechanism of shoulder movements and a plea for the recognition of "zero position" of glenohumeral joint. Clin Orthop 1983;173:3–10.

45. Taylor J, Stone R, Mullin MJ, et al. Comprehensive Sports Injury Management: From Examination Of Injury to Return to Sport. 2nd ed. Austin: PRO-ED, 2003.

46. Townsend H, Jobe FW, Pink M, et al. Electomyographic analysis of the glenohumeral muscles during a baseball rehabilitation program. Am J Sports Med 1991;19: 264–272.

47. Wallace DA, Salem GJ, Salinas R, et al. Patellofemoral joint kinetics while squatting with and without an external load. J Orthop Sports Phys Ther April 2002; 32:4;141–148.

48. White AA, Panjabi MM. Clinical Biomechanics of the Spine. 2nd ed. Philadelphia: Lippincott, 1990.

49. Wilk KE, Arrigo CA. Interval sport programs for the shoulder. In: Andrews JR, Wilk KE, eds. The Athlete's Shoulder, New York: Churchill Livingstone, 1994.

50. Wilk KE, Davies GJ, Mangine RE, et al. Patellofemoral disorders: a classification system and clinical guidelines for nonoperative rehabilitation. J Orthop Sports Phys Ther 1998;28(5):307–322.

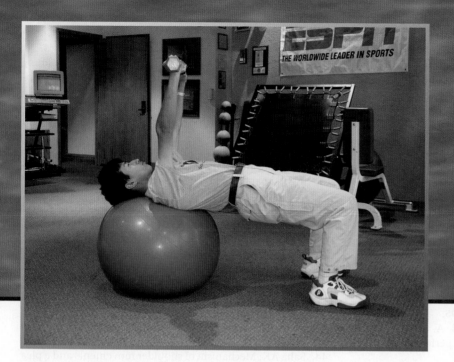

Ergogenic Aids

JOSÉ ANTONIO
TIM ZIEGENFUSS
RON MENDEL

Introduction

Ergogenic aids are substances (including nutrients, nutritional supplements, and drugs) that improve athletic performance. Nutritional ergogenic aids include substances that contain fats, carbohydrates, proteins, vitamins, and/or minerals. Fats, carbohydrates, and proteins provide energy (calories) to produce adenosine triphosphate (ATP). Vitamins and minerals regulate energy-producing metabolic pathways. Nutritional supplements are nutrients in a concentrated form. Drugs can have an effect on cellular function that can directly or indirectly improve performance.

Numerous substances have been studied in the quest for improved athletic performance. The conditions under which a substance might have a positive effect vary depending on metabolic requirements of the exercise as well as the environmental conditions. The list of ergogenic aids that do not work would be endless. This chapter focuses on several ergogenic aids that have been shown to have a positive effect under specific conditions.

BRANCHED-CHAIN AMINO ACIDS

Amino acids are the building blocks of proteins. The amino acids leucine, isoleucine, and valine are collectively known as the **branched-chain amino acids (BCAAs)**. Supplementation with BCAAs does not appear to improve short-term exercise performance but may reduce muscle breakdown during clinical conditions of wasting (e.g., starvation, postsurgery, burns, etc.) and periods of prolonged exercise (13,88,111). According to the "central fatigue hypothesis," during prolonged exercise, the plasma levels of BCAAs decrease and levels of fatty acids increase. The increase in fatty acids causes an increase in the levels of free tryptophan, which is a precursor to serotonin, a neurotransmitter that causes feelings of sleepiness and depression. In other words, decreases in BCAAs during prolonged exercise can, in theory, increase the mental effort necessary to perform. Use of BCAAs as an ergogenic aid may attenuate the increase in serotonin, thus reducing perceived exertion and mental fatigue during prolonged exercise (13–15). Although there is some support for these effects during prolonged cycling, marathon running, and time trials, an equal number of studies have shown no effect from BCAA supplementation. Since the side effects from BCAAs appear to be minimal, individuals competing in events lasting 2 or more hours, especially events in the heat, may wish to experiment with repeated liquid doses of BCAAs. One approach that has yielded positive effects is to ingest a total of 5 to 10 g of BCAAs dissolved in 1 L of fluid (i.e., drinking 150 mL of the solution every 10 to 20 minutes) (16,74).

Men and women who ingest approximately 10 to 15 g of BCAAs per day (5 to 7 g leucine, 3 to 4 g isoleucine, and 3 to 4 g valine) for at least 30 days increase their lean body mass more than do matched controls (27,96). One of the underlying mechanisms behind these effects appears to be the ability of BCAAs to increase protein synthesis during recovery from resistance exercise (74).

One interesting aspect of BCAAs that has only recently been explored is their potential effect on weight loss. During a moderate-protein (1.5 g/kg of body weight per day), lower-carbohydrate (100 to 200 g/day) diet, the increased intake of BCAAs (especially leucine) is thought to have positive effects on muscle protein synthesis, insulin signaling, and sparing of glucose use by stimulation of the glucose-alanine cycle. This leads to more fat loss and a greater sparing of lean tissue compared to an isoenergetic, higher-carbohydrate diet (83). Additional research into the effects of BCAAs on changes in body composition is warranted.

 BCAAs may have positive ergogenic effects related to their anticatabolic effect; however, fairly large doses must be consumed to achieve this.

CAFFEINE

Caffeine is a bitter white alkaloid ($C_8H_{10}N_4O_2$) often derived from tea or coffee. A huge volume of research on caffeine is available. Perhaps the most commonly consumed drug in the United States, caffeine is an effective ergogenic aid. It may promote lipolysis (1,6,30,61,69,71,115,127,170), stimulate the central nervous system (19,29,41, 72,87,97,126), and act as a performance-enhancing aid for many types of athletic activity (7–10,33, 34,38,41,42,65,70,95,107,138). Both older (65 to 80 years of age) and younger (19 to 26 years of age) men show a similar thermogenic response to caffeine ingestion. Older men, however, show a smaller increase in fatty acid availability after a caffeine challenge (6). Caffeine ingestion has been shown to stimulate both lipolysis and energy expenditure (1). It is not clear whether the lipolytic effect of caffeine is associated with increased lipid oxidation or futile cycling between triglycerides and free fatty acids (FFAs). Also, it is not known whether the effects of caffeine are mediated via the sympathetic nervous system.

Caffeine can also act as a potent ergogenic aid. Caffeine has been removed from the World Anti-Doping Agency's (WADA) banned list (169). Ingesting caffeine (5 mg/kg body weight) can significantly increase exercise time to exhaustion (9). Caffeine ingestion can also improve maximal anaerobic power (2) and sprint-swimming performance in trained swimmers (32). Table 18.1 lists the caffeine content of various beverages.

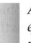 *A large volume of data supports the ergogenic effects of caffeine as well as its thermogenic properties.*

TABLE 18.1	CAFFEINE CONTENT OF VARIOUS PRODUCTS (91, 129)	
PRODUCT	SERVING	MILLIGRAMS OF CAFFEINE
Starbucks (tall) Coffee	12 oz	375
Red Bull	12 oz	120
Mountain Dew	12 oz	55
Diet Coke	12 oz	45
Dr. Pepper	12 oz	41
Sunkist Orange	12 oz	41
Starbucks Espresso	1 oz	35
Coca-Cola Classic	12 oz	34
Nestea Sweetened Iced Tea	12 oz	26
Barqs Root Beer	12 oz	22
Hot Chocolate	12 oz	8

Data for colostrum supplementation support daily doses ranging from 20 to 60 g to enhance performance as well as to promote gains in lean body mass.

COLOSTRUM

Colostrum is a component of human breast milk or cow's milk, found at its highest concentration 2 to 3 days after a female gives birth. It is a rich source of protein, antibodies, and growth factors. Several compelling studies demonstrate an ergogenic effect of colostrum supplementation (4,21–24,35,62,75). Such supplementation (20 g/per day for 8 weeks) combined with aerobic and heavy resistance training significantly increased bone-free lean body mass (mean increase of 1.49 kg) compared to whey protein (4).

Another investigation demonstrated the potential ergogenic effects of colostrum supplementation by comparing the effects of bovine colostrums to whey protein powder. Using a randomized, double-blind, placebo-controlled parallel design, 51 males completed 8 weeks of resistance and plyometric training while consuming 60 g/day of bovine colostrum or concentrated whey protein powder. By week 8, peak vertical jump power and peak cycle power were significantly greater in the colostrum group as opposed to the whey protein group. Interestingly, there were no differences between groups with regard to alactic anaerobic work capacity, 1 RM or plasma insulin-like growth factor 1 (IGF-1) (24).

CREATINE

Creatine is a naturally occurring nitrogenous compound made in the liver, kidneys, and pancreas from the amino acids arginine, glycine, and methionine. Creatine is found in relatively high amounts in meat, fish, and poultry. In fact, adults and teenagers who regularly consume these foods typically eat 1 to 2 g of creatine per day, an amount equal to its natural rate of excretion by the kidneys, where creatine is converted to creatinine. Vegetarians who do not consume meat or fish have reduced body stores of creatine. Interestingly, when these individuals are fed creatine, they retain more of it in their bodies (in comparison to nonvegetarians), suggesting that creatine might actually be "essential" to a normal diet. In a 154-lb adult male, about 120 g of creatine is found in the body, 95% of which is in skeletal muscle (145).

A large body of literature demonstrates the ergogenic properties of creatine (44,45,49–55,77, 80,81,136,137,139,140,143,144,154,155,157,160, 162). What follows is by no means a comprehensive discussion of creatine; however, it does give the reader a glimpse into this effective performance aid.

On ingestion, creatine is absorbed into the bloodstream through the small intestine and reaches peak levels 60 to 90 minutes later (145). Creatine is thought to serve at least four vital functions:

1. It stores energy that can be used to regenerate ATP.
2. It enhances energy transfer between the mitochondria and muscle fibers.
3. It serves as a buffer against intracellular acidosis during exercise.
4. It stimulates glycogenolysis (glycogen breakdown) during exercise.

Collectively, these effects underscore creatine's central role in energy metabolism and explain why this substance has been the subject of intensive study (77,154).

A common analogy used by exercise scientists is that creatine is to the weight lifter/sprinter what carbohydrate is to the distance runner. Of the well-controlled human trials on creatine, about two-thirds have shown benefits from its use. Depending on the initial fitness level of the subjects, these have included the following:

- Increased dynamic strength and power (approximately 5% to 15%)
- Increased body weight and lean body mass (approximately 2% to 5%)
- Increased sprint performance (approximately 1% to 5%)

As little as 3 days of creatine supplementation (0.35 g/kg of fat-free mass) can increase thigh muscle volume and may enhance cycle sprint performance in elite power athletes, with the effect being greater in females as sprints are repeated (171). Creatine supplementation in conjunction with heavy resistance training increased total body mass, fat-free mass, thigh volume, muscle strength, and myofibrillar protein (164,165).

In general, creatine is considered beneficial to weightlifters and athletes involved in sports requiring short, repeated bursts of high power (e.g., wrestling, rowing, sprint running/swimming/cycling, football, volleyball, soccer, ice/field hockey, lacrosse). Additionally, a growing body of evidence points to the health/medical benefits of oral administration of creatine monohydrate. For instance, creatine supplementation may slow the progression of motor neuron disease in a mouse model (66), and may improve various conditions such as mitochondrial encephalomyopathies (76); it may also protect against neuronal degeneration in amyotrophic lateral sclerosis and Huntington's disease and in chemically mediated neurotoxicity (142). Creatine may protect the immature brain from hypoxic-ischemic injury (11). Also, creatine supplementation has a "significant positive effect on both working memory (backward digit span) and intelligence (Raven's Advanced Progressive Matrices), both tasks that require speed of processing" (117). Creatine supplementation has applications that extend beyond the athletic realm. The health benefits of creatine may indeed be a positive area of research in the future.

What are the potential risks (side effects) of using creatine? The only consistently reported "side effect" in humans has been weight gain.

Despite inflammatory reports in the media of a link between creatine use and muscle cramps/pulls, dehydration/heat exhaustion, and kidney/liver disorders, these effects have not been documented by independent research. To the contrary, studies have either reported no effect (on kidney/liver function or musculotendinous stiffness) or an improved response from creatine use (a lower incidence of muscle cramps/pulls) (158). In one study of 98 athletes, long-term supplementation with creatine (up to 21 months) did not adversely affect a 69-item panel of serum, whole blood, or urinary markers of clinical health status (80).

A long-standing myth holds that creatine supplementation is harmful to the kidneys. This is clearly not the case. Neither short-, medium-, nor long-term oral creatine supplementation causes detrimental effects on the kidneys of healthy individuals (112).

In a lay article published on the Internet, a comparison of 28 creatine distributors revealed that over half were selling products containing contaminants. The overall purity of each product averaged about 90%, but there were dramatic differences in the amount of several potentially toxic impurities. Athletes considering creatine use should exercise the following precautions:

1. Do not "load." Rather than ingesting 20 to 30 g for the first 5 to 7 days and then 5 g/day thereafter, take only about 3 to 5 g daily.
2. Cycle periods of use (4 to 8 weeks) with periods of nonuse (4 weeks).
3. Purchase the product from a reputable manufacturer who is able to provide a "certificate of analysis," including all of the following information:
   - Appearance (should be white to pale cream)
   - Assay (should be at least 95% creatine)
   - Moisture content (should be less than or equal to 12.5%)
   - Residue on ignition (should be less than or equal to 1%)
   - Microbial/pathogenic contamination (should be negative for *Escherichia coli*, *Staphylococcus aureus*, and *Salmonella*)
   - Yeasts and molds (should be less than 50/g)
   - Poisons/heavy metals (should be less than 10 ppm for lead and mercury)

- Other contaminants (should be less than 3 ppm for arsenic, 30 ppm for dicyandiamide, and nondetectable for dyhydrotriazine)

Perhaps the most widely studied ergogenic aid, creatine, used for regular supplementation, has been shown to increase skeletal muscle mass and muscle fiber size and to improve anaerobic exercise performance. No evidence is available that regular creatine supplementation is harmful to otherwise healthy individuals.

ESSENTIAL AMINO ACIDS

Of the 20 amino acids used to form proteins, 8 are considered **essential amino acids (EAAs)**. Because your body does not produce them, you need to consume them in your diet. A growing body of literature demonstrates the efficacy of essential amino acid supplementation in enhancing physical performance (3,18,26,47,93,109,146, 148,149,167,168). The anabolic response to the consumption of an oral cocktail containing EAAs plus carbohydrate (EAC) before versus after heavy resistance exercise was studied (148). Six healthy subjects (three men and three women; average age 30.2 years, height 1.71 m, weight 66 kg) consumed the EAC (6 g of EAAs plus 35 g of sucrose in 500 mL water) either immediately before or after exercise (in a randomized order). The exercise bout consisted of 10 sets of eight reps of the leg press (80% of 1 RM), and 8 sets of eight reps of the leg extension (80% of 1 RM). The rest interval was about 2 minutes, with the total exercise time roughly 45 minutes. The investigators then examined phenylalanine uptake across the leg as a measure of muscle protein accretion. Over a 3-hour period, taking the EAC before exercise resulted in a net phenylalanine uptake that was about 160% greater than that noted when the EAC was taken after exercise. Furthermore, work from the same laboratory found that the nonessential amino acids are not required to stimulate protein synthesis. Finally, there is a dose-dependent effect of EAA ingestion on muscle protein synthesis (18). Thus, a relatively small dose (6 g) of EAA may confer a significant anabolic response.

The essential amino acids play a critical role in promoting skeletal muscle anabolism.

GLUCOSAMINE

Glucosamine is a combination of glutamine and glucose (amino polysaccharide). After the oral consumption of glucosamine, it is incorporated into molecules called proteoglycans, which are part of the joint cartilage. This helps maintain the integrity of the joint as well as repair damaged cartilage. Glucosamine may also stimulate chondrocytes, or cartilage-producing cells, to make new cartilage. The regular consumption of glucosamine may alleviate the signs and symptoms of osteoarthritis (OA). Glucosamine supplementation may provide some degree of pain relief and improved function in persons experiencing regular knee pain, which may be caused by prior cartilage injury and/or OA. At a dosage of 2,000 mg/day, most of the noted improvement occurs within 8 weeks (20). A meta-analysis examined clinical trials of glucosamine from January 1980 to March 2002. This study demonstrated that glucosamine (alone or in combination with chondroitin sulfate) reduced pain and damage to the knee joint. No differences were found in adverse events between placebo and glucosamine, indicating that the supplement appears to be safe (122).

Regular supplementation of glucosamine may decrease the symptoms associated with OA.

GLUTAMINE

Glutamine is the most plentiful nonessential amino acid in the human body, particularly in the plasma and skeletal muscle, and has numerous physiological functions (78). Although the body can synthesize glutamine, it does become a "conditionally" essential amino acid in cases of major trauma such as surgery. Even an intense workout or multiple intense workouts that lead to overtraining are a cause for decreased glutamine levels. Among other things, glutamine acts as a cell-volume regulator (121), anticatabolic agent, and "gut builder"; its more defined roles are as a muscle builder by stimulating muscle protein synthesis (119,120) and as an immune stimulator. Glutamine has been widely used by weight trainers owing to its muscle building potential. It has been shown not only to increase protein synthesis but also to stimulate glycogen synthesis (150). Although more research is neces-

Q & A from the Field

I am concerned about my boyfriend. He wants to lift weights every day. He is always looking in the mirror and flexing his muscles. He spends a lot of time lifting weights and his muscles are extremely well developed. He is taking lots of different supplements. What is muscle dysmorphia, and what can we do for him if he has it?

Let me offer an example. Joe, a man 5 ft, 10 in. tall with extremely hypertrophied muscles, walks over to the squat rack, his eyes focused and his concentration fierce. He is a regular at the gym and is admired for his well-developed pecs, lats so large his arms appear uncomfortably pushed inches away from his body, and powerful quads. Yet at 230 lb, Joe feels scrawny. He is embarrassed by what he perceives to be an underdeveloped body and tormented by the fear of losing what muscle he has if he doesn't work out for hours daily and follow a strict muscle-building diet. His kitchen is filled with large canisters of protein powder, a cupboard full of supplements touted to build muscles, and a scale to measure everything, but Joe is still displeased with his body.

Joe suffers from **muscle dysmorphia**, a preoccupation with his body image and the feeling that his body is not muscular enough. Like many other men who suffer from this disorder, Joe actually has a well-defined, muscular physique (57,58,84,106,108,113,114). Because of its striking similarity to other body-image distortions, muscle dysmorphia has been referred to as "reverse anorexia" or "bigorexia" and is considered to be a type of body dysmorphic disorder seen primarily in men. It is not surprising that an individual with body dysmorphia would take a lot of supplements to help him reach his goal.

Men suffering from muscle dysmorphia often lift weights for hours, pay meticulous attention to their diet, use various ergogenic aids, frequently check their bodies out in mirrors, and may spend more than 5 hours daily obsessing about their musculature. Like those who suffer from anorexia or other body-image disorders, these individuals are often depressed and may also experience anxiety, especially at the thought of anything disrupting their workout or diet regimen.

It isn't known how many men suffer from muscle dysmorphia, since large-scale studies have not been conducted. In addition, the etiology of muscle dysmorphia is unclear, though many theories have been presented; researchers believe that it may follow a psychosocial model with an underlying biological or genetic predisposition combined with social influences. The sociocultural theory is also believed to be a significant contributing factor. This view describes the societal pressures placed on men to fit media images of masculinity that include a fit, muscular physique. For years, women have been subjected to images of how a desirable female "should" look. Similarly unrealistic expectations for men, however, have become popular only in recent years.

Those who suffer from muscle dysmorphia rarely seek help for many reasons, including embarrassment over their preoccupation, the anxiety they feel at the thought of having to reduce their gym time during treatment, and the fear of a potential decrease in muscle mass once they start treatment. Proposed treatment options include cognitive behavioral therapy and the use of antidepressant medication.

—Marie Spano, MS, RD

sary, there are limited data to support its ability to increase cellular hydration and stimulate protein synthesis (5,78), leading to increases in muscle mass and strength.

Clinical evidence for the exogenous use of glutamine supplementation in critically ill patients for the maintenance of muscle mass and immune function is well supported. Glutamine's role as an ergogenic aid as it relates to immune function may be of greater significance to athletes than its ability to increase muscle mass. Glutamine use may modify the apparent immunodepression that is observed after prolonged, exhausting exercise. Following such strenuous exercise, the concentration of glutamine in the blood is severely decreased. Supplementation of glutamine in this situation may decrease the incidence of illness in these athletes (28). The influence of glutamine on time to exhaustion and power before and after a prolonged bout of exercise has been examined (110). One group ingested a carbohydrate-plus-glutamine (Glu) beverage and a placebo group ingested a carbohydrate-only beverage (Pl). The Glu group significantly increased time to exhaustion compared to Pl. Peak power in the Glu group was similar in both trials, whereas the Pl group was still significantly lower after the second trial 6 days later. Therefore, glutamine supplementation seemed to help the Glu group exercise longer and recover quicker than the Pl group.

There is a sound physiological rationale and some evidence that glutamine supplementation can have a positive impact on muscle mass and strength gains in athletes. More convincing, though, is evidence that supports exogenous glutamine supplementation for immune system function, especially with prolonged, exhausting exercise.

■ *Glutamine is an amino acid that may be needed in greater quantities during times of severe stress.*

GLYCEROL

Regular exercise can cause fluid loss that, if not replaced, can potentially compromise performance and/or the next exercise session. This is particularly true with exercise that is intense, prolonged, and performed in the heat, since high core temperatures and high sweat rates accelerate fluid loss (82,156,166). As little as a 2% to 3% loss of body weight (as fluid) can negatively impact performance, so strategies to optimize preexercise hydration have been developed. The most common method of "hyperhydration," a condition in which body water stores are temporarily elevated, is the consumption of glycerol (94,123). **Glycerol** is a clear, syrupy, liquid found in all animal and vegetable fats and oils. In contrast to drinking extra water (which is processed by the kidneys and removed within an hour), glycerol ingestion causes an increase in fluid absorption by the blood and tissues, prolonging hyperhydration for up to 4 hours (125). Because glycerol is not easily absorbed by the eyes or brain, it has also been used clinically to treat cerebral edema (swelling of the brain) and glaucoma (increased intraocular pressure from fluid buildup in the eyes). Glycerol administration causes a shift in fluid out of the brain and eyes and into the peripheral tissues. An unfortunate consequence of this effect however, is that headache and blurred vision sometimes accompany glycerol use.

Research on the effectiveness of glycerol as a performance enhancer is equivocal. Methodological differences (i.e., variations in the type and intensity of the exercise bout, environmental conditions, and dosing pattern) are difficult to control. Improvements are most likely when the exercise bout results in substantial dehydration (when the activity is intense, prolonged, and is performed under conditions of high heat and humidity). In this case, performance benefits during timed events are likely to be a few percent, which can be significant considering that many athletic events at the elite level are decided by less than 1%.

■ *Glycerol may be an additional aid for hydration.*

GREEN TEA EXTRACT

Green tea extract has a high content of caffeine and catechin polyphenols, which could increase 24-hour energy expenditure and fat oxidation in humans. **Epigallocatechin gallate (EGCG)** is a purified catechin derived from green tea and is the main active component of the biological activity of tea polyphenols. For instance, one study compared three treatments: green tea extract (50 mg caffeine and 90 mg EGCG), caffeine (50 mg), and placebo, which were ingested at breakfast, lunch, and dinner. Green tea extract resulted in a significant increase in 24-hour energy expenditure as well as a decrease in respiratory quotient, indicating a greater reliance on fatty acid oxidation. Green tea has thermogenic properties and promotes fat oxidation beyond that explained by its caffeine content. Green tea extract may play a role in the control of body composition by thermogenesis, fat oxidation, or both (43).

Interestingly, an in vitro (test tube) investigation suggests that green tea may have lipolytic activity due to its vitamin C content, which purportedly inhibits triglyceride accumulation (60). It still remains to be seen whether green tea extract is an effective ergogenic aid.

■ *EGCG is one of the active components of green tea.*

HMB

Beta-hydroxy-beta-methylbutyrate (HMB) is a natural component of fish and milk. As a breakdown product of the essential amino acid leucine, HMB is thought to increase strength and lean body mass by acting as an anticatabolic agent in muscle (i.e., decreasing muscle protein breakdown)

(78,101–104). Several studies have verified these beneficial effects, particularly in untrained men and women who consume 1.5 to 3.0 g of HMB per day, divided into two doses, for at least 4 weeks. One study suggested that its effects on strength and lean body mass can be further enhanced by coingesting creatine (Cr dose: 20 g/day for 7 days followed by 10 g/day thereafter) (73). Although the exact mechanism(s) behind its effects are unclear, one hypothesis is that HMB helps to support cholesterol synthesis in stressed muscle cells, an effect that would maintain proper cell membrane function. This effect is in contrast to those of anabolic hormones like testosterone and insulin, which, under certain conditions, increase muscle size by enhancing protein and/or glycogen synthesis. Ingestion of HMB appears to be safe and may even have beneficial effects on cardiovascular health (e.g., decreasing total cholesterol, LDL cholesterol, and blood pressure) when doses of 3 g/day are ingested for up to 8 weeks (102). To date, time-released sources of HMB do not appear to be effective (135).

HMB supplementation may have an anticatabolic effect in untrained individuals.

HYDRATION

Dehydration has negative effects on performance (132,159). Inadequate hydration can refer to either hypohydration (being dehydrated prior to exercise) or exercise-induced dehydration, which occurs during exercise. Either state of dehydration can negatively impact muscle metabolism, body temperature regulation, and cardiovascular function, with decreased exercise performance occurring with as little as a 1% to 2% reduction in body weight.

Water and commercial sports drinks can be very effective in maintaining performance or delaying the inevitable decrease in performance, especially in endurance or team sports that last longer than 1 hour. It is recommended that individuals consume a nutritionally balanced diet and drink adequate fluids in the 24-hour period prior to training or competition. The American College of Sports Medicine Position Statement on Exercise and Fluid Replacement (1996) also recommends

the consumption of about 500 mL of fluid 2 hours prior to training or competition to promote adequate hydration and allow for excretion of excess fluid. Maintaining proper hydration prior to exercise is simple and generally should not be an issue if prudent measures are followed.

Fluid replacement during exercise is extremely critical not only to exercise performance but also to health. Without proper fluid replacement during prolonged exercise or exercise in a hot and humid environment, heat-related illness and cardiovascular issues can become life-threatening. To minimize these conditions, it is recommended that water losses via sweating be replaced at a rate equal to the sweat rate (39,105). Athletes should replace the weight lost during exercise by drinking fluid. Unfortunately, individuals generally do not sufficiently replace lost fluid at a rate equal to water loss. This is referred to as "voluntary dehydration" (56). Water alone is not always sufficient to replace the fluid deficit incurred due to exercise, especially long-duration exercise with high sweat rates. Complete restoration of fluid lost during exercise cannot occur without replacement of electrolytes, primarily sodium (141).

Along with sodium, the addition of carbohydrates to fluid-replacement solutions can enhance the intestinal absorption of water (133). More importantly, though, ingestion of a carbohydrate-containing beverage during exercise will help maintain blood glucose concentration and thus delay reliance on muscle glycogen stores as well as ultimately delaying fatigue (31,36,40,98). This is especially true in sessions lasting longer than 1 hour. An optimal carbohydrate solution of 4% to 8% helps maintain blood glucose concentrations and replace fluid lost via sweating. The inclusion of carbohydrates in rehydration solutions is necessary to maintain blood glucose concentrations for optimal performance in exercise lasting longer than 1 hour. It is also important to note that fructose should not be the predominant carbohydrate in a fluid-replacement solution due to its low glycemic index and the associated relatively slow increase in blood glucose. Frequent ingestion of water and commercial sports drinks (containing electrolytes and carbohydrates) during exercise is certainly one of the simplest and most beneficial ergogenic aids available.

Hydration is a critical factor governing exercise performance in the heat.

PRE- AND POSTWORKOUT NUTRITION

Strenuous exercise, whether aerobic or anaerobic, can reduce various energy substrates [glycogen, protein, stored phosphagens (ATP, phosphocreatine), intracellular triglycerides], increase muscle protein breakdown, damage cell membranes, cause fluid loss, and temporarily impair immune function. The manner in which these physiological changes occur and how they respond to different interventions has provided clues to researchers as to what to eat and when with regard to optimizing performance.

Assuming that body hydration and muscle glycogen levels are adequate, a successful preexercise strategy is to provide a small amount of carbohydrate (25 to 50 g) along with 6 g of essential amino acids (or 40 g of complete protein) approximately 15 minutes prior to resistance training (146–148). This specific combination of carbohydrates and essential amino acids has been shown to increase muscle protein synthesis 160% more than ingesting the same cocktail postexercise (154). In this case, the exercise bout was for the lower body only (i.e., 10 sets of eight reps of leg press at 80% of 1 RM and 8 sets of eight reps of leg extension at 80% of 1 RM). Interestingly, research from the same lab found that adding nonessential amino acids to the mix does not increase protein synthesis. In other words, only the essential amino acids are needed to promote anabolic processes in muscle (18).

Nutrition during the postexercise period accomplishes three goals: (a) it puts the brakes on protein degradation, (b) it increases muscle protein synthesis, and (c) it rapidly initiates the process of muscle glycogen regeneration. An "optimal" food/beverage has yet to be identified. Based on research conducted over the past few years (13–16, 27,74,88,96,111), however, a carbohydrate-to-protein ratio that ranges from 4:1 to approximately 1:1 may expedite recovery as well as enhance muscle glycogen synthesis *and* net protein status (46, 48,67,68,146–148,161). Athletes should use a lower ratio of carbohydrates to protein when the volume of work (sets times reps) being performed is low, and a higher ratio when the volume of work being performed is high. Practically, this means that athletes interested in increasing lean body mass as well as muscular strength and power should consume a postworkout beverage containing at least 100 cal and as much as 500 cal (and a combination of protein and carbohydrate). It is critical to consume this immediately after training or competition.

Anecdotally, many athletes find that adding 3 to 5 g of creatine and 5 to 10 g of BCAAs to their pre- and/or postworkout beverages provides an enormous benefit.

 Consuming a combination of carbohydrate and protein immediately after exercise will expedite recovery and perhaps improve subsequent performance.

OTHER POTENTIAL ERGOGENIC AIDS

Ergogenic aids will always be a part of sports and athletic performance. A number of additional ergogenic aids become popular from time to time. Myostatin blockers, for example, have been purported to enhance muscle hypertrophy.

Nitric oxide stimulators (arginine and arginine alpha-ketoglutarate) are currently popular to build muscle mass. Up to now, controlled research studies have not demonstrated a benefit from this supplement.

The focus of this chapter has been on legal ergogenic aids, although illegal substances such as anabolic-androgenic steroids are commonly used (Box 18.1).

Q & A from the Field

I've been hearing a lot of talk about using myostatin blockers. I am not familiar with these. What are they, and how effective are they? Do they pose any dangers?

I have seen these supplements in health food stores; they have been marketed with claims that they bind to serum myostatin and inhibit it. Myostatin causes muscle atrophy and wasting. Therefore, myostatin blockers could basically remove the inhibition of muscle growth and allow unlimited potential in muscle mass. One study has recently shown that *Cystoseira canariensis*, a brown sea algae that is the active ingredient in myostatin blockers, does exhibit binding specificity for serum myostatin (118). We have recently shown that *C. canariensis* binds myostatin; however, when combined with heavy weight training, 1,200 mg/day of *C. canariensis* had no effect in reducing the level of serum myostatin or in preferentially increasing muscle strength and mass and decreasing fat mass (163). Therefore, the results from this study suggest that there is no apparent anabolic benefit from ingesting myostatin-blocking supplements.

Myostatin appears to negatively regulate skeletal muscle growth. In the blood, myostatin appears to work in part by slowing down and inhibiting the growth of muscle.

Recent studies with adult rodents showed that antibodies were created against myostatin, increasing total body mass, muscle mass, muscle size, and absolute muscle strength (17). The implication is that a myostatin blocker could conceivably provide benefits as an ergogenic aid or in the treatment of patients with muscle-wasting diseases.

—Darryn Willoughby, PhD, CSCS, FISSN,
Baylor University

Q & A from the Field

A friend in my class says he is taking a supplement containing nitric oxide. He says he has gained 10 lb of muscle in a month. What does research say about nitric oxide stimulators (arginine and arginine alpha-ketoglutarate)? Is there any evidence that they might help athletes gain muscle mass?

The problem here is that you have some fairly complex physiology being thrown around about nitric oxide without any substantive human data showing an effect on exercise performance or body composition. For instance, we know that arginine is an amino acid that participates in the maintenance of muscle and lean tissue throughout the body. It can be converted into ornithine, another amino acid. Its presence can stimulate the release of certain endogenous anabolic hormones, such as growth hormone and insulin-like growth factor. There is supposedly a better-absorbed form of arginine on the market called arginine alpha-ketoglutarate. This supplement is marketed under various names with claims that it accelerates the body's natural production of nitric oxide (NO), vastly augmenting blood flow to muscles. It is also claimed that this product adds new muscle fibers, not muscle water, and that this addition of lean muscle combined with ingestion of the supplement will decrease body fat and enhance recovery. Unfortunately, there appear to be no scientific studies to validate any of these claims. Future research will reveal the effectiveness of this supplement.

Based on the current research, pure arginine may be better and more effective than arginine alpha-ketoglutarate. Arginine has been well researched and has many beneficial effects, especially in terms of cardiovascular health. Its main mechanism of action lies in boosting NO. NO is a signaling molecule within muscle cells that may have many anabolic effects, including increased nutrient transport and vasodilation. Arginine boosts nitric oxide by stimulating nitric oxide synthase, the enzyme that makes NO. Research suggests it may help improve exercise performance, support protein synthesis, boost growth hormone levels at higher doses, and even help replenish postworkout glycogen stores.

OKG (a salt formed from one molecule of alpha-ketoglutarate and two molecules of ornithine) is a metabolic regulator and precursor for glutamine and arginine. Glutamine promotes protein synthesis in skeletal muscle. OKG is also a precursor for other amino acids and ketoacids, which are important for protein synthesis. OKG stimulates the secretion of hormones such as insulin and human growth hormone and has an anabolic effect on muscles. It can also help with ammonia detoxification. This could be of significance, since high levels of ammonia are prevalent among body builders and other athletes. Therefore, OKG has been marketed as a sports supplement for helping to build muscle.

—Darryn Willoughby, PhD, CSCS, FISSN,
Baylor University

18.1 ANABOLIC-ANDROGENIC STEROIDS IN SPORTS

Anabolic-androgenic steroids are synthetic forms of testosterone, the primary male hormone. Testosterone is responsible for both anabolic (muscle growth) and androgenic (secondary sex characteristics) effects that begin at puberty in males. The anabolic and androgenic characteristics of the drug go hand in hand, thus the name anabolic-androgenic steroids (AASs). The androgenic properties of the drug are responsible for many of the negative side effects we have all heard about.

AASs are generally effective in promoting muscle growth. Although some forms of AASs can be obtained as a legal prescription drug for certain medical conditions, they are illegal for possession without a prescription. AASs can be prescribed for males with delayed puberty, inadequate endogenous testosterone production, and individuals with muscle-wasting diseases. AASs are against the rules of most sport governing bodies. Because of their pronounced effect on muscle size and strength, these drugs are widely used and abused by athletes, particularly in strength and power sports.

Abuse of AASs, however, can lead to potentially serious health problems, some irreversible. In addition to using AASs to improve athletic performance, many individuals are using AASs simply to improve physical appearance. Anabolic steroids come in both oral and injectable forms. Athletes, in an attempt to maximize the benefits of AAS use, will cycle the drugs rather than use them continuously. Cycling means taking multiple doses of steroids over a period of time and then going off them for a period of time before starting again. One concern is that athletes often combine several different types of steroids in an effort to maximize their effectiveness and minimize negative effects (referred to as "stacking"). Many of the studies looking at the negative effects of AAS use are looking at the effects of a prescription dose,

not a dose that is stacked and/or cycled. It is quite possible that the larger doses used by athletes would cause the side effects to be even more pronounced.

The side effects from abusing AASs may include liver tumors (usually benign), negative blood lipid changes [increases in low-density-lipoprotein (LDL) (bad) cholesterol, and decreases in high-density-lipoprotein (HDL) (good) cholesterol], fluid retention, high blood pressure, and severe acne. Since AASs are male hormones, they produce different side effects in males, females, and adolescents. In males, common side effects are shrinking testicles, reduced sperm count, infertility, baldness, gynecomastia (breast development) and an increased risk of prostate cancer. In females, anabolic steroids can cause male hair growth patterns on the face and body, male-pattern baldness, enlargement of the clitoris, and a deepened voice. Adolescents may experience premature closure of epiphyseal discs, causing stunted growth. Negative side effects are likely a result of the type of AAS used, the dose and the frequency and duration of use. Notice that males tend to develop feminine side effects and females tend to develop masculine side effects. In males, excess androgens (excess testosterone) are converted to estrogen, a primary female hormone. It is the estrogen production in males that is related to the feminine side effects. Many but not all of the side effects are reversible when the athlete stops taking AAS.

What does all this mean to the strength and conditioning professional? First of all, we should be aware that the athletes we work with may be using AASs to enhance performance or appearance. Second, we must be able to provide sound advice to athletes and parents based on the safety and legality of using AASs. Third, competition and sports should be based on the concept of fair play. The use of AASs by athletes to enhance performance crosses this line.

SUMMARY

Table 18.2 summarizes the main ergogenic aids discussed in this chapter. Strength and conditioning professionals should be aware of the various ergogenic aids potentially available to athletes. The research on a specific substance will likely always be equivocal, as the efficacy of ergogenic aids will be specific to their mechanism of action. Future research should continue to focus on both the safety and efficacy of these substances.

TABLE 18.2	SUMMARY OF ERGOGENIC AIDS				
NUTRIENT/ SUPPLEMENT	ACTIONS	DOSAGE	COMMENTS		REFERENCES
BCAA	May increase fat-free mass; anticatabolic effect; may ameliorate performance decrement.	BCAA (12–14 g/day; 50% L-leucine, 25% L-isoleucine, 25% L-valine)	High dose BCAA supplementation may be ergogenic.		27,131

TABLE 18.2	SUMMARY OF ERGOGENIC AIDS (Continued)			
NUTRIENT/ SUPPLEMENT	**ACTIONS**	**DOSAGE**	**COMMENTS**	**REFERENCES**
Caffeine	Lipolytic agent; increases mental alertness; increases thermogenesis; may enhance performance.	200–400 mg (acute dose)	No longer a banned substance; most commonly consumed drug.	1,6,71,127
Colostrum	May increase LBM; may enhance performance.	20–60 g/day for several weeks	Compared to whey protein, may be more anabolic.	4,21–24,35, 62,75
Creatine	May increase LBM; may enhance performance (i.e., sprints, 1 RM, repeated anaerobic exercise bouts, etc.).	3–5 g/day; for loading phase (if chosen), 20–25 g/day for about a week	Enormous scientific support for ergogenic effect.	12,25,44,45, 139,151–154, 157,171
EAA	May increase muscle protein accretion.	6 g (acute dose increases net muscle protein balance)	Has greater anabolic effects when taken preworkout versus postworkout.	18,93,146, 148,149,167, 168
EGCG	A component of green tea; may increase thermogenesis beyond the normal effects of caffeine.	270 mg/day	May have antioxidant and anticarcinogenic effects; data show enhanced thermogenesis.	43,59,124, 128
Glucosamine	May treat symptoms of osteoarthritis.	1500 mg of glucosamine hydrochloride (GH) and 1200 mg of chondroitin sulfate (CS) daily	May ameliorate symptoms of osteoarthritis.	134
Glutamine	Increases immune function.	6–10 g	May be more effective as immune function supporter in times of severe stress (exercise).	5
Glycerol	May increase time to exhaustion; enhance hydration status.	Preexercise glycerol ingestion (1.2 g/ kg glycerol in 26 mL/ kg solution (94)	Individual responses vary.	37,89,130
HMB	May alleviate the exercise-induced proteolysis and/or muscle damage; may increase muscle mass/function.	3 g/day	May work best in untrained individuals.	101,103
Pre- and postworkout supplements	Increase muscle mass; increase muscle glycogen repletion; increase recovery.	Supplement containing 80 g CHO, 28 g Pro, 6 g fat immediately after exercise (10 minutes)	Timing of ingestion is critical. Need to consume a carbohydrate-protein beverage immediately postexercise.	46,67,68, 85,86

(continued)

TABLE 18.2	SUMMARY OF ERGOGENIC AIDS (Continued)				
NUTRIENT/ SUPPLEMENT	**ACTIONS**	**DOSAGE**	**COMMENTS**	**REFERENCES**
		and 2 hours post-exercise (67); as little as 100 calories may help (48); 6 g of essential amino acids consumed prework-out effective (148)		
Sodium bicarbonate	Buffer the increase in H⁺ ions which increase acidity (lowers pH) and impact fatigue.	0.3 g/kg body weight	Potentially effective in maximal exercise lasting 2–5 minutes; may improve sprint performance.	92,116
Sports drinks	Carbohydrates necessary to maintain blood glucose to delay fatigue; electrolytes (sodium) helps with absorption and complete fluid restoration.	4–8% carbohydrate solution	Dehydration causes decrease in performance; may be only effective when exercise duration exceeds 1 hour; fluid and electrolyte loss due to sweat is variable and dependent upon individual sweat rates; sports drinks without added protein are inadequate for promoting skeletal muscle recovery.	63,90,100

MAXING OUT

1. A football running back for a Division I college football team asks for your advice regarding his nutrition and supplementation program. He currently eats two to three very large meals each day (lunch and dinner). He often skips breakfast because he is not hungry, and he drinks coffee. His meals are mainly fast food (e.g., burgers, fries, and regular cola) as well as pizza and beer on late-night binges. At 5 ft, 10 in. tall, weighing 200 lb, and 18 years of age, he consumes approximately 3,000 calories per day. His workouts for football are quite rigorous, and the day after a game he feels extremely lethargic. He wants to know how he can improve his diet as well as whether supplements might improve his performance and help him gain lean body mass.

2. There are literally thousands of purported ergogenic aids, all of which cannot be covered in a single chapter. Using the Internet or a library resource, investigate a substance you are aware of that is a purported ergogenic aid. Answer the following questions relative to that substance:
   a. Is there a logical "mechanism of action" by which this substance may have a positive effect on human performance?
   b. If this substance were to improve performance, what sports or events would be most likely to be improved?
   c. What information can you find regarding the effectiveness of this ergogenic aid?
   d. What information can you find regarding the safety of this ergogenic aid?

3. It is difficult to address the ethical considerations of using ergogenic aids. Most will agree that there is a line we should not cross in recommending ergogenic aids. Write your own definition of an ergogenic aid. Then make a determination of whether or not these substances should be allowed to be used by athletes under your definition:
   a. Amino acids
   b. Creatine monohydrate
   c. Concentrated glucose replacement beverage

d. Testosterone and related compounds
e. Insulin
f. Insulin-like growth factor
g. Growth hormone
h. Vitamin concentrates

i. Mineral concentrates
j. Coffee and concentrated caffeine beverages or tablets
k. Vitamin B_{12} injections
l. Protein bars

CASE EXAMPLE
Professional Boxer

BACKGROUND

You are a sports nutritionist who has been asked by a professional boxer how to best enhance his performance. He fights in the heavyweight division at 200 lb (he is 6 ft tall and 26 years old). He is preparing for an upcoming fight in 3 months and needs advice on how to improve his punching power/speed relative to nutrition. He is currently working with a top strength and conditioning specialist to improve his conditioning. This upcoming fight is 10 rounds (3-minute rounds), with 1 minute of rest between rounds.

RECOMMENDATIONS/CONSIDERATIONS

Because he is a heavyweight, he can add extra lean body mass and not worry about exceeding a weight limit. Also, he is "light" for a heavyweight boxer and likely needs more lean body mass.

IMPLEMENTATION

Descriptive Information. First get basic information such as height, weight, percentage body fat (skinfolds), age, and training history. Examine past fights to see how he fared at different body weights. Determine, if possible, whether he has an "ideal" boxing weight.

Diet Analysis. Have the subject keep a record of his food intake over the next 7 days to determine whether he is currently meeting his energy needs as well as macronutrient require-

ments. It is important to ensure an adequate intake of protein and essential fatty acids.

Supplements. Is this athlete taking any weight-gain supplements? Again, you can determine this from the interview and his food diary. Perhaps creatine monohydrate supplementation is needed.

Rest. How much rest is the athlete getting?

Conditioning Program. Is he training properly for the fight? Core training? Sports-specific training? Work with his strength and conditioning coach to answer these questions.

RESULTS

Based on the information obtained from this process, you make the following recommendations:

1. Increase daily caloric intake to 4,000 kcals/day, utilizing a weight gain supplement if needed to obtain the desired intake.
2. Maintain a protein intake of 1 g/lb of body weight per day.
3. Consume a preworkout beverage containing essential amino acids plus carbohydrate.
4. Consume a postworkout carbohydrate-protein shake to expedite recovery and promote gains in lean body mass.
5. Consume 3 to 5 g of creatine monohydrate as a daily supplement.
6. Get 7 to 8 hours of sleep every night.

REFERENCES

1. Acheson KJ, Gremaud G, Meirim I, et al. Metabolic effects of caffeine in humans: lipid oxidation or futile cycling? Am J Clin Nutr 2004;79:40–46.
2. Anselme F, Collomp K, Mercier B, et al. Caffeine increases maximal anaerobic power and blood lactate concentration. Eur J Appl Physiol Occup Physiol 1992; 65:188–191.
3. Antonio J, Sanders MS, Ehler LA, et al. Effects of exercise training and amino-acid supplementation on body composition and physical performance in untrained women. Nutrition 2000;16:1043–1046.
4. Antonio J, Sanders MS, Van Gammeren D. The effects of bovine colostrum supplementation on body composition and exercise performance in active men and women. Nutrition 2001;17:243–247.

5. Antonio J, Street C. Glutamine: a potentially useful supplement for athletes. Can J Appl Physiol 1999; 24:1–14.
6. Arciero PJ, Gardner AW, Calles-Escandon J, et al. Effects of caffeine ingestion on NE kinetics, fat oxidation, and energy expenditure in younger and older men. Am J Physiol 1995;268:E1192–1198.
7. Armstrong LE. Caffeine, body fluid-electrolyte balance, and exercise performance. Int J Sport Nutr Exerc Metab 2002;12:189–206.
8. Battram DS, Shearer J, Robinson D, Graham TE. Caffeine ingestion does not impede the resynthesis of proglycogen and macroglycogen after prolonged exercise and carbohydrate supplementation in humans. J Appl Physiol 2004;96:943–950.
9. Bell DG, McLellan TM. Effect of repeated caffeine ingestion on repeated exhaustive exercise endurance. Med Sci Sports Exerc 2003;35:1348–1354.
10. Bell DG, McLellan TM. Exercise endurance 1, 3, and 6 h after caffeine ingestion in caffeine users and nonusers. J Appl Physiol 2002;93:1227–1234.
11. Berger R, Middelanis J, Vaihinger HM, et al. Creatine protects the immature brain from hypoxic-ischemic injury. J Soc Gynecol Invest 2004;11:9–15.
12. Bermon S, Venembre P, Sachet C, et al. Effects of creatine monohydrate ingestion in sedentary and weight-trained older adults. Acta Physiol Scand 1998;164:147–155.
13. Blomstrand E, Ek S, Newsholme EA. Influence of ingesting a solution of branched-chain amino acids on plasma and muscle concentrations of amino acids during prolonged submaximal exercise. Nutrition 1996;12:485–490.
14. Blomstrand E, Hassmen P, Ek S, et al. Influence of ingesting a solution of branched-chain amino acids on perceived exertion during exercise. Acta Physiol Scand 1997;159:41–49.
15. Blomstrand E, Hassmen P, Ekblom B, Newsholme EA. Administration of branched-chain amino acids during sustained exercise—effects on performance and on plasma concentration of some amino acids. Eur J Appl Physiol Occup Physiol 1991;63:83–88.
16. Blomstrand E, Saltin B. BCAA intake affects protein metabolism in muscle after but not during exercise in humans. Am J Physiol Endocrinol Metab 2001;281: E365–E374.
17. Bogdanovich S, Krag TO, Barton ER, et al. Functional improvement of dystrophic muscle by myostatin blockade. Nature 2002;420:418–421.
18. Borsheim E, Tipton KD, Wolf SE, Wolfe RR. Essential amino acids and muscle protein recovery from resistance exercise. Am J Physiol Endocrinol Metab 2002; 283:E648–E657.
19. Boyer M, Rees S, Quinn J, et al. Caffeine as a performance-enhancing drug in rats: sex, dose, housing, and task considerations. Percept Mot Skills 2003;97:259–270.
20. Braham R, Dawson B, Goodman C. The effect of glucosamine supplementation on people experiencing regular knee pain. Br J Sports Med 2003;37:45–49; discussion 49.
21. Brinkworth GD, Buckley JD. Bovine colostrum supplementation does not affect plasma buffer capacity or haemoglobin content in elite female rowers. Eur J Appl Physiol 2004;91:353–356.
22. Brinkworth GD, Buckley JD, Bourdon PC, et al. Oral bovine colostrum supplementation enhances buffer capacity but not rowing performance in elite female rowers. Int J Sport Nutr Exerc Metab 2002;12:349–365.
23. Buckley JD, Abbott MJ, Brinkworth GD, Whyte PB. Bovine colostrum supplementation during endurance running training improves recovery, but not performance. J Sci Med Sport 2002;5:65–79.
24. Buckley JD, Brinkworth GD, Abbott MJ. Effect of bovine colostrum on anaerobic exercise performance and plasma insulin-like growth factor I. J Sports Sci 2003;21:577–588.
25. Burke DG, Chilibeck PD, Davidson KS, et al. The effect of whey protein supplementation with and without creatine monohydrate combined with resistance training on lean tissue mass and muscle strength. Int J Sport Nutr Exerc Metab 2001;11:349–364.
26. Campbell WW, Trappe TA, Jozsi AC, et al. Dietary protein adequacy and lower body versus whole body resistive training in older humans. J Physiol 2002;542:631–642.
27. Candeloro N, Bertini I, Melchiorri G, De Lorenzo A. [Effects of prolonged administration of branched-chain amino acids on body composition and physical fitness]. Minerva Endocrinol 1995;20:217–223.
28. Castell LM. Can glutamine modify the apparent immunodepression observed after prolonged, exhaustive exercise. Nutrition 2002;18:371–375.
29. Cauli O, Pinna A, Valentini V, Morelli M. Subchronic caffeine exposure induces sensitization to caffeine and cross-sensitization to amphetamine ipsilateral turning behavior independent from dopamine release. Neuropsychopharmacology 2003;28:1752–1759.
30. Cheung WT, Lee CM, Ng TB. Potentiation of the antilipolytic effect of 2-chloroadenosine after chronic caffeine treatment. Pharmacology 1988;36:331–339.
31. Coggan AR, Coyle EF. Carbohydrate ingestion during prolonged exercise: effects on metabolism and performance. Exerc Sport Sci Rev 1991;19:1–40.
32. Collomp K, Ahmaidi S, Chatard JC, et al. Benefits of caffeine ingestion on sprint performance in trained and untrained swimmers. Eur J Appl Physiol Occup Physiol 1992;64:377–380.
33. Collomp K, Candau R, Millet G, et al. Effects of salbutamol and caffeine ingestion on exercise metabolism and performance. Int J Sports Med 2002;23:549–554.
34. Conway KJ, Orr R, Stannard SR. Effect of a divided caffeine dose on endurance cycling performance, postexercise urinary caffeine concentration, and plasma paraxanthine. J Appl Physiol 2003;94:1557–1562.
35. Coombes JS, Conacher M, Austen SK, Marshall PA. Dose effects of oral bovine colostrum on physical work capacity in cyclists. Med Sci Sports Exerc 2002;34:1184–1188.
36. Costill D, Hargreaves M. Carbohydrate nutrition and fatigue. Sports Med 1992;13:86–92.
37. Coutts A, Reaburn P, Mummery K, Holmes M. The effect of glycerol hyperhydration on olympic distance triathlon performance in high ambient temperatures. Int J Sport Nutr Exerc Metab 2002;12:105–119.
38. Cox GR, Desbrow B, Montgomery PG, et al. Effect of different protocols of caffeine intake on metabolism and endurance performance. J Appl Physiol 2002;93: 990–999.

39. Coyle EF, Montain SJ. Benefits of fluid replacement with carbohydrate during exercise. Med Sci Sports Exerc 1992;24: S324–S330.

40. Coyle EF, Hagberg JM, Hurley BF, Martin WH. Carbohydrate feeding during prolonged strenuous exercise can delay fatigue. J Appl Physiol 1983;55:30–35.

41. Davis JM, Zhao Z, Stock HS, et al. Central nervous system effects of caffeine and adenosine on fatigue. Am J Physiol Regul Integr Comp Physiol 2003;284: R399–R404.

42. Doherty M, Smith PM, Davison RC, Hughes MG. Caffeine is ergogenic after supplementation of oral creatine monohydrate. Med Sci Sports Exerc 2002;34:1785–1792.

43. Dulloo AG, Duret C, Rohrer D, et al. Efficacy of a green tea extract rich in catechin polyphenols and caffeine in increasing 24-h energy expenditure and fat oxidation in humans. Am J Clin Nutr 1999;70:1040–1045.

44. Earnest CP, Snell PG, Rodriguez R, et al. The effect of creatine monohydrate ingestion on anaerobic power indices, muscular strength and body composition. Acta Physiol Scand 1995;153:207–209.

45. Eckerson JM, Stout JR, Moore GA, et al. Effect of two and five days of creatine loading on anaerobic working capacity in women. J Strength Cond Res 2004;18: 168–173.

46. Esmarck B, Andersen JL, Olsen S, et al. Timing of post-exercise protein intake is important for muscle hypertrophy with resistance training in elderly humans. J Physiol 2001;535:301–311.

47. Ferrando AA, Paddon-Jones D, Wolfe RR. Alterations in protein metabolism during space flight and inactivity. Nutrition 2002;18:837–841.

48. Flakoll PJ, Judy T, Flinn K, et al. Postexercise protein supplementation improves health and muscle soreness during basic military training in marine recruits. J Appl Physiol 2004;96:951–956.

49. Greenhaff PL. Creatine and its application as an ergogenic aid. Int J Sport Nutr 1995;5(Suppl):S100–S110.

50. Greenhaff PL. Creatine supplementation: recent developments. Br J Sports Med 1996;30:276–277.

51. Greenhaff PL. The creatine-phosphocreatine system: there's more than one song in its repertoire. J Physiol 2001;537:657.

52. Greenhaff PL, Bodin K, Soderlund K, Hultman E. Effect of oral creatine supplementation on skeletal muscle phosphocreatine resynthesis. Am J Physiol 1994;266: E725–E730.

53. Greenhaff PL, Casey A, Short AH, et al. Influence of oral creatine supplementation of muscle torque during repeated bouts of maximal voluntary exercise in man. Clin Sci (Lond) 1993;84:565–571.

54. Greenhaff PL, Nevill ME, Soderlund K, et al. The metabolic responses of human type I and II muscle fibres during maximal treadmill sprinting. J Physiol 1994; 478(Pt 1):149–155.

55. Greenhaff PL, Ren JM, Soderlund K, Hultman E. Energy metabolism in single human muscle fibers during contraction without and with epinephrine infusion. Am J Physiol 1991;260:E713–E718.

56. Greenleaf JE, Sargent F. Voluntary dehydration in man. J Appl Physiol 1965;20:719–724.

57. Gruber AJ, Pope HG Jr. Compulsive weight lifting and anabolic drug abuse among women rape victims. Comp Psychiatry 1999;40:273–277.

58. Gruber AJ, Pope HG Jr. Psychiatric and medical effects of anabolic-androgenic steroid use in women. Psychother Psychosom 2000;69:19–26.

59. Hakim IA, Harris RB, Brown S, et al. Effect of increased tea consumption on oxidative DNA damage among smokers: a randomized controlled study. J Nutr 2003; 133:3303S–3309S.

60. Hasegawa N, Niimi N, Odani F. Vitamin C is one of the lipolytic substances in green tea. Phytother Res 2002; 16(Suppl 1):S91–S92.

61. Hetzler RK, Knowlton RG, Somani SM, et al. Effect of paraxanthine on FFA mobilization after intravenous caffeine administration in humans. J Appl Physiol 1990;68:44–47.

62. Hofman Z, Smeets R, Verlaan G, et al. The effect of bovine colostrum supplementation on exercise performance in elite field hockey players. Int J Sport Nutr Exerc Metab 2002;12:461–469.

63. Holzmeister LA. Sports and energy drinks. Diabetes Self Mgtg 2003;20:96–97, 99–100, 102–103.

64. Hultman E, Soderlund K, Timmons JA, et al. Muscle creatine loading in men. J Appl Physiol 1996;81:232–237.

65. Hunter AM, St Clair Gibson A, Collins M, et al. Caffeine ingestion does not alter performance during a 100-km cycling time-trial performance. Int J Sport Nutr Exerc Metab 2002;12:438–452.

66. Ikeda K, Iwasaki Y, Kinoshita M. Oral administration of creatine monohydrate retards progression of motor neuron disease in the wobbler mouse. Amyotroph Lateral Scler Other Motor Neuron Disord 2000;1:207–212.

67. Ivy JL, Goforth HW Jr, Damon BM, et al. Early post-exercise muscle glycogen recovery is enhanced with a carbohydrate-protein supplement. J Appl Physiol 2002; 93:1337–1344.

68. Ivy JL, Res PT, Sprague RC, Widzer MO. Effect of a carbohydrate-protein supplement on endurance performance during exercise of varying intensity. Int J Sport Nutr Exerc Metab 2003;13:382–395.

69. Izawa T, Koshimizu E, Komabayashi T, Tsuboi M. [Effects of Ca^{2+} and calmodulin inhibitors on lipolysis induced by epinephrine, norepinephrine, caffeine and ACTH in rat epididymal adipose tissue]. Nippon Seirigaku Zasshi 1983;45:36–44.

70. Jacobs I, Pasternak H, Bell DG. Effects of ephedrine, caffeine, and their combination on muscular endurance. Med Sci Sports Exerc 2003;35:987–994.

71. Jiang M, Kameda K, Han LK, et al. Isolation of lipolytic substances caffeine and 1,7-dimethylxanthine from the stem and rhizome of Sinomenium actum. Planta Med 1998;64:375–377.

72. Jones HE, Griffiths RR. Oral caffeine maintenance potentiates the reinforcing and stimulant subjective effects of intravenous nicotine in cigarette smokers. Psychopharmacology (Berl) 2003;165:280–290.

73. Jowko E, Ostaszewski P, Jank M, et al. Creatine and beta-hydroxy-beta-methylbutyrate (HMB) additively increase lean body mass and muscle strength during a weight-training program. Nutrition 2001;17:558–566.

74. Karlsson HK, Nilsson PA, Nilsson J, et al. Branched-chain amino acids increase p70S6k phosphorylation in human skeletal muscle after resistance exercise. Am J Physiol Endocrinol Metab 2004;287:E1–E7.

75. Kelly GS. Bovine colostrums: a review of clinical uses. Alt Med Rev 2003;8:378–394.

76. Komura K, Hobbiebrunken E, Wilichowski EK, Hanefeld FA. Effectiveness of creatine monohydrate in mitochondrial encephalomyopathies. Pediatr Neurol 2003; 28:53–58.

77. Kraemer WJ, Volek JS. Creatine supplementation. Its role in human performance. Clin Sports Med 1999;18: 651–666, ix.

78. Kreider RB. Dietary supplements and the promotion of muscle growth with resistance exercise. Sports Medicine 1999;27:97–110.

79. Kreider RB, Ferreira M, Wilson M, Almada AL. Effects of calcium beta-hydroxy-beta-methylbutyrate (HMB) supplementation during resistance-training on markers of catabolism, body composition and strength. Int J Sports Med 1999;20:503–509.

80. Kreider RB, Melton C, Rasmussen CJ, et al. Long-term creatine supplementation does not significantly affect clinical markers of health in athletes. Mol Cell Biochem 2003;244:95–104.

81. Lambert CP, Archer RL, Carrithers JA, et al. Influence of creatine monohydrate ingestion on muscle metabolites and intense exercise capacity in individuals with multiple sclerosis. Arch Phys Med Rehabil 2003;84: 1206–1210.

82. Latzka WA, Sawka MN. Hyperhydration and glycerol: thermoregulatory effects during exercise in hot climates. Can J Appl Physiol 2000;25:536–545.

83. Layman DK, Baum JI. Dietary protein impact on glycemic control during weight loss. J Nutr 2004;134: 968S–973S.

84. Leit RA, Pope HG Jr, Gray JJ. Cultural expectations of muscularity in men: the evolution of playgirl centerfolds. Int J Eat Disord 2001;29:90–93.

85. Levenhagen DK, Carr C, Carlson MG, et al. Postexercise protein intake enhances whole-body and leg protein accretion in humans. Med Sci Sports Exerc 2002;34: 828–837.

86. Levenhagen DK, Gresham JD, Carlson MG, et al. Postexercise nutrient intake timing in humans is critical to recovery of leg glucose and protein homeostasis. Am J Physiol Endocrinol Metab 2001;280:E982–E993.

87. Lorist MM, Tops M. Caffeine, fatigue, and cognition. Brain Cogn 2003;53:82–94.

88. Madsen K, MacLean DA, Kiens B, Christensen D. Effects of glucose, glucose plus branched-chain amino acids, or placebo on bike performance over 100 km. J Appl Physiol 1996;81:2644–2650.

89. Magal M, Webster MJ, Sistrunk LE, et al. Comparison of glycerol and water hydration regimens on tennis-related performance. Med Sci Sports Exerc 2003;35: 150–156.

90. Maughan RJ, Leiper JB. Limitations to fluid replacement during exercise. Can J Appl Physiol 1999;24:173–187.

91. Mayo Clinic. Caffeine content of common beverages. Available at http://www.mayoclinic.com/health/drug-information/DR202105. Accessed June 26, 2006.

92. McNaughton L, Thompson D. Acute versus chronic sodium bicarbonate ingestion and anaerobic work and power output. J Sports Med Phys Fitness 2001;41: 456–462.

93. Miller SL, Tipton KD, Chinkes DL, et al. Independent and combined effects of amino acids and glucose after resistance exercise. Med Sci Sports Exerc 2003;35:449–455.

94. Montner P, Stark DM, Riedesel ML, et al. Pre-exercise glycerol hydration improves cycling endurance time. Int J Sports Med 1996;17:27–33.

95. Motl RW, O'Connor PJ, Dishman RK. Effect of caffeine on perceptions of leg muscle pain during moderate intensity cycling exercise. J Pain 2003;4:316–321.

96. Mourier A, Bigard AX, de Kerviler E, et al. Combined effects of caloric restriction and branched-chain amino acid supplementation on body composition and exercise performance in elite wrestlers. Int J Sports Med 1997;18:47–55.

97. Murphy JA, Deurveilher S, Semba K. Stimulant doses of caffeine induce c-FOS activation in orexin/hypocretin-containing neurons in rat. Neuroscience 2003;121: 269–275.

98. Murray R, Paul GL, Seifert JG, Eddy DE. Responses to varying rates of carbohydrate ingestion during exercise. Med Sci Sports Exerc 1991;23:713–718.

99. Nakamura T, Sugino K, Titani K, Sugino H. Follistatin, an activin-binding protein, associates with heparan sulfate chains of proteoglycans on follicular granulosa cells. J Biol Chem 1991;266:19432–19437.

100. Nicholas CW, Tsintzas K, Boobis L, Williams C. Carbohydrate-electrolyte ingestion during intermittent high-intensity running. Med Sci Sports Exerc 1999;31: 1280–1286.

101. Nissen SL, Sharp RL. Effect of dietary supplements on lean mass and strength gains with resistance exercise: a meta-analysis. J Appl Physiol 2003;94:651–659.

102. Nissen S, Sharp RL, Panton L, et al. Beta-hydroxy-beta-methylbutyrate (HMB) supplementation in humans is safe and may decrease cardiovascular risk factors. J Nutr 2000;130:1937–1945.

103. Nissen S, Sharp R, Ray M, et al. Effect of leucine metabolite beta-hydroxy-beta-methylbutyrate on muscle metabolism during resistance-exercise training. J Appl Physiol 1996;81:2095–2104.

104. Nissen S, Van Koevering M, Webb D. Analysis of beta-hydroxy-beta-methyl butyrate in plasma by gas chromatography and mass spectrometry. Anal Biochem 1990;188:17–19.

105. Noakes TD. Fluid replacement during exercise. Exerc Sport Sci Rev 1993;21:297–330.

106. Olivardia R, Pope HG Jr, Hudson JI. Muscle dysmorphia in male weightlifters: a case-control study. Am J Psychiatry 2000;157:1291–1296.

107. Paluska SA. Caffeine and exercise. Curr Sports Med Rep 2003;2:213–219.

108. Phillips KA, O'Sullivan RL, Pope HG Jr. Muscle dysmorphia. J Clin Psychiatry 1997;58:361.

109. Phillips SM, Parise G, Roy BD, et al. Resistance-training-induced adaptations in skeletal muscle protein turnover in the fed state. Can J Physiol Pharmacol 2002;80:1045–1053.

110. Piattoly T, Welsch MA. L-Glutamine supplementation: effects on recovery from exercise. Med Sci Sports Exerc 2004; 36:S127.

111. Platell C, Kong SE, McCauley R, Hall JC. Branched-chain amino acids. J Gastroenterol Hepatol 2000;15:706–717.

112. Poortmans JR, Francaux M. Long-term oral creatine supplementation does not impair renal function in healthy athletes. Med Sci Sports Exerc 1999;31:1108–1110.

113. Pope HG Jr, Gruber AJ, Choi P, et al. Muscle dysmorphia. An underrecognized form of body dysmorphic disorder. Psychosomatics 1997;38:548–557.

114. Pope HG Jr, Gruber AJ, Mangweth B, et al. Body image perception among men in three countries. Am J Psychiatry 2000;157:1297–1301.

115. Powers SK, Dodd S. Caffeine and endurance performance. Sports Med 1985;2:165–174.

116. Price M, Moss P, Rance S. Effects of sodium bicarbonate ingestion on prolonged intermittent exercise. Med Sci Sports Exerc 2003;35:1303–1308.

117. Rae C, Digney AL, McEwan SR, Bates TC. Oral creatine monohydrate supplementation improves brain performance: a double-blind, placebo-controlled, cross-over trial. Proc R Soc Lond B Biol Sci 2003;270:2147–2150.

118. Ramazov, Z, Jimenez del Rio M, Ziegenfuss T. Sulfated polysaccharides of brown seaweed Cystoseira canariensis bind to serum myostatin protein. Acta Physiol Pharmacol 2003;27:1–6.

119. Rennie MJ. Amino acid transport in heart and skeletal muscle and the functional consequences. Biochem Soc Trans 1996;24:869–873.

120. Rennie MJ. Glutamine metabolism and transport in skeletal muscle and heart and their clinical relevance. J Nutr 1996;126:1142S–1149S.

121. Rennie MJ, Low SY, Taylor PM, et al. Amino acid transport during muscle contraction and its relevance to exercise. Adv Exp Med Biol 1998;441:299–305.

122. Richy F, Bruyere O, Ethgen O, et al. Structural and symptomatic efficacy of glucosamine and chondroitin in knee osteoarthritis: a comprehensive meta-analysis. Arch Intern Med 2003;163:1514–1522.

123. Riedesel ML, Allen DY, Peake GT, Al-Qattan K. Hyperhydration with glycerol solutions. J Appl Physiol 1987; 63:2262–2268.

124. Rietveld A, Wiseman S. Antioxidant effects of tea: evidence from human clinical trials. J Nutr 2003;133: 3285S–3292S.

125. Robergs RA, Griffin SE. Glycerol. Biochemistry, pharmacokinetics and clinical and practical applications. Sports Med 1998;26:145–167.

126. Ryan L, Hatfield C, Hofstetter M. Caffeine reduces time-of-day effects on memory performance in older adults. Psychol Sci 2002;13:68–71.

127. Ryu S, Choi SK, Joung SS, et al. Caffeine as a lipolytic food component increases endurance performance in rats and athletes. J Nutr Sci Vitaminol (Tokyo) 2001; 47:139–146.

128. Saffari Y, Sadrzadeh SM. Green tea metabolite EGCG protects membranes against oxidative damage in vitro. Life Sci 2004;74:1513–1518.

129. Schardt, D, Schmidt, S. Caffeine, the inside scoop. Nutrition Action Healthletter, December, 1996.

130. Scheett TP, Webster MJ, Wagoner KD. Effectiveness of glycerol as a rehydrating agent. Int J Sport Nutr Exerc Metab 2001;11:63–71.

131. Schena F, Guerrini F, Tregnaghi P, Kayser B. Branched-chain amino acid supplementation during trekking at high altitude. The effects on loss of body mass, body composition, and muscle power. Eur J Appl Physiol Occup Physiol 1992;65:394–398.

132. Schoffstall JE et al. Effects of dehydration and rehydration on the one-repetition maximum bench press of weight-trained males. J Strength Cond Res 2001;15:102–108.

133. Schedl HP, Maughan RJ, Gisolfi CV. Intestinal absorption during rest and exercise: implications for formulating an oral rehydration solution (ORS). Med Sci Sports Exerc 1994;26:267–280.

134. Segal L, Day SE, Chapman AB, Osborne RH. Can we reduce disease burden from osteoarthritis? Med J Aust 2004;180:S11–S17.

135. Slater GJ, Jenkins D. Beta-hydroxy-beta-methylbutyrate (HMB) supplementation and the promotion of muscle growth and strength. Sports Med 2000;30:105–116.

136. Steenge GR, Verhoef P, Greenhaff PL. The effect of creatine and resistance training on plasma homocysteine concentration in healthy volunteers. Arch Intern Med 2001;161:1455–1456.

137. Stevenson SW, Dudley GA. Creatine loading, resistance exercise performance, and muscle mechanics. J Strength Cond Res 2001;15:413–419.

138. Stine MM, O'Connor RJ, Yatko BR, et al. Evidence for a relationship between daily caffeine consumption and accuracy of time estimation. Hum Psychopharmacol 2002;17:361–367.

139. Stout J, Eckerson J, Ebersole K, et al. Effect of creatine loading on neuromuscular fatigue threshold. J Appl Physiol 2000;88:109–112.

140. Stout JR, Eckerson JM, May E, et al. Effects of resistance exercise and creatine supplementation on myasthenia gravis: a case study. Med Sci Sports Exerc 2001;33: 869–872.

141. Takamata A, Mack GW, Gillen CM, Nadel ER. Sodium appetite, thirst, and body fluid regulation in humans during rehydration without sodium replacement. Am J Physiol 1994;266:R1493–R1502.

142. Tarnopolsky MA, Beal MF. Potential for creatine and other therapies targeting cellular energy dysfunction in neurological disorders. Ann Neurol 2001;49:561–574.

143. Tarnopolsky MA, MacLennan DP. Creatine monohydrate supplementation enhances high-intensity exercise performance in males and females. Int J Sport Nutr Exerc Metab 2000;10:452–463.

144. Tarnopolsky MA, Parise G, Yardley NJ, et al. Creatine-dextrose and protein-dextrose induce similar strength gains during training. Med Sci Sports Exerc 2001;33: 2044–2052.

145. Terjung RL, Clarkson P, Eichner ER, et al. American College of Sports Medicine roundtable. The physiological and health effects of oral creatine supplementation. Med Sci Sports Exerc 2000;32:706–717.

146. Tipton KD, Borsheim E, Wolf SE, et al. Acute response of net muscle protein balance reflects 24-h balance after exercise and amino acid ingestion. Am J Physiol Endocrinol Metab 2003;284:E76–E89.

147. Tipton KD, Ferrando AA, Phillips SM, et al. Postexercise net protein synthesis in human muscle from orally administered amino acids. Am J Physiol 1999;276: E628–E634.

148. Tipton KD, Rasmussen BB, Miller SL, et al. Timing of amino acid-carbohydrate ingestion alters anabolic response of muscle to resistance exercise. Am J Physiol Endocrinol Metab 2001;281:E197–E206.

149. Tipton KD, Wolfe RR. Exercise, protein metabolism, and muscle growth. Int J Sport Nutr Exerc Metab 2001; 11:109–132.

150. Varnier M et al. Stimulatory effect of glutamine on glycogen accumulation in human skeletal muscle. Am J Physiol 1995;269:E309–E315.

151. Volek JS, Duncan ND, Mazzetti SA, et al. Performance and muscle fiber adaptations to creatine supplementation and heavy resistance training. Med Sci Sports Exerc 1999;31:1147–1156.

152. Volek JS, Kraemer WJ, Bush JA, et al. Creatine supplementation enhances muscular performance during high-intensity resistance exercise. J Am Diet Assoc 1997;97: 765–770.

153. Volek JS, Ratamess NA, Rubin MR, et al. The effects of creatine supplementation on muscular performance and body composition responses to short-term resistance training overreaching. Eur J Appl Physiol 2004; 91:628–637.

154. Volek JS, Rawson ES. Scientific basis and practical aspects of creatine supplementation for athletes. Nutrition 2004;20:609–614.

155. Vorgerd M, Grehl T, Jager M, et al. Creatine therapy in myophosphorylase deficiency (McArdle disease): a placebo-controlled crossover trial. Arch Neurol 2000; 57:956–963.

156. Wagner DR. Hyperhydrating with glycerol: implications for athletic performance. J Am Diet Assoc 1999;99: 207–212.

157. Warber JP, Tharion WJ, Patton JF, et al. The effect of creatine monohydrate supplementation on obstacle course and multiple bench press performance. J Strength Cond Res 2002;16:500–508.

158. Watsford ML, Murphy AJ, Spinks WL, Walshe AD. Creatine supplementation and its effect on musculotendinous stiffness and performance. J Strength Cond Res 2003;17:26–33.

159. Webster S et al. Physiological effects of a weight loss regimen practiced by college wrestlers. Med Sci Sports Exerc 1990;22:229–234.

160. Wiedermann D, Schneider J, Fromme A, et al. Creatine loading and resting skeletal muscle phosphocreatine flux: a saturation-transfer NMR study. Magma 2001;13: 118–126.

161. Williams MB, Raven PB, Fogt DL, Ivy JL. Effects of recovery beverages on glycogen restoration and endurance exercise performance. J Strength Cond Res 2003;17: 12–19.

162. Williams MH, Branch JD. Creatine supplementation and exercise performance: an update. J Am Coll Nutr 1998;17:216–234.

163. Willoughby DS. Effects of an alleged myostatin binding supplement and heavy resistance training on serum myostatin, muscle strength and mass, and body composition. Int J Sports Nutr Exerc Metab. In press.

164. Willoughby DS, Rosene JM. Effects of oral creatine and resistance training on myogenic regulatory factor expression. Med Sci Sports Exerc 2003;35:923–929.

165. Willoughby DS, Rosene J. Effects of oral creatine and resistance training on myosin heavy chain expression. Med Sci Sports Exerc 2001;33:1674–1681.

166. Wingo JE, Casa DJ, Berger EM, et al. Influence of a pre-exercise glycerol hydration beverage on performance and physiologic function during mountain-bike races in the heat. J Athlet Train 2004;39:169–175.

167. Wolfe RR. Control of muscle protein breakdown: effects of activity and nutritional states. Int J Sport Nutr Exerc Metab 2001;11(Suppl):S164–S169.

168. Wolfe RR. Effects of amino acid intake on anabolic processes. Can J Appl Physiol 2001;26(Suppl):S220–S227.

169. World Anti-Doping Agency. The World Anti-Doping Code: The 2006 Prohibited List International Standard. Available at http://www.wada-ama.org/rtecontent/document/2006_LIST.pdf. Accessed June 26, 2006.

170. Zhang Y, Wells JN. The effects of chronic caffeine administration on peripheral adenosine receptors. J Pharmacol Exp Ther 1990;254:757–763.

171. Ziegenfuss TN, Rogers M, Lowery L, et al. Effect of creatine loading on anaerobic performance and skeletal muscle volume in NCAA Division I athletes. Nutrition 2002;18:397–402.

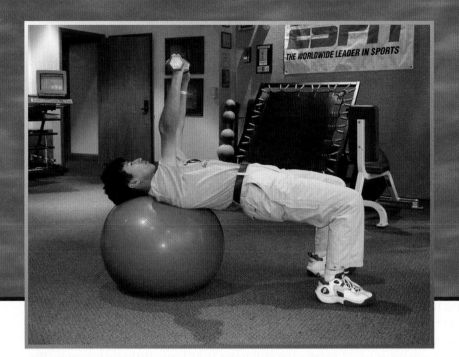

Implement Training

ALLEN HEDRICK

Introduction

In today's world of competitive athletics, a tremendous emphasis is placed on strength and conditioning as a method to improve athletic performance. More and more frequently, financial resources are being directed toward building bigger and better strength and conditioning facilities. Further, through education and professional organizations, the knowledge base of strength and conditioning coaches continues to improve.

Resistance training is viewed as a necessary aspect of the overall program designed to improve athletic performance.

SIMILARITY IN TRAINING PROGRAMS

Although there are exceptions, the majority of athletic strength and conditioning programs today emphasize free weights as their preferred training method (4,18,21,25). Further, many of those programs emphasizing free-weight training put a priority on performance of the Olympic-style exercises (17,9,19). In addition, most strength and conditioning coaches adhere to the concept of periodization, organizing their training programs into cycles so that each cycle has a specific physiological goal, with the ultimate goal being to bring their athletes to a peak at the appropriate point in the competitive calendar (2,14,15,23). Although there are variations in the periodization model from program to program, a review of training programs being used in strength and conditioning facilities across the country would likely reveal strong similarities in program design from facility to facility.

What this means is that there are a significant number of athletes training in high-quality facilities who are being directed by well-educated strength and conditioning professionals employing programs that have similarities in design. As a result, it becomes difficult to give athletes a significant competitive edge through their strength and conditioning programs. The challenge for the strength and conditioning coach is to find ways to enhance their strength and conditioning programs so that their athletes have an advantage during competition.

The majority of strength and conditioning coaches accentuate free-weight training and performance of the Olympic-style exercises following a periodized training program. As a result, it is difficult to give athletes a competitive advantage.

RELYING ON SCIENCE

The field of sports science has dramatically grown in terms of the amount of research being conducted to evaluate a wide spectrum of topics related to performance training. Because of this it is important that the strength and conditioning coach take advantage of the available information and apply it whenever possible. Certainly the majority of any training program should be based on what sports science has determined to be the best approach to

achieving the desired performance goal. For example, research tells us (5) that periodized training is superior to nonperiodized training in attempting to bring about further increases in strength and power in trained athletes. As a result, as previously mentioned, the vast majority of athletic strength and conditioning programs adhere to the concept of periodization.

 Because of the vast spectrum of research occurring in the area of sports science, the majority of any training program should be based on science.

Lack of Implement-Training Research

Areas related to training to improve athletic performance still exist that have little or no scientific evidence to support or refute them. One area of sports performance training that is lacking scientific research is the value of training with **implements** (nonstandard resistance-training tools, such as kegs and tires) other than the traditional barbell, dumbbell, or strength training machines. Based on a review of literature, little if any research has been conducted evaluating the effectiveness of training with nonstandard equipment, such as tires, logs, kegs, stones, and similar, for lack of a better term, strongman-type implements.

 One area that is lacking research is the value of performing strength training with nontraditional resistance training implements.

TRAINING PRINCIPLES

Despite this lack of research, the same principles that apply to traditional training methods can be used to guide the use of implement training. Perhaps most important is the concept of training movements, not muscle groups (13,20,22,23). That is, increases in strength and/or power will occur primarily in the movement used during training. That is why it is important to think in terms of training a specific movement and not an individual muscle.

Whenever a strength and conditioning coach considers the use of a new training mode, such as those described in this chapter, transfer specificity must be considered. This relates to the percentage of carryover from the training activity to the sport or activity for which the individual is training.

Q & A from the Field

Differences of opinion exist in the field about training modalities and the use of various implements. Many of the implements lack a solid foundation in the research literature in terms of effectiveness. Should we, as professionals, be concerned about that fact? How should we deal with questions about the lack of research when speaking with administrators, coaches, and parents?

Admittedly, there is a lack of research on many of the implements discussed in this chapter. Does that mean we must wait for that research to be done before using these implements? Not really. As long as we apply safe and effective principles of training, implement training can be safely added to any training program. To justify the exercise as related to a specific sport, the concepts of specificity and transferability can be used.

Future research will provide additional evidence related to the effectiveness of the various implements discussed in this chapter. As professionals, even though we do not need to wait on that research to utilize these innovative methods of training, we must keep up with new research and be willing to adjust our training programs accordingly. We must also consider the entire body of research on a specific topic. A single study is unlikely to "prove" or "disprove" the effectiveness of a single training implement.

Optimal training for the individual must maximize the transfer or carryover of trainable characteristics from the training activities to the specific activity or sport performance (3).

Performing a complex, multijoint movement helps establish a neural pathway so that all the muscles involved in the movement work in a synchronized pattern. An example of this is an offensive lineman exploding out from a three-point stance. The primary actions involved in this movement involve knee and hip extension, plantarflexion, shoulder flexion, and elbow extension. The movement would be similar to what occurs in flipping a tractor tire (discussed below) (24).

In contrast, the more dissimilar the movement pattern is to the target sport or activity, the less valuable such training becomes. As a result, it becomes obvious that activities such as a fireman's carry, where the athlete is carrying a heavy implement in each hand over a prescribed distance or time, does not transfer well to most athletic activities except perhaps as a method of achieving a general anaerobic training effect. Similarly, lifting heavy stones and placing them on an elevated stand, because of the risk of injury and need for strict technique, may represent time better spent in performing more traditional type training.

Although there is a lack of research evaluating implement training, the same principles that are applicable to conventional training modes can be applied to implement training.

Transferability of Implement Training to Sports Performance

On the other hand, some nontraditional training can transfer very effectively to athletic performance, and its inclusion in an athletic strength and conditioning program can be of value for two primary reasons. First, the movement pattern can be similar to the movement pattern seen during competition (for example, the movement of flipping a tire transfers well to blocking, tackling, jumping, and so on). Second, implement training increases the variation in training, reducing the physiological and psychological staleness that can arise when performing the same strength training movements repetitively.

Some nontraditional training methods can be used to effectively train sport-specific movements and provide variation in the training program.

Water-Filled Implements

One implement training method that theoretically seems as if it could be of significant value in the training programs of certain types of athletes (i.e., football, hockey, wrestling) is the use of water-filled implements. **Water-filled implements** are objects such as kegs or specially designed training logs or dumbbells where the majority of the resistance is provided by water contained within the object. Water as a form of resistance represents a unique training stimulus because it provides **active fluid resistance**; that is, the water is constantly moving during performance of the exercise and thus provides an active rather than a static resistance (10,11). Contrast that to a typical exercise where the resistance (in the form of either a weight stack or a barbell) is relatively static and therefore very little if any extraneous movement is occurring.

Unfortunately little if any research evaluates the value of training with an active fluid resistance. But applying the concept of specificity, it makes sense that training with an active fluid resistance provides a highly sport-specific method of training for certain types of athletes as compared

to lifting exclusively with a static resistance, because in many situations athletes encounter dynamic resistance in the form of an opponent as compared to a static resistance. Further, because the active fluid resistance enhances the need for stability and control, this type of training may reduce the opportunity for injury because of improved joint stability.

> *Water-filled implements give the athlete an opportunity to train against an active fluid resistance rather than the static resistance that most traditional training methods provide.*

Implement Training Should Supplement Traditional Methods

It is not being suggested that implement training become the primary form of resistance training for athletes. Whereas some people do compete in strongman competitions, it is important to remember, in using implement training with a client or an athlete, that there is a legitimate reason to do so. The physical attributes required to perform the activity, the movements that make up the activity, and the objectives of the program must all be evaluated when one is considering integrating implement training into the program (24). Barbells and dumbbells, after all, are proven tools that have been shown to be very effective at developing increases in strength and power. If the goal is to use the weight room to gain a competitive edge, however, then supplementing this traditional training with implement training may be a viable option.

> *Implement training should be used to supplement the exercises (i.e., barbell and dumbbell) that make up the traditional athletic resistance-training program.*

PROGRAM DESIGN

Examples of supplementing traditional training methods with implement training are provided in Boxes 19.1, 19.2, and 19.3. The following list provides explanations of the abbreviations used in the workouts presented in the tables below:

- TB: Total body exercise; this is one of the Olympic-style lifts or related training exercise.

REAL-WORLD APPLICATION

Unstable Resistance or Unstable Surface?

This chapter discusses several forms of implements used in training programs that provide an unstable resistance: kegs, sandbags, etc. Implements are available that provide an unstable surface or an unstable base from which the athlete is required to produce force. One question then becomes which modality is more appropriate: an unstable resistance or an unstable surface?

The answer to this question is most certainly sport-specific. One point of consideration will be the degree to which a supporting surface is "unstable" while performing sport-specific activities.

A stability ball is a common piece of equipment used in training athletes today. A "balance disk" or a "wobble board" is used in some cases to provide an unstable surface underneath a planted foot. As a strength and conditioning professional, you must be able to evaluate these exercise modalities and determine whether they are specific to the sport for which the athlete is training.

In many sports, the ground is the primary surface the athlete uses to generate ground reaction force. In some cases the ground is slippery (wet grass) or allows sliding (a clay tennis court). Is a slippery surface the same as an unstable surface? Probably not.

Although this does not mean that an unstable surface should never be used, you as a strength and conditioning professional should have a reason for using any piece of equipment. These modalities may be very useful in the rehabilitation of specific injuries. Since conditioning programs should progress from general to specific, it may be that unstable surfaces are useful in the general conditioning phase but not applicable to the sport-specific phase.

Before using an unstable surface in a sport-specific conditioning phase, evaluate the sport and have a specific rationale for using the modality.

19.1 STRENGTH CYCLE 1. HOCKEY

DATES: April 28–May 25
CYCLE: Strength 1
GOAL: To increase muscle strength because of the positive relationship between strength and power.
LENGTH: 4 weeks.
INTENSITY: Complete the full number of required repetitions on the first set only prior to increasing resistance.
PACE: *Total* body lifts performed as explosively as possible. All other exercises lift in 2 seconds, lower in 3 seconds.
REST: 2.5 minutes rest between total body lifts, 2 minutes rest between all other exercises.
SETS/REPS:

April 28–May 4: TB = 4 × 5, CL = 4 × 7, AL = 3 × 8
May 5–May 11: TB = 4 × 2, CL = 4 × 4, AL = 3 × 8
May 12–May 18: TB = 4 × 5, CL = 4 × 7, AL = 3 × 8
May 19–May 25: TB = 4 × 2, CL = 4 × 4, AL = 3 × 8

MONDAY	WEDNESDAY	FRIDAY
TOTAL BODY	**TOTAL BODY**	**TOTAL BODY**
Squat clean (**floor**) TB	DB hang clean/tire flip TB	Hang alt foot snatch TB
LOWER BODY	**LOWER BODY**	**CHEST**
Squat CL	Keg/log 1-leg squat CL	Bench press (**1 set standing**) CL
Keg lateral squat CL	Keg/log hockey lunge CL	
60-second stabilization		
TRUNK	**TRUNK**	**TRUNK**
WT decline twist push-down 3 × 15	MB trunk twist 3 × 15	WT Russian twist 3 × 15
WT reverse back ext	Keg/log straight leg dead lift	WT toe touchers 3 × 15
UPPER BACK	**CHEST**	**SHOULDERS**
MR row 2 × 8	DB/keg bench press CL	Keg shoulder press CL
		MR front raise 2 × 8
NECK	**UPPER BACK**	**NECK**
MR lat flexion 2 × 8	DB row CL	MR flex/ext 2 × 8

- CL: Core lift; this is a multijoint exercise, such as a squat.
- AL: Auxiliary lift; this is a single joint exercise such as a biceps curl.
- DB: Dumbbell; the exercise is performed with a dumbbell.
- WT: Weighted; the exercise is performed with an external resistance to provide added intensity.
- MR: Manual resistance; the exercise uses a partner as the form of resistance.
- MB: Medicine ball; the exercise is performed with a medicine ball.
- Alt: Alternating; the exercise is performed alternating legs or alternating arms (depending on the exercise being performed).
- DB/tire squat clean: On days athletes perform dumbbell hang squat cleans, they are given the opportunity to perform a tire flip. This tire flip is performed with a movement similar to the pull sequence seen during a clean.
- SB: Sandbag, the exercise is performed with a sandbag.
- KB: Kettlebell, the exercise is performed with a kettlebell.

DESCRIPTION OF SUGGESTED TRAINING IMPLEMENTS

Numerous training implements can be used to carry out a training program. The following list provides a description of some of those implements as well as guidelines for how to use them.

19.2 STRENGTH CYCLE 2. RUNNING BACKS/WIDE RECEIVERS

DATES: March 29–May 2
CYCLE: Strength 2.
GOAL: Increase muscle strength, because of the positive relationship between strength and power.
LENGTH: 5 weeks.
INTENSITY: Select a resistance that allows completion of the full number of required repetitions on the first set only prior to increasing resistance.
PACE: Total body lifts performed explosively. All other exercises lift in 2 seconds, lower in 3 seconds.
REST: 2.5 minutes rest between total body exercises, 2 minutes rest between all other sets and exercises.
SETS/REPS:

    March 29–April 4: TB = 4 × 5, CL = 4 × 6, AL = 3 × 6
    April 5–April 11: TB = 4 × 3, CL = 4 × 4, AL = 3 × 6
    April 12–April 18: TB = 4 × 5, CL = 4 × 6, AL = 3 × 6
    April 19–April 25: TB = 4 × 3, CL = 4 × 4, AL = 3 × 6
    April 26–May 2: TB = 4 × 5, CL = 4 × 6, AL = 3 × 6

MONDAY	WEDNESDAY	FRIDAY
TOTAL BODY	**TOTAL BODY**	**TOTAL BODY**
Squat clean **(floor)** TB	DB/KB hang clean/tire flip TB	Split alt ft snatch balance TB
Split alt foot jerks TB		
CHEST	**LOWER BODY**	**LOWER BODY**
Chain bench press CL	DB/KB/keg/log/SB 1-leg sqt CL	Chain squats CL
	DB/KB/keg/log/sb lat sqt CL	Keg/log/SB walking lunges CL
	Leg curl/MR leg curl AL	1 × 60-s stabilization
TRUNK	**TRUNK**	**TRUNK**
MB decline 1-arm throws 3 × 15	MB push-downs 3 × 15	WT alt V-ups/with MB 3 × 15
MR reverse back ext 3 × 12	MB twist push-downs 3 × 15	MR reverse back ext 3 × 12
SHOULDERS	**CHEST**	**UPPER BACK**
MR front raise	DB/KB/keg/log/SB incline CL	T-bar row/DB row/KB row
UPPER BACK	**ARMS**	**NECK**
Bent row CL	MR stand triceps	MR flex/ext 2 × 8
MR upright row		
NECK		
MR lateral flex 2 × 8		

Kegs

The number of **kegs** (water-filled steel drums) needed and the range of poundage required will depend on the number of athletes training with kegs at one time and the variety of keg exercises included in the training program. Think of each keg as a training station; ideally you will want no more than three athletes per keg. Certain exercises, such as a keg front raise, require a fairly light weight (e.g., 20 lb), while some athletes may be able to go as heavy as 280 to 300 lb on a keg squat.

Be aware that because of the additional balance and stability requirements, athletes will not be able to use the same amount of weight in a keg exercise that they would in performing the same exercise with a barbell. Although this may seem to compromise potential increases in strength, consider that the athletes may be building a higher level of transferable strength—that is, strength that can be used effectively during competition.

The kegs can best be filled to the desired weight by removing the cap, placing the keg on a scale, and using a hose to fill the keg with water until the desired weight is reached. A full-size keg filled with

19.3 POWER CYCLE 2. VOLLEYBALL

DATES: May 31–June 27
CYCLE: Power 2.
GOAL: Increases in muscle power, because of the positive relationship between muscle power and performance.
LENGTH: 4 weeks.
INTENSITY: Complete the full number of repetitions in good form on the first set only prior to increasing resistance.
PACE: Total body lifts performed as explosively as possible. Timed lifts performed at a pace that allows completion of the required number of repetitions in the specified time period.
REST: 3 minutes rest between total body sets and exercises, 2.5 minutes rest between all other sets and exercises.
SETS/REPS:

> May 31–June 6: TB = 5 × 2, TL = 4 × 4 at 5 seconds (1.3)
> June 7–June 13: TB = 5 × 3, TL = 4 × 6 at 9 seconds (1.5)
> June 14–June 20: TB = 5 × 2, TL = 4 × 4 at 5 seconds (1.3)
> June 21–June 27: TB = 5 × 3, TL = 4 × 6 at 9 seconds (1.5)

MONDAY	WEDNESDAY	FRIDAY
TOTAL BODY	**TOTAL BODY**	**TOTAL BODY**
Hang squat clean TB	DB/KB split alt ft alt snatch balance TB	Scoop split alt ft snatch TB
	DB hang split alt ft alt Snatch TB	Split alt ft jerks TB
LOWER BODY	**LOWER BODY**	**CHEST**
Chain squats (2 sets) CL	DB/KB/SB/log 1-leg squats TL	Chain bench press (2 sets) CL
Keg/log/SB squats (2 sets) TL	Keg/KB/SB/log arch lunge TL	Bench press (2 sets) TL
Keg/log/SB side lunge TL	60-s stabilization	DB pull-overs TL
TRUNK	**TRUNK**	**TRUNK**
Stand 2-hand bar twist 3 × 10	MB ankle chop/twist 3 × 10	MB decline two-hand arm throw 3 × 10
WT back ext 3 × 8	WT twist back ext 3 × 8	
UPPER BACK	**CHEST/SHOULDER**	**SHOULDERS**
Bar/keg/SB bent row TL	DB/KB/SB bench press TL	Keg/KB/SB shoulder press TL
ROTATOR CUFF	**ROTATOR CUFF**	**ROTATOR CUFF**
Internal rotation 2 × 12	Empty cans 2 × 12	Functional rotation 2 × 12
		MB overhead throw

water will typically weight about 160 lb. To further increase the weight of the keg, sand can be mixed with the water. Sand has the advantage of being inexpensive and, because it stays wet inside the keg, it maintains its dynamic characteristics, moving inside the keg as the exercise is performed.

To make it easier to perform exercises such as squats, lunges, or shoulder press, keg stands can be built. The purpose of these stands is to securely hold the keg in place at about shoulder height, making it easier to place the keg in the correct position to perform the desired exercise. For example, think of the keg stands as a squat rack where the bar is held in place at about shoulder height so that the athlete can place the bar on his back to perform a squat.

Most kegs are built with a handle on the top. The bottom is typically built with a lip to allow the user to grip that end of the keg more effectively. By gripping the handle at the top and using the lip at the bottom, a secure grip can be achieved. However, caution is advised in using the kegs to perform resistance-training exercises. The athlete's grip on the keg will not be as secure as it would be on a barbell or dumbbell. Further, the water will be moving inside the keg, creating a more difficult resistance to control. Care must be taken to spot very carefully when a keg exercise is being performed, and the user must remember to use a lighter resistance than would be used in performing the same exercise with a barbell.

The number of kegs needed to supplement the strength training program and the range of poundage needed in the kegs will depend on the number of athletes training with kegs at one time and the types of keg exercises to be performed. It is important to remember that exercises performed with kegs are much more difficult than the same exercises performed with barbells or dumbbells; because of this the athlete will have to reduce the training weight in performing a keg exercise as compared to the same exercise performed with a barbell or dumbbell.

Logs

Logs (6-ft "tubes" with a 12-in circumference) are also filled with water. Extending out from each tube is piping the size of a standard barbell, so that additional weight plates can be positioned on the log. The ability to change the weight of the log rapidly by adding additional plates limits the need to have a large number of logs of various weights.

Logs are designed with handles to make it easier to hold on to them. Because of the length of the logs, the water can travel a significant distance as compared to the kegs and thus enhance the dynamic nature of exercises performed with this implement.

As in the case of the kegs, athletes will not be able to perform log exercises with the same weight that they would use to perform the identical exercise with a barbell. Err on the side of caution and slowly increase the intensity of this type of training as the athlete demonstrates the ability to control the implement during exercise.

Because the logs are 6 ft long, the water encased in them has the potential to move more, thus increasing the dynamic characteristics of the exercise and the degree of difficulty of the movement.

Water-Filled Dumbbells

Water-filled dumbbells (smaller versions of the water-filled logs) are meant to be used in the same way as a typical dumbbell. Because the dumbbells are much shorter in length than the logs, the degree of water movement within them is much less. That movement still provides an additional challenge to the athlete, however, especially as the implement is being held with just one hand rather than both

hands. It provides a unique training stimulus and thus the potential to give the athlete an advantage over the competition.

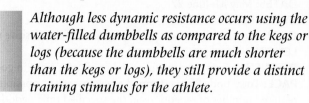

Although less dynamic resistance occurs using the water-filled dumbbells as compared to the kegs or logs (because the dumbbells are much shorter than the kegs or logs), they still provide a distinct training stimulus for the athlete.

Tires

Tires (simply used truck and heavy equipment tires) are modified so that the athlete can place additional weight to the center of the tire to adjust the resistance to his specific strength levels. Unlike the kegs, logs, and water-filled dumbbells, where a variety of exercises can be performed, the tires can only be flipped. The movement at the ankle, knee, and hip are very similar during the pull in performing a clean or flipping the tire.

Using the tires does provide some advantages. First, flipping the tire gives athletes greater variety in their training programs, which is a positive. Second, athletes may have injuries that prevent them from performing a clean (typically wrist, elbow, shoulder, or back injuries) safely and pain-free, but they can perform a tire flip without aggravating an existing injury. Finally, because there is no catch phase in flipping a tire, the athlete sometimes feels better able to concentrate on the explosion phase of the movement.

The tires provide a unique and challenging variation for athletes who regularly perform cleans or high pulls as parts of their workout.

Kettlebells

The sport of kettlebell lifting originated in Russia in the mid-19th century. Although not new, kettlebells are still unique in the United States, although they are growing in popularity. Kettlebells have been described as looking like black bowling balls with a suitcase handle attached; they normally weigh between 35 and 100 lb.

Although exercises typically performed with kettlebells can also be performed with dumbbells, kettlebells provide some unique differences. First, the handle of a kettlebell is much thicker than the handle on a dumbbell, which makes it more difficult to handle. This can challenge an athlete's grip strength. Second, the handle on a kettlebell is designed to allow it to swing freely, creating a more active resistance as compared to a typical dumbbell. This causes a greater number of stabilizer muscles to be recruited during kettlebell training as compared to dumbbell training (16).

Two of the major exercises typically performed with kettlebells are the power clean and the power snatch (6). One of the reasons these two lifts are so useful (and this is not unique to kettlebells) is the importance of training movements and not muscles (3). This guideline stresses the value of performing athletic movements during resistance training with correct postural alignment; moreover, it is not just the amount of weight lifted during training that matters but also the speed in which the movement occurs and how that transfers to athletics (3).

Exercises that can be performed with kettlebells include but are not limited to the following:

- Power cleans
- Power jerks
- Swings
- Front squats
- Military presses
- Bench presses
- Incline presses
- One-leg dead lifts
- Single-arm rows
- Swings

It is also important to note that, like dumbbell maneuvers, kettlebell exercises can be grouped together into an infinite number of routines. They can also be combined with other free- and body-weight exercises.

Chains

Chains (6 to 7 ft long weighing 12 to 20 lb apiece) are used in conjunction with a standard barbell and weight plates by hanging the chains at the ends of the barbell. When hung correctly, a portion of the chain rests on the floor underneath the barbell. As the barbell is lifted, additional links of the chain rise off the floor, adding to the total weight of the barbell. The value of this gradual increase in the amount of weight being lifted is that it occurs as the body moves into a mechanically favorably position (in certain exercises such as squat, dead lift, or bench press). Similarly, as the bar is lowered, the total weight on it is reduced as chain links collect on the floor and the body moves into a mechanically unfavorable position.

For example, in performing a parallel squat, the weakest position of the movement is at the bottom of the squat; at this position most of the chain is resting on the floor. As the person performing the squat begins to return to a standing position, he or she moves toward the strongest position and additional links are lifted off the floor, increasing the total weight on the bar (8). Using the chains in this manner progressively increases and decreases resistance throughout a movement, more closely matching the strength curve that occurs within the body. Additionally, chains oscillate and swing throughout the range of motion, causing increased involvement of stabilization muscles (3).

In performing a typical free-weight or machine exercise (depending on the design of the machine), in contrast to the varying resistance that occurs while using chains, the external resistance (weight) selected remains constant throughout an exercise. Whereas the external resistance remains constant, the force exerted by the muscle varies as the mechanical advantage of the joints involved in the movement changes as the exercise is taken through the range of motion (3).

It is hypothesized that by matching the strength curve to produce near-maximal force throughout the range of motion and increasing the need for stabilization when performing a given exercise because of the movement of the chains, the amount of transfer to a task is enhanced. A commonly used example is a football lineman, who typically during competition is in an upright position and encountering high forces from many angles. Unlike traditional barbell training, chain training results in the generation of high forces in the top quarter of the lineman's range of motion (3).

Research evaluating the effectiveness of chain squats suggests that the addition of chains offers no advantage to performing the exercise. Using electromyography (EMG) and ground reaction forces (GRF) for squats performed with barbell and plates and squats performed with barbell, plates, and chains hung on each side, no statistically significant differences were found between the training adaptations that occur from performing traditional barbell squats as compared to barbell squats with the addition of chains (3).

Although scientific evidence is lacking, anecdotal support for the use of chains for strength and power enhancement is increasing among strength coaches and athletes. With proper supervision ensuring that chain training is performed in a safe manner, chains provide coaches and lifters a low-cost, supplementary method of training that can easily be incorporated into the training program (3).

Sandbags

Sandbags are canvas bags encasing plastic bags filled with sand. They can range in weight from 25 to 100 lb or more (17). Like water-filled implements, sandbags allow room for the sand to shift, creating an active rather than a static resistance. This active resistance causes the lifter to move and adjust as he or she performs the exercise, thus increasing muscular activation and energy expenditure.

Sandbags are also very effective at increasing grip strength (12). Because the sandbags provide no convenient gripping point, they challenge the lifter's ability to grip the bag while performing a wide variety of exercises

Sandbags also have the advantage of being both inexpensive and extremely versatile (12). For a small amount of money (as compared to purchasing traditional types of resistance-training equipment) sandbags can easily be made and provide a training implement that can be used to perform a wide variety of exercises.

An additional advantage of including sandbag exercises in the training program is to add variety for the athlete. This helps to avoid the boredom that is likely to occur when the same exercises are repetitively performed with the same implements.

Because of the awkwardness of handling the sandbag, it is important to focus on good lifting posture (12). The technique used to perform the vast majority of sandbag exercises (squats, "good mornings," lunges, bench press, shoulder press, rows, and so on) is generally identical to that used to perform the same exercises with traditional types of resistance-training equipment.

DESCRIPTION OF IMPLEMENT EXERCISES AND EXAMPLES OF WORKOUTS

The following list of exercises that can be performed with the implements discussed in this chapter is not all-inclusive but offers descriptions of the implement exercises included in the sample workouts provided above. Most of the implement exercises are performed in a manner similar to the exercises performed with traditional strength training equipment.

It is important to note that Olympic-style exercises are not performed with either kegs or logs. Because of the technical difficulty of performing these types of exercises and the awkwardness of using these implements, the chance of injury while performing these types of exercises with these implements is too great. All of the Olympic-style exercises, however, can be safely performed with the water-filled dumbbells by those athletes who have good technique in performing these exercises. Remember that in all of the exercises performed with implements, the training weight must be reduced in comparison to what the athlete would use with a traditional barbell or dumbbell.

Exercise descriptions for the water-filled dumbbells are not included in this list. Movements using the water-filled dumbbells are identical to movements using standard dumbbells and so are not discussed.

Power Exercises
Dumbbell/Kettlebell Hang Cleans
Kettlebell Split Alt Foot Alt Snatch Balance
Kettlebell Hang Split Alt Foot/Alt Snatch
Tire Flip

Hip/Thigh Exercises
Chain Squat
Keg/Log/Sandbag Squat
Keg/Log Lateral Squat
Kettlebell/Keg/Log/Sandbag One-Leg Squat
Keg/Log/Sandbag Walking Lunge
Kettlebell/Keg/Log/Sandbag Hockey Lunge
Keg/Log/Sandbag Arch Lunge
Keg/Log/Sandbag Straight Leg Dead Lift

Chest Exercises
Kettlebell/Keg/Log/Sandbag Bench Press
Chain Bench Press
Keg/Log/Sandbag Incline Press

Upper Back Exercises
Kettlebell Row

Shoulder Exercises
Kettlebell/Keg/Log/Sandbag Shoulder Press

Abdominal and Lower Back Exercises
Sandbag Russian Twist
Sandbag Toe Toucher

POWER EXERCISES

Dumbbell/Kettlebell Hang Cleans

Type of Exercise

Total body/power (explosive) exercise

Muscles Used

Gluteus maximus, hamstrings (semimembranosus, semitendinosus, biceps femoris), quadriceps (vastus lateralis, vastus intermedius, vastus medialis, rectus femoris), soleus, gastrocnemius, trapezius, deltoids (anterior, medial, and posterior)

Starting Position

Grasp the two kettlebells at the handles. Assume a shoulder-width stance with the head up, the back arched, and the feet flat. The handles of the kettlebells should be held at knee height, in a palms-down position, on the lateral portion of each leg. The legs should be slightly bent, the back arched, the shoulders slightly forward of the kettlebells, and the head/eyes up (Fig. 19.1A).

Upward Movement

Initiate the movement by jumping into a fully extended hip position, then aggressively shrug the shoulders and finally pull with the arms until the kettlebells are pulled up along the outside of the rib cage to approximately sternum height (Fig. 19.1B). At this point bring the elbows up and around so that they are held up at shoulder height, pointing directly forward of the body. As the kettlebell reaches sternum height, sit back at the hips and drop into a full squat position, then return to a standing position.

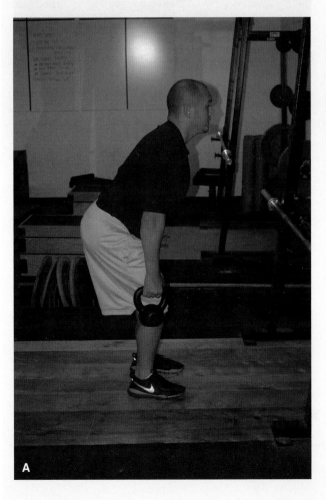

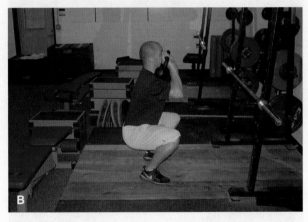

FIGURE 19.1 Kettlebell hang cleans. **A.** Starting position. **B.** Upward movement.

Kettlebell Split Alt Foot Alt Snatch Balance

Type of Exercise

Total body/power (explosive) exercise

Muscles Used

Gluteus maximus, hamstrings (semi-membranosus, semitendinosus, biceps femoris), quadriceps (vastus lateralis, vastus intermedius, vastus medialis, rectus femoris), soleus, gastrocnemius, trapezius (upper portion), deltoids (anterior, medial, and posterior), triceps brachii

Starting Position

Stand with the feet shoulder-width apart, holding the kettlebells at shoulder height with the palms facing forward (Fig. 19.2A).

Upward Movement

With a small, quick flexion and then extension of the hips, drive the kettlebells straight up while simultaneously splitting the feet front to back so that you catch the kettlebells in a lunge position with the arms fully extended overhead (Fig 19.2B). Return to the start position and repeat the movement, alternating which foot is split forward and backward at each repetition.

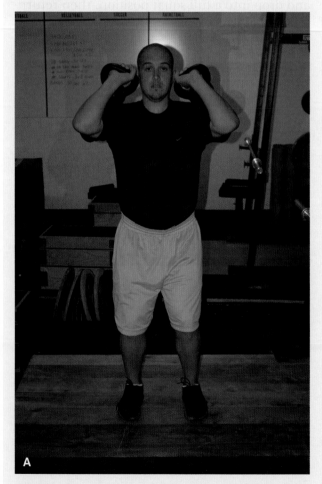
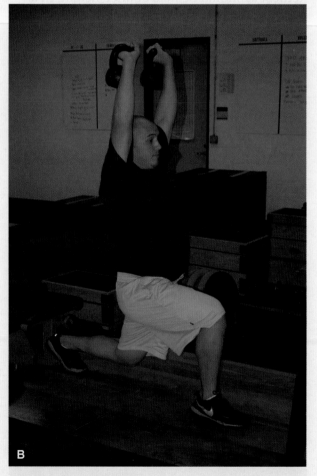

FIGURE 19.2 Kettlebell split alt foot alt snatch balance. **A.** Starting position. **B.** Upward movement.

Kettlebell Hang Split Alt Foot/Alt Snatch

Type of Exercise

Total body/power (explosive) exercise

Muscles Used

Gluteus maximus, hamstrings (semi-membranosus, semitendinosus, biceps femoris), quadriceps (vastus lateralis, vastus intermedius, vastus medialis, rectus femoris), soleus, gastrocnemius, trapezius (upper portion), deltoids (anterior, medial, and posterior), triceps brachii

Starting Position

Stand with the feet shoulder-width apart, knees slightly bent, back arched. The kettlebells should be held in a palms down position at knee height. The shoulders should be slightly forward of the kettlebells in this position (Fig. 19.3A).

Upward Movement

Quickly extend the hips, at the top of hip extension aggressively shrug the shoulders and then pull the kettlebells along the lateral portion of the rib cage. At the top of the pull, the kettlebells should be at chest height (Fig. 19.3B). At this point split the feet front to back so that you catch the kettlebells in a lunge position with the arms fully extended overhead (Fig. 19.3C). Return to the start position and repeat the movement, alternating which foot is split forward and backward at each repetition.

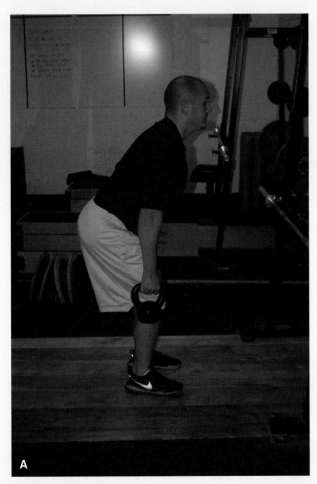
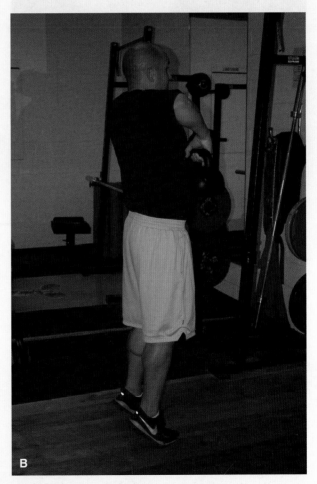

FIGURE 19.3 Kettlebell hang split alt foot/alt snatch. **A.** Starting position. **B.** Upward movement.

(continued)

Kettlebell Hang Split Alt Foot/Alt Snatch *(continued)*

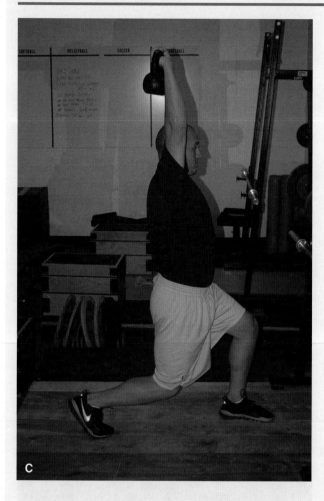

C.

FIGURE 19.3 *(continued)* Kettlebell hang split alt foot/alt snatch.
C. Ending position.

Tire Flip

Type of Exercise

Total body/power (explosive) exercise

Muscles Used

Gluteus maximus, hamstrings (semi-membranosus, semitendinosus, biceps femoris), quadriceps (vastus lateralis, vastus intermedius, vastus medialis, rectus femoris), soleus, gastrocnemius, trapezius, deltoids (anterior, medial, and posterior)

Starting Position

Place the feet about shoulder-width apart. Keeping the back arched, sit back at the hips (not allowing the knees to drift forward of the toes) and assume an underhand grip on the tire. The hands should be slightly wider than shoulder-width apart. Use the legs to lift the tire so that the hands are raised to a mid-shin position. The arms should be fully extended, the back arched, and the feet flat on the floor (Fig. 19.4A).

High Pull

Using a jumping action, explode up through the legs and flip the tire onto its side, remembering to keep the back arched through the entire movement (Fig. 19.4B). Once the tire has been flipped onto its side, step forward and aggressively push the tire onto its opposite side (Fig. 19.4C).

Tire Flip *(continued)*

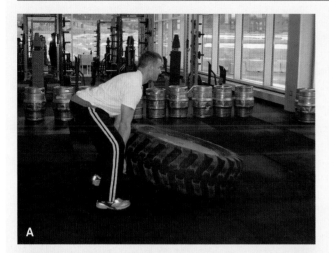

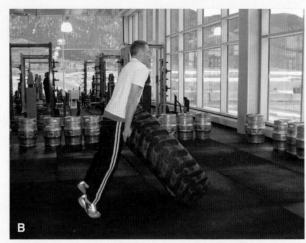

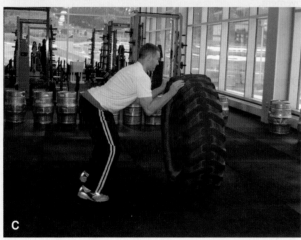

FIGURE 19.4 Tire flip. **A.** Starting position. **B.** High pull. **C.** Ending position.

HIP/THIGH EXERCISES

Chain Squat

Type of Exercise
Lower body/multijoint

Muscles Used
Gluteus maximus, quadriceps (vastus lateralis, vastus intermedius, vastus medialis, rectus femoris), hamstrings (semimembranosus, semitendinosus, biceps femoris)

Movement
This exercise is performed identically to a normal barbell squat. The only difference is that lifting chains are attached to either end of the barbell (Fig 19.5A,B).

(continued)

Chain Squat *(continued)*

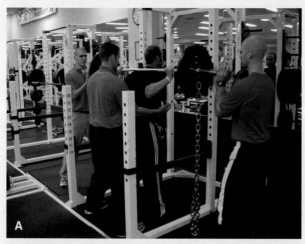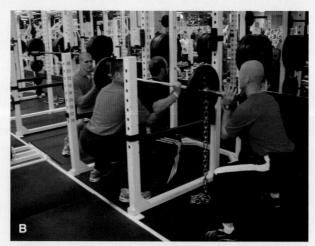

FIGURE 19.5 Chain squats. **A.** Starting position. **B.** Downward movement.

Keg/Log/Sandbag Squat

Type of Exercise

Lower body/multijoint

Muscles Used

Gluteus maximus, quadriceps (vastus lateralis, vastus intermedius, vastus medialis, rectus femoris), hamstrings (semimembranosus, semitendinosus, biceps femoris)

Starting Position

Place the keg, log, or sandbag on the back, as in performing barbell squats. Place the feet about shoulder-width apart (Fig. 19.6A).

Downward Movement

Keeping the back arched, initiate the movement by sitting back at the hips, not allowing the knees to drop forward of the toes. Continue to sit back until the mid-thigh has achieved a position parallel to the floor (Fig. 19.6B). Maintaining an arched back position, return to the starting position.

Keg/Log/Sandbag Squat *(continued)*

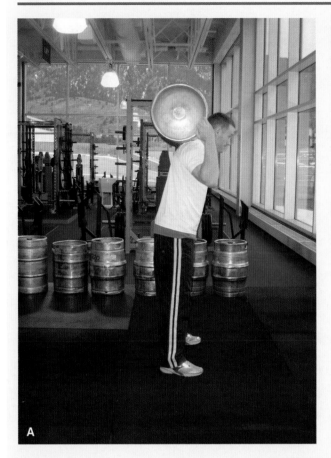

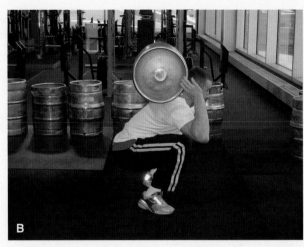

FIGURE 19.6 Keg squat. **A.** Starting position. **B.** Downward movement.

Keg/Log Lateral Squat

Type of Exercise

Lower body/multijoint

Muscles Used

Gluteus maximus, quadriceps (vastus lateralis, vastus intermedius, vastus medialis, rectus femoris), hamstrings (semimembranosus, semitendinosus, biceps femoris), hip abductors, hip adductors

Starting Position

Place the keg or log on the back, as in performing barbell squats. Place the feet 10 to 12 in. wider than shoulder width (Fig. 19.7A).

Downward Movement

Keeping the left knee straight and the left foot planted, flex the right knee while sitting back at the hips and moving the hips laterally to the right (Fig. 19.7B). Return to the starting position and alternate the movement to the opposite side until the required number of repetitions have been performed (Fig. 19.7C).

Alternate Movement: Keg/Log/ Sandbag Side Lunge

Place the keg, log, or sandbag on the back, as in performing barbell squats. Place the feet about shoulder-width apart. Step directly laterally with the right foot through a comfortable range of motion. Keeping the left knee straight and the left foot planted, flex the right knee while sitting back at the hips and moving the hips laterally to the right. Return to the starting position and alternate the movement to the opposite side until the required number of repetitions have been completed.

(continued)

Keg/Log Lateral Squat *(continued)*

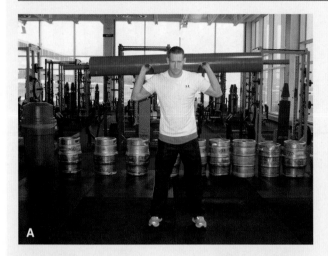

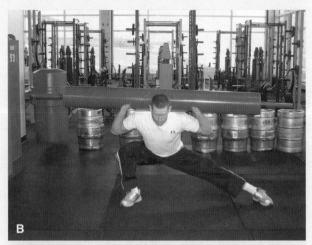

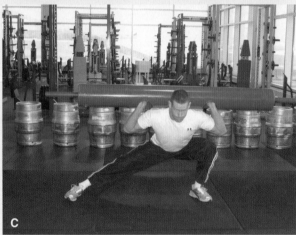

FIGURE 19.7 Log lateral squat. **A.** Starting position. **B.** Downward movement, right leg. **C.** Downward movement, left leg.

Kettlebell/Keg/Log/Sandbag One-Leg Squat

Type of Exercise
Lower body/multijoint

Muscles Used
Gluteus maximus, quadriceps (vastus lateralis, vastus intermedius, vastus medialis, rectus femoris), hamstrings (semimembranosus, semitendinosus, biceps femoris), hip abductors, hip adductors

Starting Position
Hold the kettlebells at arm's length directly underneath the shoulders or place the keg, log, or sandbag on the back, as in performing barbell squats. Stand about a stride's length away from a utility bench. Reach back with one leg and place the foot on the bench (Fig. 19.8A).

Downward Movement
Keeping the back arched initiate the movement by sitting back at the hips, not allowing the knee to drip forward of the toes on the forward foot. Continue to sit back until the mid thigh has achieved a parallel position (Fig 19.8B). Maintain an arched back position and return to the starting position. Repeat with the opposite leg.

Kettlebell/Keg/Log/Sandbag One-Leg Squat *(continued)*

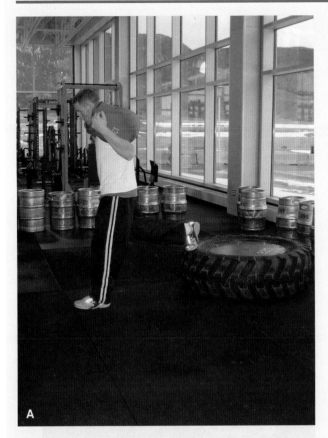

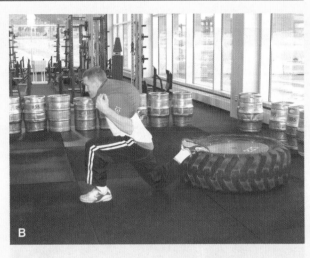

FIGURE 19.8 Sandbag one-leg squat. **A.** Starting position. **B.** Downward movement.

Keg/Log/Sandbag Walking Lunge

Type of Exercise

Lower body/multi-joint

Muscles Used

Gluteus maximus, iliopsoas, quadriceps (vastus lateralis, vastus intermedius, vastus medialis, rectus femoris), hamstrings (semi-membranosus, semitendinosus, biceps femoris), soleus, gastrocnemius

Starting Position

Place the keg, log, or sandbag on the back, as in performing barbell squats (Fig. 19.9A).

Downward Movement

Take an exaggerated stride with the right leg and then lower the body so that the right knee is behind the toes on the right foot and the left leg is bent with the left knee just off the floor (Fig 19.9B). From that bottom position, stride forward in one continuous movement with the left leg and take an exaggerated stride with the left leg; the right leg is bent and the right knee is just off the floor (Fig. 19.9C). It is important to keep the back arched during the entire performance of this exercise.

(continued)

Keg/Log/Sandbag Walking Lunge *(continued)*

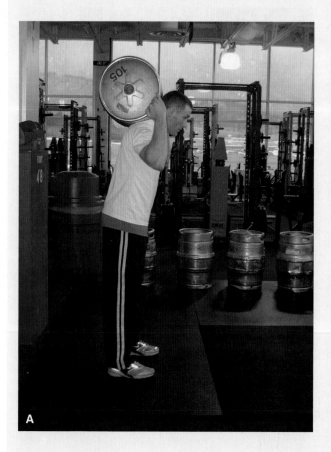

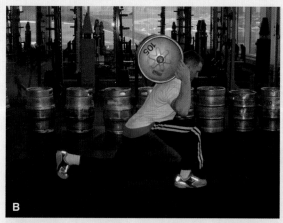

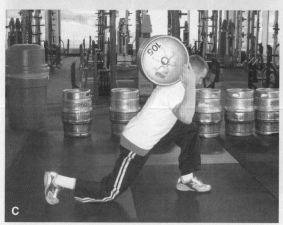

FIGURE 19.9 Keg walking lunge. **A.** Starting position. **B.** Downward movement, right leg. **C.** Downward movement, left leg.

Kettlebell/Keg/Log/Sandbag Hockey Lunge

Type of Exercise
Lower body/multijoint

Muscles Used
Gluteus maximus, quadriceps (vastus lateralis, vastus intermedius, vastus medialis, rectus femoris), hamstrings (semimembranosus, semitendinosus, biceps femoris), hip abductors, hip adductors

Starting Position
Start with the dumbbell lunge before progressing to other implements. Hold the dumbbells or kettlebells at arm's length directly underneath the shoulders, or place the keg, log, or sandbag on the back, as in performing barbell squats.

Downward Movement
Take an exaggerated stride with the right leg, stepping forward so that the right foot is 14 to 16 in. wider than the right shoulder and then lower the body so that the right knee is behind the toes on the right foot and the left leg is bent with the left knee just off the floor (Fig 19.10A). From that bottom position, stride forward in one continuous movement with the left leg and take an exaggerated stride with the left leg, as described above; the right leg is bent and the right knee is just off the floor (Fig 19.10B). It is important to keep the back arched during the entire performance of this exercise.

Kettlebell/Keg/Log/Sandbag Hockey Lunge *(continued)*

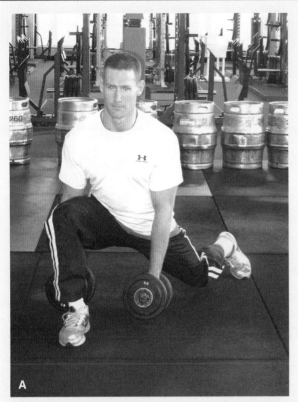 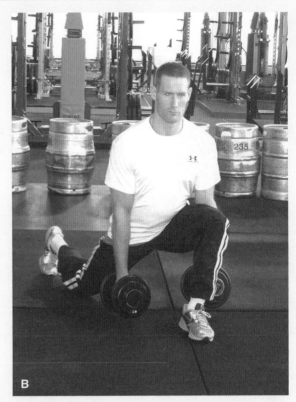

FIGURE 19.10 Dumbbell lunge. **A.** Downward movement, right leg. **B.** Downward movement, left leg.

Keg/Log/Sandbag Arch Lunge

Type of Exercise

Lower body/multi-joint

Muscles Used

Gluteus maximus, quadriceps (vastus lateralis, vastus intermedius, vastus medialis, rectus femoris), hamstrings (semimembranosus, semitendinosus, biceps femoris), hip abductors, hip adductors

Starting Position

Place the keg, log, or sandbag on the back, as in performing barbell squats. Place the feet about shoulder-width apart (Fig 19.11A).

Downward Movement

Imagine an arch on the floor in front of where you are standing. Starting a stride length away, directly lateral of the right foot and ending a stride length away, directly lateral of the left foot. initiate the movement by lunging directly laterally with the right foot to the right edge of the arch while keeping the right knee behind the toes on the right foot and the left leg straight (Fig 19.11B). Return to the starting position. Alternate lunging with each leg, gradually working from one corner of the arch to the opposite corner of the arch with each step (Fig 19.11C). The number of steps and the placement of the foot on each step will depend on the number of required repetitions.

(continued)

Keg/Log/Sandbag Arch Lunge *(continued)*

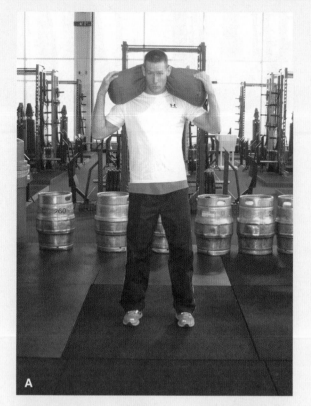

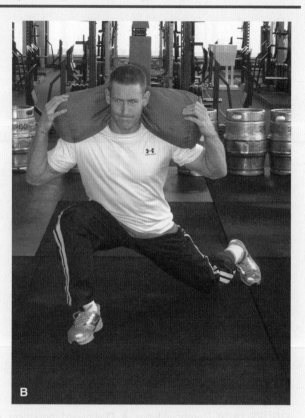

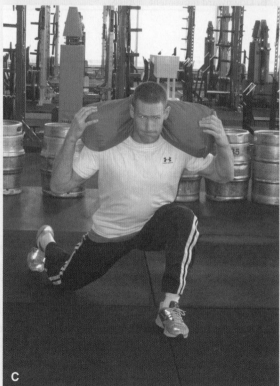

FIGURE 19.11 Sandbag arch lunge. **A.** Starting position. **B.** Downward movement, right leg. **C.** Downward movement, left leg.

Keg/Log/Sandbag Straight Leg Dead Lift

Type of Exercise
Lower body/single-joint

Muscles Used
Gluteus maximus, erector spinae, hamstrings (semimembranosus, semitendinosus, and biceps femoris)

Starting Position
Squat down and, keeping the back arched, pick up the keg, log, or sandbag. Holding the implement at arm's length in front of the body, bend the knees slightly (Fig 19.12A).

Downward Movement
Maintain a slight knee bend and arch the back, then bend forward at the hips and lower the implement to a point just short of touching the floor directly underneath the feet (Fig 19.12B). Return to the starting position.

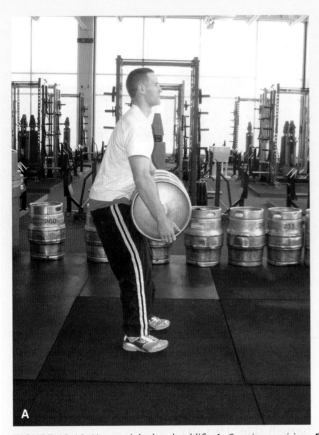
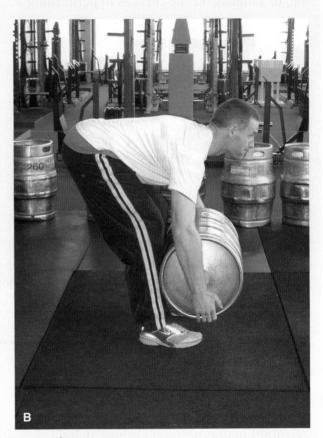

FIGURE 19.12 Keg straight-leg dead lift. **A.** Starting position. **B.** Downward movement.

CHEST EXERCISES

Kettlebell/Keg/Log/Sandbag Bench Press

Type of Exercise

Upper body/multijoint

Muscles Used

Pectoralis major, pectoralis minor, deltoid (anterior), serratus anterior, triceps brachii

Starting Position

Lie down on a flat utility bench, feet on the floor and buttocks on the bench. Place the keg, log, or sandbag on the chest as in performing a barbell bench press and grip the implement, or grasp the kettlebells as in performing a dumbbell bench press (Fig. 19.13A).

Upward Movement

Fully extend the arms, keeping the buttocks on the bench and the feet flat on the floor (Fig. 19.13B). Lower under control. The spotter(s) must be diligent in assisting the lifter during performance of this exercise.

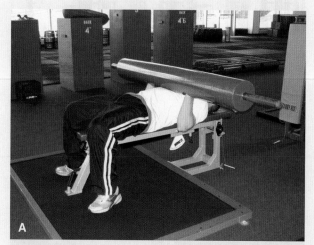
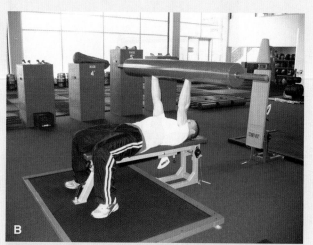

FIGURE 19.13 Log bench press. **A.** Starting position. **B.** Upward movement.

Chain Bench Press

Type of Exercise

Upper body/multijoint

Muscles Used

Pectoralis major, pectoralis minor, deltoid (anterior), serratus anterior, triceps brachii

Starting Position

Lie down on a flat utility bench, as you would for a normal barbell bench press (Fig. 19.14A).

Upward Movement

This exercise is performed identically to a normal bench press. The only difference is that lifting chains are attached to the ends of the barbell (Fig. 19.14B).

Chain Bench Press *(continued)*

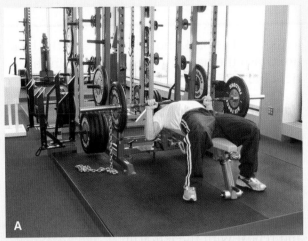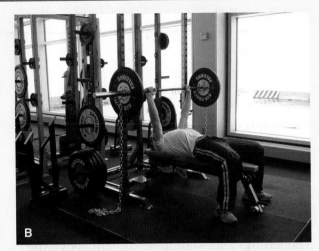

FIGURE 19.14 Chain bench press. **A.** Starting position. **B.** Upward movement.

Keg/Log/Sandbag Incline Press

Type of Exercise
Upper body/multijoint

Muscles Used
Pectoralis major, pectoralis minor, deltoid (anterior), serratus anterior, triceps brachii

Starting Position
Lie down on an incline bench, feet on the floor and buttocks on the bench. Place the keg, log or sandbag on the chest as in performing a barbell incline press and grip the implement (Fig. 19.15A).

Upward Movement
Fully extend the arms, keeping the buttocks on the bench and the feet flat on the floor (Fig. 19.15B). Lower under control. The spotter(s) must be diligent in assisting the lifter during the performance of this exercise.

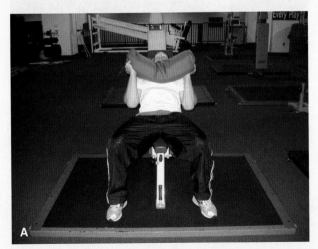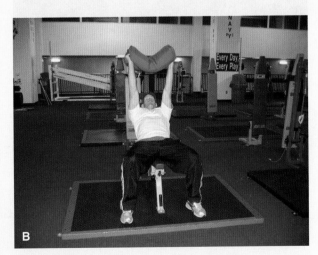

FIGURE 19.15 Sandbag incline press. **A.** Starting position. **B.** Upward movement.

UPPER BACK EXERCISES

Kettlebell Row

Type of Exercise

Upper body/multijoint

Muscles Used

Latissimus dorsi, middle trapezius, rhomboids, teres major, posterior deltoid, biceps brachii, brachialis, brachioradialis

Starting Position

Place the left knee on an exercise bench, with the palm of the left hand flat on the bench. The left hip joint should be straight above the left knee. The back should be flat and the head up. Grasp the handle of the kettlebell in the right hand (Fig. 19.16A).

Upward Movement

Shrug the right shoulder backwards toward the ceiling, seeing how high you can lift the kettlebell without bending the right elbow. At the top of the shrug, finish by pulling the kettlebell with the right arm to the outside of the rib cage (Fig 19.16B). Reverse the position and repeat with the left arm.

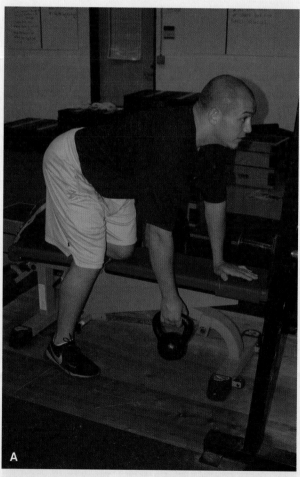
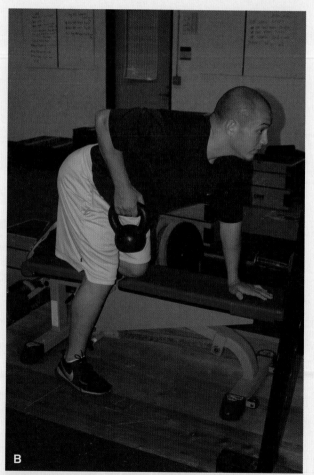

FIGURE 19.16 Kettlebell row. **A.** Starting position. **B.** Upward movement.

SHOULDER EXERCISES

Kettlebell/Keg/Log/Sandbag Shoulder Press

Type of Exercise

Upper body/multijoint

Muscles Used

Deltoid (anterior and medial), trapezius (upper portion), serratus anterior, triceps brachii

Starting Position

Grip the keg, log, or sandbag high on the chest, or grasp the kettlebells as in performing

a dumbbell shoulder press. Stand with feet shoulder-width apart (Fig. 19.17A).

Upward Movement

Press the implement directly overhead until the arms are fully extended (Fig. 19.17B), then lower under control. It is important to not lean back while performing the exercise; the back should remain straight. Lower through the full comfortable range of motion.

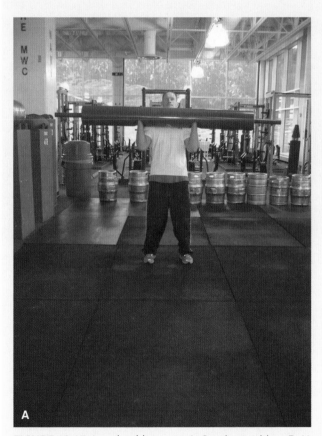
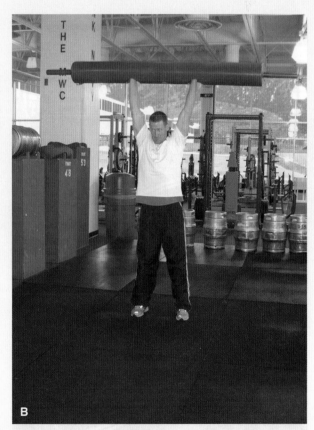

FIGURE 19.17 Log shoulder press. **A.** Starting position. **B.** Upward movement.

ABDOMINAL AND LOWER BACK EXERCISES

Sandbag Russian Twist

Type of Exercise
Trunk

Muscles Used
Rectus abdominis, obliquus externus abdominis, obliquus internus abdominis, transverse abdominis

Starting Position
Assume a seated position on a back extension bench, the feet between the rollers and the upper body leaning back moderately. Grasp the sandbag and hold it at arm's length directly in front of the body (Fig. 19.18A).

Side-Twist Movement
Twist through a full comfortable range of motion to the right, keeping the arms long and the head pointed directly toward the sandbag (Fig. 19.18B). Rotate to the left through a full comfortable range of motion (Fig. 19.18C) and repeat for the required number of times.

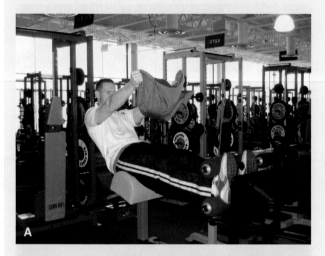

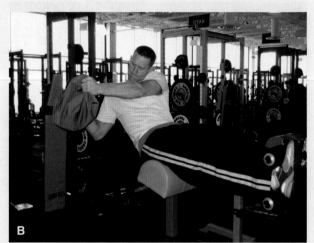

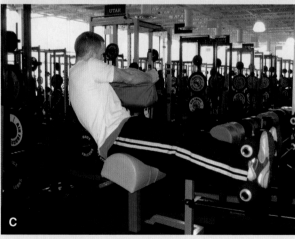

FIGURE 19.18 Sandbag Russian twist. **A.** Starting position. **B.** Side twist, right. **C.** Side twist, left.

Sandbag Toe Toucher

Type of Exercise

Trunk

Muscles Used

Rectus abdominis, obliquus externus abdominis, tensor fascia lata

Starting Position

Lie with your back on the floor. Keep the legs straight and lift them up so the feet are just short of being directly over the hips. Grasp the sandbag in both hands (Fig. 19.19A).

Upward Movement

Elevate the upper back off the floor, crunching the sandbag up toward the toes (Fig. 19.19B).

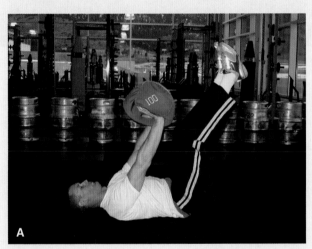 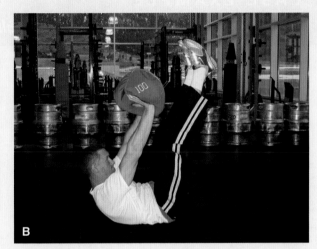

FIGURE 19.19 Sandbag toe-toucher. **A.** Starting position. **B.** Upward movement.

SUMMARY

Although there are exceptions, most athletic strength and conditioning programs emphasize free weights as the preferred training methods for their athletes. Further, many of these programs put a priority on the performance of Olympic-style exercises in a periodized training program.

Research evaluating the benefits of training with implements is lacking. Despite this lack of research, the same principles that apply to conventional training modes can be applied to implement training. Perhaps most important is the concept of training movements and not muscle groups. That is because increases in strength or power will occur primarily in the movement used during training.

One benefit of implement training is that the movement pattern during training can be similar to the movement pattern seen during competition. Implement training also increases the variation in training, reducing physiological and psychological staleness.

Water as a form of resistance provides a unique training stimulus because water is an active resistance rather than a static resistance that traditional resistance-training modes provide. We are not suggesting, however, that implement training should become the primary mode of resistance training. Rather, implement training should be used to supplement traditional barbell and dumbbell training. Implements discussed in this chapter include kegs, logs, water-filled dumbbells, tires, kettlebells, chains, and sandbags.

MAXING OUT

1. You are introducing a new implement in your conditioning program for baseball players. Name the implement, briefly discuss how you will introduce it into the conditioning program over the next 4 weeks, briefly describe the exercises you will use with the implement to perform, and explain how you expect this form of training to benefit your athletes.

2. In evaluating the athletic ability of a high school basketball player, his coach tells you he needs better balance and stability. He is already performing resistance training using a standard free-weight resistance. Would you consider using a training modality that incorporates an active fluid resistance? Why or why not?

3. Some of the athletes in your program are complaining of low back pain. The only significant change in the program is an increase in the volume and intensity of power cleans over the past 2 weeks. Would you consider tire flipping as an alternative to power cleans? Why or why not?

CASE EXAMPLE

Designing a Program for a College Football Running Back

BACKGROUND

You are charged with designing a conditioning program for a 6-ft, 215-lb sophomore Division I running back. His test results are as follows:

a. Bench press—370 lb
b. Squat—500 lb
c. Clean—330 lb
d. Forty-yard dash—4.5 seconds
e. Vertical jump—38 in

He is very committed to his strength and conditioning program and rarely misses a training session. Despite his impressive test results, he is looking for ways to improve his athletic performance; his position coach feels that he needs to develop more functional strength to reach his potential as a football player. What are some training techniques that could be used to help this athlete achieve his goals?

RECOMMENDATIONS/CONSIDERATIONS

With his superior strength levels, it is doubtful that further enhancement of these would have a positive effect on performance. For example, he could focus on increasing his squat from 500 to 525 lb, but it is not certain that this would have the effect of improving his on-the-field performance.

IMPLEMENTATION

What might be more effective at improving performance is the integration of water-filled-implement exercises into his training program, giving him the opportunity to train using an active fluid resistance. For example, exercises such as keg bench press (to help pass blocking and straight arm capabilities) and log lunges (to help him maintain balance during contact) could be worked into his training program to help improve his athletic performance, converting his "weight-room strength" to "functional strength."

RESULTS

The athlete was successfully able to incorporate fluid-resistance implements into his training program. Because his strength levels were relatively high from the pretest, there were only small or no gains in absolute strength. The athlete did progress in his ability to lift and control an active fluid resistance, increasing in intensity as the program progressed. These gains are difficult to measure in terms of increases in traditional lifts and difficult to correlate with performance.

REFERENCES

1. Allerheiligen B. In-season strength training for power athletes. Strength Cond J 2003;25(3):23–28.
2. Baker D. Applying the in-season periodization of strength and power training for football. Strength Cond 1998;20(2):18–24.
3. Berning JM, Coker CA, Adams KJ. Using chains for strength and conditioning. Strength Cond J 2004;26(5):80–84.
4. Brooks TJ. Women's collegiate gymnastics: a multifactorial approach to training and conditioning. Strength Cond J 2003;25(2):23–37.
5. Brown L, Greenwood M. Periodization Essentials and Innovations in Resistance Training Protocols. Strength Cond J 2005;27(4):80–85.
6. Davies J. KB Power, Part 1: the KB Power Clean. Kettlebell.com. The Ultimate Online Strength Resource. Available at http://www.kettlebell.com/training/jdavies/articles/kbpowerclean.html. Accessed June 5, 2006.
7. DeGarmo R. University of Nebraska in-season resistance training for horizontal jumper. Strength Cond J 2000;22(3):23–26.
8. Ebben WP. Electromyographic and kinetic analysis of traditional, chain, and elastic band squats. Journal of Strength Cond Res 2002;16(4):547–550.
9. Gadeken SB. Off-season strength, power, and plyometric training for Kansas State volleyball. Strength Cond J 1999;21(5):49–55.
10. Hedrick A. Using uncommon implements in the training programs of athletes. Strength Cond 2003;25(4):18–22.
11. Hedrick A. Athlete strongman. Pure Power 2003;3(5):66–74.
12. Henkin J. Effective sandbag training. Bodybuilding.com. Available at http://www.bodybuilding.com/fun/henkin37.htm. Accessed June 5, 2006.
13. Keogh J. Lower body resistance training: increasing functional performance with lunges. Strength Cond J 1999;21(1):67–72.
14. Kirksey B, Stone MH. Periodizing a college sprint program: theory and practice. Strength Cond 1998;20(3):42–47.
15. Kraemer WJ, Vescovi JD, Dixon P. The physiological basis of wrestling: implications for conditioning programs. Strength Cond J 2004;26(2):10–15.
16. Mahler M. The power of kettlebell training: time to train like a man again. Vegsource.com. Available at http://www.vegsource.com/articles2/mahler_kettlebell.htm. Accessed June 5, 2006.
17. Mannie K. Sandbag training. Coach Athl Dir, March 2004.
18. Murlasits Z, Langley J. In-season resistance training for high school football. Strength Cond J 2002;24(4):65–68.
19. Parakh AA, Domowitz FR. Strength training for men's and women's ice hockey. Strength Cond J 2000;22(6):42–45.
20. Pollitt D. Sled dragging for hockey training. Strength Cond J 2003;25(5):7–16.
21. Rosene JM. In-season, off-ice conditioning for minor league professional ice hockey players. Strength Cond J 2002;24(1):22–28.
22. Siff MC. Functional training revisited. Strength Cond J 2002;24(5):42–46.
23. Szymanski DJ, Fredrick GA. College baseball/softball periodized torso program. Strength Cond J 1999;21(4):42–47.
24. Waller M, Townsend R. Strongman events and strength and conditioning programs. Strength Cond J 2003;25(5):44–52.
25. Young W, Pryor J. Resistance training for short sprints and maximum-speed sprints. Strength Cond J 2001;23(2):7–13.

Sample Mission, Goals, and Objectives

MISSION

The strength and conditioning program will empower athletes and coaches to optimize their capabilities—and thereby achieve excellence—through learning and applying fundamentally sound principles.

PHILOSOPHY

Winning is the art—and training is the science—of systematic preparation. Smart hard work is the common denominator. Sound priorities and positive, proactive leadership are the basis of success.

■ Athletics is an integral part of the overall educational process, but academics come first.
■ Encourage scholarship and sportsmanship.
■ Apply professional guidelines in daily practice, as established by the
  ● National Strength and Conditioning Association and NSCA Certification Commission,
  ● National Board for Professional Teaching Standards,
  ● Center for Research on Education, Diversity and Excellence, and
  ● Learner-Centered Principles Work Group of the American Psychological Association.
■ Lead by guiding rather than ruling.
  ● Project influence and insight with a positive, proactive attitude and example.
    ■ Cultivate an atmosphere where smart, hard work—and fun—are a way of life.
    ■ Earn loyalty and cooperation by encouraging discipline and teamwork to evolve naturally.
    ■ Encourage individuals to set their own goals and monitor their progress as they work toward them.

    ■ Avoid resorting to forceful measures that create resistance or elicit negative counter-reactions.
  ● Use a simple, direct approach.
    ■ Clearly and concisely explain the evidence or principle-based reasons for everything we do.
    ■ Plan the process so that athletes can focus on managing the tasks.
  ● Reinforce the concept that strength and conditioning is a weapon as well as a foundation.
    ■ *Competitiveness* . . . We must challenge ourselves to excel, because leadership and teamwork are how ordinary people achieve extraordinary goals.
    ■ *Confidence* . . . We must believe in ourselves and expect to win.
    ■ *Fundamentals* . . . We must be fundamentally sound and execute our assignments with precision.
    ■ *Tenacity* . . . We must have an aggressive "make it happen" mentality, being willing to take calculated risks and to attack our opponents with relentless effort.
    ■ *Think!* . . . We must be situation-smart; maintain our poise and focus at all times; and eliminate mental errors and foolish penalties.
  ● Keep it clean.
  ● Maintain open lines of communication.
  ● Apply andragogical—rather than pedagogical—principles whenever possible.
    ■ Facilitate self-directed, performance-centered learning rather than instructor-dependent teaching; use didactic instruction methods only when necessary.
    ■ Augment the athlete's need to know by appealing to internal motivators (self-esteem, recognition, quality of life, self-confidence, and self-actualization).
    ■ Challenges should be designed with achievable solutions as well as the potential for

correctable errors in order to stimulate meaningful reflection and processing.

■ Learning is most effective when tasks are immediately relevant and levels of authenticity, complexity, uncertainty, self-direction, and self-adjustment are maximized.

Fundamental Principles

These training principles are straightforward and interdependent. The operative concept is to optimize the trade-off between fitness and fatigue by emphasizing quality of work—and recovery—over quantity and in turn maximize each athlete's abilities without exceeding his or her adaptive capabilities.

■ *Accommodation.* The biological response to constant stimuli decreases with repeated application. Novel/beneficial stressors yield supercompensation; whereas monotonous/detrimental stressors yield stagnation or decay.

■ *Continuity and Reversibility.* The body's homeostatic mechanisms upregulate corresponding systems in response to training and downregulate them in response to detraining.

■ *Individuality.* The same method(s) and/or technique(s) elicit unique responses in each athlete due to genetic differences, training status, and environmental factors.

■ *Progressive Overload.* Supernormal stressors should be progressively applied—while also allowing for adequate restoration—in order to improve fitness. The quality of both workload and recovery has priority over quantity and is optimized via cyclic increases in training intensity and decreases in volume.

■ *Specificity.* Adaptation becomes increasingly specific to imposed demands as fitness improves. Generalized tasks should be progressively replaced with specialized ones that dynamically correspond to the biomechanical, coordinative, and metabolic demands of the sport:

● The exercise menu should be prioritized such that the most functional movements—i.e., those yielding the greatest training/learning effects—are emphasized.

● Learning and training effects are optimized by making tasks progressively more challenging to control, direct, and stabilize (where appropriate), as well as by increasing workload.

■ *Synergy.* Movement qualities (i.e., strength, speed, flexibility, endurance) are integrated and stress responses are systemic rather than isolated in nature. Complementary or contrasting stimuli should be planned and implemented to exploit their cumulative and interactive effects.

■ *Variability.* Adaptive responses to strenuous loading become manifest during subsequent unloading periods. Summated training effects are realized—and accommodation is avoided—via fluctuation (rather than linear progression) in training load and content.

There is no mystery or secret about how to apply these principles. The only trick is to balance the contrasting needs for fluctuation (according to the law of variability) versus stability (to satisfy the demand for specificity).

Practical Implications

Effectiveness, efficiency, and safety are top priorities at all times. In order to assure a high level of professionalism, the strength and conditioning staff will:

■ Achieve and maintain expertise in the competencies defined in the NSCA Certification Commission's *National Study of the Certified Strength and Conditioning Specialist* and apply professional practice knowledge that is evidence-based as well as principle-based in daily practice.

■ Achieve and maintain the Certified Strength and Conditioning Specialist (CSCS) credential; fulfill the NSCA Certification Commission's Continuing Education Program requirements and apply its Code of Ethics in daily practice.

■ The name of the game is *speed-strength*—the ability to apply force rapidly and/or at high velocities. Speed is the result of explosive force but is often mistakenly believed to be independent of (or incompatible with) strength. It is important to understand that they are interrelated, because speed of execution and technical precision are fundamental goals of athletics.

This concept can be defined in terms of basic movement mechanics:

■ *Impulse = force × time.* The execution of skillful, explosive athletic tasks requires peak force application for a very short time (i.e., typically about 0.1 to 0.2 seconds, whereas absolute maximum force development requires 0.6 to 0.8 seconds). Continuous, prolonged application of force is not the answer. Brief, explosive force production is, and is what separates the best from the rest.

■ *Power = force × velocity*. A critical power output is required to perform any task, especially in athletics. Depending on the movement, power production usually peaks at 30% to 50% of maximum force and/or velocity. This does not mean that we should abandon heavy resistance training but does mean that the range of productive workloads extends well beyond the "slow squeeze" zone.

■ *Force = mass × acceleration*. This is the most deceptively simple of these laws. Once the weight is determined, peak force (relative to one's strength capabilities) and motoneural activity are generated only if it is maximally accelerated through the power position or sticking point. In all cases, exercise range of motion should therefore be considered an acceleration path.

Functional strength is expressed in terms of acceleration, execution time, or velocity. This has two implications with respect to training effect and athleticism: First, the intent to move explosively is more important than actual velocity achieved. Full volitional effort—i.e., a deliberate attempt to maximally accelerate the resistance, even if it is too heavy to move rapidly—yields the greatest neuromuscular activation and subsequent adaptive response. Second, rate, direction, and amplitude of force production are equally important (and trainable). Their brief application in certain parts of the movement is more important than sustained application throughout its entire distance or duration.

Every repetition is an opportunity to produce a certain impulse or power output. There are several interdependent ways to achieve this: emphasizing basic movements that have the greatest training effects, alternating between "heavy" and "explosive" execution; using equipment that challenges the athlete to control, direct, and stabilize it; rest-pausing as needed to execute each rep at full power; and progressively cycling the workload on a periodic 3- to 4-week basis in order to summate training effects and avoid accommodation.

Muscles act in functional task groups and should be targeted via force transmission and summation through—rather than isolation within—the kinetic chain. A critical impulse (i.e., force within given time) and power output (i.e., velocity with given resistance) must be achieved in order to perform skillful/explosive athletic tasks. Strength training is no exception, and in all cases movement range of motion should be considered an acceleration path. The only distinction is whether the object is accelerated through the sticking region or the entire movement (e.g., in order to launch it ballistically).

Training activities should be prioritized according to their *dynamic correspondence* with the demands of the sport: Their basic mechanics, but not necessarily outward appearance, should be specific to those occurring in competition. Rate and time of peak force production (impulse) and dynamics of effort (power) are especially important criteria. Other considerations include amplitude and direction of movement, accentuated region of force application, and regime of muscular work. This concept is analogous to the motor learning principle of *practice specificity* with respect to sensorimotor, processing, and contextual effects on skill acquisition, retention, and transfer.

Technical execution is determined by biomechanical principles:

■ Optimum path of acceleration
■ Initial force
■ Concentration/distribution of force
■ Coordination of impulse (deceleration/acceleration)
■ Reaction (movement/countermovement)
■ Conservation of momentum (angular velocity/moment of inertia)

Workloads should be designed to target the neuromuscular and neuroendocrine systems and in turn upregulate every system in the body. Emphasis should be placed on skillful athletic movements that transfer motor control/learning effects to the athlete's "coordinative abilities":

■ Orientation
■ Differentiation
■ Reactive ability
■ Rhythm
■ Balance
■ Combinatory ability
■ Adaptive ability

The greater the exertion in basic movements, the higher the production of endogenous hormones (as well as activity and number of tissue receptors): moderate weights for high reps and high-intensity endurance activities in general tend to maximize the somatotropic response; whereas heavy weights for low reps and brief maximal efforts in general tend to maximize the testosterone response.

Quality of effort has priority over quantity and is interdependent with recovery. Fitness and fatigue are a trade-off, and there is a threshold of diminishing returns beyond which the athlete's effort is diluted and recoverability/adaptability are compromised. Training effect, not strength or speed demonstration, is the underlying objective.

Optimal results are achieved by virtue of a long-term plan with cyclic workload variation. Specialized strength and endurance training methods should be implemented on a periodic 3- to 4-week basis in order to summate training effects and avoid accommodation.

In summary, fitness is a means toward an end: to develop complementary abilities and skills and thereby couple effort with execution. Power, flexibility, agility, speed, and endurance are the elements of athleticism. Each of these qualities is trainable, but they are interdependent parts of a larger whole and must therefore be trained collectively. None is a separate entity, nor is any one more important than another.

Sample Policies and Procedures

WEIGHT-ROOM REGULATIONS

■ The weight room is an equal-access working facility solely for the use of current varsity athletes and athletic staff.

■ Consult the posted schedule for team weight-room times and contact the strength and conditioning staff in advance if you are unable to attend your scheduled workout. Athletes may work out during their reserved time or during open/unreserved times, but not during another team's scheduled time (unless prior arrangements have been made).

■ Proper team-issued attire—including shirts and shoes—is required at all times. No spikes, cleats, bare feet, or open-toe/unlaced footwear are permitted. Each team's policies regarding apparel and appearance (as well as conduct) are in effect in the weight room.

■ Think safety! Respect platforms and power racks as work stations, not loitering/jaywalking areas. Use equipment correctly; use collars and spotter(s) on free-weight exercises; use proper form; and never sacrifice technique for weight.

■ Take pride in the weight room and keep it in order. It is each athlete's responsibility to pick up after a workout. Keep equipment in its proper location (do not rearrange or remove). Strip bars, rack weights correctly, and replace all items when done. Equipment is to be kept off the floor (except for the platforms) and properly racked when not in use.

■ Food, open beverage containers, glass, or tobacco of any kind are not permitted in the weight room. Sport bottles may be used throughout the weight room, but cups must remain at the beverage machine.

■ The telephone and stereo are available for use with permission from the strength and conditioning staff. Music with profane or obscene lyrics is inappropriate in the weight room. Wearing of headphones is not allowed.

■ Consult with the strength and conditioning staff regarding any questions, concerns, or suggestions. Failure to observe posted regulations and schedules may result in suspension or termination of weight-room privileges at the discretion of the strength and conditioning staff.

■ Provide positive, proactive leadership and strive for excellence. No excuses or alibis—do the right thing and do it right!

ENFORCEMENT POLICIES AND PROCEDURES

The strength and conditioning staff will conduct itself in a professional manner at all times. Always explain policies and procedures and answer questions, keeping in mind that every situation sets a precedent. There cannot be exceptions to posted regulations or schedules:

■ Direct the athlete to the posted regulations and/or schedules. If an athlete claims that these are new or unfamiliar, do not hesitate to point out that there is a reason for each one, they are posted in plain sight, and they were explained during orientation.

■ In the case of a minor offense, use a discretionary 1-2-3 approach:
  ● *First incident:* Approach the athlete politely.
  ● *Second incident:* Caution the athlete firmly.
  ● *Third incident:* Take action.

■ In taking disciplinary action, that is, in the case of repeated minor offenses or one or more major offenses, once again use a 1-2-3 approach:
  ● *First* action: Inform the athlete that his or her weight-room privileges are being suspended for the remainder of the day (or week).
  ● *Second action:* Inform the athlete that his or her weight-room privileges are being suspended for the remainder of the week (or month).

- *Third action:* Inform the athlete that his or her weight-room privileges are being suspended for the remainder of the month, season, semester or academic year if necessary.

■ Record any such disciplinary incident(s) and/or action taken on a weight-room incident report. Inform the respective team coach of the situation, scheduling a three-way follow-up meeting in order to resolve it.

The strength and conditioning staff will maintain loyalty, cooperation, and discipline in the varsity weight room, keeping in mind that our leverage with athletes is limited by the fact that we do not control depth charts or playing time. However, we will not be placed in a position where we must resolve attitude/compliance problems or conflicts without the direct support of the respective head coach. In dealing with a defiant or disrespectful athlete, the strength and conditioning staff reserve the right to suspend or terminate his or her weight-room privileges until the team coach addresses the situation satisfactorily.

■ Give athletes an opportunity to govern themselves—and thereby prevent or resolve problems internally—by recruiting the input of the team captain. Use these situations to facilitate the captain's role as "player coach."

■ When challenged by a noncompliant athlete, focus on the issue or behavior rather than the person's character. Maintain control of the situation and take prudent and reasonable steps to defuse it. Use disciplinary measures with discretion while protecting your ability to take further measures if necessary (until the head coach can intervene).

■ If a team coach is not immediately available, the strength and conditioning staff reserve the right to contact campus police in order to remove problematic individuals from the weight room if necessary.

HOURS OF OPERATION

Weight room hours of operation are Monday through Friday, 7:00 a.m. to noon and 1:00 p.m. to 7:00 p.m. during the academic year; 2:00 p.m. to 7:30 p.m. during the summer. With a limited staff and ongoing equipment upgrades, all attempts will be made to eliminate scheduling conflicts and make strength and conditioning programs and services accessible to all committed sports.

PROGRAMMING AND SCHEDULING

The strength and conditioning staff's commitment to each respective sport will be determined first and foremost by that team's commitment to continuous, long-term training:

■ *Access to strength and conditioning facilities, programs, and services is a varsity athlete privilege.* The respective coach and his or her athletes are expected to accept responsibility for improving their levels of strength and conditioning during each phase of the off season—including the summer—as well as for maintaining them during the season. The strength and conditioning staff cannot redirect its time and effort away from athletes who are committed to the program toward those who need to be retaught and retrained due to lack of commitment. Such individuals will be assigned to a workout program consisting of machines and/or body-weight exercises that do not require technique instruction and pose minimal risk of injury. At the discretion of the strength and conditioning staff, use of free-weight equipment and/or access to the varsity weight room may be disallowed until it is justified by the individual's compliance and work ethic.

■ *Because of the futility of discontinuous training, the strength and conditioning staff reserve the right to suspend or terminate programming and scheduling privileges for athletes or teams who fail to demonstrate a continuous, year-round commitment.* Those who do not participate—or whose attendance or work ethic is unsatisfactory—during certain segments of the year will forfeit their privileges. These individuals or teams will be responsible for implementing their own training programs, be delegated to open/unreserved times, and yield the right-of-way on equipment.

■ *The strength and conditioning staff will not be placed in a position of competing rather than cooperating with team coaches.* If the team coaching staff chooses to introduce its own training program during certain segments of the year, the strength and conditioning staff will defer full program responsibility for the entire year. This includes design as well as implementation: the respective coaches will oversee all aspects of instruction/supervision at every workout. The strength and conditioning staff's involvement will be limited to offering the varsity weight room as a place to do this, so that we may focus on working with teams whose coaches collaborate with us and whose athletes comply with our programs on a year-round basis.

For those teams fulfilling the first set of requirements, scheduling and programming priority will be based on the following criteria:

- In-season segment versus out-of-season segment
- Needs and demands of each sport with respect to performance enhancement and injury prevention:
  - Collision/contact versus noncollision/non-contact
  - Ballistic/weight-bearing versus nonballistic/non-weight-bearing
  - High impulse/power versus low impulse/power
- Space allowance of 100 ft² per athlete

A tentative schedule will be circulated to all coaches and staff prior to each segment and a meeting will be scheduled with each committed coach to plan workout times and programs. In situations where multiple teams request the same time, different options should be considered:

- Afternoons are generally very competitive times, especially after 3 p.m. Mornings should be considered whenever feasible.
- If afternoons are the only realistic option, groups can be scheduled concurrently as needed. Starting times can be staggered if necessary (e.g., at 20- to 30-minute intervals). This minimizes the competition for platforms and other primary pieces of equipment and improves the strength and conditioning staff's ability to supervise large groups.
- In each case, the respective coaching staff should be asked to assist in supervising their team's workout.

Once completed, the varsity workout schedule will be posted and distributed to all athletic coaches and staff. Coaches will be asked to post/circulate the schedule to their athletes as well.

There is a potential problem with unscheduled walk-in workouts during peak afternoon hours. Athletes from each respective team will be permitted access to the weight room during their scheduled team session and during unreserved or below-capacity times. There is usually adequate open time to allow some flexibility for all teams, but athletes will not be allowed to walk in during another team's reserved workout without prior approval from the strength and conditioning staff.

Athletes who are given permission to work out on another team's reserved time (due to class or other scheduling conflicts) will be delegated to equipment/exercises where they will not interfere with the reserved team's workout and will yield the right-of-way on all equipment.

TEAM ORIENTATION

The first scheduled team workout(s) of each training segment or semester consists of an orientation session, including the following:

- Staff introductions.
- The posted team workout schedule, rationale, and "capacity/below capacity" policies and procedures.
- Regulations. In most cases it is not necessary to insult the athletes' intelligence by reading the rules to them one by one. However, it is important to draw attention to the fact that there is a reason for each one that is ultimately based on effectiveness, efficiency, and/or safety:
  - Discuss basic weight-room courtesy, pointing out rules or policies that are frequently bent, broken, or otherwise problematic.
  - Facilitate the captain's role as "player coach" in order to give each team the opportunity to govern itself in the weight room.
  - Team policies as set by each head coach are in effect while in the weight room.
  - In the case of teams who do not incorporate strength and conditioning regulations into their policy manual, it may be necessary to distribute a written performance contract (e.g., including principles, regulations, and/or the "train smart" checklist).
- The strength and conditioning program's purpose, fundamental principles, and practical implications.
- The team's—and each individual athlete's—responsibility to improve their levels of preparation during each phase of the off season (including the summer) and to maintain them with the season.
- Train-smart checklist: "Think like a person of action—act like a person of thought"
  - *Access to strength and conditioning facilities, programs, and services is a varsity athlete's privilege.* The same proactive attitude, effort, and execution are expected on as well as off the field.

- *It is understood that academics come first and that scheduling conflicts arise.* Each athlete is responsible for notifying the strength and conditioning staff in advance in order to schedule a makeup workout (or be excused in the event of serious illness/injury).

- *Distinguish between the discomfort of exertion and the pain of injury.* Every athlete can expect to be hurt or otherwise limited at some point, and there are alternatives for every movement. Injuries or other problems mean that we adapt, improvise, or modify—not skip—exercises or workouts (unless indicated by the sports medicine staff).

- *Think safety!* Platforms and racks are work stations, not loitering/jaywalking areas.

- *Work with an attentive spotter—and use appropriate safety equipment (e.g. power racks)—when performing movements where free weights are supported on the trunk or moved over the head/face.* Olympic lifts are an exception to the spotter rule and should be performed on an 8- by 8-ft platform that is clear of people and equipment.

- *Plan each workout in advance, and keep accurate records on your work sheets to track your progress.*

- *Our objective is training effect, not strength demonstration.* We are not training to be powerlifters, weightlifters, or sprinters, although we have borrowed many of their concepts and methods.

- *Do your workout in the prescribed manner and sequence.* When and how each task is executed is as important as what we are doing.

- *Use warm-up sets as a technique/range-of-motion drill.* Submaximal workloads do not offer an opportunity to go through the motions.

- *Use the technique that allows you to maximize effort and results (e.g., power pull versus clean; low-bar versus high-bar squat).* This is not optional when failure to do so hinders progress.

- *Rest-pause as needed to execute each rep at full power.* Accelerate through the power position/sticking point; do not reduce weight unless you cannot get the first rep with good form.

- *Use between-set recovery time wisely.* Take about 6 minutes to stretch between primary (multi-joint) exercise sets. Alternate secondary (two-joint) exercises. Superset or circuit tertiary (one-joint) exercises.

■ *Regardless of how well our program is planned, it is only as good as your ability to recover from and adapt to it.* Maximize your gains—and conserve energy and time—with efficient effort. Avoid diluting the quality of work performed and decreasing the ability of the athlete to recover and adapt to the training stimulus by sacrificing days off or performing additional work.

■ *In conjunction with sound training, nutrition and sleep are your most important means of recovery and restoration.* You will not achieve optimal training effects—or fully recover and adapt—without a rational diet and stable sleep-wake cycle. Optimal fitness is a specialized state of health, and training cannot offset a poor lifestyle.

■ The equipment situation
   - Rationale for existing setup and planned upgrades (i.e., emphasis on rugged/versatile equipment and athletic, powerful movements)
   - Equipment-specific rules posted at certain stations

■ The specific team workout.

Sample Strength and Conditioning Professional Standards and Guidelines*

1. PREPARTICIPATION SCREENING & CLEARANCE

Standard 1.1 Strength & Conditioning professionals must require athletes to undergo health care provider screening and clearance prior to participation, in accordance with instructions specified by the *AAFP-AAP-AMSSM-AOSSM-AOASM Preparticipation Physical Evaluation Task Force* (15), the AHA & ACSM (6,11,12), as well as relevant governing bodies and/or their constituent members [e.g., the NCAA (16) for collegiate athletes; state legislatures, or individual state high school athletic associations/ districts for scholastic athletes]. In recreational activity programs, Strength & Conditioning professionals must require participants to undergo preparticipation screening and clearance in accordance with AHA & ACSM recommendations (6,11,12). For children, the clearance decision must include a determination or certification than the child has reached a level of maturity allowing participation in such activities as addressed in the *Participation in Strength & Conditioning Activities by Children* standards statement (refer to item 8).

Guideline 1.1 Strength & Conditioning professionals should cooperate with a training participant's health care providers at all times, and provide service in the participant's best interest according to instructions specified by such providers.

2. PERSONNEL QUALIFICATIONS

Guideline 2.1 The Strength & Conditioning practitioner should acquire a bachelor's or master's degree from a regionally accredited college or uni-

*Excerpted from Plisk SS (chair), Brass MS, Eickhoff-Shemek J, Epley B, Herbert DL, Owens J, Pearson DR, Wathen ND/ National Strength & Conditioning Association. *Strength & Conditioning Professional Standards & Guidelines*. Colorado Springs, CO: NSCA, 2001.

versity (verification by transcript or degree copy) in one or more of the topics comprising the *Scientific Foundations* domain identified in the *Certified Strength & Conditioning Specialist (CSCS) Examination Content Description* (13) or in a relevant subject. An ongoing effort should also be made to acquire knowledge and skill in the other content areas.

Guideline 2.2 The Strength & Conditioning practitioner should achieve and maintain professional certification(s) with continuing education requirements and a code of ethics, such as the CSCS credential offered through the NSCA Certification Commission. Depending on the practitioner's scope of activities, responsibilities, and knowledge requirements, relevant certifications offered by other governing bodies may also be appropriate.

Guideline 2.3 The productivity of a Strength & Conditioning staff, as well as learning and skill development of individual members, should be enhanced by aligning a "performance team" comprised of qualified practitioners with interdependent expertise and shared leadership roles. Once the team is assembled, respective activities and responsibilities from the *Practical/Applied* domain identified in the *Certified Strength & Conditioning Specialist (CSCS) Examination Content Description* (13)— as well as appropriate liaison assignments—should be delegated according to each member's particular *Scientific Foundations* expertise.

3. PROGRAM SUPERVISION & INSTRUCTION

Standard 3.1 Strength & Conditioning programs must provide adequate and appropriate supervision with well-qualified and trained personnel, especially during peak usage times. In order to ensure maximum health, safety, and instruction, Strength & Conditioning professionals must be present during Strength & Conditioning activities, have a clear view of the entire facility (or at least the zone being supervised by each practitioner) and the athletes in it, be physically close enough to the athletes under their care to be able to see and clearly communicate with them, and have quick access to those in need of spotting or assistance.

Standard 3.2 In conjunction with appropriate safety equipment (e.g., power racks), attentive spotting must be provided for athletes performing activities where free weights are supported on the trunk or moved over the head/face.*

Guideline 3.1 Strength & Conditioning activities should be planned—and the requisite number of qualified staff (refer to item 2) should be available—such that recommended guidelines for minimum average floor space allowance per athlete (100 sq ft^2), professional-to-athlete ratios (1:10 junior high school, 1:15 high school, 1:20 college), and number of athletes per barbell or training station ($\leq$ 3) is achieved during peak usage times (4,5,8–10). Younger participants, novices, or special populations engaged in such Strength & Conditioning activities should be provided with greater supervision (refer to item 8). Strength & Conditioning practitioners and their employers should work together toward a long-term goal of matching the professional-to-athlete ratio in the Strength & Conditioning facility to each sport's respective coach-to-athlete ratio.

4. FACILITY & EQUIPMENT SETUP, INSPECTION, MAINTENANCE, REPAIR, & SIGNAGE

Standard 4.1 Exercise devices, machines, and equipment—including free weights—must be assembled, set up, and placed in activity areas in full accordance with manufacturer's instructions, tolerances, and recommendations and with accompanying safety signage, instruction placards, notices, and warnings posted or placed according to ASTM standards (2,3) so as to be noticed by users prior to use.

*Refer to Earle RW, Baechle TR. Resistance training and spotting techniques. In: Baechle TR, Earle RW, eds. *National Strength & Conditioning Association. Essentials of Strength Training & Conditioning.* 2nd ed. Champaign IL: Human Kinetics, 2000:343–388.

In the absence of such information, professionals must complete these tasks in accordance with authoritative information available from other sources.

Standard 4.2 Prior to being put into service, exercise devices, machines, or free weights must be thoroughly inspected and tested by Strength & Conditioning professionals to ensure that they are working and performing properly and as intended by the manufacturer.

Standard 4.3 Exercise machines, equipment and free weights must be inspected and maintained at intervals specified by manufacturers. In the absence of such specifications, these items must be regularly inspected and maintained according to the Strength & Conditioning practitioner's professional judgment.

Standard 4.4 Exercise devices, machines, equipment and free weights that are in need of repair, as determined by regular inspection or as reported by users, must be immediately removed from service and locked "out of use" until serviced and repaired and be reinspected and tested to ensure that they are working and performing properly before being returned to service. If such devices are involved in incidents of injury, legal advisors or risk managers must be consulted for advice prior to service/repair or destruction.

Guideline 4.1 Strength & Conditioning professionals and their employers should ensure that facilities are appropriate for Strength & Conditioning activities. Factors to be reviewed and approved prior to activity include, but are not limited to, floor surfaces, lighting, room temperature and air exchanges (10).

Guideline 4.2 Manufacturer-provided user's manuals, warranties, and operating guides should be preserved and followed (refer to item 6).

Guideline 4.3 All equipment, including free weights, should be cleaned and/or disinfected regularly as deemed necessary by staff. Users should be encouraged to wipe down skin-contact surfaces after each use.

5. EMERGENCY PLANNING & RESPONSE

Standard 5.1 Strength & Conditioning professionals must be trained and certified in current guidelines for cardiopulmonary resuscitation (CPR) established by AHA/ILCOR (1) as well as universal precautions for preventing disease transmission established by the CDC (7) and OSHA (14). First Aid training/certification is also necessary if Sports Medicine personnel (e.g., MD or ATC) are not immediately available during Strength & Conditioning activities. New staff engaged in Strength & Conditioning activities must comply with this standard within six (6) months of employment.

Standard 5.2 Strength & Conditioning professionals must develop a written, venue-specific emergency response plan to deal with injuries and reasonably foreseeable untoward events within each facility. The plan must be posted at strategic areas within each facility and practiced and rehearsed at least quarterly. The emergency response plan must be initially evaluated (e.g., by facility risk managers, legal advisors, medical providers, and/or off-premises emergency response agencies) and modified as necessary at regular intervals. As part of the plan, a readily accessible and working telephone must be immediately available to summon on-premises and/or off-premises emergency response resources.

Guideline 5.1 The components of a written and posted emergency response plan should include planned access to a physician and/or emergency medical facility when warranted, including a plan for communication and transportation between the venue and the medical facility; appropriate and necessary emergency care equipment on site that is quickly accessible; and a thorough understanding of the personnel and procedures associated with the plan by all individuals.

6. RECORDS & RECORD KEEPING

Guideline 6.1 In conjunction with written policies and procedures, Strength & Conditioning professionals should develop and maintain various records, including manufacturer-provided user's manuals, warranties, and operating guides; equipment selection, purchase, installation, setup, inspection, maintenance, and repair records; personnel credentials; professional standards, and guidelines; safety policies and procedures, including a written emergency response plan (refer to item 5); training logs, progress entries and/or activ-

ity instruction/supervision notes; injury/incident reports, preparticipation medical clearance, and return-to-participation clearance documents. In settings where participants are not otherwise required to sign protective legal documents (e.g., informed consent, agreement to participate, waiver) covering all athletically related activities, the Strength & Conditioning professional should have such legal documents prepared for athletes under his or her care. These records should be preserved and maintained for a period of time determined by professional legal advice and consultation.

7. EQUAL OPPORTUNITY & ACCESS

Standard 7.1 Strength & Conditioning professionals and their employers must provide facilities, training, programs, services, and related opportunities in accordance with all laws, regulations, and requirements mandating equal opportunity, access, and nondiscrimination. Such federal, state, and possibly local laws and regulations apply to most organizations, institutions, and professionals. Discrimination or unequal treatment based upon race, creed, national origin, sex, religion, age, handicap/disability, or other such legal classifications is generally prohibited.

8. PARTICIPATION IN STRENGTH & CONDITIONING ACTIVITIES BY CHILDREN

Guideline 8.1 Children under seven (7) years of age should not be permitted to engage in Strength & Conditioning activities with free weights or exercise devices/machines in facilities designed for use by adults and adolescents and should be denied access to such training areas. Other forms of Strength & Conditioning activities may be beneficial for such children and should be recommended according to the practitioner's professional judgment and with a greater degree of instruction and supervision than that supplied to adolescents and adults. Children participating in such activities should be cleared as specified in the NSCA's "Standard for Preparticipation Screening & Clearance" (refer to item 1).

Guideline 8.2 Children between seven (7) and fourteen (14) years of age who have reached a level of maturity allowing participation in specified Strength & Conditioning activities, as determined and certified by their medical care provider (or by the Strength & Conditioning professional acting in concert with a child's medical care provider), and after clearance for participation as specified in the NSCA's "Standard for Preparticipation Screening & Clearance" (refer to item 1), should be individually assessed by the Strength & Conditioning professional in conjunction with the child's parent(s)/guardian(s)/custodian(s) and health care provider(s) to determine if such children may engage in such activities in areas containing free weights and exercise devices/machines generally used by adults and older children. If so permitted, such activities should be developed and implemented according to the practitioner's professional judgment, in conjunction with the child's health care provider(s), and with a greater degree of instruction and supervision than that supplied to adolescents and adults.

Guideline 8.3 Children fourteen (14) years of age and older who, according to the Strength & Conditioning practitioner's professional judgment, have reached a level of maturity allowing them to engage in specified Strength & Conditioning activities (provided that they have been cleared for participation as specified in the NSCA's "Standard for Preparticipation Screening & Clearance"; refer to item 1), may engage in such activities in areas containing free weights and exercise devices/machines generally used by adults, and with a greater degree of instruction and supervision than that supplied to adult populations while training.

9. SUPPLEMENTS, ERGOGENIC AIDS, & DRUGS

Standard 9.1 Strength & Conditioning professionals must not prescribe, recommend, or provide drugs, controlled substances or supplements that are illegal, prohibited, or harmful to athletes for any purpose including enhancing athletic performance, conditioning, or physique. Only those substances that are lawful and have been scientifically proven to be beneficial—or at least not harmful—may be recommended or provided to athletes by Strength & Conditioning professionals.

REFERENCES

1. American Heart Association in collaboration with the International Liaison Committee on Resuscitation. Guidelines 2000 for cardiopulmonary resuscitation and emergency cardiovascular care: international consensus on science. Circulation 2000;102(8 Suppl).
2. American Society for Testing and Materials. ASTM Standard Consumer Safety Specification for Stationary Exercise Bicycles: Designation F1250-89. West Conshohocken PA: ASTM, 1989.
3. American Society for Testing and Materials. ASTM Standard Specification for Fitness Equipment and Fitness Facility Safety Signage and Labels: Designation F1749-96. West Conshohocken PA: ASTM, 1996.
4. Armitage-Johnson S. Providing a safe training environment: part I. Strength and Conditioning 1994;16(1): 64–65.
5. Armitage-Johnson S. Providing a safe training environment: part II. Strength and Conditioning 1994;16(2):34.
6. Balady GJ (chair), Chaitman B, Driscoll D, et al for the American Heart Association & American College of Sports Medicine. Recommendations for cardiovascular screening, staffing and emergency policies at health/fitness facilities. Circulation 1998;97(22): 2283–2293; Med Sci Sports Exerc 1998;30(6):1009–1018.
7. Centers for Disease Control & Prevention/U.S. Department of Health & Human Services. Perspectives in disease prevention and health promotion update: universal precautions for prevention of transmission of human immunodeficiency virus, hepatitis B virus, and other bloodborne pathogens in health-care settings. MMWR 1988;37(24):377–388.
8. Hillmann A, Pearson DR. Supervision: the key to strength training success. Strength and Conditioning 1995;17(5): 67–71.
9. Jones L. U.S. Weightlifting Federation. USWF Coaching Accreditation Course: Club Coach Manual. Colorado Springs, CO: USWF, 1991.
10. Kroll W. Structural and functional considerations in designing the facility, part I. NSCA J 1991;13:1;51–58.
11. Maron BJ (chair), Thompson PD, Puffer JC, et al for the American Heart Association. Cardiovascular preparticipation screening of competitive athletes. Circulation 1996; 94(4):850–856; Med Sci Sports Exerc 1996;28(12): 1445–1452.
12. Maron BJ (chair), Thompson PD, Puffer JC, et al for the American Heart Association. Cardiovascular preparticipation screening of competitive athletes: addendum. Circulation 1998;97(22):2294.
13. NSCA Certification Commission. Certified Strength and Conditioning Specialist (CSCS) Examination Content

Description. Lincoln, NE: NSCA Certification Commission, 2000.

14. Occupational Safety and Health Administration. U.S. Department of Labor. OSHA Regulations (Standards-29 CFR) 1910.1030: Blood-Borne Pathogens. Washington, DC: OSHA, 1996.

15. Preparticipation Physical Evaluation Task Force. American Academy of Family Physicians, American Academy of Pediatrics, American Medical Society for Sports Medicine, American Orthopaedic Society for Sports Medicine and American Osteopathic Academy of Sports Medicine. Preparticipation Physical Evaluation. 2nd ed. New York: McGraw-Hill, 1996.

16. Schluep C, Klossner DA, eds. National Collegiate Athletic Association. 2003–04 NCAA Sports Medicine Handbook. 16th ed. Indianapolis, IN: NCAA, 2003.

Sample Strength and Conditioning Performance Team Development*

A team is "a small number of people with complementary skills who are committed to a common purpose, performance goals, and approach for which they hold themselves mutually accountable" (2). Teams are preferable to single-leader groups when there is a need for collective work products (i.e., multiple skills, judgments, and experiences) by members working together in real time, shifting leadership roles, and mutual as well as individual accountability. In contrast, single-leader/hierarchical work groups are appropriate when the sum of independent workers' contributions is adequate, singular rather than shared leadership is effective, task(s) and corresponding solution(s) are familiar, workers' skills can be applied productively without interaction (other than sharing information), and speed and efficiency have priority over extra performance results (1,2).

Extraordinarily demanding challenges are the driving forces behind high-performance teams. Common features of such teams include the following (1,2):

■ Members are committed to a clear mission, common approach, collaboration, and mutual accountability and responsibility.
■ Expectations and goals are high but achievable, and performance evaluation is based on results.
■ Roles are interdependent; leadership is shared; abilities, experiences, expertise, knowledge, skills and talents are complementary; contribution, participation and influence are balanced.
■ Effective task performance is facilitated by encouraging and rewarding creativity, innovation and risk taking in all decision making or problem solving activities.

In aligning a strength and conditioning staff, the "performance team" concept can be applied by hiring practitioners with expertise and formal education in one or more of the topics comprising the "scientific foundations" domain (3) or a related subject. Once the team is assembled, corresponding activities and responsibilities comprising the "practical/applied" domain (3)—as well as liaison assignments—can be delegated. In addition to exploiting greater collective expertise, this approach provides each practitioner with an opportunity to augment knowledge and skill acquisition in areas outside of his/her specialty. The strength and conditioning coordinator is still ultimately responsible for overseeing all aspects of the program and determining appropriate utilization of associates/assistants in the provision of safe, effective and efficient service. Specific duties and responsibilities can be assigned according to specialty areas or subdisciplines, in much the same way a sport coaching staff typically has offensive/defensive coordinators, liaison assignments, etc. Table D.1 provides an example of how to align a strength and conditioning performance team.

*Modified from Plisk SS (chair), Brass MS, Eickhoff-Shemek J, Epley B, Herbert DL, Owens J, Pearson DR, Wathen ND/ National Strength & Conditioning Association. *Strength & Conditioning Professional Standards & Guidelines.* Colorado Springs, CO: NSCA, 2001.

TABLE D.1	EXAMPLE OF STRENGTH AND CONDITIONING PERFORMANCE TEAM ALIGNMENTS	
SCIENTIFIC FOUNDATIONS— EDUCATION/EXPERTISE	**PRACTICAL AND APPLIED ACTIVITIES/RESPONSIBILITIES**	**LIAISON ASSIGNMENT(S)**
Exercise/sport anatomy; biomechanics	Exercise technique Testing and evaluation Rehabilitation and reconditioning*	Exercise and sport science faculty Team coaches Sports medicine team
Exercise/sport physiology	Program design Testing and evaluation	Exercise and sport science faculty Team coaches
Exercise/sport nutrition	Nutritionist	Exercise and sport science faculty
Exercise/sport pedagogy	Program design Exercise technique Organization and administration	Exercise and sport science faculty Athletic administration
Exercise/sport psychology; motor learning	Exercise technique Rehabilitation and reconditioning*	Exercise and sport science faculty Sports medicine team
Training methodology	Program design Organization and administration	Exercise and sport science faculty Athletic administration
Kinesiology; physiotherapy; sports medicine	Rehabilitation and reconditioning*	Sports medicine team

*One area to carefully consider is that of a rehabilitation and reconditioning specialist—i.e., a member of the performance team who works specifically with injured/modified athletes to reduce risk of reinjury and facilitate return to full activity. Due to such athletes' increased need for care, it is impractical—especially during peak usage times—for practitioners to work with injured or modified participants while simultaneously instructing/supervising larger groups. In some situations, the strength and conditioning and sports medicine facilities are adjacent (or shared), with natural crossover in respective activities and responsibilities. In many others, however, they are separated; and there is an opportunity to improve interaction, communication, and resulting provision of care for injured/modified athletes. In either case, the rehabilitation and reconditioning specialist would be an appropriate choice for liaison between the strength and conditioning and sports medicine staff.

REFERENCES

1. Katzenbach JR, Beckett F, Dichter S, et al. Real Change Leaders. New York: Times Books/Random House, 1995: 217–224.
2. Katzenbach JR, Smith DK. The Wisdom of Teams. Boston: Harvard Business School, 1993.
3. NSCA Certification Commission. Certified Strength and Conditioning Specialist (CSCS) Examination Content Description. Lincoln, NE: NSCA Certification Commission, 2000.

Sample Emergency Care and Planning*

EMERGENCY CARE AND COVERAGE

Reasonable attention to all possible preventive measures will not eliminate sports injuries. Each scheduled practice or contest of an institution-sponsored intercollegiate athletics event, as well as all out-of-season practices and skills sessions, should include an emergency plan. Like student-athlete well-being in general, a plan is a shared responsibility of the athletics department; administrators, coaches, and medical personnel should all play a role in the establishment of the plan, procurement of resources, and understanding of appropriate emergency response procedures by all parties. Components of such a plan should include the following:

1. The presence of a person qualified and delegated to render emergency care to a stricken participant
2. The presence or planned access to a physician for prompt medical evaluation of the situation, when warranted
3. Planned access to early defibrillation.
4. Planned access to a medical facility, including a plan for communication and transportation between the athletics site and the medical facility for prompt medical services when warranted. Access to a working telephone or other telecommunications device, whether fixed or mobile.
5. All necessary emergency equipment should be at the site or quickly accessible. Equipment should be in good operating condition, and personnel must be trained in advance to use it properly. Additionally, emergency information about the student athlete should be available both at campus and while traveling for use by medical personnel.

6. An inclement weather policy that includes provisions for decision making and evacuation plans (see Guideline 1d).
7. A thorough understanding by all parties, including the leadership of visiting teams, of the personnel and procedures associated with the emergency-care plan.
8. Certification in cardiopulmonary resuscitation techniques (CPR), first aid, and prevention of disease transmission (as outlined by OSHA guidelines) should be required for all athletics personnel associated with practices, competitions, skills instruction, and strength and conditioning. New staff engaged in these activities should comply with these rules within 6 months of employment.
9. A member of the institution's sports medicine staff should be empowered to have the unchallengeable authority to cancel or modify a workout for health and safety reasons (i.e., environmental changes), as he or she deem appropriate.

EMERGENCY ACTION PLAN EXAMPLE TEMPLATE

Reprinted from: National Athletic Trainers' Association. Available online: http://www.nata.org/committees/cuatc/cuatc_emergency/cuatc_emergency.htm.

Acknowledgment

The following emergency action plan and emergency protocols were developed by Ron Courson, Director of Sports Medicine, University of Georgia, and the University of Georgia Sports Medicine staff. These documents are designed to serve as examples and/or provide a starting point for institutional development of individualized emergency plans for all athletics activities. The National Athletic Train-

*Modified from Klossner DA, ed., and the National Collegiate Athletic Association. Guideline 1c. 2005–06 NCAA Sports Medicine Handbook. 18th ed. Indianapolis IN: NCAA, 2005.

ers' Association College and University ATCs committee recommends that each institution have a written venue specific emergency action plan which is reviewed and rehearsed on a regular basis; encourage institutional ownership in the emergency action plan; and require CPR, first aid, BBP, and emergency plan training for all coaches and strength and conditioning personnel. The emergency action plan should be approved by the medical director and shared with all individuals who may be involved in emergency care (i.e., athletic administration, coaches, athletic trainers, student athletic trainers, EMS, campus police, etc.). The institution may also elect to develop emergency protocols for specific categories of emergency care. All protocols should be approved by the medical director. Emergency protocols should be based on the level of training and expertise of medical staff, availability of appropriate equipment, and recognition of local and state statutes and ordinances.

Introduction

Emergency situations may arise at anytime during athletic events. Expedient action must be taken in order to provide the best possible care to the sport participant of emergency and/or life threatening conditions. The development and implementation of an emergency plan will help ensure that the best care will be provided.

As emergencies may occur at anytime and during any activity, the athletic association must be prepared. Athletic organizations have a duty to develop an emergency plan that may be implemented immediately when necessary and to provide appropriate standards of emergency care to all sports participants. As athletic injuries may occur at any time and during any activity, the sports medicine team must be prepared. This preparation involves formulation of an emergency plan, proper coverage of events, maintenance of appropriate emergency equipment and supplies, utilization of appropriate emergency medical personnel, and continuing education in the area of emergency medicine and planning. Hopefully, through careful preparticipation physical screenings, adequate medical coverage, safe practice and training techniques and other safety avenues, some potential emergencies may be averted. However, accidents and injuries are inherent with sports participation, and proper preparation on the part of the sports medicine team should enable each emergency situation to be managed appropriately.

Components of the Emergency Plan

These are the basic components of this plan:

1. *Emergency Personnel.* With athletic association practice and competition, the first responder to an emergency situation is typically a member of the sports medicine staff, most commonly a certified athletic trainer. A team physician may not always be present at every organized practice or competition. The type and degree of sports medicine coverage for an athletic event may vary widely, based on such factors as the sport or activity, the setting, and the type of training or competition. The first responder in some instances may be a coach or other institutional personnel. Certification in cardiopulmonary resuscitation (CPR), first aid, prevention of disease transmission, and emergency plan review is required for all athletics personnel associated with practices, competitions, skills instruction, and strength and conditioning. Copies of training certificates and/or cards are maintained in the athletic training facility. The development of an emergency plan cannot be complete without the formation of an emergency team. The emergency team may consist of a number of healthcare providers including physicians, emergency medical technicians, certified athletic trainers; student athletic trainers; coaches; managers; and, possibly, bystanders. Roles of these individuals within the emergency team may vary depending on various factors such as the number of members of the team, the athletic venue itself, or the preference of the head athletic trainer.

2. *Emergency Communication.* Communication is the key to quick emergency response. Athletic trainers and emergency medical personnel must work together to provide the best emergency response capability and should have contact information such as telephone tree established as a part of preplanning for emergency situations. Communication prior to the event is a good way to establish boundaries and to build rapport between both groups of professionals. If emergency medical transportation is not available on site during a particular sporting event, then direct communication with the emergency medical

system at the time of injury or illness is necessary. Access to a working telephone or other telecommunications device, whether fixed or mobile, should be assured. The communications system should be checked prior to each practice or competition to ensure proper working order. A backup communication plan should be in effect should there be failure of the primary communication system. The most common method of communication is a public telephone. However, a cellular phone is preferred if available. At any athletic venue, whether home or away, it is important to know the location of a workable telephone. Prearranged access to the phone should be established if it is not easily accessible.

3. *Emergency Equipment.* All necessary emergency equipment should be at the site and quickly accessible. Personnel should be familiar with the function and operation of each type of emergency equipment. Equipment should be in good operating condition, and personnel must be trained in advance to use it properly. Emergency equipment should be checked on a regular basis and its use rehearsed by emergency personnel. The emergency equipment available should be appropriate for the level of training for the emergency medical providers. Creating an equipment inspection log book for continued inspection is strongly recommended. It is recommended that a few members of the emergency team be trained and responsible for the care of the equipment. It is important to know the proper way to care for and store the equipment as well. Equipment should be stored in a clean and environmentally controlled area. It should be readily available when emergency situations arise.

4. Roles of first responder
5. Venue directions with map
6. Emergency action plan checklist for nonmedical emergency

Roles within the Emergency Team

There are four basic roles within the emergency team. The first and most important role is establishing safety of the scene and immediate care of the athlete. Acute care in an emergency situation should be provided by the most qualified individual on the scene. Individuals with lower credentials should yield to those with more appropriate training. The second role, EMS activation, may be necessary in situations where emergency transportation is not already present at the sporting event. This should be done as soon as the situation is deemed an emergency or a life-threatening event. Time is the most critical factor under emergency conditions. Activating the EMS system may be done by anyone on the team. However, the person chosen for this duty should be someone who is calm under pressure and who communicates well over the telephone. This person should also be familiar with the location and address of the sporting event. The third role, equipment retrieval, may be done by anyone on the emergency team who is familiar with the types and location of the specific equipment needed. Student athletic trainers, managers, and coaches are good choices for this role. The fourth role of the emergency team is that of directing EMS to the scene. One member of the team should be responsible for meeting emergency medical personnel as they arrive at the site of the emergency. Depending on ease of access, this person should have keys to any locked gates or doors that may slow the arrival of medical personnel. A student athletic trainer, manager, or coach may be appropriate for this role.

1. Establish scene safety and immediate care of the athlete.
2. Activation of the Emergency Medical System. Making the call:
   - 911 (if available)
   - Notify campus police
   - Telephone numbers for local police, fire department, and ambulance service
   Providing information:
   - Name, address, telephone number of caller
   - Nature of emergency, whether medical or nonmedical (if nonmedical, refer to the specific checklist of the emergency action plan)
   - Number of athletes
   - Condition of athlete(s)
   - First aid treatment initiated by first responder
   - Specific directions as needed to locate the emergency scene
   - Other information as requested by dispatcher

3. Emergency equipment retrieval.
4. Direction of EMS to scene.

In forming the emergency team, it is important to adapt the team to each situation or sport. It may also be advantageous to have more than one individual assigned to each role. This allows the emergency team to function even though certain members may not always be present.

Medical Emergency Transportation

Emphasis is placed at having an ambulance on site at high-risk sporting events. EMS response time is additionally factored in when determining on site ambulance coverage. The athletic association coordinates on-site ambulances for [list specific activities]. Ambulances may be coordinated on-site for other special events/sports. Consideration is given to the capabilities of transportation service available (i.e., Basic Life Support or Advanced Life Support) and the equipment and level of trained personnel on board the ambulance. In the event that an ambulance is on site, there should be a designated location with rapid access to the site and a cleared route for entering/exiting the venue. In the event of an emergency, the 911 system will still be utilized for activating emergency transport.

In the medical emergency evaluation, the primary survey assists the emergency care provider in identifying emergencies requiring critical intervention and in determining transport decisions. In an emergency situation, the athlete should be transported by ambulance, where the necessary staff and equipment is available to deliver appropriate care. Emergency care providers should refrain from transporting unstable athletes in inappropriate vehicles. Care must be taken to ensure that the activity areas are supervised should the emergency care provider leave the site in transporting the ath-

lete. Any emergency situations where there is impairment in level of consciousness (LOC); airway, breathing, or circulation (ABC); or there is neurovascular compromise should be considered a "load and go" situation and emphasis placed on rapid evaluation, treatment, and transportation. In order to provide the best possible care, transportation to one of the utilized medical facilities is based upon the strengths of each facility. All cardiac and vascular emergencies are to be transported to [list specific hospital/medical center], and all other types of injuries are to be transported to [list specific hospital/medical center].

Nonmedical Emergencies

Refer to the laminated emergency action plan checklist and follow the instructions for the following non-medical emergencies: fire, bomb threats, severe weather, and violent or criminal behavior. [List specific police/public safety, fire department, and hospital/medical center] should be on standby at high risk sporting events.

Conclusion

The importance of being properly prepared when athletic emergencies arise cannot be stressed enough. An athlete's survival may hinge on how well trained and prepared athletic healthcare providers are. It is prudent to invest athletic department ownership in the emergency plan by involving the athletic administration and sport coaches as well as sports medicine personnel. The emergency plan should be reviewed at least once a year with all athletic personnel, along with CPR and first aid refresher training. Through development and implementation of the emergency plan, the athletic association helps ensure that the athlete will have the best care provided when an emergency situation does arise.

Sample Protective Legal Documents*

The following provides general legal information. Protective legal documents should not be adopted or used in any context without individualized legal advice.

TYPES OF PROTECTIVE LEGAL DOCUMENTS

Institutions such as universities/colleges and high schools often require athletes to read and sign some type of protective legal document(s) prior to participation in athletically related activities, including strength and conditioning. These documents can help protect the institution and its employees from potentially costly legal claims and lawsuits. The law involving protective legal documents is quite complex, however, and understanding their function and the specific legal protection they provide is often confusing.

Several types of protective legal documents exist. Three that are commonly used in the health/fitness field may be applicable in strength and conditioning settings: *informed consent, agreement to participate,* and *waiver.* Each provides protection from lawsuits arising from certain types of injuries that can occur while participating in activities, as explained below.

CAUSES OF INJURY ASSOCIATED WITH PHYSICAL ACTIVITY

Cotten and Cotten (1) describe three causes of injury associated with physical activity: *inherent risks, negligence,* and *extreme forms of conduct.*

Inherent Risks

As the term implies, these risks are inherent in the activity. Generally, injuries caused by inherent risks are accidental in nature, not preventable, and no one's fault. The *informed consent* and *agreement to participate* documents provide the best legal protection for lawsuits arising from such injuries. Although actual sections and content of protective documents vary (and depend on state law), the following are generally included in informed consent and agreement to participate documents:

Informed consent

- Purpose of the activity
- Risks of the activity*
- Benefits of the activity
- Confidentiality
- Inquiries
- Signatures

Agreement to participate

- Nature of the activity
- Possible consequences of injury*
- Behavioral expectations of the participant
- Condition of the participant
- Concluding statement
- Signatures

A section within each of these documents is devoted to informing the participant of the potential risks, including those inherent in the activity. It is important that this section carefully describes these risks (e.g., types of accidents that might occur and the consequences of these accidents), and that the language used is understandable to the person who will be signing it. This provides an "assumption of risk" defense, i.e., the participant knew and fully understood the risks, appreciated the risks, and voluntarily assumed them. In gen-

---

*Reprinted from Eickhoff-Shemek J. Distinguishing protective legal documents. *ACSM Health Fit J* 2001;5(3): 27–29.

*Note: "Assumption of risk" language.

eral, the law does not allow individuals to recover compensation for injuries resulting from assumed risks.

Negligence

Injuries can be caused by negligence, i.e., failure to act as reasonable and prudent professional would act under the circumstances. Participants can be injured by negligent acts of the Strength and Conditioning staff (e.g., failure to inspect/maintain exercise equipment, failure to provide CPR or first aid when needed). A *waiver* document—also called a *prospective release*—provides the best legal protection for lawsuits arising from injuries caused by negligence. Once again, whereas the actual sections and content of such documents vary depending on state law, waiver documents generally include exculpatory clause; description of risks ("assumption of risk" language); indemnification language (may not be valid); severability clause; affirmation of legal capacity; and signatures.

The "exculpatory clause" is a key section within the waiver explicitly stating that the participant releases the strength and conditioning facility for any liability associated with negligence by the facility or its employees. This clause, which must be written very carefully to be enforceable, provides evidence that the participant gave up (waived) his or her right to file a negligence lawsuit against the facility. However, the exculpatory clause does not provide protection from lawsuits arising from injuries due to inherent risks; and an "assumption of risk" section is often added to the waiver for this purpose.

Extreme Forms of Conduct

Injuries can also be caused by extreme forms of conduct (often referred to as gross negligence, willful and wanton conduct, or reckless conduct). For example, if the strength and conditioning staff had prior knowledge of an existing danger or risk but took no corrective action to help prevent resulting injuries, this failure to act would most likely constitute an extreme form of conduct. Generally, no documents can provide legal protection for grossly negligent or reckless conduct. A few states may allow the use of a waiver to protect from such conduct, but most do not (1).

MAKING PROTECTIVE LEGAL DOCUMENTS ENFORCEABLE

Protective legal documents, signed by participants prior to their participation in strength and conditioning programs and services, can provide a good defense for the strength and conditioning facility after an injured participant files a claim or lawsuit. A variety of factors should be considered in order for these forms to be legally enforceable (1–3):

■ A lawyer who is knowledgeable about the law regarding protective documents must review your protective legal documents to help ensure they are written properly and reflect the law in your state.

■ *Informed consent* and *waiver* documents are contracts, and can only be signed by adults because minors cannot enter into a contract. *Agreement to participate* documents are not contracts and therefore can be signed by adults as well as minors.

■ The exculpatory clause used in a *waiver* is not allowed in an *informed consent* or *agreement to participate*. If an exculpatory clause is added to an agreement to participate for adults, it then becomes a waiver.

■ The exculpatory clause used in a *waiver* is not enforceable in medical or research settings, or in certain states (Virginia, Montana, Louisiana) where they are against public policy. In educational settings such as a college/university, the general rule is that waivers are against public policy for required activities but may be enforceable for voluntary activities.

■ *Informed consent* documents used in medical settings must be administered prior to a patient having any kind of medical procedure. If the informed consent is not written or administered properly, the health care provider (and medical facility) could be found negligent for not informing the patient of particular risks. This also applies in research settings, because subjects must be properly informed of risks through informed consent (note that this point is applicable in strength and conditioning settings where athletes participate as human subjects in research studies).

■ All documents must be administered properly. For example, participants should have ample time to read them, and a well-trained employee should verbally explain the document to each participant.

■ Protective documents must be stored in a secure place for the amount of time consistent with the statue of limitations, which may be up to 4 years in some states.

The choice of document or combination of documents to use is a very important decision. In situations where strength and conditioning activities are not covered in the employing institution's legal documentation, strength and conditioning professionals should consult with a qualified lawyer to assist with these decisions and to review—or write—the documents prior to implementation. Because legal advice and consultation can be quite expensive, Strength and Conditioning professionals may reduce costs by "drafting" their own legal documents using information from applicable resources [e.g., refer to Cotten and Cotten (1) for examples of *agreement to participate* and *waiver* documents; and Herbert and Herbert (3) for examples of *informed consent* documents]. These resources should be shared with your lawyer when he or she reviews the drafts and makes the final document revisions.

Written protective documents provide important evidence when a lawsuit occurs. For example, if a strength and conditioning facility is sued for negligence, but has evidence that the injured party signed a properly written and administered waiver, this document provides the evidence needed to seek summary judgment (i.e., a pretrial motion in which the judge can dismiss the case because, as a matter of law, there is no issue to be tried in a court of law). In this situation, the legal document protects the facility from a potentially costly negligence lawsuit.

REFERENCES

1. Cotten DJ, Cotten MB. Legal Aspects of Waivers in Sport, Recreation and Fitness Activities. Canton, OH: PRC Publishing, 1997.
2. Eickhoff-Shemek J. Distinguishing protective legal documents. ACSM Health Fit J 2001;5(3):27–29.
3. Herbert DL, Herbert WG. Legal Aspects of Preventive, Rehabilitative and Recreational Exercise Programs, 3rd ed. Canton, OH: PRC Publishing, 1993.

Index

Page numbers followed by f denote figures; those followed by t denote tables